Dentistry: Contemporary Insights

Dentistry: Contemporary Insights

Editor: Graham Jones

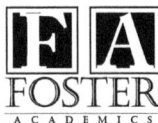

FA FOSTER
ACADEMICS

www.fosteracademics.com

www.fosteracademics.com

F A
FOSTER
ACADEMICS

Cataloging-in-Publication Data

Dentistry : contemporary insights / edited by Graham Jones.
    p. cm.
Includes bibliographical references and index.
ISBN 978-1-63242-613-0
1. Dentistry. 2. Oral medicine. 3. Teeth. I. Jones, Graham.
RK51 .D46 2019
617.6--dc23

Foster Academics,
118-35 Queens Blvd., Suite 400,
Forest Hills, NY 11375, USA

ISBN 978-1-63242-613-0 (Hardback)

Contents

Preface

Dentistry is a branch of medicine concerned with the treatment and prevention of oral diseases, including the diseases of the teeth, conditions of the soft tissues of the mouth and disorders of the supporting structures. The correction of any malformation of the jaw, birth anomalies of the oral cavity including cleft palate and misalignment of the teeth is also treated within the domain of dentistry. It has a number of subspecialties, such as orthodontics, periodontics, prosthodontics, endodontics, maxillofacial pathology, oral and maxillofacial radiology, etc. Orthodontics encompasses the correction and prevention of the malocclusion of the teeth and dentofacial incongruities. The diagnosis, treatment and prevention of diseases of the periodontal tissues, such as jaws, gums and related contiguous structures, which surround the teeth and support it falls under the domain of periodontics. The correction of any condition to restore oral function and appearance by the replacement of contiguous tissues and replacement of missing teeth with prostheses and other artificial substitutes is under the scope of prosthodontics. This book attempts to understand the multiple branches that fall under the discipline of dentistry and how such concepts have practical applications. The various studies that are constantly contributing towards advancing technologies and evolution of this field are examined in detail. Students, researchers, experts and all associated with dentistry will benefit alike from this book.

This book is the end result of constructive efforts and intensive research done by experts in this field. The aim of this book is to enlighten the readers with recent information in this area of research. The information provided in this profound book would serve as a valuable reference to students and researchers in this field.

At the end, I would like to thank all the authors for devoting their precious time and providing their valuable contribution to this book. I would also like to express my gratitude to my fellow colleagues who encouraged me throughout the process.

Editor

Alveolar Crestal Approach for Maxillary Sinus Membrane Elevation with <4 mm of Residual Bone Height

Jae Won Jang, Hee-Yung Chang, Sung-Hee Pi, Yoon-Sang Kim, and Hyung-Keun You ⓘⒹ

Department of Periodontology, School of Dentistry, Wonkwang University, 344-2 Shinyong-dong, Iksan, Jeonbuk 54538, Republic of Korea

Correspondence should be addressed to Hyung-Keun You; hkperio@wku.ac.kr

Academic Editor: Saso Ivanovski

Introduction. For maxillary sinus membrane elevation (MSME), the lateral window approach and crestal approach are available, and high success rates have been achieved with low residual bone height as a development of technology. *Objective.* To evaluate MSME using the crestal approach with a rotary-grind bur (RGB (including reamer or sinus bur)) in patients with residual bone height of <4 mm. *Materials and Methods.* Ten implants were placed in 10 patients with residual bone height of <4 mm, by sinus elevation using an RGB. The implant stability quotient (ISQ) was measured immediately after implant placement (ISQ 1) and before taking impression for the final prosthesis (ISQ 2). The extent of marginal bone loss was measured on periapical radiographs. *Results.* The mean residual bone height before implant placement was 3.41 ± 0.53 mm; no complications, including membrane perforation, severe postoperative pain, or discomfort, occurred either during or after surgery. The mean ISQ 1 was 63.4 ± 12.1, whereas the mean ISQ 2 was 77.6 ± 5.8. The mean marginal bone resorption was 0.23 ± 0.18 mm on periapical radiographs. *Conclusions.* MSME using the crestal approach with an RGB is a reliable technique for implant placement in sites where available bone is insufficient.

1. Introduction

A reduction in alveolar bone, through sinus pneumatization in the maxillary posterior area, is commonly encountered after tooth extraction. Maxillary sinus membrane elevation (MSME) is an essential procedure to recover the appropriate bone height for implant treatment and has become a generalized clinical technique used by many dentists in recent years.

For MSME, the lateral window approach and the alveolar crestal approach through the extraction socket are both available; operations using either of these techniques have yielded high implant success rates [1, 2]. In previous studies, the lateral window approach has been reported to elevate the maxillary sinus by up to 10–12 mm, which is greater elevation than that provided by the alveolar crestal approach (2.5–5.7 mm); notably, the lateral window approach is generally used in cases with low residual bone height (≤4-5 mm) [3–6]. However, the lateral window approach is technically more difficult than the alveolar crestal approach

and is more likely to cause postoperative complications, including pain and swelling [7]. Moreover, it has a sinus membrane perforation rate of 12–40%, which is higher than that of the alveolar crestal approach (2.2–6.7%) [4–6, 8–12].

Since the alveolar crestal approach was introduced, several studies have reported high survival rates following the use of this technique [4, 13–16]. The osteotome technique, which avoids membrane perforation, has led to significant advances in implant treatment; however, there are disadvantages associated with the osteotome technique [3, 5], the most significant of which is that the patient may experience headaches and postoperative dizziness that result from aggressive mallet tapping [17].

To overcome these problems, instruments designed to grind the bone without perforating the membrane—rather than fracturing the maxillary cortical bone via mallet tapping—have been developed [6, 17, 18]. Compared with traditional methods, this method reportedly confers advantages to both the operator and the patient, as it is simple

TABLE 1: Patient characteristics.

Patient	Age (years)	Sex	Medical history	Smoking
1	63	Male	Myocardial infarction (15 years ago)	No
2	71	Female	Hypertension	No
3	54	Female	Unremarkable	3-4 per day
4	67	Female	Hypertension	No
5	38	Male	Unremarkable	No
6	51	Male	Hypertension	No
7	42	Female	Unremarkable	3-4 per day
8	47	Female	Unremarkable	No
9	55	Female	Hyperlipidemia	No
10	54	Female	Hyperlipidemia	No

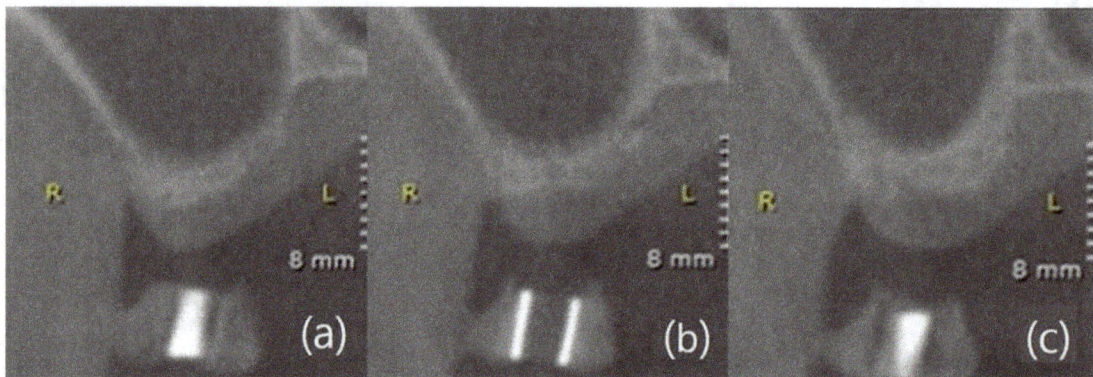

FIGURE 1: Residual bone height measurement method. Average value derived from (a) mesial, (b) central, and (c) distal aspects of the stent on computed tomography coronal view.

to perform and is associated with fewer postoperative complications [17, 19, 20]. This method of smoothly grinding the bone may enable the membrane to be elevated in a stable manner, even in areas with short residual bone height.

The objective of the present study was to assess the postoperative outcomes following MSME via the alveolar crestal approach, using a rotary-grind bur (RGB (including reamer or sinus bur)) in the maxillary posterior area of patients with residual bone heights <4 mm.

2. Materials and Methods

2.1. Participants.
The present study included individuals who underwent implant placement with MSME via the alveolar crestal approach using an RGB; these individuals were recruited from among a group of patients who visited the Department of Periodontology at Wonkwang University Dental Hospital (Jeonbuk, South Korea) and who had residual bone height <4 mm in the maxillary posterior area. Patients with anatomical structures that would interfere with the use of alveolar crestal approach, such as sinus septum, were excluded from this study. The study was approved by the Institutional Review Board (IRB) of Wonkwang University Dental Hospital (WKDIRB 201702-01). A total of 10 patients (three males and seven females) participated in the study, and a total of 10 implants were placed using the alveolar crestal approach. The age of the participants ranged between 38 and 71 years (mean, 54.2 years) (Table 1). Although two participants were smokers, they were instructed

to abstain from smoking for 2 weeks before and 2 months after the procedure.

Residual bone height was measured as the distance from the alveolar crest to the sinus floor on the coronal view of a cone beam computed tomography (CT) image; it was expressed as the average value derived from the mesial, central, and distal aspects of the stent on the CT image (Figure 1).

2.2. Surgical Method.
The surgical site was sterilized, and infiltration anesthesia was administered using 2% lidocaine hydrochloride with epinephrine (1 : 1,00,000; Yuhan, Korea). After a crestal incision was made, full-thickness elevation was performed. The Crestal Approach Sinus Kit (CAS, Osstem Implant, Korea) and Dentium Advanced Sinus Kit (DASK, Dentium, Korea) were used, according to the manufacturer's instructions and the previous study [17]. Briefly, after using a pilot drill, a 2.0 mm twist drill was used to drill 1-2 mm shorter than the remaining alveolar bone height. Ø2.8 and Ø3.1 CAS drills with stopper were sequentially used to completely grind the cortical bone. Stopper systems with 1 mm increments were particularly useful when the bone height was not sufficient. If decortication of the sinus floor could not be achieved readily using the CAS drill alone, an additional drill from the DASK was used. The speed of the drill was maintained at 400~600 rpm during the process. The sensation of a slight drop suddenly occurred when the sinus floor was completely grinded. Round shape of the drill top of CAS drill or

TABLE 2: Surgical attributes for each patient.

Patient	Surgical site	Residual bone height (mm)	Graft material	ISQ 1	ISQ 2	Method
1	#26	3.09	MBCP	75	83	2-stage
2	#16	3.82	OCS-B	68	83	2-stage
3	#16	3.56	OCS-B	52	73	2-stage
4	#17	2.62	MBCP	65	68	2-stage
5	#16	3.72	OCS-B	68	77	2-stage
6	#16	3.78	OCS-B	74	84	2-stage
7	#16	2.37	ICB + MBCP	42	74	2-stage
8	#27	3.70	MBCP	N/A	72	1-stage
9	#16	3.77	ICB + OCS-B	N/A	84	2-stage
10	#17	3.67	OCS-B	N/A	78	1-stage

ISQ 1: implant stability quotient measured during implant placement; ISQ 2: implant stability quotient measured immediately before impression taking for the final prosthesis; N/A: not applicable.

diamond-coated drill in DASK can minimize the possibility of puncturing the sinus membranes. Sinus membrane perforation was checked using the Valsalva maneuver. The depth gauge with round tip in the kit was placed on the margin of the osteotomy, and the sinus membrane was carefully gently detached. To fully elevate membranes to the desired height, the bone graft was filled with bone carrier, and the bone graft was pushed into the sinus with bone condenser with stopper. A bone spreader was then used to laterally spread the bone graft material. Repeating this process, the membrane was sufficiently elevated by the bone graft material (1-2 mm longer than the implant length). We used MBCP (biphasic calcium phosphate, Biomatlante, France), OCS-B (deproteinized bovine bone, NIBEC, Korea), and ICB (allogenic cancellous bone, Rocky Mountain Tissue Bank, Aurora, CO, USA) alone or in combination (Table 2). SLA-surface implants (TS III, US II, Osstem Implant, Korea), with diameters of 4.0-5.0 mm and lengths of 8.5-10.0 mm, were used. Depending on the primary stability, implant placement was performed via a 1- or 2-stage technique. Suturing was performed using nonabsorbable sutures (4-0 Ethilon; Ethicon, OH, USA) (Figures 2 and 3).

A healing period of 6 months was permitted in the 1-stage technique; in contrast, a second surgery was performed after 4-6 months of healing in the 2-stage technique. The implant stability quotient (ISQ) was measured twice: once after implant placement (ISQ 1) and once immediately before impression taking of the final prosthesis (ISQ 2).

2.3. Evaluation of Marginal Bone Resorption after Final Prosthesis Loading. After loading the final prosthesis, the patients were instructed to make regular visits to the Department of Periodontology and Prosthodontics at 3- to 6-month intervals. During these visits, marginal bone resorption at the mesial and distal aspects of the implant was measured from parallel periapical radiographs; mean bone resorption values were recorded.

3. Results

A total of 10 implants were placed in 10 patients (Table 2). The mean residual bone height before implant placement was 3.41 ± 0.53 mm (range: 2.37-3.82 mm). Perforation of the sinus membrane did not occur during the procedures, and the patients experienced no severe pain, swelling, or discomfort after the procedure. Of 10 implants, eight were placed via the 2-stage technique, while two were placed via the 1-stage technique. From implant placement to final prosthesis loading, a mean healing period of 5.0 ± 0.8 months was observed (range: 4-6 months). The mean ISQ 1 was 63.4 ± 12.1, while the mean ISQ 2 increased to 77.6 ± 5.8 (Table 2).

The mean follow-up observation period after final prosthesis loading was 12.0 ± 9.4 months (range: 4-34 months); during this period, no gingival inflammation, radiolucency, or implant mobility was observed. The mean marginal bone resorption was 0.23 ± 0.18 mm (range: 0.00-0.48 mm), as measured on periapical radiographs (Table 3, Figure 4).

4. Discussion

In the present study, successful outcomes were achieved via the alveolar crestal approach, using an RGB for MSME in patients who exhibited residual bone height of <4 mm. Although the number of patients was small and patients with systemic diseases were included in the study, our results demonstrated that implant treatment can be successfully performed using the alveolar crestal approach, even at lower alveolar bone heights.

For ISQ values measured immediately after implant placement, Patel et al. [21] reported a mean ISQ of 68.9 ± 1.6 for the lateral window approach, with a residual bone height of 3.0-7.9 mm. Additionally, Lai et al. [22] reported a mean ISQ of 68.0 using the osteotome technique, with a residual bone height of 4-8 mm. In the present study, the mean ISQ 1 was 63.4 ± 12.1, which was slightly lower than the mean ISQ reported in previous studies; however, the final value (77.6 ± 5.8 (ISQ 2)) was stable and demonstrated an appropriate value for osseointegration. In addition, in a patient with residual bone height of 2.37 mm and type 4 bone quality, the ISQ markedly increased from 42 to 74. As all patients exhibited a residual bone height of <4 mm, satisfactory stability may thus be achieved using an RGB; we suspect that even when primary stability is poor because of low alveolar bone height, sufficient osseointegration can still be achieved

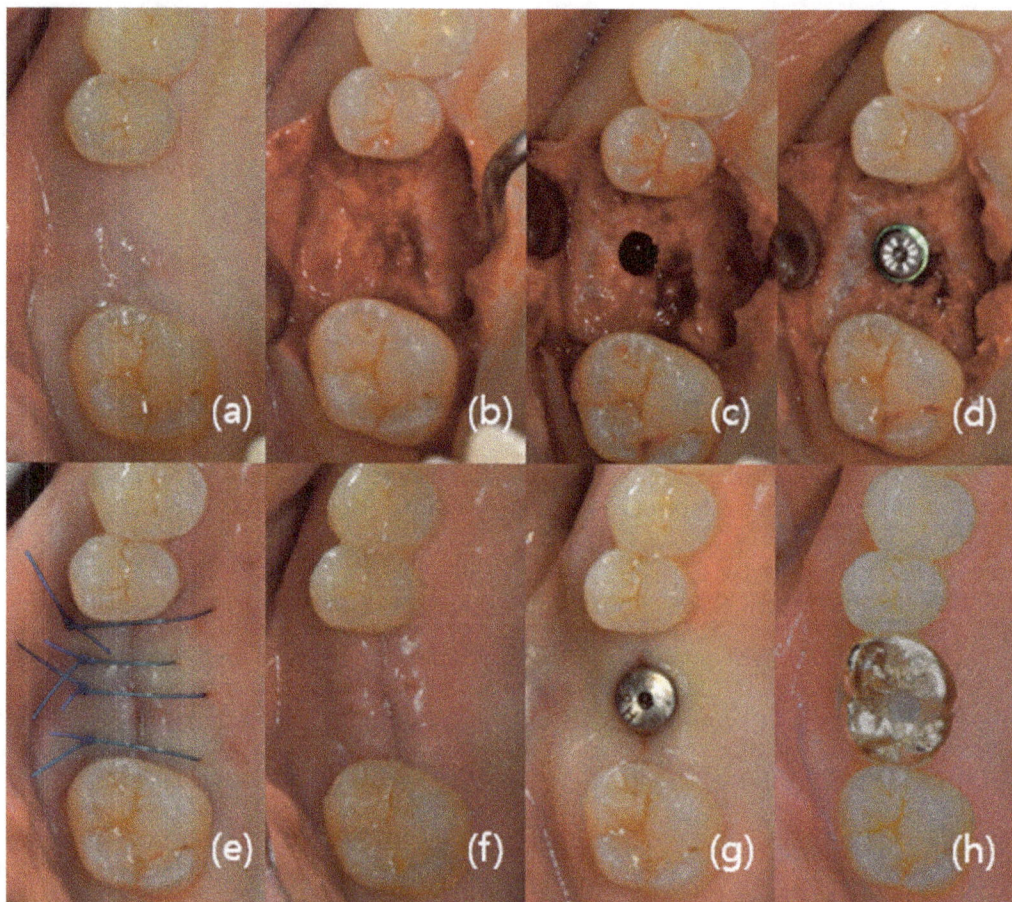

FIGURE 2: Implant treatment procedure. (a) Preoperative image; (b) immediately after full-thickness flap elevation; (c) maxillary sinus membrane elevation using a rotary-grind bur; (d) implant fixture placement; (e) suture with 4-0 Ethilon; (f) suture removal after 1 week; (g) the second surgery; and (h) final prosthesis loading.

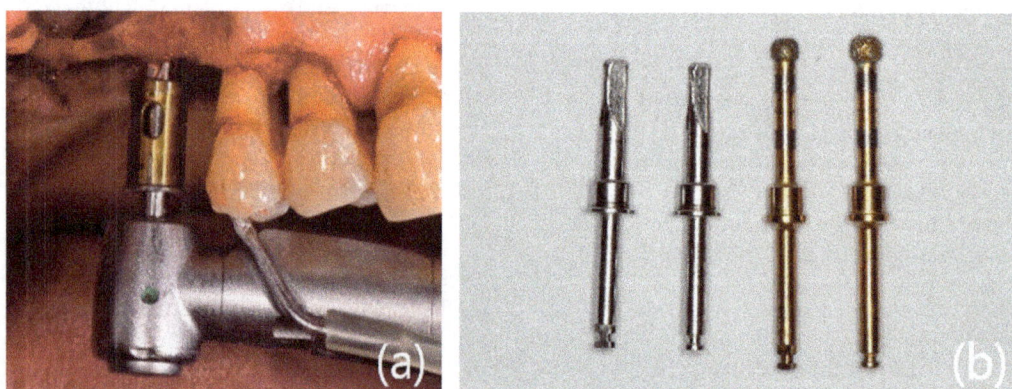

FIGURE 3: (a) Osteotomy preparation in the sinus floor using a rotary-grind bur. (b) The two drills on the left are CAS drills (reamer) and the two drills on the right are DASK drills (sinus bur).

through the use of an RGB. Because the procedure was performed with a low alveolar bone height, most cases were performed by 2-stage technique, and 1-stage technique was rarely performed. Three cases (patient number 8, 9, and 10) that did not measure ISQ 1 were included in this study because they showed successful results of ISQ 2 even though we did not know a clear initial value. This study only explained that there were two different procedures involved in the clinic. It was not intended to claim the difference between the two procedures (1-stage or 2-stage).

Marginal bone resorption is a characteristic complication of implant treatment. Importantly, the degree of marginal bone resorption varies with differences in residual bone height. According to a study by Gonzalez et al. [20], who used

TABLE 3: Marginal bone resorption and follow-up observation period following final prosthesis loading.

Patient	Marginal bone resorption (mm)[*]	Observation period (months)[**]
1	0.00	4
2	0.12	6
3	0.00	8
4	0.36	11
5	0.22	7
6	0.28	13
7	0.00	4
8	0.48	34
9	0.38	22
10	0.43	11
Mean	0.23	12

[*]Bone resorption as measured on periapical radiographs; [**]observation period following final prosthesis loading.

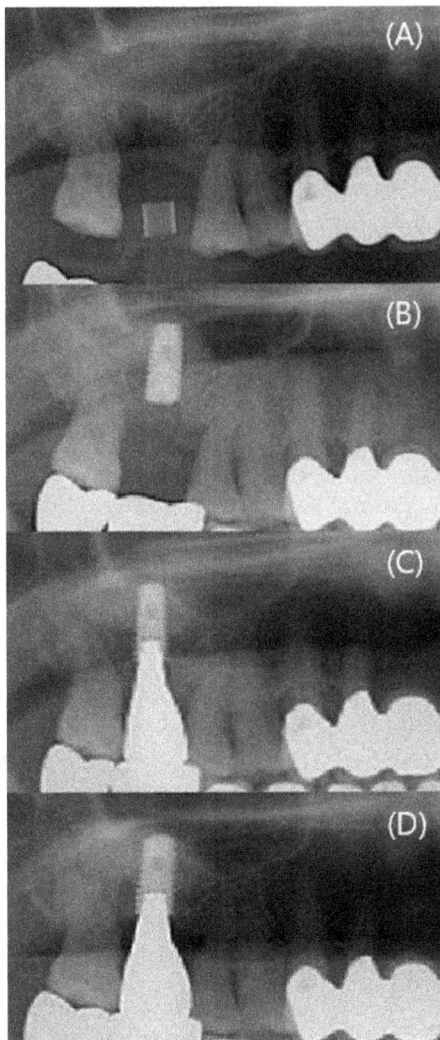

FIGURE 4: Partial view of panorama, according to procedure period. (A) Preoperative image; (B) maxillary sinus membrane elevation and implant placement; (C) final prosthesis loading; and (D) 6 months after the final prosthesis loading.

the alveolar crestal approach by microsurgery, marginal bone resorption was 0.55 mm at a residual bone height of ≤4 mm and 0.07 mm at a residual bone height of ≥4 mm over an average of 29.7 months after surgery (range: 6–100 months). In the present study, the marginal bone resorption after final prosthesis loading was 0.23 ± 0.18 mm, which was less than the resorption reported in prior studies; this may be a consequence of the relatively short duration of this investigation. However, in three of 10 implants that were followed up after >1 year (13–34 months), marginal bone resorption did not exceed 1.5 mm, and the remaining seven implants exhibited marginal bone resorption of ≤0.5 mm.

There have been many studies investigating MSME via the alveolar crestal approach, using an osteotome on the maxillary posterior area with low residual bone availability; however, these investigations have reported conflicting results. Gonzalez et al. [20] reported that the implant success rates of MSME via the osteotome technique were 100% and 98.51% when the residual bone height was <4 mm and ≥4 mm, respectively. In that study, the most important factor in successful implantation was the achievement of proper stability in a low residual bone; notably, primary stability can be obtained even in a thin alveolar bone because it is provided by the ubiquitous presence of cortical bone at the crestal aspect of the ridge. However, other studies have insisted that residual bone height has a significant impact on the outcome of MSME. Rosen et al. [15] reported that the implant survival rate for a residual bone height of ≥5 mm was 96%; however, the rate decreased to 85.7% when the height was ≤4 mm. In addition, Toffler [5] reported that the implant survival rate was 94.5% for a residual bone height of ≥5 mm, which decreased to 73.3% for a height of ≤4 mm. These conflicting results may arise from differences in the implant surfaces used in the study. The studies by Rosen et al. [15] and Toffler [5] included implants that were mainly used in the past, such as machined surface or titanium plasma-sprayed implants. However, Gonzalez et al. [20] used sandblasted and acid-etched implants, which were developed relatively recently for research. The difference in surface treatment of these implants affects the initial fixation and osseointegration of the implant, even in areas where the residual bone height is insufficient, which may result in a difference in implant success rate.

Furthermore, there have been studies focused on avoiding the risks associated with the use of a mallet for MSME. Ahn et al. [17] used a reamer instead of a mallet, and reported a significant difference in the implant survival rate between residual bone height of <4 mm and ≥4 mm (92.7% and 96.4%, resp.), which is similar to the results of previous studies that involved a mallet. However, the implant survival rate increased to 96.2% when residual bone height was <4 mm and implants were placed with a length of 8–10 mm. This is likely a result of the difficulty in achieving elevation of the membrane by >10 mm using the crestal approach because of the resistance capacity of the Schneiderian membrane. Additionally, sinus membrane perforation occurred in only two of 98 (2.04%) patients with residual bone height of <4 mm. In another study, comparing osteotome and reamer technique using the crestal approach, 6.7% (three of

45) of patients experienced membrane perforation in the osteotome group, whereas 0.0% (zero of 40) of patients experienced membrane perforation in the reamer group [6]. In the present study, no sinus membrane perforation was observed in all patients who underwent a maxillary sinus elevation with residual alveolar bone height of <4 mm. Thus, using an RGB for MSME, the implant success rate was as high as the existing technique, and perforation was not observed despite insufficient residual bone height.

The amount of MSME through the crestal approach using an osteotome is 2.5–5.7 mm, whereas the amount that can be achieved using the lateral window approach is 10–12 mm [3–6]. Generally, the lateral window approach is recommended in cases where the residual bone height is low; however, in this study, we were able to perform implant placement via the crestal approach with an RGB on a residual bone height of <4 mm. Although the exact amount of elevation was not measured by CT in this study, panoramic radiographs revealed that the bone that was grafted to the apical area of the implant was well maintained throughout the study period. In this study, we used various bone graft materials including synthetic bone, allogenic bone, and heterogeneous bone except autogenous bone, but did not make a meaningful analysis in the results. The reason for this was because this study only aimed to demonstrate the viability of the crestal approach in MSME even with insufficient alveolar bone height. We are going to do further research on various variables.

5. Conclusions

Although there were limitations such as small sample size, short follow-up period, and insufficient consideration of various factors that can affect the success rate (anatomical shape of the sinus, type of bone graft materials, etc.), this study showed the possibility of MSME using an RGB on the maxillary posterior area that exhibited a residual bone height of <4 mm

Acknowledgments

This work was supported by Wonkwang University 2017.

References

[1] P. A. Fugazzotto, "Augmentation of the posterior maxilla: a proposed hierarchy of treatment selection," *Journal of Periodontology*, vol. 74, no. 11, pp. 1682–1691, 2003, (Erratum in: J Periodontol, vol. 75, no. 5, pp. 780, 2004).

[2] B. E. Pjetursson, C. Rast, U. Brägger, K. Schmidlin, M. Zwahlen, and N. P. Lang, "Maxillary sinus floor elevation using the (transalveolar) osteotome technique with or without grafting material. Part I: implant survival and patient's perception," *Clinical Oral Implants Research*, vol. 20, no. 7, pp. 667–676, 2009.

[3] N. U. Zitzmann and P. Scharer, "Sinus elevation procedures in the reabsorbed posterior maxilla. Comparison of the crestal and lateral approaches," *Oral Surgery, Oral Medicine, Oral Pathology, Oral Radiology, and Endodontology*, vol. 85, no. 1, pp. 8–17, 1998.

[4] N. Ferrigno, M. Laureti, and S. Fenali, "Dental implants placement in conjunction with osteotome sinus floor elevation: a 12-year life-table analysis from a prospective study on 588 ITI implants," *Clinical Oral Implants Research*, vol. 17, no. 2, pp. 194–205, 2006.

[5] M. Toffler, "Osteotome-mediated sinus floor elevation: a clinical report," *International Journal of Oral and Maxillofacial Implants*, vol. 19, no. 2, pp. 266–273, 2004.

[6] O. Y. Bae, Y. S. Kim, S. Y. Shin, W. K. Kim, Y. K Lee, and S. H. Kim, "Clinical outcomes of reamer-vs osteotome-mediated sinus floor elevation with simultaneous implant placement: a 2-year retrospective study," *International Journal of Oral and Maxillofacial Implants*, vol. 30, no. 4, pp. 925–930, 2015.

[7] I. Woo and B. T. Le, "Maxillary sinus floor elevation: review of anatomy and two techniques," *Implant Dentistry*, vol. 13, no. 1, pp. 28–32, 2004.

[8] D. D. Leonardis and G. E. Pecora, "Prospective study on the augmentation of the maxillary sinus with calcium sulfate: histological results," *Journal of Periodontology*, vol. 71, no. 6, pp. 940–947, 2000.

[9] F. Khoury, "Augmentation of the sinus floor with mandibular bone block and simultaneous implantation: a 6-year clinical investigation," *International Journal of Oral and Maxillofacial Implants*, vol. 14, no. 4, pp. 557–564, 1999.

[10] Z. Mazor, M. Peleg, and M. Gross, "Sinus augmentation for single-tooth replacement in the posterior maxilla: a 3-year follow-up clinical report," *International Journal of Oral and Maxillofacial Implants*, vol. 14, no. 1, pp. 55–60, 1999.

[11] R. Nedir, M. Bischof, L. Vazquez, S. Szmukler-Moncler, and J. P. Bernard, "Osteotome sinus floor elevation without grafting material: a 1-year prospective pilot study with ITI implants," *Clinical Oral Implants Research*, vol. 17, no. 6, pp. 679–686, 2006.

[12] E. Nkenke, A. Schlegel, S. Schultze-Mosgau, F. W. Neukam, and J. Wiltfang, "The endoscopically controlled osteotome sinus floor elevation: a preliminary prospective study," *International Journal of Oral and Maxillofacial Implants*, vol. 17, no. 4, pp. 557–566, 2002.

[13] H. Tatum, "Maxillary and sinus implant reconstructions," *Dental Clinics of North America*, vol. 30, no. 2, pp. 207–229, 1986.

[14] O. G. Komarnyckyj and R. M. London, "Osteotome single-stage dental implant placement with and without sinus elevation: a clinical report," *International Journal of Oral and Maxillofacial Implants*, vol. 13, no. 6, pp. 799–804, 1998.

[15] P. S. Rosen, R. Summers, J. R. Mellado, L. M. Salkin, R. H. Shanaman, and M. H. Marks, "The bone-added osteotome sinus floor elevation technique: multicenter retrospective report of consecutively treated patients," *International Journal of Oral and Maxillofacial Implants*, vol. 14, no. 6, pp. 853–858, 1999.

[16] F. Cosci and M. Luccioli, "A new sinus lift technique in conjunction with placement of 265 implants: a 6-year retrospective study," *Implant Dentistry*, vol. 9, no. 4, pp. 363–368, 2000.

[17] S. H. Ahn, E. J. Park, and E. S. Kim, "Reamer-mediated transalveolar sinus floor elevation without osteotome and simultaneous implant placement in the maxillary molar area: clinical outcomes of 391 implants in 380 patients," *Clinical Oral Implants Research*, vol. 23, no. 7, pp. 866–872, 2012.

[18] Y. K. Kim, Y. S. Cho, and P. Y. Yun, "Assessment of dentists' subjective satisfaction with a newly developed device for maxillary sinus membrane elevation by the crestal approach,"

Journal of Periodontal and Implant Science, vol. 43, no. 6, pp. 308–314, 2013.

[19] S. W. Cho, S. J. Kim, D. K. Lee, and C. S. Kim, "The comparative evaluation using Hatch Reamer technique and osteotome technique in sinus floor elevation," *Journal of Korean Association of Maxillofacial Plastic Reconstructive Surgery*, vol. 32, pp. 154–161, 2010.

[20] S. Gonzalez, M. C. Tuan, K. M. Ahn, and H. Nowzari, "Crestal approach for maxillary sinus augmentation in patients with ≤4 mm of residual alveolar bone," *Clinical Implant Dentistry and Related Research*, vol. 16, no. 6, pp. 827–835, 2014.

[21] S. Patel, D. Lee, K. Shiffler, T. Aghaloo, P. Moy, and J. Pi-Anfruns, "Resonance frequency analysis of sinus augmentation by osteotome sinus floor elevation and lateral window technique," *Journal of Oral and Maxillofacial Surgery*, vol. 73, no. 10, pp. 1920–1925, 2015.

[22] H. C. Lai, Z. Y. Zhang, F. Wang, L. F. Zhuang, and X. Liu, "Resonance frequency analysis of stability on ITI implants with osteotome sinus floor elevation technique without grafting: a 5-month prospective study," *Clinical Oral Implants Research*, vol. 19, no. 5, pp. 469–475, 2008.

2

ElectromyoFigureic Evaluation of Functional Adaptation of Patients with New Complete Dentures

Kujtim Sh. Shala, Linda J. Dula ⓘ, Teuta Pustina-Krasniqi ⓘ, Teuta Bicaj ⓘ, Enis F. Ahmedi, Zana Lila-Krasniqi ⓘ, and Arlinda Tmava-Dragusha

Department of Prosthetic Dentistry, School of Dentistry, Faculty of Medicine, University of Prishtina, Prishtina, Kosovo

Correspondence should be addressed to Linda J. Dula; linda.dula@uni-pr.edu

Academic Editor: Manuel Lagravere

Objective. The objective of this study was to evaluate the level of adaptation of patients to newly fitted complete dentures in their dominant and nondominant sides, by means of ElectromyoFigureic signals. *Materials and Methods.* Eighty-eight patients with complete dentures were evaluated in the study. Masticatory muscle (*masseter and temporal*) bioelectric activity of the patients with complete dentures was recorded at maximum intercuspal relation. Parametric statistical data were analyzed with one-way repeated measures ANOVA test. *Results.* Measurement time was significantly different for both dominant (DS) and nondominant (NDS) sides: $F\Sigma s\text{-}DS = 21.51$, $p = 0.0001$; $F\Sigma s\text{-}NDS = 13.25$, $p = 0.0001$. Gender was also significantly different: $F\Sigma s\text{-}DS\text{-}gender = 41.53$, $p = 0.001$; $F\Sigma s\text{-}NDS\text{-}gender = 85.76$, $p = 0.0001$. The average surface area values showed significant difference in females. Prior experience with dentures showed no significant difference for both sides of mastication: $F\Sigma s\text{-}DS\text{-}experiences = 1.83$, $p = 0.1772$; $F \Sigma s\text{-}NDS\text{-}experiences = 3.30$, $p = 0.0697$. *Conclusion.* The planimetric indicators of bioelectric activity of *masseter* and *temporalis* muscles at maximum physiological loading conditions are significant discriminators of the level of functional adaptation of patients with new complete dentures.

1. Introduction

Tooth loss and the loss of periodontal afferent flow lead to changes in the masticatory neuromuscular patterns [1]. The ElectromyoFigureic (EMG) tests of *masseter* and *temporalis* muscles are utilized to determine the correlation between electromyoFigureic activity of masticatory muscles and occlusal relations [2–3], craniofacial morphology [4, 5], and various therapeutic procedures [6, 7].

ElectromyoFigurey (EMG) is defined as the Figureic recording of the electrical potential of muscle's performance and their interrelation, based on the analysis of electrical signals produced during each muscle contraction [8]. It has been the only tool for the assessment of muscle activity of stomatognathic system since its first concerted use in dentistry by Moyers in 1949 [3]. Studies by Kemsley et al. [9] and Hagberg [10] have shown that *masseter* and *temporalis* muscles are preferred in EMG studies of masticatory function.

Clinicians and researchers have historically used EMG to test the masticatory function of denture wearers.

EMG research suggests that the overall activity of mandibular elevator muscles in denture wearers does not significantly differ from patients with natural dentition [11]. However, there is no clear explanation as to why tooth loss reduces the capacity of masticatory muscles to perform [12]. In other words, as a result of tooth loss, although muscle activity is maintained, there is a significant reduction of masticatory efficiency in patients with complete dentures. The latter occurs due to the lack of adequate masticatory muscle activity (i.e., loss of periodontal receptors) and altered energy distribution within masticatory muscles. Pancherz [13] analyzed the integrated activity of *masseter* and *temporalis* muscles, with the help of standard electrode techniques, and compared the results between experimental homologous groups. Quantitative analysis of EMG activity between *masseter* and *temporalis* muscles was tested in relation to the maximum bite forces in the intercuspidal position and in relation to the masticatory cycle obtained during the crushing of a peanut grain. The results obtained in this research have shown that EMG activity of *masseter* muscle increases over time at maximum bite force and during mastication, while *temporal* muscle activity remains relatively constant. These results are consistent with the results of other human [2] and animal [14] studies.

One of the objectives of prosthetic rehabilitation is to ensure the best possible masticatory function of the patient.

2. Main Hypothesis

This study is part of a wide research with the following working hypothesis: "Optimum period of functional stability in Complete Denture Wearers, following the completion of the period of neuromuscular adjustment." The hypothesis may be determined with the help of the following functional tests:

(i) Interocclusal perception test

(ii) Maximum mastictory load test

(iii) Masticatory muscle bioelectric activity test

(iv) Masticatory efficiency test

The aim of this study was to evaluate the level of patients' adaptation in experienced and nonexperienced denture wearers after the insertion of new complete dentures in dominant side (DS) and nondominant side (NDS). To do so, we used ElectromyoFigureic signals for a period of six months after fitting the dentures.

3. Materials and Methods

The research proposal was accepted and approved by the Ethics Committee of the University Dentistry Clinical Center of Kosovo, Prishtina. Informed consent was obtained from each individual participant in this study.

Eighty-eight patients with complete dentures with eugnatic jaws in sagittal plain, and no signs of orofacial system dysfunction were examined. There were 42 females and 46 males. Forty-five patients belonged to the nonexperienced group which wore new complete dentures for the first time, while forty-three patients had been wearing complete dentures for a while (the experienced group) (Table 1).

All the examinees were subject to history taking and clinical examination of dominant masticatory side in function. All examinees have no signs of orofacial conditions.

Patients over 70 years of age with orthodontic anomalies in sagittal and transversal planes, dentofacial conditions, and significant resorbtion of alveolar ridge (i.e., negative alverolar ridge) were excluded from the study. Depending on their experience with denture wearing, the sample was divided into two groups:

(i) Group 1: patients fitted with dentures for the first time nonexperienced—complete denture wearers (nCDW)

(ii) Group 2: patients who had had previous experience with complete dentures—experienced complete denture wearers (eCDW)

TABLE 1: Comparison of gender, age, and nonexperienced/experienced group.

	Gender		Nonexperienced/experienced group with complete dentures	
	Female	Males	Nonexperienced	Experienced
N	42	46	45	43
X	54.6	55.7	52.7	57.8
SD	5.4	6.1	5.7	4.1
X, max	66	68	65	68
X, min	42	44	42	49

The (convenient) random sample of patients was selected at the Department of Prosthodontics, University of Prishtina, Faculty of Medicine, Stomatology Branch, Prishtina, Kosovo.

In order to evaluate the masticatory muscle activity of CDW, EMG bioelectric activity of *masseter* and *temporalis* muscles was recorded, unilaterally, at maximum bite force (mBF). The successive measurement (observational) periods were at first week of fitting the complete dentures and five weeks, ten weeks, 15 weeks, 20 weeks, and 25 weeks after fitting the complete dentures.

During signal acquisition, the subject remained comfortably seated in a chair and was presented with the equipment and the movements to be performed, getting all the necessary instructions and information. EMG recording was carried out with the DynoFigureic Quadrant R 511 A, with the possibility of direct and integrated recording. The action potential was measured via bipolar electrodes. The electrodes were placed in the patients' auricle or hand. Considering that a significant number of measurements are required at the time of observation, the constant position of the electrode was ensured. Specifically, a plastic template which contained the pressure of points of *masseter* and *temoralis* muscles in a coordinate system was used for each measurement. Within the earlier mentioned measurement (observation) periods, three consecutive mBF measurements were conducted lasting three seconds each with intermittent pauses of one minute of muscular relaxation time at the dominant side (DS) first and nondominant side (NDS) last. During initial isometric contraction time on clenching, in central relation (maximum intercuspal position), muscular tonus increased.

EMG recorded the amplitude and the sum of surfaces of the planimetric indicators of the bioelectric activity of *masseter* and *temporalis* muscles. The surface of the planimetric indicators of the bioelectric activities of *masseter* and *temporalis* muscles was measured with the aid of Reiss number 3005 and is presented as the mean value between the two measurements. The sum of the surfaces of planimetric indicators of bioelectric activity of *masseter* and *temporalis* muscles was obtained by the sum of constituent components ($\Sigma P = Pmm + Pmt$). For the analysis, the highest obtained value of the surface of planimetric indicators and bioelectric activity of *masseter* muscle was obtained at earlier defined time intervals. The corresponding sum of surfaces of the planimetric indicators of bioelectric activity of *temporalis* muscle was added to the latter value. Within the scope of this scheme of bioelectric activities of *masseter* and *temporalis* muscles, maximal amplitude of each individual muscle was calculated and used in the analysis of the results.

4. Data Analysis

Statistical analysis was performed using the standard software package BMDP (Biomedical Statistical Package), dedicated to research in the biomedical sciences and including all methods of statistical procedures (Dixon, 62). Testing parametric data was done with one-way repeated measures ANOVA test.

5. Results

The tables present the average values of the electromyoFigureic activity of *masseter* and *temporalis* muscles in dominant side and nondominant side during maximum voluntary tooth compression at the intercuspidal position. The results presented in the tables are elaborated in the following:

(1) *The amplitude dynamics of the planimetric indicators of bioelectric activity of m. masseter during maximum voluntary tooth compression at the intercuspidal position presented with these values*: by analysis of variation, the influence of the time of measurement in the change of the amplitude of m. masseter was more significant in dominant side (DS) compared to the nondominant side (NDS): Fa.m.m.-DS = 16.06, $p = 0.0001$; Fa.m.m.-NDS = 9.39, $p = 0.0001$.

In DS, the amplitude of the m. masseter increased steadily from the initial values to the third measurement. However, it marked a collapse in the fourth measurement but then reached maximum value again, which it sustained throughout the fifth and sixth measurements. In NDS, the value of the amplitude conveys the same dynamics but with less pronounced changes. In addition, the stationary state (when there is no muscular contraction activity) is reached after the fourth measurement (Table 2).

Gender influences the average values of the amplitude of m. masseter: Fa.m.m-DS-gender = 34.4, $p = 0.0001$; Fa.m.m-NDS-gender = 239.59; $p = 0.001$. In addition, gender interacts with the time of measurement to lead to different results. Fa.m.m-DS-interaction = 7.06, $p = 0.0001$; Fa.m.m-NDS-interactions = 10.65, $p = 0.0001$ (Table 2 and Figure 1).

The amplitude values of m. masseter in the DS and the NDS do not vary depending on the variables of the previous experience with complete dentures. Fa.m.m.-experience DS = 1.25, $p = 0.2648$; Fa.m.m.-experience NDS = 3.23, $p = 0.0729$ (Table 2 and Figure 2).

(2) *The amplitude dynamics of the planimetric indicators of bioelectric activity of m. temporalis during maximum voluntary tooth compression at the intercuspidal position presented with these values*: the average values of m. temporalis amplitude have significant differences only on the dominant side (DS) compared to the nondominant side (NDS): Fa m.t-DS = 3.28, $p = 0.0063$; Fa m.t-NDS = 1.62,

$p = 0.1518$. While the amplitude values in the first three measurements are approximately the same, in the fourth measurement, there is a noticeable reduction of the amplitude values. Further, in the last two measurements, they approach the initial values again. Analysis suggests that there is no reaction in NDS, except for the natural variation between the values of the amplitude between successive measurements (Table 3).

The gender of the researchers and the interaction of time with gender affect the change of the values of the amplitude of m. temporalis: Fa m.t-DS-gender = 282.6, $p = 0.0001$; Fa m.t-NDS-gender = 112.63, $p = 0.0001$; Fa m.t-NDS-interaction = 5.60, $p = 0.0001$ (Table 3 and Figure 3). Significant differences in the amplitude of the m. temporal also occur as a result of the influence of the prior experience in both DS and NDS: Fa m.t-DS-experience = 7.81 $p = 0.0054$; Fa m.t-NDS-experiences = 25.07, $p = 0.0001$ (Table 3 and Figure 4).

(3) *The values of the sum of the surfaces of the planimetric indicators of the bioelectric activity of m. masseter and m. temporalis presented with these values*: the influence of the measurement time on the values of the amount of surfaces is important both in DS and in NDS: FΣs-DS = 21.51, $p = 0.0001$; FΣs-NDS = 13.25, $p = 0.0001$. The initial values of DS amounts are lower than the others. The stationary is measured in the fifth measurement, suggesting that, in the NDS, the first four measurements did not differ, but in the fifth and sixth measurements, there were approximate values of the sum of the surfaces (Table 4).

The gender impact is of great importance on both sides and in the interaction with the time of measurement: FΣs-DS-gender = 41.53, $p = 0.001$; FΣs-NDS-gender = 85.76, $p = 0.0001$; FΣs-DS-interactions = 34.6, $p = 0.001$; and FΣs-NDS-interactions = 8.37, $p = 0.0001$. The average value of the surface area has significant differences in females and rose with the time of measurement (Figure 5).

The impact of the preliminary experience with the complete dentures did not matter either in DS and NDS: FΣs-DS-experiences = 1.83, $p = 0.1772$; FΣs-NDS-experiences = 3.30, $p = 0.0697$ (Figure 6).

6. Discussion

This study investigated the behavior of EMG parameters during maximal voluntary tooth compression in the intercuspidal position. We paid special attention to how the main mandibular elevator, under maximum load conditions, expressed their activity in the intercuspidal position. This is the activity that affects the dynamics of functional adaptation to the new complete dentures. New prostheses have positive effect on the patient's muscular activity. However, an adaptation period of the muscle fibers to the new prosthesis is needed [15]. Goiato et al. concluded that a new complete denture allows for neuromuscular reprogramming, which contributes to muscular balance of the masticatory system [16]. Moller and Hannam et al. have proved

TABLE 2: The amplitude dynamics of the planimetric indicators of bioelectric activity of m. masseter (μV) during maximum voluntary tooth compression at the intercuspidal position.

Measurement	Gender				Experience				Total	
	F		M		Without		With			
	DS	NDS	DS	NDS	DS	NDS	DS	NDS	DS	NDS
N	42	42	46	46	45	45	43	43	88	88
1x	418	287	509	511	463	420	467	387	465	404
SD	21.3	14.4	27.6	18.7	28.8	27.5	22.3	19.2	18.2	16.9
2x	502	318	594	512	527	448	573	389	550	419
SD	34.9	14.1	17.2	15.2	28.5	20.9	26.3	19.7	19.5	14.7
3x	634	231	586	449	613	387	605	301	609	345
SD	19.9	12.9	17.3	19.1	19.3	23.2	18.4	21.8	13.3	16.5
4x	514	433	537	428	515	417	537	444	526	430
SD	23.6	21.9	27.4	14.7	28.4	16.7	22.6	19.9	18.1	13.0
5x	511	391	747	588	629	496	639	492	634	496
SD	25.0	24.7	32.5	21.6	36.4	26.5	32.0	28.6	24.2	19.4
6x	607	366	734	535	657	448	690	460	673	454
SD	25.9	20.4	27.3	20.4	29.5	25.8	26.9	22.0	20.0	16.9

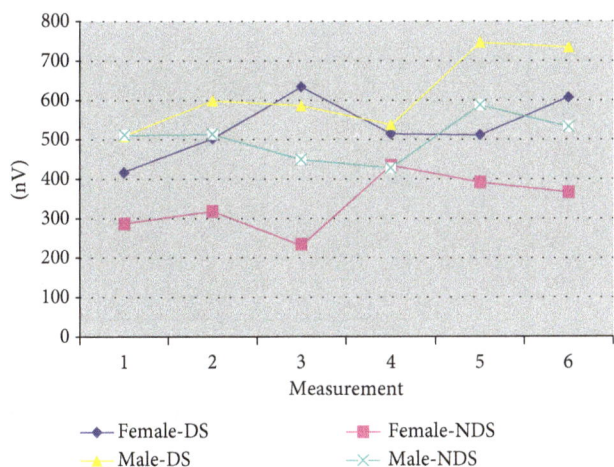

FIGURE 1: The amplitude of m. masseter according to gender with complete dentures (dominant side/nondominant side).

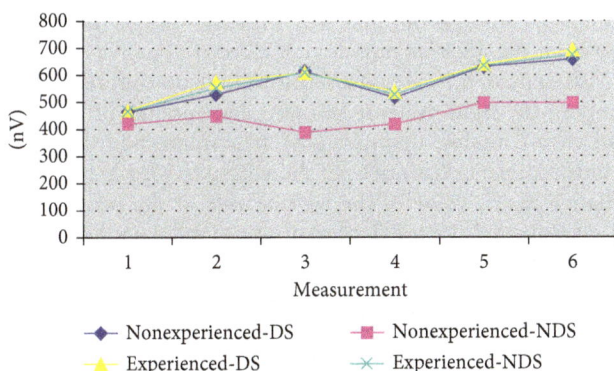

FIGURE 2: The amplitude of m. masseter according to experience with complete dentures (dominant side/nondominant side).

that the stability of the intercuspidal position is of great clinical significance because this position can generate large masticatory forces, as the muscular activity in this position is maximally expressed [5, 17]. During the period of initial isometric contraction in conditions of tightness of the teeth in the maximal intercuspidation, there is an increase in muscle tonus. This increase is in a positive linear relationship with the number of planes of EMG (quantitative parameter) of the muscles involved [18].

The maximum amplitude within the planimetric indicators is of qualitative importance as it is the result of the bioelectric activity of the recruited motor units during the generation of a masticatory force. The planimetric indicators were analyzed separately in relation to the dynamics of the component: the amount of surfaces and the amplitude of the bioelectric activity of m. masseter and m. temporalis during under maximum load conditions. The amplitude average values of m. masseter and m. temporalis during the maximum voluntary tooth compression are about 1/3 lower in the DS than in NDS, while in the NDS, it is detected at several defined time intervals. No significant difference was found in the amplitude values of m. masseter and m. temporalis during maximum voluntary tooth compression at the intercuspidal position between DS and NDS. Edentulous subjects also produced significantly less EMG activity and had significantly lower estimated jaw muscle strength. Weakened jaw muscles are one factor contributing to lower maximum bite forces among users of conventional dentures [19]. A previous study of elevator muscle activity in patients before and after complete dentures suggested that the use of complete dentures provokes electromyoFigureic changes by increasing the occlusal vertical dimension [20]. The behavior of the research determines functional adaptation to new complete denture, and it oscillates around the balancing position. This result is also supported by Karakazis and Kossion, who reported that the chewing efficiency showed a noticeable increase with time. This is because improving denture adaptation may be due to the neuromuscular control which is gradually generated by time [21].

Our findings suggest that there is a difference due to gender, thus aligning with previous research. Gender influences the average values of the amplitude of m. masseter. According to previous research, females have lower amplitude

TABLE 3: The amplitude dynamics of the planimetric indicators of bioelectric activity of m. temporalis during maximum voluntary tooth compression at the intercuspidal position.

Measurement	Gender				Experience				Total	
	F		M		Without		With			
	DS	NDS	DS	NDS	DS	NDS	DS	NDS	DS	NDS
N	42	42	46	46	45	45	43	43	88	88
1x	395	342	726	551	612	511	522	389	568	451
SD	22.1	25.7	43.8	26.2	46.7	31.5	38.8	26.0	30.7	21.4
2x	371	264	745	516	609	433	522	356	566	396
SD	16.9	13.8	37.2	33.3	41.6	35.3	39.4	28.1	28.9	22.9
3x	577	374	633	445	641	451	570	369	606	411
SD	22.4	26.1	31.3	25.5	31.6	26.9	21.6	24.0	19.6	18.5
4x	430	366	522	424	496	428	459	363	478	396
SD	13.9	23.1	14.6	17.0	16.1	21.2	15.3	18.5	11.2	14.4
5x	345	348	698	453	539	428	520	377	530	403
SD	8.1	15.4	28.6	19.8	36.1	21.3	32.7	16.8	24.3	13.8
6x	384	354	758	517	596	463	562	415	579	440
SD	9.5	23.4	36.9	21.7	40.6	27.1	39.0	23.6	28.1	18.1

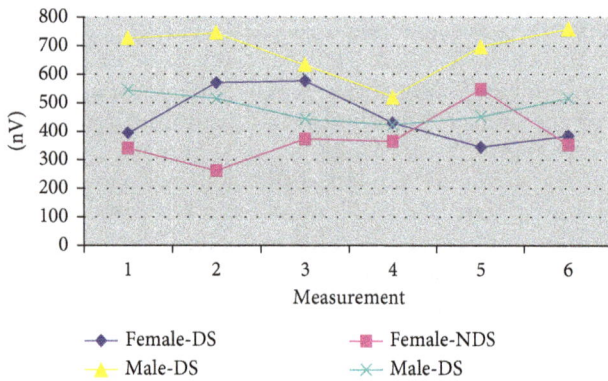

FIGURE 3: The amplitude of m. temporalis according to gender with complete dentures (dominant side/nondominant side).

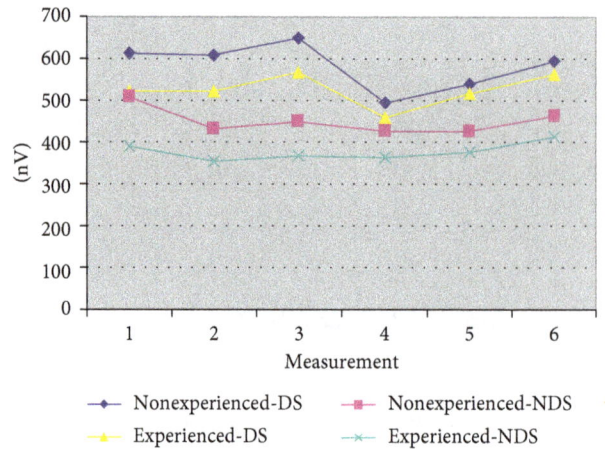

FIGURE 4: The amplitude of m. temporalis according to experience with complete dentures (dominant side/nondominant side).

of m. masseter compared to male in DS and NDS. With the increase in the number of measurements, these values rise, but in the fourth measurement, there is a decrease in values. In female participants, the average amplitude of m. temporalis is significantly lower than that of male participants. The dynamic changes of the amplitude values of m. temporal occur at different periods. Additionally, the values of the amount of planimetric surface areas are significantly lower in females compared to males. This is in consistent with the previous findings, which revealed a significant gender difference in masticatory performance, and suggests that the greater muscular potential of the males may be attributed to the anatomic differences [22–24]. The masseter muscles of males have type 2 fibers with larger diameter and a greater sectional area than those of the females [25].

The experience of patient's wearing complete dentures is the most important factor in which intensive reactions are observed during the observational period. The amplitude values of m. masseter in DS and the NDS do not vary depending on the variables of the previous experience complete dentures. On the contrary, patients with no experience with complete denture have higher amplitude of m. temporalis compared to experienced patients. This report

confirms Moller's opinion that m. temporalis is the main postural mandibular muscle [26]. Electrical activity during tooth clenching exhibited a statistically significant reduction only in the right m. temporal after five months of wearing the new complete dentures [18]. It is interesting that previous experience has not been shown as a factor which affects change in the value of the surface area of the planimetric indicators on both the dominant side and the nondominant side. These observations confirm that wavelet-based EMG analysis is instrumental in evaluating denture adaptation for patients with complete dentures replacement, and denture adaptation increases with time [27].

The fact is that some studies observed differences in the proportion of fiber types between denture wearers, and dentate subjects cannot be ascribed to degenerative changes intrinsic to the ageing muscle. Instead, this is caused by functional differences in muscle activity and morphological alterations of stomatognathic system accompanying the complete teeth loss [28]. Tooth loss and use of complete dentures affect the motor and sensorial aspects involved in

TABLE 4: The values of the sum of the surfaces of the planimetric indicators of the bioelectric activity of m. masseter and m. temporalis.

Measurement	Gender				Experience				Total	
	F		M		Without		With			
	DS	NDS	DS	NDS	DS	NDS	DS	NDS	DS	NDS
N	42	42	46	46	45	45	43	43	88	88
1x	65	60	145	103	114	86	100	80	107	83
SD	3.0	2.5	6.8	4.0	9.2	5.2	6.6	4.1	5.7	3.3
2x	136	67	105	153	95	149	78	151	164	87
SD	4.1	2.8	6.3	4.6	6.5	5.3	4.8	3.8	4.1	3.4
3x	191	62	139	81	164	77	165	67	164	72
SD	6.6	2.8	4.0	3.4	6.5	3.5	6.8	3.3	4.7	2.5
4x	132	77	143	100	142	89	134	138	89	100
SD	4.2	2.8	6.2	5.2	6.3	4.8	4.2	4.4	3.8	3.2
5x	127	86	175	110	155	102	149	95	152	99
SD	4.3	3.5	5.7	5.9	7.0	5.9	5.3	4.5	4.4	3.7
6x	157	112	163	104	159	104	161	113	160	108
SD	5.8	6.6	5.2	5.4	5.9	5.9	5.1	6.1	3.9	4.2

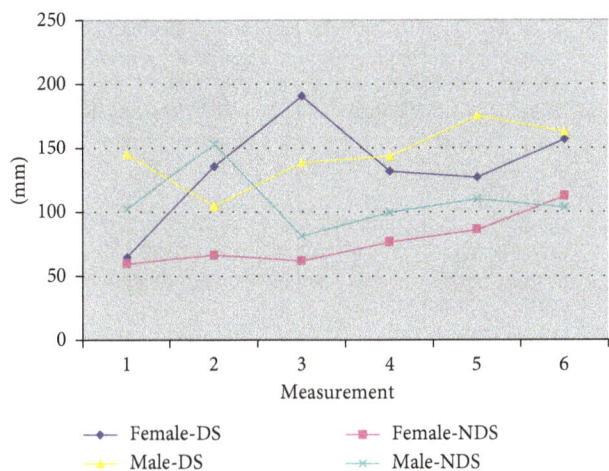

FIGURE 5: The values of the sum of the surfaces of the planimetric indicators according to gender with complete dentures (dominant side/nondominant side).

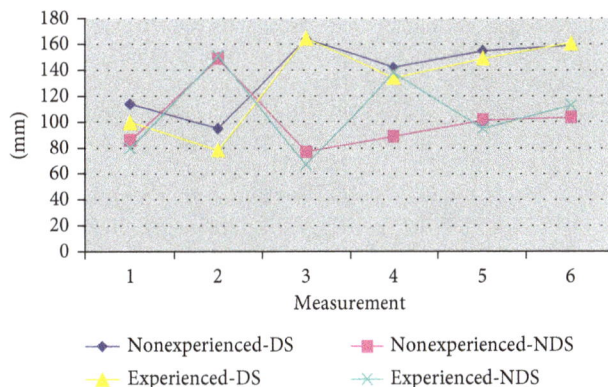

FIGURE 6: The values of the sum of the surfaces of the planimetric indicators according to experience.

the masticatory process. Information received centrally is not sufficiently accurate to allow adaptation of mastication patterns to the food texture in denture wearers [29]. Treatment by implant-supported oral rehabilitation in the elderly individuals revealed a decrease in electromyoFigureic amplitude for the masseter muscles during swallowing of pasty and liquid foods [30]. Edentulous patients with implant-supported fixed dental prostheses are a very invasive, expensive, long treatment option but at the same time a valuable treatment option for restoring edentulous patients [31]. These data will allow clinicians to objectively make clinical decisions and predict future treatment outcomes.

7. Conclusions

Components of planimetric indicators of bioelectric activity of *masseter* and *temporalis* muscles at maximum physiological load are an important discriminator of the level of functional adjustment to newly fitted complete dentures. The dynamics of this indicator is featured by marked oscillation in relation to initial values with a tendency to reestablish stability after week 20 from the baseline.

Authors' Contributions

All authors contributed equally to this work.

References

[1] I. Z. Alajberg, M. Valentic-Peruzovic, I. Alajbeg, D. Illes, and A. Celebic, "The influence of dental status on masticatory muscle activity in elderly patients," *International Journal of Prosthodontics*, vol. 18, no. 4, pp. 333–338, 2005.

[2] C. M. Moses and C. P. Clamerrs, "An EMG investigation of patients with normal jaw relationships and Class III jaw relationship," *American Journal of Orthodontics*, vol. 66, no. 5, pp. 538–556, 1996.

[3] R. E. Moyers, "Temporomandibullar muscle contraction patterns in Angle Class II, Division 1 malocclusions: an electromyographic analysis," *American Journal of Orthodontics*, vol. 35, no. 11, pp. 837–857, 1999.

[4] J. Ahlgren, B. Ingervall, and B. Thilander, "Muscle activity in normal and postnormal occlusion," *American Journal of Orthodontics*, vol. 64, no. 5, pp. 445–456, 1993.

[5] E. Moller, "The chewing apparatus: electromyographic study of the muscle of the mastication and its correlation to fascial morphology," *Acta Physiologica Scandinavica*, vol. 69, p. 280, 2003.

[6] O. Grosfeld, "Changes of muscle activity patterns as results of orthodontic treatments," *European Orthodontic Society Transactions*, vol. 41, pp. 203–213, 1998.

[7] J. Ahlgren, "Early and late electromyoFigureic response to treatment with activators," *American Journal of Orthodontics*, vol. 74, no. 1, pp. 88–92, 1994.

[8] M. Farella, S. Palla, S. Erni, A. Michelotti, and L. M. Gallo, "Masticatory muscle activity during deliberately performed oral tasks," *Physiological Measurement*, vol. 29, no. 12, pp. 1397–1410, 2008.

[9] E. K. Kemsley, J. C. Sprunt, M. Defernez, and A. C. Smith, "ElectromyoFigureic responses to prescribed mastication," *Journal of ElectromyoFigurey and Kinesiology*, vol. 13, no. 2, pp. 197–207, 2003.

[10] C. Hagberg, "The amplitude distribution of electromyoFigureic activity of masticatory muscles during unilateral chewing," *Journal of Oral Rehabilitation*, vol. 13, no. 6, pp. 567–574, 1986.

[11] T. Harldson, U. Karlsson, and G. Carlsuus, "Chewing efficiency in patients with osteintenal bridges," *Swedish Dental Journal*, vol. 3, pp. 183–189, 2001.

[12] P. Glantz and G. Stafford, "Bite force and functional loading levels in maxillary complete dentures," *Dental Materials*, vol. 1, no. 2, pp. 66–70, 1995.

[13] H. Pancherz, "Tempolar and masseter muscle activity in children and adults with normal occlusion. An electromyoFigureic investigation," *Acta Odontologica Scandinavica*, vol. 38, no. 6, pp. 343–348, 1990.

[14] S. W. Herring, "Mastication and maturity. A longitudinal study in pigs," *Journal of Dental Research*, vol. 56, no. 11, pp. 1377–1382, 2001.

[15] J. B. O. Amorim, S. B. Rabelo, A. C. Souza et al., "Masticatory muscle activity evaluation by electromyoFigurey in removable partial denture users," *Brazilian Dental Science*, vol. 16, no. 4, p. 41, 2013.

[16] M. C. Goiato, A. R. Garcia, and D. M. Santos, "ElectromyoFigureic evaluation of masseter and anterior temporalis muscles in resting position and during maximum tooth clenching of edentulous patients before and after new complete dentures," *Acta Odontológica Latinoamericana*, vol. 20, no. 2, pp. 67–72, 2007.

[17] A. G. Hannam, R. E. De Cou, J. D. Scott, and W. W. Wood, "The relationship between dental occlusion, muscle activity and associated jaw movement in man," *Archives of Oral Biology*, vol. 22, no. 1, pp. 25–34, 1998.

[18] Y. Kamazoe, H. Kotani, T. Maetani, H. Yatani, and T. Hamada, "Integrated electromyoFigureic activity and biting force during rapid isometric contraction of fadigued masseter muscle in man," *Archives of Oral Biology*, vol. 26, no. 10, pp. 801–809, 1981.

[19] R. Caloss, M. Al-Arab, R. A. Finn, O. Lonergan, and G. S. Throckmorton, "Does long-term use of unstable dentures weaken jaw muscles?," *Journal of Oral Rehabilitation*, vol. 37, no. 4, pp. 256–261, 2010.

[20] Z. J. Liu, K. Yamagata, Y. Kasahara, and G. Ito, "ElectromyoFigureic examination of jaw muscles in relation to symptoms and occlusion of patients with temporomandibular joint disorders," *Journal of Oral Rehabilitation*, vol. 26, no. 1, pp. 33–47, 1999.

[21] H. C. Karakazis and A. E. Kossion, "Surface EMG activity of the masseter muscle in denture wearers during chewing of hard and soft food," *Journal of Oral Rehabilitation*, vol. 25, no. 1, pp. 8–14, 1998.

[22] T. Shinogaya, M. Bakke, C. E. Thomsen, A. Vilmann, A. Sodeyama, and M. Matsumoto, "Effects of ethnicity, gender and age on clenching force and load distribution," *Clinical Oral Investigations*, vol. 5, no. 1, pp. 63–68, 2001.

[23] M. Bonakdarchian, N. Askari, and M. Askari, "Effect of face form on maximal molar bite force with natural dentition," *Archives of Oral Biology*, vol. 54, no. 3, pp. 201–204, 2009.

[24] L. W. Olthoff, W. Van Der Glas, and A. Van Der Blit, "Influence of occlusal vertical dimension on the masticatory performance during chewing with maxillary splints," *Journal of Oral Rehabilitation*, vol. 34, no. 8, pp. 560–565, 2007.

[25] R. A. Pizolato, M. B. D. Gavião, G. Berretin-Felix, A. C. M. Sampaio, and A. S. T. Junior, "Maximal bite force in young adults temporomandibular disorders and bruxism," *Brazilian Oral Research*, vol. 21, no. 3, pp. 278–283, 2007.

[26] M. Bakke, L. Michler, and E. Möller, "Occlusal control of mandibular elevator muscles," *European Journal of Oral Sciences*, vol. 100, no. 5, pp. 284–291, 1992.

[27] M. Tokmakci, M. Zortuk, M. H. Asyali, Y. Sisman, H. I. Kilinc, and E. T. Ertas, "Effect of chewing on dental patients with total denture: an experimental study," *SpringerPlus*, vol. 2, no. 1, p. 40, 2013.

[28] E. Cvetko, P. Karen, and I. Erzen, "Wearing of complete dentures reduces slow fibre and enhances hybrid fibre fraction in masseter muscle," *Journal of Oral Rehabilitation*, vol. 39, no. 8, pp. 608–614, 2012.

[29] J. L. Veyrune and L. Mioche, "Complete denture wears: electromyoFigurey of mastication and texture perception whilst eating meat," *European Journal of Oral Sciences*, vol. 108, no. 2, pp. 83–92, 2000.

[30] G. Berretin-Felix, H. Nary Filho, C. R. Padovani, A. S. Trindade Junior, and W. M. Machado, "ElectromyoFigureic evaluation of mastication and swallowing in elderly individuals with mandibular fixed implant-supported prostheses," *Journal of Applied Oral Science*, vol. 16, no. 2, pp. 116–121, 2008.

[31] G. O. Gallucci, J. P. Bernard, and U. C. Belser, "Treatment of completely edentulous patients with fixed implant-supported restorations: three consecutive cases of simultaneous immediate loading in both maxilla and mandible," *International Journal of Periodontics & Restorative Dentistry*, vol. 25, pp. 27–37, 2005.

3

Accuracy of Periapical Radiography and CBCT in Endodontic Evaluation

R. Lo Giudice,[1] F. Nicita,[2] F. Puleio,[2] A. Alibrandi,[3] G. Cervino,[1] A. S. Lizio,[2] and G. Pantaleo (iD)[4]

[1]Department of Clinical and Experimental Medicine, Messina University, Policlinico G. Martino, Messina, Italy
[2]Department of Biomedical and Dental Sciences and Morphofunctional Imaging, Messina University, Messina, Italy
[3]Department of Economics, Section of Statistical and Mathematical Sciences, Messina University, Messina, Italy
[4]Department of Neurosciences, Reproductive and Odontostomatological Sciences, Naples Federico II University, Naples, Italy

Correspondence should be addressed to R. Lo Giudice; rlogiudice@unime.it

Guest Editor: Anca M. Vitalariu

Introduction. A radiological evaluation is essential in endodontics, for diagnostic purposes, planning and execution of the treatment, and evaluation of the success of therapy. The periapical radiography is nowadays the main radiographic investigations used but presents some limits as 3D anatomic alteration, geometric compression, and possible anatomical structures overlapping that can obscure the area of interest. CBCT (cone beam computed tomography) in endodontics allows a detailed assessment of the teeth and surrounding alveolar anatomy for endodontic diagnosis, treatment planning, and follow-up. *Objective.* The purpose of this study was to evaluate the accuracy of CBCT in comparison with conventional intraoral radiographs used in endodontic procedures. *Materials and Methods.* Statistical analysis was performed on 101 patients with previous endodontic treatments with the relative radiographic documentation (preoperative, postoperative, and follow-up intraoral X-ray) that had underwent at CBCT screening for surgical reasons. The CBCT scans were evaluated independently by two operators and compared with the corresponding periapical images. *Results.* Our analysis shows that the two radiological investigations statistically agree in 100% of cases in the group of patients without any endodontic sign. In the group of patients with an endodontic pathology, detected with CBCT, endodontic under extended treatments (30.6%), MB2 canals in nontreated maxillary molars (20.7%), second canals in nontreated mandibular incisors (9%), root fractures (2.7%), and root resorption (2.7%) were not always visible in intraoral X-ray. Otherwise, positivity in the intraoral X-ray was always confirmed in CBCT. A radiolucent area was detected in CBCT exam in 46%, while the intraoral X-ray exam was positive only in 18%. *Conclusions.* Our study shows that some important radiological signs acquired using CBCT are not always visible in periapical X-ray. Furthermore, CBCT is considered as a II level exam and could be used to solve diagnostic questions, essential to a proper management of the endodontic problems.

1. Introduction

Radiology is essential in endodontics for diagnostic purposes, planning and execution of the treatment, and evaluation of the success of therapy [1].

Until few years ago, the main radiographic investigations used in the endodontic treatment were periapical radiography and, for a general evaluation, orthopantomography.

The conventional radiographic techniques show some limits. These include the following:

(i) *Anatomic 3D compression.* The conventional radiography gives a two-dimensional image, obliging the operator to perform many X-rays with different projections in numerous cases in order to obtain a complete display of the teeth and nearby tissues anatomy [2, 3].

(ii) *Geometric alteration.* For an accurate anatomy reproduction, the image receptor should be parallel to the longitudinal tooth axis and the radiogenic font perpendicular to them. An overangulated or downangulated radiography reduces or increases the roots' length and the tooth dimension, and it can determine diagnostic omissions of periradicular pathologies [4–6]. The distortion degree of the anatomic structures could range from 3.4% for the periapical radiography to more than 14% for OPT (orthopantomography) [7].

(iii) *Anatomic obstacles.* Some anatomic structures can obscure the area of interest causing a difficult radiological interpretation of the images [8]. So, in the routine clinical practice, there are some cases in which the conventional radiography does not give sufficient information on the pathological conditions, anatomic shapes of the structures, and positional relations.

Ex vivo and in vivo studies confirm that two-dimensional radiology presents clear limits in the periapical lesion diagnoses [9, 10].

One of the factors that highly influence the lesion recognition is bone thickness. Indeed, it has been established that, in an intraoral radiogram, the lesions which involve only the bone medullary component may pass unobserved because of the overhead cortical lines up to the radiolucent area [11–13].

Moreover, two-dimensional images sometimes do not allow to detectthe real number of root canals with consequences on the success rate [14, 15].

The modern systems of digital radiographic imaging introduced relevant improvements in endodontics. The quality of the image is highly important in endodontics because it makes easier the accurate interpretation of the endodontic anatomy, and in particular, the detection of possible canal curvatures, as well as the postoperatory evaluation and long-term result of the endodontic treatment [16–18].

The CBCT permitted a detailed three-dimensional evaluation of the teeth, maxillofacial skeletal district, and relation among anatomical structures [19, 20].

The CBCT in endodontics not only gives a three-dimensional evaluation of the region of interest but also an appropriate resolution of images that allows a detailed analysis of tooth and surrounding alveolar anatomy.

The guidelines of the European Society of Endodontology suggest the use of CBCT in endodontics in limited cases as follows [21]:

(i) Periapical pathology diagnosis in presence of contradictory (not specific) signs and/or symptoms

(ii) To confirm the causes of nonodontogenic pathology

(iii) Maxillofacial trauma evaluation and/or treatment quality

(iv) The extremely complex root canal anatomy evaluation before endodontic orthograde retreatment

(v) The evaluation of the causes of the endodontic failure in surgical endodontic treatment planning

(vi) Evaluation and/or management of radicular resorption.

Therefore, CBCT can be a powerful instrument in endodontic diagnosis, as well as in the treatment planning and follow-up.

At the same time, the decision to expose a patient to a CBCT investigation must be done evaluating risk/benefit ratio in each case, which is determined by the necessity to obtain the optimal endodontic treatment management [22, 23].

The purpose of this study is to compare the accuracy of CBCT imaging with periapical radiographs in the interpretation of clinical endodontic situations.

2. Materials and Methods

2.1. Patient Selection. Our research has been conducted on patients treated between 2015 and 2018 in the Department of Dentistry of Messina University. The selection was performed according to the following inclusion criteria:

(1) Execution of three-dimensional X-ray examination (CBCT) for surgical reasons

(2) Presence of at least one tooth previously endodontically treated, with the relative radiographic documentation (pre- and post-operative intraoral X-ray and the follow-up X-ray between 3 and 6 months)

(3) Radiographic quality of the images adequate for the evaluation of the periapical status of the teeth.

One hundred and one patients satisfied these criteria and have been submitted for further evaluation.

The CBCT images have been done by using an extraoral radiographic hybrid system (MyRay Hyperion X9 Pan/Ceph/CBCT Scanner).

The equipment accomplishes the reconstruction of three-dimensional mold of the volume examined.

Then, the image is transferred to a computer real time and visualized and saved with the iRYS Software.

2.2. Radiographic Evaluation. All the images have been endodontically evaluated separately, by two operators selected as experienced endodontists with more than 10 years of clinical practice and II level master in Endodontics, not directly involved in the patients' treatment planning.

The operators have analyzed each tooth and the periapical structures, highlighting all the images with possible endodontic relevance.

For the CBCT images, the radiolucency should be visible at least in two image plans (0.5 mm thickness).

The CBCT scans have been compared to the corresponding intraoral control X-ray.

For each detected periapical lesion, we evaluated for the following:

(1) Under extended endodontic treatments

(2) Nontreated canals (MB2 canal in maxillary molars and lingual canal in mandibular incisors)

(3) Root fractures

(4) Resorptions.

2.3. *Statistical Analysis.* The selected patients were divided into two groups:

(i) Patients without endodontic pathology in the radiographic documentation at the end of the endodontic treatment and in CBCT

(ii) Patients with an endodontic pathology in intraoral X-ray and/or CBCT.

All the data have been evaluated through preliminary descriptive analysis.

The clinical-statistical evaluations were relevant to the following:

(i) Absence of lesion in CBCT, Absence of lesion in Rx

(ii) Presence of lesion in CBCT, Absence of lesion in X-ray

(iii) Presence of lesion in CBCT, Presence of lesion in X-ray

(iv) Absence of lesion in CBCT, Presence of lesion in X-ray.

Presence/absence of a periapical radiolucent area and diagnostic concordance between periapical X-ray and CBCT, considering the following the four possible combinations.

The presence of an endodontic pathology or incorrect treatment associated with a periapical radiolucency and the incidence of the diagnostic investigation on the detection of individual clinical situations.

The chi-square test was performed to compare the accuracy of intraoral radiographs and CBCT scans in the detection of periapical lesions and/or endodontic pathologies.

To evaluate diagnostic matching degree between the two instrumental exams, Cohen's kappa coefficient was considered with the following values [24]:

(i) ≤0.2: bad

(ii) 0.21–0.4: sufficient

(iii) 0.41–0.6: not bad

(iv) 0.61–0.8: good

(v) 0.81–1: excellent.

The statistical analysis was conducted by using SPSS 17.0 for Windows operating system. A P value <0.05 was considered statistically significant.

3. Results

The statistical analysis of 111 periapical radiographic images and CBCT showed that signs of endodontic relevance were not present in 34.2% (group A #38). In 65.8% of cases, these signs were observed in the radiological diagnosis exams (group B #73).

In particular, the following diagnostic elements were identified (Table 1):

(i) 34 cases of endodontic under extended treatments (30.6%)

TABLE 1: Comparison of diagnostic evidences detection between CBCT and intraoral X-ray.

Diagnostic evidences	CBCT	Intraoral Rx	Total (%)
Root fractures	3	/	2.7
Underextended endodontic treatments	34	34	30.6
Internal/external root reabsorption	3	/	2.7
Lack of superior molar's MB2 treatment	23	/	20.7
Lack of a inferior incisor's lingual canal	10	/	9

(ii) 23 cases of MB2 canals nontreated maxillary molars (20.7%) (Figure 1)

(iii) 10 cases of second canals nontreated mandibular incisors (9%)

(iv) 3 cases of root fractures (2.7%)

(v) 3 cases of internal or external root resorption (2.7%).

In group B, 70% of the cases had developed a periapical lesion. The radiolucent area was found in the CBCT exam in 51 cases on 111 (46%), while the endoral X-ray exam was positive only in 20 cases (18%) (Figure 2).

The prevalence of endodontic under extended therapy in the context of the examined trends is 34 cases on 111 (30.06%). In the 100% of cases, there was diagnostic agreement between endoral X-ray and CBCT.

The chi-square test reveals the existence of a perfect statistic concordance between the two diagnostic exams. The K Cohen's coefficient highlights an excellent agreement (1000) among the surveys performed by using endoral X-ray and CBCT.

The distribution of periapical radiolucency detected in association with the correspondent endodontic pathology is summarized in Table 2.

The chi-square test highlights a significant association between the two diagnostic exams in detecting the presence of radiolucent area and under extended endodontic treatments. Moreover, the K Cohen coefficient reports the values 0.411 and 1000, respectively, for periapical lesion and underextended treatments. The data obtained from the two analysis performed are described in Table 3.

4. Discussion

The presence of an apical periodontitis represents an important prognostic factor [25, 26].

However, it was demonstrated that periapical lesions are visible on radiography only when the periapical pathology determines a 30%–50% loss of bone structure [27].

The intraoral images technique shows many evident limitations related to a bidimensional representation of three-dimensional structures and often gives insufficient information about the dimension, extension, and position of the periapical lesion [2].

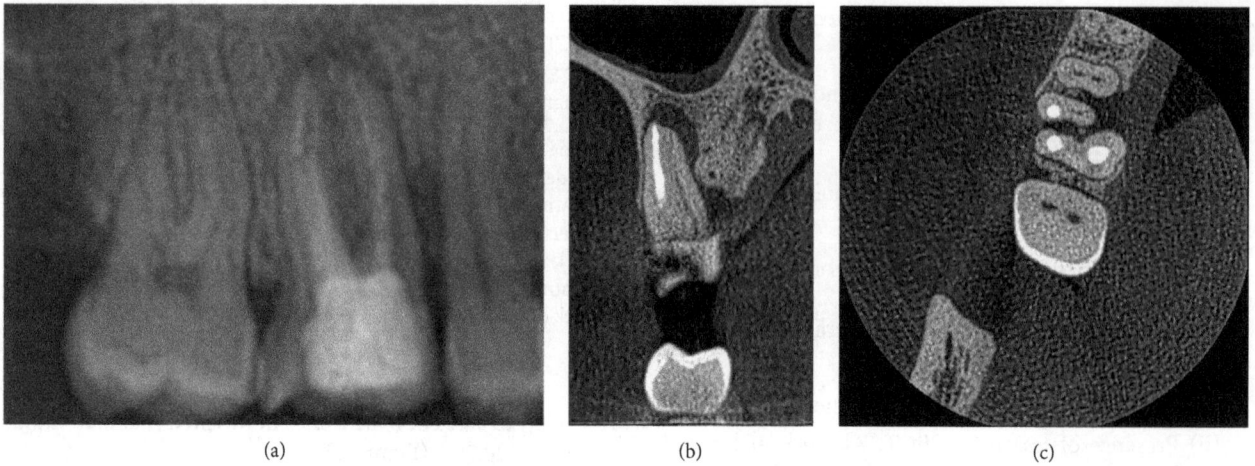

Figure 1: Endodontic treatment 1.6. (a) Periapical X-ray: apex endodontic treatment and periapical radiolucency. (b) CBCT sagittal section: apex endodontic treatment MB, untreated MB2, and periapical radiolucency. (c) CBCT transversal section: untreated MB2.

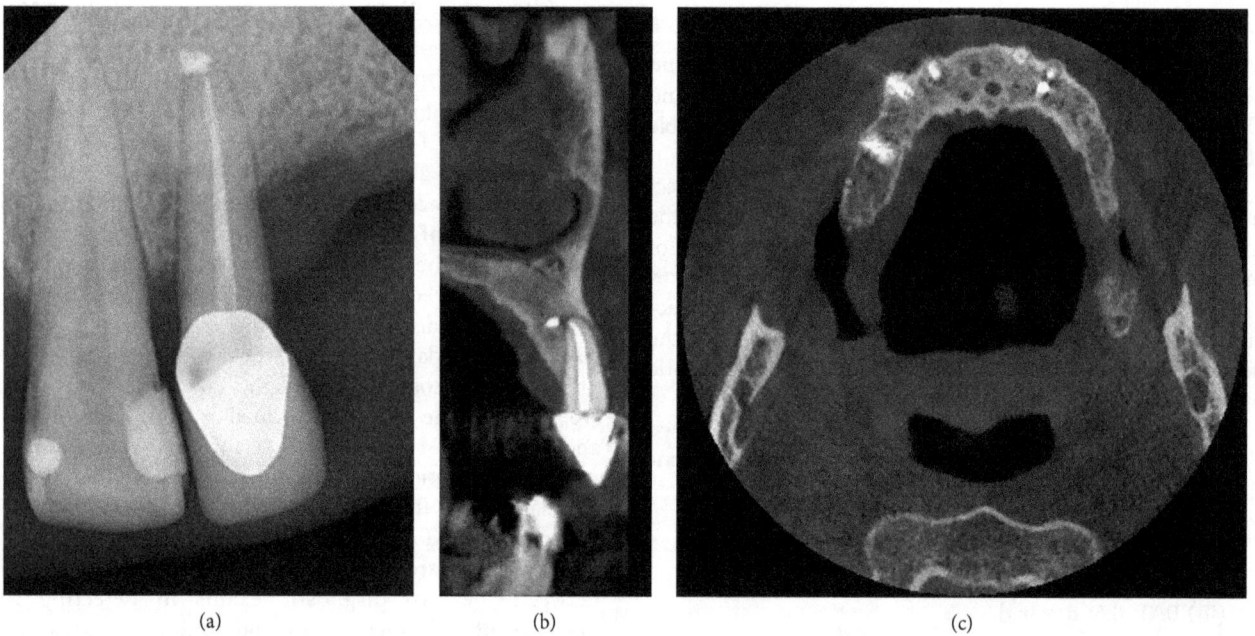

Figure 2: Endodontic treatment 2.2. (a) Periapical X-ray: endodontic overfilling and no periapical radiolucency. (b) CBCT sagittal cross section: apex endodontic treatment, over filling, and periapical radiolucency. (c) CBCT transversal section: over filling and periapical radiolucency.

Table 2: Comparison periapical lesions detection related to different endodontic and iatrogenic pathologies.

Diagnostic evidences	Periapical lesions (CBCT)	Periapical lesions (X-ray)
Under extended endodontic treatment	31	11
Nontreated MB2 canals	11	5
Nontreated lingual canals	7	4
Root fractures	1	—
Int/ext reabsorption	1	—
Total	51	20

Nowadays, the intraoral examination represents the routine investigation for the diagnosis formulation, the planning of treatment, and the evaluation of success [28].

The introduction of cone beam computed tomography (CBCT) scanning determined important advantages for the diagnosis of endodontic pathology.

TABLE 3: Statistical analysis: association between CBCT and intraoral Rx results in diagnosis of radiolucent areas and under-extended treatments.

	Pearson's chi-square	Cohen's kappa
Radiolucent area	28.701/0.000	0.411/0.000
Under-extended treatments	111.000/0.000	1/0.000

Our descriptive analysis shows that the two radiological investigations (CBCT and intraoral X-ray) agree in 100% of cases in the group of patients without any endodontic sign (A group).

However, the presence of an endodontic pathology or an incorrect treatment, associated or not to a periapical radiolucency, was not always visible in intraoral X-ray.

On the contrary, positivity in the periapical X-ray was always detectable in CBCT. This fact is confirmed by recent studies which showed how CBCT gives more accurate information in the survey of endodontic signs [29–31], avoiding anatomic structure overlapping [32, 33].

Our research points out that the periapical lesions detected in the context of all the examined CBCT scans are 51 cases. Only in 20 cases the diagnostic agreement was recorded between the two instrumental exams. Even Cheung et al. and Venskutonis et al. reported, respectively, an improvement of 63% and of 57.1% on the periapical lesions quality detection with CBCT [31, 34].

In addition, Cohen's kappa coefficient shows a decent agreement between the endoral X-ray and CBCT surveys, in spite of a relevant percentage of diagnostic discordance (27.9%).

Therefore, although CBCT is obviously more reliable in identifying signs of endodontic relevance than conventional radiography, the latter retains an effective validity.

In vitro studies have shown the greater reliability of CBCT images compared to conventional endoral X-ray in the pathology diagnosis of endodontic relevance such as root fracture, root perforation, and resorption [8, 30, 35, 36].

Our study highlights that, only in CBCT, scans are detected: root fractures (2.7%) and resorption (2.7%).

Regarding the iatrogenic errors, we have noticed the missing treatment of MB2 (20.7%) and the lingual canal of the lower incisors (9%).

In case of underextended endodontic therapies, there is a total diagnostic agreement between endoral X-ray and CBCT.

Our analysis shows that endodontic underextended treatments are more frequently associated with a periapical lesion than other endodontic diseases (31 out of 51 cases). Furthermore, some radiolucent lesions associated with no treatment of MB2 and/or mandibular incisors' lingual canal are also evident in the X-ray, despite the presence of the untreated canals which has been ascertained only in CBCT scans.

5. Conclusions

Our research shows that many of the endodontic signs obtained from the analysis of CBCT images are not resulted in the corresponding intraoral radiographs. The use of two-dimensional radiology therefore shows clear limits that can be overcome by 3D examinations.

Cone beam is therefore indispensable in all those cases in which a discrepancy between the clinical examination and the diagnostic evidence that can be objected to the intraoral radiographic examination is observable.

To perform a 3D examination, it is essential that the radiation dose is kept "at the lowest level reasonably obtainable" and that the FOV is limited only to the region of interest [37, 38].

However, the use of intraoral radiographs in different projections may increase the possibility of a correct diagnosis compared to a single radiograph.

Consequently, the CBCT remains a second level survey to be used adequately exploiting the system potential (correct FOV settings, mAs, appropriate kVp, and selection of the definition parameters) according to the ALADA concept (dosage as low as acceptable from the point of diagnostic view).

References

[1] C. Reit, K. Petersson, and O. Molven, *Diagnosis of Pulpal and Periradicular Disease. Textbook of Endodontology*, pp. 9–18, Blackwell Publishing Ltd., Oxford, UK, 1st edition, 2003.

[2] P. Velvart, H. Hecker, and G. Tillinger, "Detection of the apical lesion and the mandibular canal in conventional radiography and computed tomography," *Oral Surgery, Oral Medicine, Oral Pathology, Oral Radiology, and Endodontology*, vol. 92, no. 6, pp. 682–688, 2001.

[3] G. Lo Giudice, V. Nigrone, A. Longo, and M. Cicciù, "Supernumerary and supplemental teeth: case report," *European Journal of Paediatric Dentistry*, vol. 9, no. 2, pp. 97–101, 2008.

[4] J. Forsberg and A. Halse, "Radiographic simulation of a periapical lesion comparing the paralleling and the bisecting-angle techniques," *International Endodontic Journal*, vol. 27, no. 3, pp. 133–138, 1994.

[5] G. Lo Giudice, F. Lipari, A. Lizio, G. Cervino, and M. Cicciù, "Tooth fragment reattachment technique on a pluri traumatized tooth," *Journal of Conservative Dentistry*, vol. 15, no. 1, pp. 80–83, 2012.

[6] G. Lo Giudice, A. Alibrandi, F. Lipari et al., "The coronal tooth fractures: preliminary evaluation of a three-year follow-up of the anterior teeth direct fragment reattachment technique without additional preparation," *Open Dentistry Journal*, vol. 11, no. 1, pp. 266–275, 2017.

[7] F. Lazzerini, D. Minorati, R. Nessi, M. Gagliani, and C. M. Uslenghi, "The measurement parameters in dental radiography: a comparison between traditional and digital techniques," *La Radiologia Medica*, vol. 91, pp. 364–369, 1996.

[8] S. B. Paurazas, J. R. Geist, F. E. Pink, M. M. Hoen, and H. R. Steiman, "Comparison of diagnostic accuracy of digital

imaging by using CCD and CMOS-APS sensors with E-speed film in the detection of periapical bony lesions," *Oral Surgery, Oral Medicine, Oral Pathology, Oral Radiology, and Endodontology*, vol. 89, no. 3, pp. 356–362, 2000.

[9] E. G. Jorge, M. Tanomaru-Filho, M. Gonvalves, and J. M. Tanomaru, "Detection of periapical lesion development by conventional radiography or computed tomography," *Oral Surgery, Oral Medicine, Oral Pathology, Oral Radiology, and Endodontology*, vol. 106, no. 1, pp. e56–e61, 2008.

[10] F. W. G. Paula-Silva, M.-K. Wu, M. R. Leonardo, L. A. B. da Silva, and P. R. Wesselink, "Accuracy of periapical radiography and cone beam computed tomography in diagnosing apical periodontitis using histopathological findings as a gold standard," *Journal of Endodontics*, vol. 35, no. 7, pp. 1009–1012, 2009.

[11] S. Patel, A. Dawood, F. Mannocci, R. Wilson, and T. Pitt Ford, "Detection of periapical bone defects in human jaws using cone beam computed tomography and intraoral radiography," *International Endodontic Journal*, vol. 42, no. 6, pp. 507–515, 2009.

[12] P. Tsai, M. Torabinejad, D. Rice, and B. Azevedo, "Accuracy of cone-beam computed tomography and periapical radiography in detecting small periapical lesions," *Journal of Endodontics*, vol. 38, no. 7, pp. 965–970, 2012.

[13] Y. Gao, M. Haapasalo, Y. Shen, H. Wu, H. Jiang, and X. Zhou, "Development of virtual simulation platform for investigation of the radiographic features of periapical bone lesion," *Journal of Endodontics*, vol. 36, no. 8, pp. 1404–1409, 2010.

[14] S. Patel, "New dimensions in endodontic imaging: part 2. Cone beam computed tomography," *International Endodontic Journal*, vol. 42, no. 6, pp. 463–475, 2009.

[15] Q.-H. Zheng, Y. Wang, X.-D. Zhou, Q. Wang, G.-N. Zheng, and D.-M. Huang, "A cone-beam computed tomography study of maxillary first permanent molar root and canal morphology in a Chinese population," *Journal of Endodontics*, vol. 36, no. 9, pp. 1480–1484, 2010.

[16] K. H. Versteeg, G. C. Sanderink, F. C. van Ginkel, and P. F. van der Stelt, "Estimating distances on direct digital images and conventional radiographs," *Journal of American Dental Association*, vol. 128, no. 4, pp. 439–443, 1997.

[17] Z. Mohammadi, L. Giardino, F. Palazzi et al., "Effect of sodium hypochlorite on the substantivity of chlorhexidine," *International Journal of Clinical Dentistry*, vol. 6, no. 2, pp. 173–178, 2013.

[18] G. Lo Giudice, A. Lizio, R. Lo Giudice et al., "The effect of different cleaning protocols on post space: a SEM study," *International Journal of Dentistry*, vol. 2016, Article ID 1907124, 7 pages, 2016.

[19] H. M. Pinsky, S. Dyda, R. W. Pinsky, K. A. Misch, and D. P. Sarament, "Accuracy of three-dimensional measurements using CBCT," *Dentomaxillofacial Radiology*, vol. 35, no. 6, pp. 410–416, 2006.

[20] G. Lo Giudice, G. Iannello, A. Terranova, R. Lo Giudice, G. Pantaleo, and M. Cicciù, "Transcrestal sinus lift procedure approaching atrophic maxillary ridge: a 60-month clinical and radiological follow-up evaluation," *International Journal of Dentistry*, vol. 2015, Article ID 261652, 8 pages, 2015.

[21] S. Patel, C. Durack, F. Abella et al., "European society of endodontology position statement: the use of CBCT in endodontics," *International Endodontic Journal*, vol. 47, no. 6, pp. 502–504, 2014.

[22] S. Patel, C. Durack, F. Abella, H. Shemesh, M. Roig, and K. Lemberg, "Cone beam computed tomography in endodontics—a review," *International Endodontic Journal*, vol. 48, pp. 3–15, 2015.

[23] M. M. Bornstein, R. Lauber, P. Sendi, and T. von Arx, "Comparison of periapical radiography and limited cone-beam computed tomography in mandibular molars for analysis of anatomical landmarks before apical surgery," *Journal of Endodontics*, vol. 37, no. 2, pp. 151–157, 2011.

[24] D. G. Altman, *Practical Statistics for Medical Research*, Chapman & Hall/CRC, London, UK, 1991.

[25] S. Patel, R. Wilson, A. Dawood, F. Foschi, and F. Mannocci, "The detection of periapical pathosis using digital periapical radiography and cone beam computed tomography-part 2: a 1-year post-treatment follow-up," *International Endodontic Journal*, vol. 45, no. 8, pp. 711–723, 2012.

[26] G. Lo Giudice, G. Matarese, A. Lizio et al., "Invasive cervical resorption: a case series with 3-year follow-up," *International Journal of Periodontics and Restorative Dentistry*, vol. 36, no. 1, pp. 102–109, 2016.

[27] I. B. Bender and S. Seltzer, "Roentgenographic and direct observation of experimental lesions in bone. Part I," *Journal of American Dental Association*, vol. 62, no. 2, pp. 152–160, 1961.

[28] D. A. Tyndall and S. Rathore, "Cone-beam CT diagnostic applications: caries, periodontal bone assessment, and endodontic applications," *Dental Clinics of North America*, vol. 52, no. 4, pp. 825–841, 2008.

[29] M. B. Vizzotto, P. F. Silveira, N. A. Arús, F. Montagner, B. P. Gomes, and H. E. da Silveira, "CBCT for the assessment of second mesiobuccal (MB2) canals in maxillary molar teeth: effect of voxel size and presence of root filling," *International Endodontic Journal*, vol. 46, no. 9, pp. 870–876, 2013.

[30] C. Durack, S. Patel, J. Davies, R. Wilson, and F. Mannocci, "Diagnostic accuracy of small volume cone beam computed tomography and intraoral periapical radiography for the detection of simulated external inflammatory root resorption," *International Endodontic Journal*, vol. 44, no. 2, pp. 136–147, 2011.

[31] G. S. Cheung, W. L. Wei, and C. McGrath, "Agreement between periapical radiographs and cone-beam computed tomography for assessment of periapical status of root filled molar teeth," *International Endodontic Journal*, vol. 46, no. 10, pp. 889–895, 2013.

[32] K. M. Low, K. Dula, W. Bürgin, and T. von Arx, "Comparison of periapical radiography and limited cone-beam tomography in posterior maxillary teeth referred for apical surgery," *Journal of Endodontics*, vol. 34, no. 5, pp. 557–562, 2008.

[33] E. Soğur, H. G. Gröndahl, B. G. Baksı, and A. Mert, "Does a combination of two radiographs increase accuracy in detecting acid-induced periapical lesions and does it approach the accuracy of cone-beam computed tomography scanning?," *Journal of Endodontics*, vol. 38, no. 2, pp. 131–136, 2012.

[34] T. Venskutonis, P. Daugela, M. Strazdas, and G. Juodzbalys, "Accuracy of digital radiography and cone beam computed tomography on periapical radiolucency detection in endodontically treated teeth," *Journal of Oral and Maxillofacial Research*, vol. 5, no. 2, p. e1, 2014.

[35] M. Varshosaz, M. A. Tavakoli, M. Mostafavi, and A. A. Baghban, "Comparison of conventional radiography with cone beam computed tomography for detection of vertical root fractures: an in vitro study," *Journal of Oral Science*, vol. 52, no. 4, pp. 593–597, 2010.

[36] T. Venskutonis, G. Juodzbalys, O. Nackaerts, and L. Mickeviciene, "Influence of voxel size on the diagnostic ability of cone-beam computed tomography to evaluate

4

Morse Taper Connection Implants Placed in Grafted Sinuses in 65 Patients: A Retrospective Clinical Study with 10 Years of Follow-Up

Francesco Mangano,[1] **Renata Bakaj,**[1] **Irene Frezzato,**[2] **Alberto Frezzato,**[2]
Sergio Montini,[3] **and Carlo Mangano**[4]

[1]Department of Medicine and Surgery, University of Insubria, 21100 Varese, Italy
[2]Private Practice, 45100 Rovigo, Italy
[3]Private Practice, 22019 Tremezzo, Italy
[4]Department of Dental Science, Vita Salute S. Raffaele University, 20132 Milan, Italy

Correspondence should be addressed to Francesco Mangano; francescoguidomangano@gmail.com

Academic Editor: Luigi Canullo

Purpose. To investigate the 10-year survival and complication rates of Morse taper connection implants (MTCIs) placed in grafted sinuses. *Methods.* This study reports on patients treated with maxillary sinus augmentation (with the lateral window technique (LWT) or the transalveolar osteotomy technique (TOT)) and installed with MTCIs supporting fixed restorations (single crowns (SCs) and fixed partial dentures (FPDs)), in two dental clinics. The outcomes of the study were the 10-year implant survival and complication rates. *Results.* Sixty-five patients (30 males and 35 females) with a mean age of 62.7 (±10.2) years were installed with 142 MTCIs: 79 fixtures were inserted with the LWT and 63 were placed with the TOT. After ten years, five implants failed, for an overall survival rate of 96.5%. Three implants failed in the LWT group, for a survival rate of 96.3%; two implants failed in the TOT group, for a survival rate of 96.9%. The 10-year incidence of biologic complications was 11.9%. Prosthetic complications were all technical in nature and amounted to 7.6%. *Conclusions.* MTCIs seem to represent a successful procedure for the prosthetic restoration of the grafted posterior maxilla, in the long term. This study was registered in the ISRCTN registry with number ISRCTN30772506.

1. Introduction

In the posterior maxilla, sinus pneumatisation with ageing [1] and postextraction alveolar crest resorption [2] can severely affect the amount of bone volume, jeopardizing a successful osseointegration, unless a reconstructive osseous surgery is performed to sustain a functional and aesthetic implant-supported restoration [3].

Currently, bone volume increase in the posterior maxilla is mainly obtained by maxillary sinus floor augmentation [4–6]. This surgical procedure was found to be reliable and it can be performed according to two major techniques: the lateral window approach [7], which is still the most common method, and the transalveolar osteotomy technique [8, 9].

Many variables should be taken into consideration by the clinician before choosing the surgical technique, such as the residual bone quantity [9], the type of grafting material [10–12], the use of barrier membranes [13], the implant insertion timing in relation to grafting (one- or two-stage approach) [14, 15], and the type of implants to be placed. The one-stage approach consists of simultaneous implant placement into the augmented sinus graft [14], while the two-stage method involves implant insertion secondary to reconsolidation of the bone graft [15].

Morse taper connection implants (MTCIs) represent a valid treatment option for restoring partially and completely edentulous patients, as demonstrated by several long-term follow-up studies [16–19].

In MTCIs, the implant-abutment connection relies on the "cold welding" achieved through frictional resistance between the surfaces of the abutment and the implant [18, 20]. If the taper angle is less than 2°, the connection is called "self-locking" [17, 20].

Although several studies have confirmed that the use of MTCIs yields excellent survival and success rates [16–19, 21–23], there are currently no clinical studies on the long-term outcomes of MTCIs placed in the grafted sinuses.

In light of the above, the purpose of this retrospective clinical study was to investigate the 10-year survival and complication rates of MTCIs placed in grafted sinuses via the lateral window technique or the transalveolar osteotomy technique.

2. Materials and Methods

2.1. Patient Population. We conducted a retrospective clinical study on patients that have been treated with maxillary sinus augmentation (with the lateral window or the transalveolar osteotomy technique) and with fixed prosthetic restorations (SCs and FPDs) supported by MTCIs, in the period from January 2003 to August 2006, in two private dental clinics (located in Gravedona, Como, Italy, and in Padua, Italy, resp.).

Patients selected for the present study were identified through the records of two dental clinics; these records included all information about each enrolled patient (patient-related information: systemic health, age at surgery, gender, smoking habit, and oral hygiene) and each implant-supported restoration placed (implant-related information: position, premolar or molar; length and diameter; restoration-related information: type of prosthesis, SC or FPD; date of deliveries). The customized records included all information about any implant failure and/or biological/prosthetic complication that occurred during the 10-year follow-up.

Patients were excluded from the present retrospective study in case of (1) systemic diseases or ongoing treatments/conditions that may contraindicate intervention (uncontrolled diabetes, immunocompromised states, chemo/radiotherapy of the head/neck region, treatment with amino-bisphosphonates, psychiatric disorders, and abuse of drugs/alcohol); (2) oral diseases (nontreated periodontal disease and active/chronic/persistent sinus infections); (3) nonacceptance or inability to attend the 10-year follow-up clinical/radiographic examination for different reasons (death, hospitalization, and transferring to another country or city).

All of the enrolled patients were requested to return to the dental clinic and to attend a 10-year control follow-up clinical/radiographic examination. Patients who did not accept to attend the 10-year follow-up control, as well as patients who could not attend it, were excluded from the present study. All included patients read and signed a written consent form for inclusion in this retrospective study. Approval of the Ethics Committee at University of Insubria was obtained for this study; the Helsinki Declaration of 1975, as revised in 2008, was followed. In addition, the study was registered in the publicly available ISRCTN clinical studies registry, a trial registry recognized by the WHO, with number ISRCTN30772506.

2.2. Implant Design and Surface Characterization. The implants used were screw-shaped and made of grade-5 titanium alloy (Leone Implants®, Florence, Italy). Their surfaces were blasted with 350 μm Al_3O_2 particles and acid-etched with HNO_3, producing a R_a value (the peak-valley distance of surface irregularities) of 2.5 μm [24] (Figure 1). The implant-abutment connection is based on a Morse taper with an angle of 1.5° combined with an internal hexagon [16–19, 21] (Figure 2).

2.3. Preoperative Work-Up. Each patient underwent a primary investigation within a complete medical examination of the hard and soft oral tissues and panoramic radiographs. Where needed, computed tomography (CT) scans were requested, in selected patients. CT datasets were acquired and then converted into DICOM format. DICOM files were used to obtain a three-dimensional reconstruction of the jaws in implant navigation software, which showed the anatomic tissues including residual bone volume, thickness/density of the cortical and cancellous bone, ridge angulations, and also possible sinus pathology. Each implant site was carefully assessed. An accurate evaluation of the edentulous ridges using casts and diagnostic wax-up were included in the preoperative workups.

2.4. Surgery. Patients were instructed to rinse with 0.2% chlorhexidine mouthwash (Chlorhexidine®; OralB, Boston, MA) for 1 minute twice daily, two days before surgery, and also for 1 minute prior to the surgery. All patients received prophylactic antibiotic therapy of 2 g of amoxicillin + clavulanic acid 1 hour before the surgery. After surgery, they continued taking antibiotics twice daily for 6 days. All patients were treated under local anaesthesia using 4% articaine with adrenaline 1 : 100000.

When the lateral window technique (LWT) was used, the surgeon proceeded as follows. In order to expose the maxillary sinus lateral side, a horizontal crestal incision and two vertical incisions were performed in the buccal mucosa, in order to raise a mucoperiosteal flap. Using piezosurgery equipment under continuous saline irrigation, it was possible to outline a bone window approximately 1.5 × 1.5 cm in size. The sinus mucosa was separated from the bony surface of the sinus floor with an elevator and the bony window fragment removed. Great effort was made to prevent disruption of the Schneiderian membrane; when this occurred, a collagen barrier was used to contain the graft. After the elevation of the Schneiderian membrane was completed, the gap created between the maxillary alveolar process and the new sinus floor was filled with coral-derived porous hydroxyapatite (Biocoral®, Biocoral Inc., Saint Gonnery, France) blocks. These blocks were shaped and modelled by the surgeon, who also used porous hydroxyapatite granules to completely fill in the spaces between the porous material blocks and residual bone crest. The granules were interspersed with tetracycline powder to obtain a local antibiotic effect and moistened with

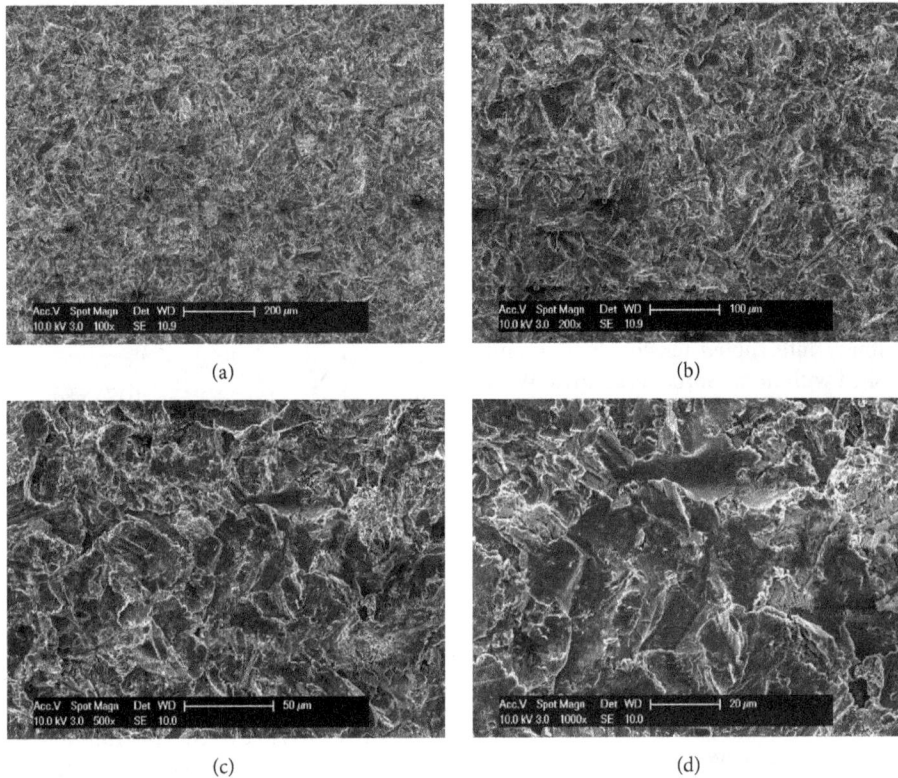

FIGURE 1: The sandblasted-acid-etched surface of the implants used in this study, at different magnification: (a) ×100; (b) ×200; (c) ×500; (d) ×1000. Implant surface was treated with a sandblasting process producing an average roughness R_a of 2.5 μm: fixtures were blasted with alumina particles. Sandblasting was followed by a decontamination treatment series, including a passivation process with nitric acid.

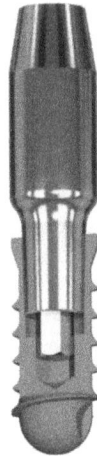

FIGURE 2: The implants used in this study featured a cone Morse taper interference-fit (TIF) locking-taper, with a taper angle of 1.5°, combined with an internal hexagon.

physiological saline solution so that this mixture could be easily moulded to fit the gaps. The sinus window was then sealed with the bony window fragment, covered by a collagen membrane and the mucosa sutured with non-absorbable sutures. When using a two-stage approach, the healing period for grafted sinuses was 6 months before implant placement. Conversely, in the one-stage approach, simultaneous implant insertion was performed. Implant placement was performed

as follows. Spiral drills of increasing diameter were used under constant irrigation, to prepare the implant site. All implants were placed at the bone crest level.

When the transalveolar osteotomy technique (TOT) was used, the surgeons proceeded as follows. A horizontal crestal incision with minimal lateral releases was performed to expose all implant sites. A mucoperiosteal flap was elevated. The preparation of the site was performed with a speed reducing gear handpiece under copious saline irrigation. Using the aforementioned drill sequence, the palatal osseous lid was removed and the Schneiderian membrane was meticulously lifted by means of the sequential use of osteotomes and a metal mallet. After the elevation was completed, the sinus cavity was grafted with coral-derived hydroxyapatite granules, mixed with tetracycline powder. The material was packed into the cavity and the implant was placed. The fixture was tightly screwed by means of a hand ratchet until it came into alignment with the crest of alveolar bone. Excessive graft material particles were removed and the flap was repositioned. Primary interrupted tension-free wound closure was accomplished with nonabsorbable sutures. With the transalveolar osteotomy technique, the implants were submerged for a minimum healing period of 3 months before beginning the prosthetic phases.

2.5. Healing Period, Second-Stage Surgery, and Prosthetic Restoration.
Postoperative pain was controlled in all patients with 100 mg nimesulide intake every 12 hours for 2 days and detailed oral hygiene instructions were given, including mouth rinses with 0.2% chlorhexidine for 7 days. Sutures were removed around 8–10 days after the surgery.

The submerged healing period lasted around 3–9 months (lateral window technique, two-stage approach = 6 + 3 months; lateral window technique, one-stage approach = 3 months; transalveolar osteotomy technique = 3 months). A second surgery was performed to accede to the healed implants and to place the healing abutments. After two weeks, impressions were taken and, one week later, the provisional restorations were provided. The provisional restorations remained in situ for 3 months, before placing definitive restorations. All definitive restorations (SCs and FPDs) were ceramometallic and cemented with a temporary oxide-eugenol cement.

2.6. Implant Survival and Complications.
Implants were classified as "surviving" when still functioning at the final follow-up.

Conversely, all implants that were lost and/or had to be removed (for implant mobility due to absence and/or loss of osseointegration in absence of infection, for recurrent/persistent peri-implantitis, and for implant body fracture) were considered as "failed."

In addition, all biologic and prosthetic complications registered during the entire follow-up period were considered. Among the biologic complications, loss of the graft, sinus infection, peri-implant mucositis, and peri-implantitis were considered [25]. Among the prosthetic complications, all mechanical complications (i.e., complications affecting the prefabricated implant components at the implant-abutment interface such as abutment loosening and abutment fracture) and all technical complications (i.e., complications affecting the superstructures made by the dental technician, such as loss of retention, ceramic chipping/fracture, and fracture of the metallic framework of restoration) were considered [26].

All data were carefully analysed in a statistical software package. Means and standard deviations, ranges,

TABLE 1: Patient distribution.

	Number of patients (%)	*p
Gender		
Males	30 (46.2%)	0.535
Females	35 (53.8%)	
Age at surgery		
20–39 years	2 (3.1%)	
40–59 years	21 (32.3%)	<0.0001
60–79 years	42 (64.6%)	
Smoking habit		
Yes	15 (23.1%)	<0.0001
No	50 (76.9%)	
Oral hygiene		
Satisfactory	35 (53.8%)	0.535
Not satisfactory	30 (46.2%)	
Total	65 (100%)	—

*p = Chi-square test.

and confidence intervals were calculated for the available quantitative variables (patients' age). Absolute and relative frequency distributions were calculated for all the available qualitative variables. The distribution of the patients (by gender, age at surgery, smoking, and oral hygiene habits) and the distribution of the implants (by sinus augmentation technique, position, length and diameter, and type of supported restoration) were investigated, and a Chi-square test (with level of significance set at 0.05) was used to calculate the differences in distribution between the groups. Finally, implant survival and complications were calculated using the implant as a statistical unit.

3. Results

3.1. Patients Enrolled and Implants Placed.
Sixty-five patients were enrolled in this study: 30 males (30/65: 46.2%) and 35 females (35/65: 53.8%) with an average age of 62.7 ± 10.2 years (median 66, range 38–79, 95% CI: 60.3–65.1). Most of the enrolled patients (42/65 patients, 64.6%) were between the ages of 60 and 79 at surgery, whereas 21 (21/65, 32.3%) were between the ages 40 and 59 and only two patients (2/65: 3.1%) were between the ages of 20 and 39 years. Fifteen patients (15/65: 23.1%) were smokers. Among all patients, 35 (35/65: 53.8%) had satisfactory oral hygiene with low plaque score levels and 30 patients (30/65: 46.2%) had unsatisfactory oral hygiene levels. The distribution of the patients by gender, age at surgery, smoking habit, and oral hygiene is reported in Table 1.

As twelve patients required bilateral maxillary sinus augmentation, the number of sinus augmentation procedures amounted to 77. Forty-five of these procedures were performed with the lateral window technique and 32 were performed with the transalveolar osteotomy technique.

In total, 142 implants were placed: 79 (79/142: 55.6%) were inserted with the lateral window technique and 63 (63/142: 44.4%) were placed with the transalveolar osteotomy technique. With regard to the distribution of the implants,

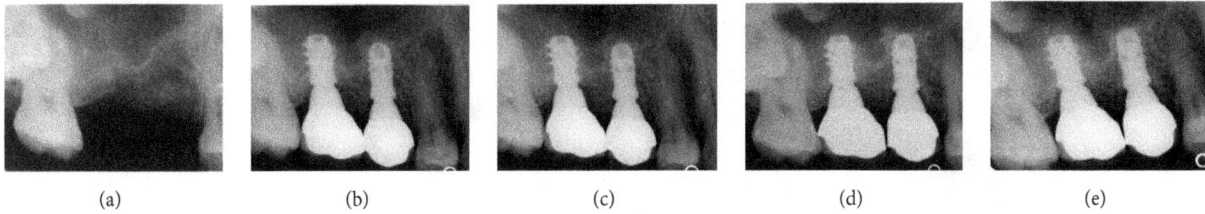

FIGURE 3: Two implants (#15 and #16) inserted with the transalveolar osteotomy technique: (a) preoperative rx; (b) radiographic control at the delivery of final restorations; (c) radiographic control 1 year after implant placement; (d) radiographic control 5 years after implant placement; (e) radiographic control 10 years after implant placement.

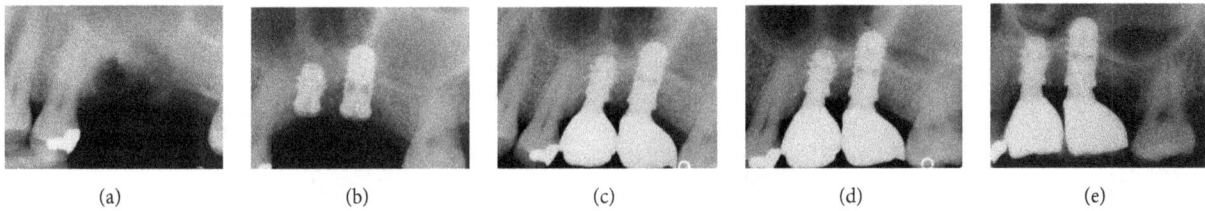

FIGURE 4: Two implants (#25 and #26) inserted with the transalveolar osteotomy technique: (a) preoperative rx; (b) the implants placed after the sinus elevation with the Summers technique; (c) radiographic control 1 year after implant placement; (d) radiographic control 5 years after implant placement; (e) radiographic control 10 years after implant placement.

55 (55/142: 38.7%) were premolars and 87 (87/142: 61.3%) were molars; the most frequent length was 10 mm (49/142 fixtures, 34.5%), followed by 8 mm (35/142 implants, 24.7%), 12 mm (32/142 implants, 22.5%), and 14 mm (26/142 implants, 18.3%). The most frequently used diameter was 4.1 mm (75/142 fixtures, 52.8%), followed by 4.8 mm (43/142 fixtures, 30.3%) and 3.3 mm (24/142 fixtures: 16.9%). Finally, with regard to the prosthetic restoration, as 44 fixtures were used to support SCs, and 98 fixtures were used to support FPDs, the final prosthetic restorations amounted to 44 SCs and 47 FPDs (43 FPDs were supported by two implants and 4 FPDs were supported by three implants, resp.). The distribution of the fixtures by surgical technique, position, length, diameter, and type of supported restoration is reported in Table 2.

3.2. Implant Survival and Complications. At the end of the study, 10 years after implant placement, only five implants failed (5/142), for an overall survival rate of 96.5% (Figures 3–5). Three implants failed in the lateral window group (3/79), for a survival rate of 96.3%. Two implants failed in the transalveolar osteotomy group (2/63), for a survival rate of 96.9%. Three of the failed implants were removed during the second-stage surgery, because they showed clinical mobility due to absence of osseointegration. These failures occurred before the connection of the prosthetic abutment and were therefore defined as "early" failures. Conversely, two implants failed in the same patient due to recurrent peri-implant infection and were removed due to massive bone loss 6 years after placement. All information regarding the failed implants is summarized in Table 3.

With regard to biologic complications, one patient experienced infection and loss of the graft after sinus augmentation with the lateral window technique, probably due to an undetected perforation of the Schneiderian membrane. This

TABLE 2: Implant distribution.

	Number of implants (%)	*p
Sinus augmentation technique		
Lateral window technique	79 (55.6%)	0.179
Transalveolar osteotomy technique	63 (44.4%)	
Position		
Premolars	55 (38.7%)	0.007
Molars	87 (61.3%)	
Length		
8 mm	35 (24.7%)	
10 mm	49 (34.5%)	0.045
12 mm	32 (22.5%)	
14 mm	26 (18.3%)	
Diameter		
3.3 mm	24 (16.9%)	
4.1 mm	75 (52.8%)	<0.0001
4.8 mm	43 (30.3%)	
Restoration		
SC	44 (31.0%)	<0.0001
FPD	98 (69.0%)	
Total	142 (100%)	—

*p = Chi-square test.

sinus was surgically revisited and cleaned. This intervention was followed by a prolonged systemic antibiotic treatment and a healing period of 6 months and subsequent successful augmentation. Conversely, no biologic complications were found for the implants placed according to the transalveolar osteotomy technique.

In addition, nine implants (9/142: 6.3%) suffered from a reversible inflammation of the peri-implant soft tissues

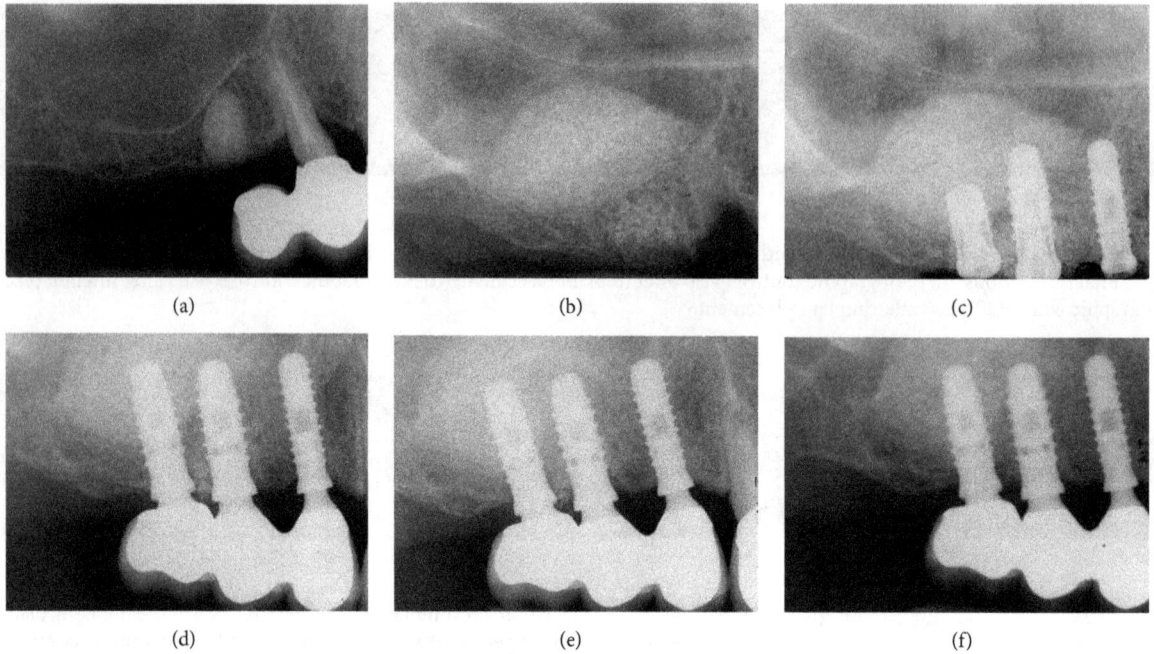

FIGURE 5: Three implants (#14, #15, and #16) inserted with the lateral window technique. (a) preoperative rx; (b) periapical rx after the sinus augmentation procedure according to Tatum; (c) 6 months later the implants are inserted; (d) radiographic control at the delivery of the final restoration; (e) radiographic control 5 years after implant placement; (f) radiographic control 10 years after implant placement.

TABLE 3: Failed implants.

Gender	Age	Smoke	Hygiene	Procedure	Position	Type	Reason/timing
Male	46	No	Poor	LWT	Premolar	4.1×10	Failure to osseointegrate after 3 months
Male	66	Yes	Good	LWT	Premolar	4.1×10	Failure to osseointegrate after 3 months
Female	59	No	Good	LWT	Molar	4.8×8	Failure to osseointegrate after 3 months
Female	66	Yes	Poor	TOT	Premolar	4.1×12	Peri-implantitis after 6 years
Female	66	Yes	Poor	TOT	Molar	4.8×10	Peri-implantitis after 6 years

(peri-implant mucositis) with exudation and discomfort, but without radiographic evidence of bone loss. Eight implants (8/142: 5.6%) suffered from infection of the hard and soft tissues (peri-implantitis) with associated peri-implant marginal bone loss. Among these implants, however, only two were lost due to untreatable, recurrent peri-implantitis with advanced bone loss; the other five implants were treated with professional oral hygiene and in these cases failure was avoided. Overall, the 10-year incidence of biologic complications affecting implants was 11.9%.

Finally, with regard to prosthetic complications, no mechanical (i.e., at the implant-abutment interface) complications were registered; however, seven restorations (4 SCs and 3 FPDs) experienced ceramic chipping/fractures, which required intervention from the dental technician. The prosthetic complications amounted to 7.6% (7/91 prosthetic restorations).

4. Discussion

It has been broadly proven that maxillary sinus augmentation is a highly successful and predictable method of obtaining sufficient bone height for posterior maxillary implant placement [3–6, 10].

In an interesting systematic review, which included studies with at least 3 years of follow-up, 18 articles for the LWT (6,500 implants in 2,149 patients) and 7 for the TOT (1,257 implants in 704 patients) were selected [5]. The overall implant survival was 93.7% and 97.2% for the LWT and the TOT, respectively [5].

These outcomes were confirmed by more recent reviews of the current literature [3, 4]. In fact, Duttenhoefer et al. conducted a meta-analysis to study the influence of various treatment modalities (surgical technique, timing of implant placement, grafting materials, and use of membranes) on the implant survival in the grafted maxillary sinus [3]. This review included 122 publications on 16268 dental implants inserted in grafted sinuses [3]. At the end of this work, no differences were found in the implant survival with respect to each surgical approach, grafting material and implant type. However, the application of membranes showed a positive influence on the long-term implant outcomes, independently of other cofactors [3].

In this retrospective study, we have evaluated the 10-year implant survival and complication rates of MTCIs placed in grafted sinuses using two different surgical techniques (the LWT or the TOT). In accordance with the aforementioned literature, a satisfactorily high implant survival rate was found for both LWT (96.3%) and TOT (96.9%).

Different clinical studies have suggested that autogenous bone is the best reconstructive material, because of its osteogenic, osteoconductive, and osteoinductive properties [27, 28].

However, in recent clinical studies, bone substitutes such as allogeneic [29], xenogenic [11], and synthetic grafts [30, 31] and composite materials [32] have also been successfully employed in maxillary sinus augmentation.

Starch-Jensen et al. found that the 5-year implant survival rate after sinus elevation with autogenous bone graft or bovine bone mineral was 97% and 95%, respectively [4], and the reduction in vertical height of the augmented sinus with the two materials was the same. In this review, similarly high survival rates were found for implants, regardless of the grafting material used [4]. High implant stability, high patient satisfaction, and limited peri-implant marginal bone loss were found [4].

In another review of the literature, Danesh-Sani et al. confirmed that bone substitutes (allografts, xenografts, and synthetic materials) were good alternatives to autogenous bone, avoiding the disadvantages related to autografts (morbidity rate and limited availability) [10].

Here, we used a coral-derived porous hydroxyapatite for maxillary sinus augmentation. In accordance with a previous report [30], the present study has noted excellent results with the use of coralline calcium phosphates for grafting of the maxillary sinus.

It must be pointed out that, recently, the role and the importance of the grafting material has been partially revisited [33]. In a review on clinical studies with a follow-up period of 48 to 60 months, the implant survival rate was 99.6% for surgeries conducted with graft material and 96% for surgeries performed without it [33]. These results suggest that sinus lift can be a safe and predictable treatment procedure with low complication rates, irrespective of the use of biomaterials [33].

Recent studies have reported excellent survival and success rates for sinus grafting and implant placement in both one- and two-stage protocols [14, 15].

A noteworthy systematic review revealed that the placement of implants in combination with sinus elevation is a predictable procedure, showing high implant survival rates with low incidence of complications [6].

Once again, our present study seems to be in accordance with the current literature. In fact, excellent survival rates were found with the LWT, with both staged and simultaneous implant placement.

The choice of simultaneous implant placement and grafting procedure is generally highly influenced by the residual crestal bone height, which must be sufficient to provide adequate primary implant stability [9]. A recent literature review investigated the correlation between the amount of remaining crestal alveolar bone before sinus augmentation and implant survival. The findings indicated that a residual bone height of less than 4 mm may influence the survival/success rates of fixtures placed in combination with sinus elevation using osteotomes [9].

Comparable studies obtained findings that support a positive influence of rough surfaces on osseous integration in the posterior maxilla [34].

In a recent systematic review for implant survival in maxillary sinus augmentation, implants with rough surfaces displayed a higher survival rate (97.6%; 95% CI: 96.7–98.5%) than implants with machined surfaces (89.4%; 95% CI: 83.0–95.8%), within no correlation or influence from the graft type [35].

These results were also confirmed by a previous review of the literature, in which dental implants placed in the posterior augmented maxilla showed an average survival rate of 92.6% [36]. The use of rough-surfaced implants and particulate bone resulted in an increased implant survival rate (94.5%) and the use of a membrane to cover the graft increased the survival rate to 98.6% [36].

In the present study, in accordance with the aforementioned research, the use of sandblasted MTCIs guaranteed excellent implant survival and success rates. Moreover, only a few biologic (11.9%) and prosthetic (7.6%) complications were reported in our present long-term retrospective study.

All implants with screw type connections show a microgap of variable dimensions (40–100 μm) at the interface between the implant and the abutment [37]. Scientific evidence suggests that bacterial leakage and colonization of this microgap may be responsible for inflammatory cell recruitment and activation at the corresponding bone level, causing the development of marginal bone loss [37].

Provided that the absence of the microgaps is associated with reduced inflammation and bone loss, an efficient seal against microbial penetration may be provided by MTCIs [20, 38]. Indeed, this screwless connection reduces the microgap (1–3 μm) dimensions at the implant-abutment interface with a tight closure against the fixture; thus it contributes to a minimal level of peri-implant inflammation [20, 38].

In addition, no prosthetic complications were reported at the implant-abutment interface in our present study. This is similar to results from previous studies on MTCIs [16–20].

The stability of the implant-abutment connection is key for the long-term success of an implant-supported prosthetic restoration [16–19]. In addition, it may contribute to a more favourable load distribution into the bone [20, 39] and therefore to a reduction of the marginal bone loss around implants in the long term. This hypothesis needs further investigation, but, if correct, MTCIs may reduce micromovements at the implant-abutment interface, preventing crestal bone loss [39].

Moreover, MTCIs inherently have "platform switching" [40]. With platform switching, any potential microgap between the implant and the abutment (which harbours bacteria, responsible for toxin production) is displaced horizontally and away from the bone, with the possibility of reducing inflammation and of minimizing bone loss [40]. This aspect may further improve the long-term outcomes of Morse taper connection implants, reducing the incidence of biologic complications. In addition, a larger space exists for the organization of thick soft tissues, that can further protect the bone from resorption [40].

Our present study has limits. First, it is a retrospective clinical study, and the retrospective design is not the best way to investigate the long-term outcomes of dental implants (in fact, a prospective study design would be preferable, but the best solution to draw more specific conclusions about a treatment procedure would certainly be a randomized clinical trial). Second, our conclusions are based on a limited number of patients. Further, long-term prospective clinical studies (or even better, randomized clinical trials) on a larger sample of patients are therefore needed, to confirm the positive outcomes emerging from our present clinical study.

5. Conclusions

Within the limits of the present clinical study (retrospective design and limited number of patients enrolled), it can be stated that MTCIs represent a successful procedure for the prosthetic restoration of the grafted posterior maxilla, with both LWT and TOT, in the long term. In fact, a 10-year overall implant survival rate of 96.5% was found. Three implants failed in the lateral window group (3/79), for a survival rate of 96.3%, and two implants failed in the transalveolar osteotomy group (2/63), for a survival rate of 96.9%. A low incidence of biologic complications was reported in this study, in the long term (11.9%). In addition, the high mechanical stability of MTCIs likely contributed to the limited amount of prosthetic complications observed in this study (7.6%).

References

[1] F. Wagner, G. Dvorak, S. Nemec, P. Pietschmann, M. Figl, and R. Seemann, "A principal components analysis: how pneumatization and edentulism contribute to maxillary atrophy," *Oral Diseases*, vol. 23, no. 1, pp. 55–61, 2017.

[2] S. Bechara, R. Kubilius, G. Veronesi, J. T. Pires, J. A. Shibli, and F. G. Mangano, "Short (6 mm) dental implants versus sinus floor elevation and placement of longer (≥10 mm) dental implants: a randomized controlled trial with a 3-year follow-up," *Clinical Oral Implants Research*, pp. 1–11, 2016.

[3] F. Duttenhoefer, C. Souren, D. Menne, D. Emmerich, R. Schön, and S. Sauerbier, "Long-term survival of dental implants placed in the grafted maxillary sinus: systematic review and meta-analysis of treatment modalities," *PLoS ONE*, vol. 8, no. 9, Article ID e75357, 2013.

[4] T. Starch-Jensen, H. Aludden, M. Hallman, C. Dahlin, A. Christensen, and A. Mordenfeld, "A systematic review and meta-analysis of long-term studies (five or more years) assessing maxillary sinus floor augmentation," *International Journal of Oral and Maxillofacial Surgery*, 2017.

[5] M. Del Fabbro, S. S. Wallace, and T. Testori, "Long-term implant survival in the grafted maxillary sinus: a systematic review," *The International Journal of Periodontics & Restorative Dentistry*, vol. 33, no. 6, pp. 773–783, 2013.

[6] B. E. Pjetursson, W. C. Tan, M. Zwahlen, and N. P. Lang, "A systematic review of the success of sinus floor elevation and survival of implants inserted in combination with sinus floor elevation: part I: lateral approach," *Journal of Clinical Periodontology*, vol. 35, no. 8, pp. 216–240, 2008.

[7] H. Tatum Jr., "Maxillary and sinus implant reconstructions," *Dental Clinics of North America*, vol. 30, no. 2, pp. 207–229, 1986.

[8] R. Summers, "A new concept in maxillary implant surgery: the osteotome technique," *Compendium*, vol. 15, no. 1, pp. 152–162, 1994.

[9] C. Călin, A. Petre, and S. Drafta, "Osteotome-mediated sinus floor elevation: a systematic review and meta-analysis," *The International Journal of Oral & Maxillofacial Implants*, vol. 29, no. 3, pp. 558–576, 2014.

[10] S. A. Danesh-Sani, S. P. Engebretson, and M. N. Janal, "Histomorphometric results of different grafting materials and effect of healing time on bone maturation after sinus floor augmentation: a systematic review and meta-analysis," *Journal of Periodontal Research*, vol. 52, no. 3, pp. 301–312, 2016.

[11] F. Wang, W. Zhou, A. Monje, W. Huang, Y. Wang, and Y. Wu, "Influence of healing period upon bone turn over on maxillary sinus floor augmentation grafted solely with deproteinized bovine bone mineral: a prospective human histological and clinical trial," *Clinical Implant Dentistry and Related Research*, vol. 19, no. 2, pp. 341–350, 2017.

[12] M. P. Ramírez-Fernández, J. L. Calvo-Guirado, J. E. Maté-Sánchez del Val, R. A. Delgado-Ruiz, B. Negri, and C. Barona-Dorado, "Ultrastructural study by backscattered electron imaging and elemental microanalysis of bone-to-biomaterial interface and mineral degradation of porcine xenografts used in maxillary sinus floor elevation," *Clinical Oral Implants Research*, vol. 24, no. 5, pp. 523–530, 2013.

[13] A. Barone, M. Ricci, R. F. Grassi, U. Nannmark, A. Quaranta, and U. Covani, "A 6-month histological analysis on maxillary sinus augmentation with and without use of collagen membranes over the osteotomy window: Randomized clinical trial," *Clinical Oral Implants Research*, vol. 24, no. 1, pp. 1–6, 2013.

[14] M. Silvestri, P. Martegani, F. D'Avenia et al., "Simultaneous sinus augmentation with implant placement: Histomorphometric comparison of two different grafting materials. a multicenter double-blind prospective randomized controlled clinical trial," *International Journal of Oral and Maxillofacial Implants*, vol. 28, no. 2, pp. 543–549, 2013.

[15] N. F. Erdem, A. Ciftci, and A. H. Acar, "Three-year clinical and radiographic implant follow-up in sinus-lifted maxilla with lateral window technique," *Implant Dentistry*, vol. 25, no. 2, pp. 214–221, 2016.

[16] F. Mangano, J. A. Shibli, R. L. Sammons, G. Veronesi, A. Piattelli, and C. Mangano, "Clinical outcome of narrow-diameter (3.3 mm) locking-taper implants: a prospective study with 1 to 10 years of follow-up," *The International journal of oral & maxillofacial implants*, vol. 29, no. 2, pp. 448–455, 2014.

[17] F. Mangano, A. Macchi, A. Caprioglio, R. L. Sammons, A. Piattelli, and C. Mangano, "Survival and complication rates of fixed restorations supported by locking-taper implants: a prospective study with 1 to 10 years of follow-up," *Journal of Prosthodontics*, vol. 23, no. 6, pp. 434–444, 2014.

[18] F. G. Mangano, J. A. Shibli, R. L. Sammons, F. Iaculli, A. Piattelli, and C. Mangano, "Short (8 mm) locking-taper implants supporting single crowns in posterior region: a prospective clinical study with 1-to 10-years of follow-up," *Clinical Oral Implants Research*, vol. 25, no. 8, pp. 933–940, 2014.

[19] C. Mangano, F. Iaculli, A. Piattelli, and F. Mangano, "Fixed restorations supported by Morse-taper connection implants: a retrospective clinical study with 10–20 years of follow-up," *Clinical Oral Implants Research*, vol. 26, no. 10, pp. 1229–1236, 2015.

[20] G. Sannino and A. Barlattani, "Mechanical evaluation of an implant-abutment self-locking taper connection: finite element analysis and experimental tests," *The International Journal of Oral & Maxillofacial Implants*, vol. 28, no. 1, pp. e17–e26, 2013.

[21] F. Mangano, I. Frezzato, A. Frezzato, G. Veronesi, C. Mortellaro, and C. Mangano, "The effect of crown-to-implant ratio on the clinical performance of extra-short locking-taper implants," *Journal of Craniofacial Surgery*, vol. 27, no. 7, pp. 675–681, 2016.

[22] K. Ö. Demiralp, N. Akbulut, S. Kursun, D. Argun, N. Bagis, and K. Orhan, "Survival rate of short, locking taper implants with a plateau design: a 5-year retrospective study," *BioMed Research International*, vol. 2015, Article ID 197451, 8 pages, 2015.

[23] R. A. Urdaneta, S. Rodriguez, D. C. McNeil, M. Weed, and S.-K. Chuang, "The effect of increased crown-to-implant ratio on single-tooth locking-taper implants," *The International Journal of Oral & Maxillofacial Implants*, vol. 25, no. 4, pp. 729–743, 2010.

[24] L. Marinucci, S. Balloni, E. Becchetti et al., "Effect of titanium surface roughness on human osteoblast proliferation and gene expression in vitro," *International Journal of Oral and Maxillofacial Implants*, vol. 21, no. 5, pp. 719–725, 2006.

[25] T. Albrektsson, L. Canullo, D. Cochran, and H. De Bruyn, ""Peri-implantitis": a complication of a foreign body or a man-made "disease". facts and fiction," *Clinical Implant Dentistry and Related Research*, vol. 18, no. 4, pp. 840–849, 2016.

[26] G. E. Salvi and U. Brägger, "Mechanical and technical risks in implant therapy," *International Journal of Oral & Maxillofacial Implants*, vol. 24, pp. 69–85, 2009.

[27] B. Al-Nawas and E. Schiegnitz, "Augmentation procedures using bone substitute materials or autogenous bone—a systematic review and meta-analysis," *European Journal of Oral Implantology*, vol. 7, supplement 2, pp. S219–S234, 2014.

[28] W. S. Khan, F. Rayan, B. S. Dhinsa, and D. Marsh, "An osteoconductive, osteoinductive, and osteogenic tissue-engineered product for trauma and orthopaedic surgery: how far are we?" *Stem Cells International*, Article ID 236231, 2012.

[29] S. P. Xavier, E. R. Silva, A. Kahn, L. Chaushu, and G. Chaushu, "Maxillary sinus grafting with autograft versus fresh-frozen allograft: a split-mouth evaluation of bone volume dynamics," *The International Journal of Oral & Maxillofacial Implants*, vol. 30, no. 5, pp. 1137–1142, 2015.

[30] C. Mangano, F. Iaculli, A. Piattelli et al., "Clinical and histologic evaluation of calcium carbonate in sinus augmentation: a case series," *The International journal of periodontics & restorative dentistry*, vol. 34, no. 2, pp. e43–e49, 2014.

[31] C. Mangano, B. Sinjari, J. A. Shibli, and et al., "A Human clinical, histologic, histomorphometrical, and radiographical study on biphasic ha-beta-tcp 30/70 in maxillary sinus augmentation," *Clinical Implant Dentistry and Related Research*, vol. 17, no. 3, pp. 610–618, 2015.

[32] F. G. Mangano, L. Tettamanti, R. L. Sammons et al., "Maxillary sinus augmentation with adult mesenchymal stem cells: a review of the current literature," *Oral Surgery, Oral Medicine, Oral Pathology and Oral Radiology*, vol. 115, no. 6, pp. 717–723, 2013.

[33] L. D. Silva, V. N. de Lima, L. P. Faverani, M. R. de Mendonça, R. Okamoto, and E. P. Pellizzer, "Maxillary sinus lift surgery—with or without graft material? a systematic review," *International Journal of Oral and Maxillofacial Surgery*, vol. 45, no. 12, pp. 1570–1576, 2016.

[34] J. A. Shibli, J. T. Pires, A. Piattelli et al., "Impact of different implant surfaces topographies on peri-implant tissues: an update of current available data on dental implants retrieved from human jaws," *Current Pharmaceutical Biotechnology*, vol. 18, no. 1, pp. 76–84, 2017.

[35] M. Del Fabbro, M. Bortolin, S. Taschieri, G. Rosano, and T. Testori, "Implant survival in maxillary sinus augmentation. an updated systematic review," *Journal of Osteology and Biomaterials*, vol. 1, no. 2, pp. 69–79, 2010.

[36] S. S. Wallace and S. J. Froum, "Effect of maxillary sinus augmentation on the survival of endosseous dental implants: a systematic review," *Annals of Periodontology*, vol. 8, no. 1, pp. 328–343, 2003.

[37] A. P. Ricomini Filho, F. S. D. F. Fernandes, F. G. Straioto, W. J. da Silva, and A. A. del Bel Cury, "Preload loss and bacterial penetration on different implant-abutment connection systems," *Brazilian Dental Journal*, vol. 21, no. 2, pp. 123–129, 2010.

[38] S. Dibart, M. Warbington, M. F. Su, and Z. Skobe, "In vitro evaluation of the implant-abutment bacterial seal: the locking taper system," *International Journal of Oral and Maxillofacial Implants*, vol. 20, no. 5, pp. 732–737, 2005.

[39] C. M. Schmitt, G. Nogueira-Filho, H. C. Tenenbaum et al., "Performance of conical abutment (Morse Taper) connection implants: a systematic review," *Journal of Biomedical Materials Research A*, vol. 102, no. 2, pp. 552–574, 2014.

[40] L. Canullo, M. Caneva, and M. Tallarico, "Ten-year hard and soft tissue results of a pilot double-blinded randomized controlled trial on immediately loaded post-extractive implants using platform-switching concept," *Clinical Oral Implants Research*, pp. 1–11, 2016.

5

Antibacterial Effects of Natural Herbal Extracts on *Streptococcus mutans*: Can they be Potential Additives in Dentifrices?

Spoorthi Banavar Ravi,[1] **Sudarshini Nirupad,**[2]
Prashanthi Chippagiri,[3] **and Rohit Pandurangappa**[1]

[1]*School of Dentistry, International Medical University, No. 126, Jalan 19/155B, Bukit Jalil, Kuala Lumpur, Malaysia*
[2]*Oral Pathology, Dr. Syamala Reddy Dental College Hospital and Research Centre, SGR College Main Road, Marathahalli Post, Bangalore, Karnataka, India*
[3]*Faculty of Dentistry, MAHSA University, Kuala Lumpur, Malaysia*

Correspondence should be addressed to Spoorthi Banavar Ravi; drspoorti@gmail.com

Academic Editor: Izzet Yavuz

Background. Many plants or herbs exhibit potent antimicrobial activity against various microorganisms. They have no side effects and presumably act against and modulate the factors that are crucial for microbial survival or their activity. *Streptococcus mutans* is a pioneer bacteria implicated in dental caries. This study aims to evaluate the antimicrobial activity of garlic bulbs, pudina leaves, and mango and eucalyptus twig extracts on *Streptococcus mutans* by evaluating their zone of inhibition and determining their minimum inhibitory concentration (MIC). *Methods.* Microbiological assay (well diffusion method) to determine zone of inhibition against pure forms of *Streptococcus mutans* was performed. The antibacterial effects of methanolic extracts of mango twigs, eucalyptus twigs, pudina leaves, and garlic bulbs were studied. Test compounds were further evaluated for their MIC. *Results.* Extracts derived from mango and eucalyptus twigs showed significant antibacterial effects at test concentrations. Pudina and garlic extracts did not show any significant antibacterial effects at similar concentrations. Upon further evaluation of the 2 positive compounds for their MIC, mango twigs demonstrated more antimicrobial potential than eucalyptus twigs at a lower concentration. *Conclusion.* Our observations indicated that the mango twig extracts possess higher antibacterial effects against *Streptococcus mutans* than other compounds at specific test concentration.

1. Introduction

Dental caries is a chronic microbial disease affecting humans in all parts of the world [1, 2]. *mutans* group of streptococci, being the active cause of caries [3, 4], produce weak organic acids after fermenting carbohydrates, or a byproduct resulting in demineralization of the tooth structure [5, 6]. Preventing and controlling dental caries has been a great challenge. For ages many prophylactic agents have been used to prevent dental caries such as antibiotics, plant and herb derived compounds, mouth washes, tooth pastes, gels, varnishes, and the caries vaccines [7]. One such method practiced from an age-old time is use of natural herbs especially by rural people to clean their teeth. In our study, we aimed at evaluating the antimicrobial potential of natural herbs like garlic (*Allium sativum*), pudina (*Mentha arvensis*), mango (*Mangifera indica*) twigs, and *Eucalyptus* (*globulus* Labill., nilgiri) twigs on *S. mutans*.

2. Materials and Methods

The materials procured for this in vitro test compounds were garlic lobes, pudina leaves, mango twigs, and eucalyptus twigs. The test bacteria were *Streptococcus mutans* ATCC 2517 (American-type culture collection). Mueller Hinton agar plate and Tecan plate reader were used.

2.1. Preparation of Alcoholic Extract of Test Compound.

Preparation of alcoholic extract of each test compound was done using 10 g of dried and powdered material added to 50 ml methanol and incubated at 50°C for 4 hours and then filtered through Whatman filter paper. The supernatant was dried at 80°C. A thick paste was obtained that yielded approximately 5–7% of extracts; that is, for 10 g of test compound it yielded 0.5–0.7 g or 500–700 mg of extract. The stock preparation was done using 100 mg/ml in methanol. Standardization was based on the NCCLS (National Committee for Clinical Laboratory Standards) method. The microorganisms, *Streptococcus mutans* (ATCC 2517), were obtained from American-type culture collection, USA. The inoculum was cell suspension prepared from cultures grown on trypticase soy broth adjusted to 1.2×10^5. The positive control was chlorhexidine mouth wash-0.2% [8–11] and ciprofloxacin 250 mg [12] and the negative control was methanol.

The test was carried out in two steps, that is, evaluation of antimicrobial activity by evaluating zone of inhibition by well diffusion method and determination of minimum inhibitory concentration (MIC) as per NCCLS method [13, 14].

2.1.1. Evaluation of Antimicrobial Activity by Zone of Inhibition by Well Diffusion Method.

100 μl inoculum of test bacterial cultures was inoculated on Mueller Hinton agar plates (90 mm). The test compounds (1 mg and 2 mg, 10–20 μL) and test drugs chlorhexidine (40 μg, 20 μL) and ciprofloxacin (2.5 μg, 20 μL) were impregnated on 5 mm wells. The plates were incubated at 35°C for 24–48 hours and observed for zone of inhibition around the well.

2.1.2. Determination of MIC (Minimum Inhibitory Concentration) as per NCCLS Method.

The test bacteria, that is, *Streptococcus mutans* (ATCC 25175), and the test compounds, that is, methanolic extract of eucalyptus twigs and mango twigs, were used at the concentration of 16–1024 μg/ml by twofold dilution method in Mueller Hinton broth. Test drugs were Ciprofloxacin and Chlorhexidine used at the concentrations of 0.25–16 μg/ml and 4–256 μg/ml, respectively, by twofold dilution method in Mueller Hinton agar broth. The test compounds and the test drugs (positive control) were diluted for 8 different concentrations by 2-fold dilution method [8, 9]. Ninety ml drug or test compounds of different test concentration was mixed with 10 ml inoculum in 96-well plates in triplicate. The control used was 90 ml Mueller Hinton agar without drug mixed with 10 ml inoculum, all incubated at 35°C. The bacterial test plates were observed after 24–48 hours. Optical density (OD) of 600 nm was measured in a Tecan plate reader. MIC (minimum inhibitory concentration) was determined at 50% inhibition of OD as compared with control.

3. Results

The zone of inhibition was observed against positive controls and test sample after incubating at 35°C for 24–48 hours (Figure 1). The mango and eucalyptus twig extracts clearly showed larger zone of inhibition in comparison with

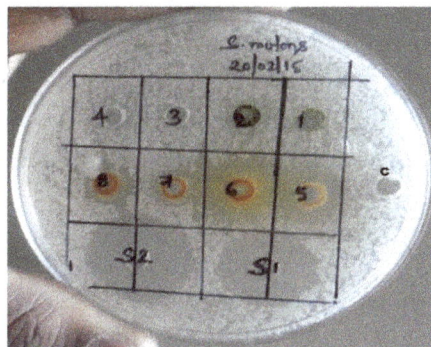

FIGURE 1: Inhibitory activity of test samples on *Streptococcus mutans*. Test extracts: (1) pudina (1 mg/well), (2) pudina (2 mg/well), (3) garlic (1 mg/well), (4) garlic (2 mg/well), (5) mango (1 mg/well), (6) mango (2 mg/well), (7) eucalyptus (1 mg/well), (8) eucalyptus (2 mg/well), S1: chlorhexidine (40 μg/well), S2: ciprofloxacin (2.5 μg/well), and C: methanol control (negative).

TABLE 1: Inhibitory activity of Test samples on Streptococcus mutans.

Test compound	Concentration (mg/Well)	Zone of inhibition (in mm) Test organisms *Streptococcus mutans*
Pudina	1	—
	2	—
Garlic	1	—
	2	—
Mango extract	1	13.5 ± 0.5
	2	16.0 ± 1.0
Eucalyptus extract	1	9.5 ± 0.5
	2	11.25 ± 0.25
Chlorhexidine	0.040	20.0 ± 0.0
Standard ciprofloxacin	0.0025	23.5 ± 0.5

other test compounds at particular concentration, as indicated/summarized in Figure 1 and Table 1. Mango twig and eucalyptus twig extracts were further evaluated to know their minimum inhibitory concentration (MIC). This was done along with determination of minimum inhibitory concentration of standards (ciprofloxacin and chlorhexidine) against *Streptococcus mutans*. The MIC observed for ciprofloxacin was at concentration of 0.5 μg/ml and the percentage of inhibition was 79.28 and MIC for chlorhexidine was at concentration of 4.00 μg/ml and the percentage of inhibition noted was 87.50 (Table 2). The MIC recorded for mango twig extract was at concentration 256 μg/ml and the percentage of inhibition was 50.70 and MIC for eucalyptus extract was at concentration 1024 μg/ml and the percentage of inhibition was 90.90 (Table 3, Figures 2 and 3).

4. Discussion

Dental caries is an irreversible chronic disease initiated by *Streptococcus mutans*, a Gram-positive, facultative anaerobic

TABLE 2: Minimum inhibitory concentration of ciprofloxacin and chlorhexidine against *Streptococcus mutans*.

Ciprofloxacin concentration (μg/ml)	% inhibition	Chlorhexidine concentration (μg/ml)	% inhibition
0.00	0.00	0.00	0.00
0.25	48.91	4.00	87.50
0.5	79.28	8.00	88.27
1.0	81.00	16.00	91.24
2.0	88.30	32.00	94.79
4.0	88.05	64.00	95.05
8.0	94.49	128.00	96.64
16.00	92.65	256.00	97.71
0.00	81.00	0.00	88.27
MIC	0.5	MIC	<4

TABLE 3: Minimum inhibitory concentration of mango and eucalyptus twigs extract against *Streptococcus mutans*.

Concentrations (μg/ml)	% inhibition	
	Mango twigs extract	Eucalyptus twig extracts
00	00	0.00
16	0.00	0.00
32	18.52	0.00
64	21.71	0.00
128	30.57	0.00
256	50.70	4.35
512	79.23	40.55
1024	88.62	90.90
MIC	256	1024

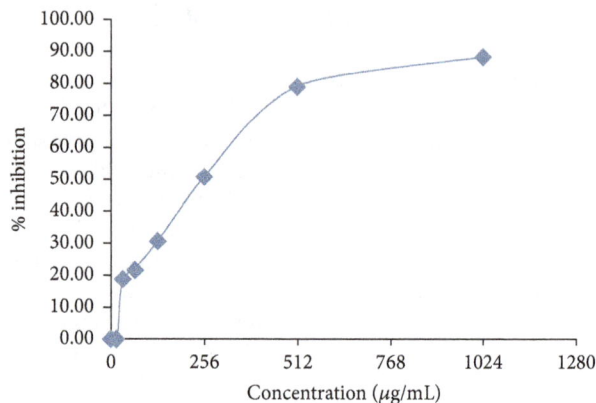

FIGURE 2: Inhibitory activity of mango twigs extracts against *S. mutans*.

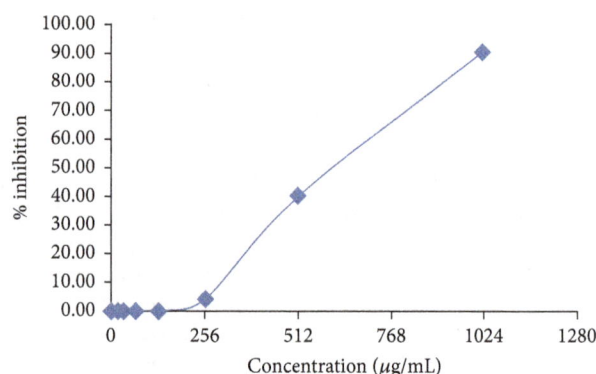

FIGURE 3: Inhibitory activity of eucalyptus twigs extracts against *S. mutans*.

microorganism [15]. Preventing and controlling dental caries have been a great challenge for decades. The garlic extract (*Allium sativum*) can inhibit growth of both Gram-positive and Gram-negative bacteria. The garlic cloves consist of sulfur containing chemicals like allicin, alliin, and ajoene [16]. When the garlic cloves are cut or crushed they release the enzyme alliinase which converts alliin to allicin and allicin is responsible for antibacterial activity [8]. The anticariogenicity of garlic extract was evaluated in previous studies and can inhibit the bacterial growth only when used at higher concentration [8, 9, 15, 17]. Pudina or mint leaves are widely used in food and medicines for their flavor and antibacterial effect. Mint leaves are comprised of menthol, menthone, methyl esters, and terpenoids which are responsible for antibacterial effect [18]. Menthol, being the chief component [19], is used in essential oils and ointments [20]. The antibacterial activity of alcoholic extract of pudina leaves was previously evaluated by Chaudhary et al. at three different concentrations, 5%, 10%, and 50%. The zone of inhibition was seen at 10% and 50% concentrations [10]. In another study, the alcoholic extract of mint leaves at 10 mg/ml was more active against microorganism [12]. Antibacterial properties of alkaloid extracts from *Callistemon citrinus* and *Vernonia adoensis*

against *Staphylococcus aureus* and *Pseudomonas aeruginosa* were evaluated by Mabhiza et al. in 2016 and they reported that alkaloids may serve as potential courses of compounds that can act as lead compounds for the development of plant-based antibacterials and/or their adjunct compounds [21]. In our study, to evaluate the antibacterial effect on *Streptococcus mutans* we used garlic lobes (*Allium sativum*) and pudina leaves (*Mentha arvensis*) alcoholic extract at 1 mg/ml and 2 mg/ml concentrations; both the test compounds did not show any antibacterial effect against the cariogenic bacteria. The reason for this could be the low concentration of test extracts that were used (1 to 2 mg/ml).

Mohammed used eucalyptus leaves and revealed that methanolic extract of *Eucalyptus spathulata* leaves was more effective in inhibiting *Streptococcus mutans* compared to gentamycin and nystatin [22]. *Eucalyptus spathulata* twig consists of ketones like juglone, regiolone, sterol, and flavonoid comprising antibacterial potential [23]. We used methanolic extract of eucalyptus twigs that demonstrated antimicrobial activity against *Streptococcus mutans* compared to garlic lobes extract and pudina leaves extract.

The *Mangifera indica* consists of tannins, bitter gum, and resins [24]. The tannins and resins have astringent effect on mucous membrane; they protect enamel by forming layer on it. Prashant et al. used mango twigs as one of the test compounds to test the antimicrobial activity of *Strepto-coccus mutans*, *Streptococcus salivarius*, *Streptococcus mitis*, and *Streptococcus sanguis*. At 50% concentration it showed maximum zone of inhibition on *Streptococcus mitis* [25]. In our study when we used mango (*Mangifera indica*) and *Eucalyptus* (*globulus* Labill.) twig extract, at concentrations of 1 mg/ml and 2 mg/ml, the mango twig extract showed highest zone of inhibition compared to extract of eucalyptus twig. When further evaluated for minimum inhibitory concentration, mango twig extract showed inhibitory activity at minimum concentration of 256 μg/ml compared to eucalyptus twig methanolic extract which was 1024 μg/ml.

The tested compounds *Mangifera indica* and eucalyptus that showed highest antibacterial activity at minimum concentration can be incorporated in oral rinses, dentifrices, cavity liners, and varnishes to improve oral hygiene and cleanliness. These are easily available and are economical.

The effectiveness of chitosan shell toothpaste white shrimp (*Litopenaeus vannamei*) in reducing *Streptococcus mutans* in cases of early childhood caries was evaluated by Achmad and Ramadhany [26], by counting the number of colonies formed before and after using the toothpaste. Their results indicated a significant reduction of the number of colonies of *Streptococcus mutans* in the case of early childhood caries. Widyagarini et al. [27] in 2016 tried to identify serotypes c and e *Streptococcus mutans* in child-mother pairs and determine the relationship between serotype of *S. mutans* and dental caries in plaque samples. There was no significant relationship between serotype c/e *S. mutans* and child-mother caries score.

The limitations of our study include that this study was conducted in vitro with the extracts of mango and eucalyptus twigs. The duration of the contact of such extracts with the microorganisms in the oral cavity in vivo is not clear; hence further studies comparing the prevalence of dental caries among users and nonusers of such extracts from the twigs should help elucidate the picture. The tested compounds can be further tested to know their minimal bactericidal concentrations (MBC) to comprehensively understand their efficacy against the most dreaded bacteria causing the dental caries.

5. Conclusion

The results of our study indicate that the mango twigs possess the antibacterial effect even at low concentration against the most cariogenic bacteria *Streptococcus mutans*. It appears that it may be possible to combat *Streptococcus mutans* to increase the efficacy of the oral hygiene practices by incorporating the mango and eucalyptus twig extracts into dentifrices. However, studies simulating in vivo situations more closely are required to get a clear understanding.

References

[1] J. D. Bader, D. A. Shugars, and A. J. Bonito, "Systematic reviews of selected dental caries diagnostic and management methods," *Journal of Dental Education*, vol. 65, no. 10, pp. 960–968, 2001.

[2] J. Walter, "Role of Streptococcus mutans in human dental decay," *Microbiological Reviews*, vol. 50, pp. 353–380, 1986.

[3] R. A. Whiley and D. Beighton, "Current classification of the oral streptococci," *Oral microbiology and immunology*, vol. 13, no. 4, pp. 195–216, 1998.

[4] S. Hamada and H. D. Slade, "Biology, immunology, and cario-genicity of *Streptococcus mutans*," *Microbiology and Molecular Biology Reviews*, vol. 44, no. 2, pp. 331–384, 1980.

[5] E. A. M. Kidd and O. Fejerskov, "What constitutes dental caries? Histopathology of carious enamel and dentin related to the action of cariogenic biofilms," *Journal of Dental Research*, vol. 83, no. C, pp. C35–C38, 2004.

[6] JD. Featherstone, "The continuum of dental caries-evidence for a dynamic disease process," *Journal of Dental Research*, vol. 83, pp. 39–42, 2004.

[7] F. Chen and D. Wang, "Novel technologies for the prevention and treatment of dental caries: a patent survey," *Expert Opinion on Therapeutic Patents*, vol. 20, no. 5, pp. 681–694, 2010.

[8] M. M. Fani, J. Kohanteb, and M. Dayaghi, "Inhibitory activity of garlic (Allium sativum) extract on multidrug-resistant Strep-tococcus mutans," *Journal of Indian Society of Pedodontics and Preventive Dentistry*, vol. 25, no. 4, pp. 164–168, 2007.

[9] B. Houshmand, F. Mahjour, and O. Dianat, "Antibacterial effect of different concentrations of garlic (*Allium sativum*) extract on dental plaque bacteria," *Indian Journal of Dental Research*, vol. 24, no. 1, pp. 71–75, 2013.

[10] N. J. Chaudhary, C. G. A. Krishnan, K. Thanveer, and H. Shah, "Anti-microbial effect of Pudina extract on streptococcus mutans: in vitro study," *Journal of International Oral Health*, vol. 4, no. 3, pp. 45–49, 2012.

[11] B. R. Chandrashekar, R. Nagarajappa, R. Singh, and R. Thakur, "An in vitro study on the anti-microbial efficacy of ten herbal extracts on primary plaque colonizers," *Journal of Young Pharmacists*, vol. 6, no. 4, pp. 33–39, 2014.

[12] D. J. Sunitha, P. Shilpa, A. S. Madhusudan, and S. V. Ravindra, "An in vitro antimicrobial activity of few plant extracts on dental caries microorganisms," *International Journal of Applied pharmaceutical sciences and Biological Sciences*, vol. 1, no. 3, pp. 294–303, 2012.

[13] National Committee for Clinical Laboratory Standards (NCCLS), "Reference method for broth dilution antifungal susceptibility testing of yeasts: approved standard," in *NCCLS document M27-A*, vol. 20, p. 24, NCCLS, Wayne, PA, USA, 1997.

[14] National Committee for Clinical Laboratory Standards (NCCLS), "National committee for clinical laboratory standards (nccls) methods for dilution antimicrobial susceptibility tests for bacteria that grow aerobically," in *NCCLS document M7-A6*, NCCLS, Wayne, PA, USA, 6th edition, 2003.

[15] A. M. Fatemeh, H. Soraya, A. Y. Mohammad, P. Jalal, and S. Javad, "Antibacterial effect of eucalyptus (*globulus Labill*) and garlic (*Allium sativum*) extracts on oral Cariogenic bacteria," *Journal of Microbiology Research and Reviews*, vol. 1, no. 2, pp. 12–17, 2013.

[16] S. Ankri and D. Mirelman, "Antimicrobial properties of allicin from garlic," *Microbes and Infection*, vol. 1, no. 2, pp. 125–129, 1999.

[17] K. Sulafa and M. R. E.-S. Jinan, "Garlic extracts and acidogenicity of mutans streptococci," *e-Journal of Dentistry Jan*, vol. 3, no. 1, 2013.

[18] T. K. Mohanta, J. K. Patra, S. K. Rath, D. K. Pal, and H. N. Thatoi, "Evaluation of antimicrobial activity and phytochemical screening of oils and nuts of Semicarpus anacardium," *L.f. Scientific Research and Essay 2007*, vol. 2, no. 11, pp. 486–490, 2007.

[19] M. Akram, "Menthaarvensis Linn.: a review article," *Journal of Medicinal Plants Research*, vol. 5, no. 18, pp. 4499–4503, 2011.

[20] P. Agarwal, L. Nagesh, and Murlikrishnan, "Evaluation of the antimicrobial activity of various concentrations of Tulsi (Ocimum sanctum) extract against Streptococcus mutans: An in vitro study," *Indian Journal of Dental Research*, vol. 21, no. 3, pp. 357–359, 2010.

[21] D. Mabhiza, T. Chitemerere, and S. Mukanganyama, "Antibacterial Properties of Alkaloid Extracts from Callistemon citrinus and Vernonia adoensis against Staphylococcus aureus and Pseudomonas aeruginosa," *International Journal of Medicinal Chemistry and Analysis*, vol. 2016, pp. 1–7, 2016.

[22] N. A. Mohammed, "In vitro, antimicrobial activity of leaves extracts of eucalyptus spathulata against streptococcus mutans and candida albicans," *Journal of Al Rafidain University College*, vol. 33, pp. 1–6, 2014.

[23] K. Takarada, R. Kimizuka, N. Takahashi, K. Honma, K. Okuda, and T. Kato, "A comparison of the antibacterial efficacies of essential oils against oral pathogens," *Oral microbiology and immunology*, vol. 19, no. 1, pp. 61–64, 2004.

[24] S. A. Muhammad and A. Muhammad, "Significance of chewing sticks (Miswaks) in oral hygiene from a pharmacological viewpoint," *JPMA*, pp. 89–95, 1981.

[25] G. M. Prashant, G. N. Chandu, K. S. Murulikrishna, and M. D. Shafiulla, "The effect of mango and neem extract on four organisms causing dental caries: Streptococcus mutans, Streptococcus salivavius, Streptococcus mitis, and Streptococcus sanguis: An in vitro study," *Indian Journal of Dental Research*, vol. 18, no. 4, pp. 148–151, 2007.

[26] H. Achmad and Y. F. Ramadhany, "Effectiveness of Chitosan Tooth Paste from White Shrimp (Litopenaeusvannamei) to Reduce Number of Streptococcus Mutans in the Case of Early Childhood Caries," *Journal of International Dental and Medical Research*, vol. 10, no. 2, pp. 358–363, 2017.

[27] A. Widyagarini, H. Sutadi, and S. B. Budiardjo, "Serotype c and e streptococcus mutans from dental plaque of child-mother pairs with dental caries," *Journal of International Dental and Medical Research*, vol. 9, pp. 339–344, 2016.

6

Survey of Screw-Retained versus Cement-Retained Implant Restorations in Saudi Arabia

Alaa Makke, Abdulwahed Homsi, Montaha Guzaiz, and Abdulrahman Almalki

Oral and Maxillofacial Department, Faculty of Dentistry, Umm Al-Qura University, Mecca, Saudi Arabia

Correspondence should be addressed to Abdulrahman Almalki; atmalki@hotmail.com

Academic Editor: Patricia Pereira

Introduction. Implant-supported prostheses are currently the standard treatment for the replacement of missing teeth and deficiencies. Implant restorations can either be screw-retained, cement-retained, or both. The implant retention system type is typically chosen during the treatment plan. The primary purpose of this study is to investigate the frequency of implant restoration retention systems. *Materials and Methods.* A five-page questionnaire was sent to private institutes, educational institutes, and governmental hospitals that provide dental services. The data were analyzed using descriptive statistics. *Results.* Prior to distribution, the surveys were proofread and pilot-tested at the Faculty of Dentistry at Umm Al-Qura University. The surveys were mailed to three groups: private institutes, educational institutes, and governmental hospitals. In total, 120 surveys were distributed and 87 surveys were returned, for a response rate of 73%. This included thirty-six surveys (41.4%) from private institutes, twenty-two surveys (25.3%) from educational institutes, and twenty-nine surveys (33.3%) from governmental hospitals. *Conclusions.* In general, Astra was cited as the most widely used implant system. In addition, cement-retained restorations were more frequently used than screw-retained restorations. However, dental implant failure was more frequently associated with cement-retained restorations than with screw-retained restorations.

1. Introduction

Implant-supported prostheses are currently the standard treatment for the replacement of missing teeth and deficiencies to enhance tooth function, for convenience, and for appearance [1]. An implant fixed prosthetic part can be screwed and/or cemented to the dental implant. The implant retention system type is typically chosen during the dental treatment plan, when the advantages and disadvantages of each system are considered [2]. In this context, patient preference may influence the retention system choice [3].

Screw-retained systems are preferred for a prosthesis with multiple abutments, due to the retrievability that allows for the removal of the prosthesis for cleaning and repair. In addition, screw-retained prosthesis tends to have less marginal misfits at the crown implant interface [4, 5]. However, the screw-retained system shows higher rates of complications (e.g., screw loosening, fracturing, and esthetic considerations) when the implants are improperly positioned [6].

Cement-retained systems are ideal for esthetic purposes. They may provide an advantage in compensating for the unfavorable angulation of an implant. Other advantages include fabrication simplicity, a decrease in laboratory complications, and less stress on bone tissue compared to the screw-retained systems [7, 8]. However, the cement-retained systems are sensitive and need more care to avoid excess cement, which can lead to surrounding soft tissue inflammation [9].

As there is currently no consensus about the ideal type of retention system for implant restorations [10], the primary purpose of this study is to investigate the frequency of implant restoration retention systems.

2. Materials and Methods

In April of 2017, a five-page questionnaire was sent to dental institutions, schools, and hospitals that provide dental services in different regions of Saudi Arabia. A total of 120 surveys were sent to 21 dental institutions. The questionnaire asked the respondents for general information, including their city, email address, institution/school, and

TABLE 1: Survey questions.

(1) Please indicate your city.

(2) Please indicate your E-mail.

(3) Please indicate your institute.

(4) Please indicate your specialty.

(5) What implant system(s) is/are used in your practice?

(6) What is your role in implant treatment? (surgical part/prosthetic part)

(7) What retention systems do you use in your practice?

(8) Do the lab technicians limit your decisions in retention systems?

(9) What material(s) do you use to fill the access hole of the abutment screw?

(10) What cement(s) do you use for the final cementation of the implant restorations?

(11) From your practice, which retention systems are more frequently associated with failure?

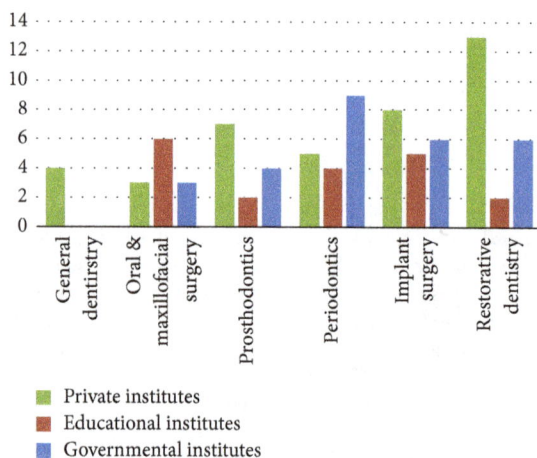

FIGURE 1: Clinician specialty of respondents.

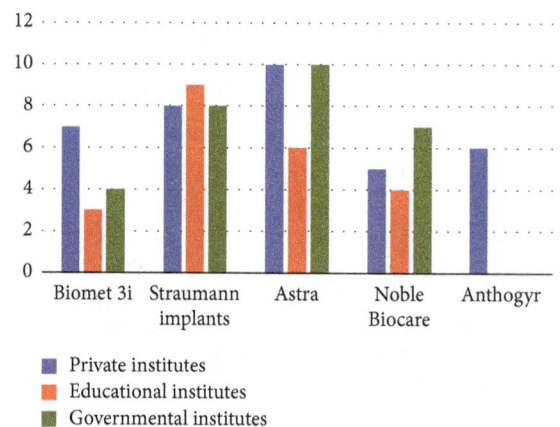

FIGURE 2: Implant manufacturers products: Biomet 3i, Inc. (Palm Beach Gardens, Florida); Astra Tech, Inc. (Waltham, Mass); Nobel Biocare AB (Göteborg, Sweden); Straumann USA, LLC (Andover, MA); and Anthogyr (Sallanches, France).

their specialty. The survey included a total of eleven questions (Table 1).

All questions were of a multiple choice format and allowed the respondent to choose multiple answers. The questions were proofread and pilot-tested at the Faculty of Dentistry at Umm Al-Qura University by a prosthodontic staff member prior to distribution. The surveys were mailed to people in three groups: private institutes, educational institutes, and governmental hospitals. Data were analyzed with descriptive statistics using Microsoft Excel, version 15.19.1.

3. Results

In total, 120 surveys were distributed and 87 surveys were returned, for a response rate of 73%. This included thirty-six surveys (41.4%) from private institutes, twenty-two surveys (25.3%) from educational institutes, and twenty-nine surveys (33.3%) from governmental hospitals. Clinician specialty of the respondents included restorative dentistry (n = 21 (24.14%)), implant surgery (n = 19 (21.84%)), periodontics (n = 18 (20.69%)), prosthodontics (n = 13 (14.94%)), oral and maxillofacial surgery (n = 12 (13.79%)), and general dentistry (n = 4 (4.60%)) (Figure 1).

3.1. Private Institutes. Private institute respondents revealed five commonly used implant manufacturers: Astra TECH implant system (n = 10 (28%)), Straumann dental implant system (n = 8 (22%)), Biomet 3i dental implant system (n = 7 (19%)), Anthogyr implants system (n = 6 (17%)), and Noble Biocare implant system (n = 5 (14%)) (implant manufacturer information is presented in Figure 2).

Twenty-six (72%) respondents reported that the role of the clinicians in dental implant treatment was in both surgical and prosthetic treatments. Ten (28%) respondents reported that their role was limited to either surgical or prosthetic treatment (Figure 3).

Thirty-one (86%) respondents used cement-retained prosthetics in their practice more than screw-retained prosthetics, while 3 (8%) respondents reported that it depended on the case (Figure 4). Furthermore, laboratory production limits the clinician's decision in retention system type by 62% (N = 22); 38% (N = 14) reported no limitations (Figure 5).

For the access hole filling material, our study revealed that twenty-six (72%) respondents used the light cure composite resin, filled partially with cotton pellets; six (17%) respondents used the resin-modified glass ionomer, partially filled

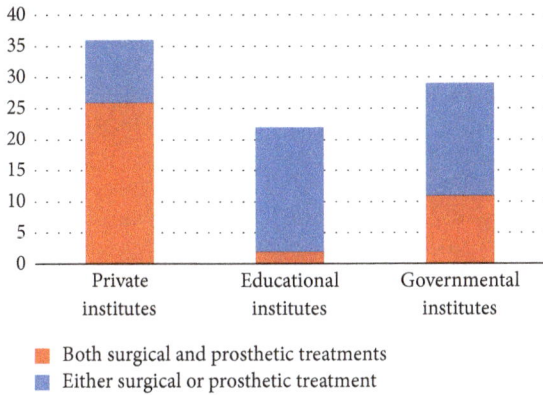

FIGURE 3: Role of the clinicians in a dental implant treatment.

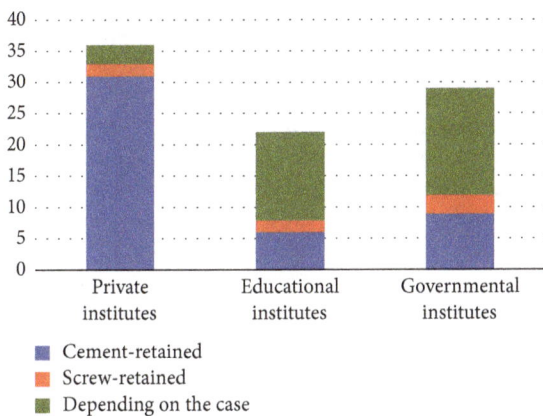

FIGURE 4: Type of retention system.

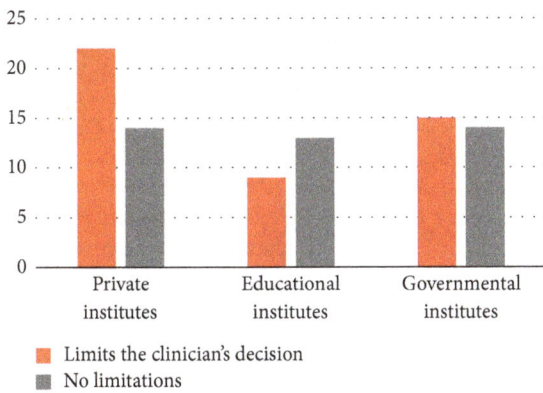

FIGURE 5: Role of the laboratory production.

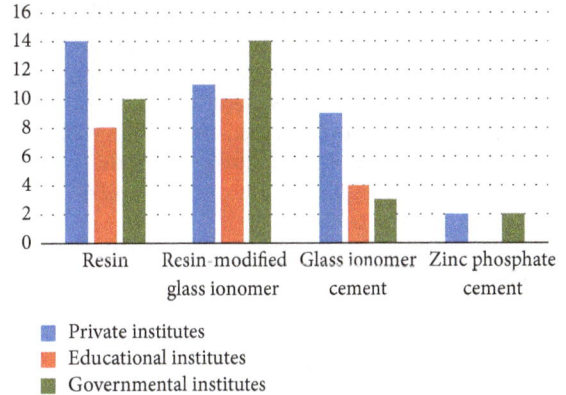

FIGURE 6: Definitive cementation material for the final implant restorations.

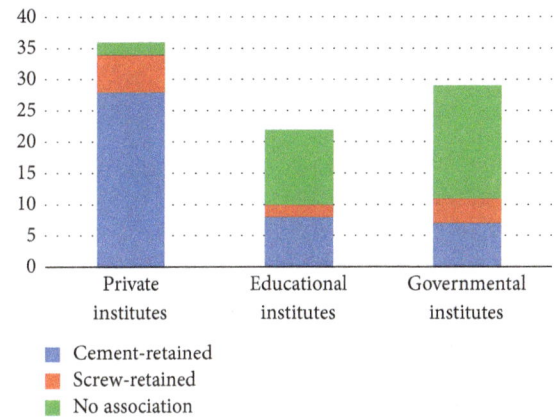

FIGURE 7: Failure of dental implants with an association with a retention system.

with cotton pellets, and four (11%) respondents used the light cure temporary filling, partially filled with cotton pellets.

The most frequently used luting agent for the definitive cementation of the implant restorations was resin (n = 14 (39%)), followed by a resin-modified glass ionomer (n = 11 (31%)), glass ionomer cement (n = 9 (26%)), and zinc phosphate cement (n = 2 (1%)) (Figure 6).

The last survey question asked about the failure rate of the dental implants, in association with the retention system. The results reveal that 28 (78%) respondents reported that

the cement-retained restoration more frequently resulted in a dental implant failure, while 6 (17%) respondents reported that the failure was associated with the screw-retained system. Moreover, 2 (6%) respondents reported no association between the retention system and the implant failure (Figure 7).

3.2. Educational Institutes. Educational institute respondents revealed four commonly used implant manufacturers for dental school implants: Straumann dental implant system (n = 9 (41%)), Astra Tech implant system (n = 6 (27%)), Nobel Biocare implant system (n = 4 (18%)), and Biomet 3i dental implant system (n = 3 (14%)) (Figure 2).

Twenty (92%) respondents reported that the role of the clinicians in a dental implant treatment was limited to either a surgical or prosthetic treatment. Only two (8%) respondents reported their role in a dental treatment as both surgical and prosthetic (Figure 3).

Fourteen (64%) respondents reported that the retention system they used depended on the case. Six (27%) respondents preferred cement-retained rather than screw-retained prosthetics (Figure 4). Furthermore, the laboratory production limited the clinician's decision in the retention system by 41% (n = 9), while 59% (n = 13) reported no limitations (Figure 5). In relation to access hole filling material, our study reported that twelve (55%) respondents used the light cure composite resin, filled partially with cotton pellets, eight (36%) respondents used the resin-modified glass ionomer, partially filled with cotton pellets, and two (9%) respondents used the light cure temporary filling, partially filled with cotton pellets.

The most frequently used luting agent for the definitive cementation of implant restorations was the resin-modified glass ionomer (n = 10 (45%)), followed by resin (n = 8 (36%)) and glass ionomer cement (n = 4 (18%)) (Figure 6).

The last survey question asked about the failure of the dental implant in association with the retention system. 12 (55%) respondents reported that there was no association between the retention system and the dental implant failure, while 8 (36%) respondents reported that the failure was more frequently associated with cement-retained restorations. Only two (9%) respondents stated that it was more frequently associated with screw-retained restorations (Figure 7).

3.3. Governmental Hospitals. In total, 38% of the surveys were from governmental hospital workers that provided dental services. The results revealed four commonly used implant manufacturers: Astra Tech implant system (n = 10 (34%)), Straumann dental implant system (n = 8 (28%)), Nobel Biocare implant system (n = 7 (24%)), and Biomet 3i dental implant system (n = 4 (14%)) (Figure 2).

Eighteen (62%) respondents reported that the role of the clinicians in a dental implant treatment was limited to either surgical or prosthetic treatment. Eleven (38%) respondents reported their role in dental treatment as both surgical and prosthetic treatments (Figure 3).

Seventeen (59%) respondents reported that the use of the retention system depended on the case, while nine (31%) respondents preferred cement-retained systems to screw-retained systems (Figure 4). Furthermore, the laboratory production limits the clinician's decision in the retention system by 52% (N = 15); 48% (N = 14) reported no limitations (Figure 5). In terms of access hole filling material, our study reported that fifteen (52%) respondents used the light cure composite resin, filled partially with cotton pellets, nine (31%) respondents used the resin-modified glass ionomer, partially filled with cotton pellets, and five (17%) respondents used the light cure temporary filling, partially filled with cotton pellets.

The most frequently used luting agent for the definitive cementation of implant restorations was the resin-modified glass ionomer (n = 14 (48%)), followed by resin (n = 10 (34%)), glass ionomer cement (n = 3 (10%)), and zinc phosphate cement (n = 2 (7%)) (Figure 6).

The last survey question asked about the failure of the dental implant in association with the retention system. 18 (62%) respondents reported that there was no association between the retention system and the dental implant failure. 7 (24%) respondents reported that the failure was more frequently associated with cement-retained restorations. Only four (14%) respondents stated that is was more frequently associated with screw-retained restorations (Figure 7).

4. Discussion

The results of this study indicate that people working in a variety of specialty areas are involved in implant treatment. In addition, a wide range of implant manufacturer products and a wide range of implant retention protocols and cementation materials are used in their practice. This study also revealed commonly used implant manufacturers and techniques among dental clinicians in Saudi Arabia.

Tarica et al. [11] found that the most commonly used implant manufacturers in USA were Nobel Biocare, Biomet 3i, and Straumann. In Saudi Arabia, the most common implant systems were Astra, Straumann, Nobel Biocare, and Biomet 3i. Other implant companies include Dentium, Bego, Axiom, RePlant Implant, and BioHorizons.

Most dental clinicians in Saudi Arabia followed the American style in implant placement, while the role of the clinicians in implant treatment varied from one institute to another. In a private institute, the role of the clinicians was to perform both the surgical and prosthetic treatment. In an educational institute or governmental hospital, this was not the case. Perhaps this is due to restricted policies in educational and governmental hospitals in Saudi Arabia. In addition, it may be that a variety of specialties exist in governmental hospitals and educational institutes, which limits the clinicians to perform duties beyond their capabilities.

In a systematic review, a comparison was conducted between the cement-retained versus screw-retained restoration for marginal bone loss. Overall, the cement-retained restoration provided fewer prosthetic complications and a higher implant survival rate than screw-retained [12] restorations. In this study, the respondents were asked which retention protocols were used in their practice. The answer varied between the institutes. In general, cement-retained restorations were more frequently used than screw-retained restorations. The next survey question asked the respondents about the lab technicians' influence on the implant treatment. The results showed a variation among institutes. In private institutes, the lab technicians limited the retention systems selection. This may be due to the cement-retained restorations being relatively inexpensive to fabricate, requiring fewer laboratory skills and providing a better esthetic outcome [13]. On the other hand, the educational institute and governmental hospitals are totally funded by the government, which means that the cost of the fabrications is not present in the equation.

The sealing of the access hole of the screw-retained restorations is generally conducted with a partial filling with a cotton pellet and composite resin restoration. In a private institute, they rarely used the amalgam restoration to fill the hole. Most institutions used the resin-modified glass ionomer, resin cement, glass ionomer cements, and zinc phosphate cement. Their agreement in cement materials for definitive cementation indicates that the same cements are selected, due to convenience, familiarity, and cost. Some studies have shown that the cement used for natural dentation does not necessarily correlate with the cement used in dental implant restoration [14, 15].

The last survey question asked about the association between dental implant failure and retention systems. In general, respondents considered the cement-retained dental implant to be more often associated with dental implant failure. The educational institute respondents stated that the dental implant failure was not associated with the retention systems. In a systematic review conducted by Lemos et al. [12], the cement-retained implant resulted in less marginal bone loss when compared with screw-retained implants.

Screw loosening is a major problem with screw-retained restorations [16, 17]. The incidence of screw loosening was 65% for single tooth implant restoration [16], whereas the incidence of unretained cemented implant restoration was less than 5% [18]. However, it is possible to leave excess cement around the implant restoration, which leads to local inflammation and peri-implant disease, due to the microbiota populating the excess cement [19, 20].

However, this study also confirmed further investigation to expand the sample size. This may lead to more in-depth knowledge about the reasons behind implant failure.

5. Conclusions

Within the limitations of this study, the findings illustrate that Astra was cited as the most widely used implant system. In addition, cement-retained restorations were more frequently used than screw-retained restorations. Moreover, resin modified glass ionomer cement was most frequently used for definitive cementation. However, dental implant failures were more commonly associated with cement-retained restoration as compared to screw-retained restorations.

References

[1] J. Pennington and S. Parker, "Improving quality of life using removable and fixed implant prostheses.," *Compendium of continuing education in dentistry (Jamesburg, N.J. : 1995)*, vol. 33, no. 4, pp. 268–276, 2012.

[2] P. V. B. da Rocha, M. A. Freitas, and T. de Morais Alves da Cunha, "Influence of screw access on the retention of cement-retained implant prostheses," *The Journal of Prosthetic Dentistry*, vol. 109, no. 4, pp. 264–268, 2013.

[3] T. D. Taylor, J. R. Agar, and T. Vogiatzi, "Implant prosthodontics: current perspective and future directions," *The International Journal of Oral & Maxillofacial Implants*, vol. 15, no. 1, pp. 66–75, 2000.

[4] R. Shadid and N. Sadaqa, "A comparison between screw- and cement-retained implant prostheses. A literature review," *Journal of Oral Implantology*, vol. 38, no. 3, pp. 298–307, 2012.

[5] N. A. Tosches, U. Brägger, and N. P. Lang, "Marginal fit of cemented and screw-retained crowns incorporated on the Straumann (ITI)® dental implant system: An in vitro study," *Clinical Oral Implants Research*, vol. 20, no. 1, pp. 79–86, 2009.

[6] M. Aglietta, V. I. Siciliano, M. Zwahlen et al., "A systematic review of the survival and complication rates of implant supported fixed dental prostheses with cantilever extensions after an observation period of at least 5 years," *Clinical Oral Implants Research*, vol. 20, no. 5, pp. 441–451, 2009.

[7] E. M. Da Silva, C. U. F. De Sá Rodrigues, D. A. Dias, S. Da Silva, C. M. Amaral, and J. A. Guimarães, "Effect of toothbrushing-mouthrinse-cycling on surface roughness and topography of nanofilled, microfilled, and microhybrid resin composites," *Operative Dentistry*, vol. 39, no. 5, pp. 521–529, 2014.

[8] B. P. Tonella, E. P. Pellizzer, R. Ferraço, R. M. Falcón-Antenucci, P. S. P. De Carvalho, and M. C. Goiato, "Photoelastic analysis of cemented or screwed implant-supported prostheses with different prosthetic connections," *Journal of Oral Implantology*, vol. 37, no. 4, pp. 401–410, 2011.

[9] M. Korsch, B.-P. Robra, and W. Walther, "Predictors of excess cement and tissue response to fixed implant-supported dentures after cementation," *Clinical Implant Dentistry and Related Research*, vol. 17, pp. e45–e53, 2015.

[10] P. Vigolo, S. Mutinelli, A. Givani, and E. Stellini, "Cemented versus screw-retained implant-supported single-tooth crowns: A 10-year randomised controlled trial," *European Journal of Oral Implantology*, vol. 5, no. 4, pp. 355–364, 2012.

[11] D. Y. Tarica, V. M. Alvarado, and S. T. Truong, "Survey of United States dental schools on cementation protocols for implant crown restorations," *Journal of Prosthetic Dentistry*, vol. 103, no. 2, pp. 68–79, 2010.

[12] C. A. Lemos, V. E. de Souza Batista, D. A. Almeida, J. F. Santiago Júnior, F. R. Verri, and E. P. Pellizzer, "Evaluation of cement-retained versus screw-retained implant-supported restorations for marginal bone loss," *The Journal of Prosthetic Dentistry*, vol. 115, no. 4, pp. 419–427, 2016.

[13] T. M. Hofstede, C. Ercoli, and M. E. Hagan, "Alternative complete-arch cement-retained implant-supported fixed partial denture.," *The Journal of Prosthetic Dentistry*, vol. 82, no. 1, pp. 94–99, 1999.

[14] A. Alvarez-Arenal, I. Gonzalez-Gonzalez, H. deLlanos-Lanchares, A. Brizuela-Velasco, and J. Ellacuria-Echebarria, "The selection criteria of temporary or permanent luting agents in implant-supported prostheses: In vitro study," *The Journal of Advanced Prosthodontics*, vol. 8, no. 2, pp. 144–149, 2016.

[15] A. Mansour, C. Ercoli, G. Graser, R. Tallents, and M. Moss, "Comparative evaluation of casting retention using the ITI solid abutment with six cements," *Clinical Oral Implants Research*, vol. 13, no. 4, pp. 343–348, 2002.

[16] T. Jemt, B. Lindén, and U. Lekholm, "Failures and complications in 127 consecutively placed fixed partial prostheses supported by Brånemark implants: From prosthetic treatment to first annual checkup," *The International Journal of Oral & Maxillofacial Implants*, vol. 7, no. 1, pp. 40–44, 1992.

[17] T. Jemt, W. R. Laney, D. Harris et al., "Osseointegrated implants for single tooth replacement: A 1-year report from a multicenter prospective study," *The International Journal of Oral & Maxillofacial Implants*, vol. 6, no. 1, pp. 29–36, 1991.

[18] A. Singer and V. Serfaty, "Cement-retained implant-supported fixed partial dentures: A 6-month to 3-year follow-up," *The International Journal of Oral & Maxillofacial Implants*, vol. 11, no. 5, pp. 645–649, 1996.

[19] W. Chee, D. A. Felton, P. F. Johnson, and D. Y. Sullivan, "Cemented versus screw-retained implant prostheses: which is better?" *The International journal of oral & maxillofacial implants*, vol. 14, no. 1, pp. 137–141, 1999.

[20] K. S. Hebel and R. C. Gajjar, "Cement-retained versus screw-retained implant restorations: Achieving optimal occlusion and esthetics in implant dentistry," *Journal of Prosthetic Dentistry*, vol. 77, no. 1, pp. 28–35, 1997.

7

Association between the Anatomy of the Mandibular Canal and Facial Types: A Cone-Beam Computed Tomography Analysis

Rudyard dos Santos Oliveira (ID), **Arlete Maria Gomes Oliveira, José Luiz Cintra Junqueira, and Francine Kühl Panzarella**

Imaging and Oral Radiology, "São Leopoldo Mandic" College, Campus of Campinas, Campinas, SP, Brazil

Correspondence should be addressed to Rudyard dos Santos Oliveira; dr.rudyardoliveira@gmail.com

Academic Editor: Manuel Lagravere

We evaluated the anatomical variations of the mandibular canal associated with various facial types, age, sex, and side of the face studied. We analyzed 348 hemimandibles in subjects without a history of trauma, lesions in the lower arch, or orthognathic or repair surgery in the posterior mandible. Facial type was determined using the VERT index. The canal path was classified as Type 1 (a large, single structure passing very close to the root tips); Type 2 (a canal passing closest to the mandibular base); and Type 3 (a canal present in the posterior mandibular region, with a lower canal running through the mandibular branch, reaching the anterior region). Bifid canals (type 3) were classified into four categories according to the course and number of mandibular canals. The brachyfacial and mesofacial types presented a Type 1 canal in 95.5% ($n = 166$) of subjects, in dolichofacial types, 68.2% ($n = 45$) presented a Type 2 canal, while in the mesofacial type, a lower prevalence of the bifid mandibular canal was observed (13.0%, $n = 23$) than in the other facial types. The bifid canal showed significant association with facial type only ($p < 0.05$), but no significant association was observed with the anterior loop type ($p > 0.05$). Facial type is significantly associated with the path and morphological variations of the mandibular canal, independently of the side of the face studied, age, and sex.

1. Introduction

The mandibular canal is present as a single conduit in most individuals, but may vary with regard to shape (oval, round, or pear-shaped) and whether an accessory canal can be identified (canal bifurcation). Many dentists are unaware of these anatomical variations and thus cannot identify them in radiographic images. Consequently, this can lead to peri- and postsurgical complications, as well as implant planning failure, as it is difficult to predict the exact position of the inferior alveolar nerve [1].

Such anatomical variations, along with operator technique, are a cause of failed inferior alveolar nerve block anesthesia. For instance, an individual who received anesthesia on two separate occasions, but who on both occasions experienced only partial anesthesia of the mandible, was found to have bilateral bifid mandibular canals on radiological examination; this anatomical variation may have affected the results of anesthesia procedures [2].

Thus, identification of bifid mandibular canals may help to prevent complications that can have serious consequences during surgery in the mandibular region. A previous study set out to identify variations of bifid mandibular canals, using computed tomography (CT) scans. From this systematic evaluation of anatomical jaw variations, the authors concluded that bifid mandibular canals are not uncommon; thus, it is important to recognize this anatomical variation prior to performing surgical procedures involving the mandible, and that their presence can be confirmed by three-dimensional imaging techniques [3].

A recent study investigated 603 digital panoramic radiographs of fully dentate patients, with complete root formation. The facial types of these individuals were assessed using cephalometric analysis, based on the VERT index of

Ricketts et al. [4], using standard lateral radiographs and sex. The bilateral path of the mandibular canal, assessed on the panoramic radiographs, was classified into three types according to the definition of Nortjé et al. [5]. In Type 1 canals, the mandibular canal was positioned a maximum of 2 mm from the apex of the third molars; in Type 2 canals, the mandibular canal was midway between the root apex of the third molars and the base of the jaw; and in Type 3 canals, the mandibular canal was positioned a maximum of 2 mm from the cortical bone of the jaw base. They showed that there were more Type 2 canals ($p = 0.0012$) and fewer Type 1 ($p = 0.0336$) canals in female than in male patients, but that there were no associations of canal types with facial types. They therefore concluded that facial type is not associated with the path of the mandibular canal [6].

Nevertheless, the shape, size, and symmetry of other craniofacial structures vary according to the facial type. Verification of different facial types is therefore important for treatment planning in several clinical areas. The facial pattern is a major factor in growth prediction and orthodontic planning. Facial types are described as dolichofacial (vertical growth), mesofacial (balanced growth), and brachyfacial (horizontal growth). There is a positive correlation between the height and average distance from the alveolar process to the upper wall of the mandibular canal. Tall individuals have longer bones than those who are shorter, which can contribute to this correlation [7].

The objective of this study was to evaluate the anatomical variations in the mandibular canal associated with the respective facial types, age, sex, and side of the face studied, using cone-beam computed tomography (CBCT) images and to compare our findings with those of previous studies that used panoramic radiographs.

2. Materials and Methods

This study was conducted in accordance with the guidelines established by Resolution 466/12 of the National Council of Ministry of Health and approved by the Research Ethics Committee under Protocol CAAE 58066016.5.0000.5374.

An observational retrospective study was performed using a convenience sample. A total of 174 cases of extended-face cone-beam computed tomography (CBCT) images were analyzed. The scans were all obtained using the same I-Cat® CBCT scanner (Imaging Science, Hatfield, PA, USA) with the following protocol: field-of-view 20×16 cm, 0.25 mm voxels, and 20 s, 120 kVp, and 36 mA. The images were assigned to three main groups according to facial type: Group 1, brachyfacial; Group 2, mesofacial; and Group 3, dolichofacial. Patients were divided into two subgroups according to sex (M, male; F, female), and a further subdivision was made according to the side studied: D, right; E, left.

Then, the mandibular canals were classified according to Carter and Keen [8]. In Type 1, the inferior alveolar nerve was a single, large structure located in a bony canal that passed very close to the root tips. In Type 2, the inferior alveolar nerve ran closer to the mandibular base, and the main nerve has small branches that penetrate the root tips. In Type 3, the main branch of the nerve innervates the

posterior region of the mandible, while a lower branch traverses the mandible to the anterior region (Figure 1).

Bifid canals (Type 3) were further classified according to Langlais et al. [9]. Type I canals consist of unilateral or bilateral channels that fork in the mandible, extending to the third molar or adjacent region. Type II channels are also unilateral or bilateral channels that fork in the mandible, but the branches extend along the main channel and rejoin within the mandible body. Type III channels are a combination of the first two categories: the branch of the bifurcated canal extends to the third molar and the surrounding area as in Type I, while the other extends along the main channel, and the branches remain within the mandibular body on the other side, as in Type II. Type IV consists of two channels originating from independent mandibular foramina (Figure 2).

In a review by Greenstein and Tarnow [10], the inferior alveolar nerve was described as presenting different morphologies in the mental foramen region. Type A has an anterior loop without any anterior extension (incisive canal). Type B shows the absence of a loop and an anterior extension, while Type C shows the presence of an anterior loop and an anterior extension. To evaluate these variations in the mental foramen region, we followed the schematic shown in Figure 3.

CBCT images were included if they had been obtained due to an indication for orthodontic evaluation and were acquired with the extended face protocol. Images were excluded if they included only the maxillary and mandibular arches. Images that had artifacts that prevented visualizing of the mandibular canal and images of patients with a history of trauma, injuries to the lower teeth, orthognathic surgery, or reconstruction of the posterior mandible were excluded.

To standardize tomographic measurement for classification of facial types and for analysis of the mandibular canal, we performed a pilot study to train the examiner (a radiologist with more than 2 years of experience). We ranked the facial types and mandibular canal types in 30 randomly selected scans and repeated the analyses after 30 days. The results were subjected to analysis of intraexaminer agreement. The intraclass correlation coefficient showed good intraexaminer reliability (kappa = 0.91).

The trained examiner then used Dolphin Imaging Software® version 11.0 (Dolphin Imaging System, Chatsworth, CA, USA) to assess facial type and OnDemand3d® software (CyberMed, Seoul, South Korea) to assess anatomical variations of the mandibular canal in a darkened room.

To determine the facial type, the VERT index of Ricketts et al. [4] was used for cephalometric analysis. Five angular variables were used. (1) The angle of the facial axis (N-BA) (Pt-Gn) is the angle formed by the basion-nasion line with the line of the pterygoid point to the cephalometric gnathion, measured at the posterior angle. The standard angle is $90°$, with a standard deviation of $+3°$, and remains constant with age. (2) The angle of the face or facial depth (E-Or) (N-POG) is the angle formed by the Frankfurt plane and the facial plane. The normal value is $87°$, which decreases with age at $0.3°$ per year. (3) The mandibular plane angle (Go-Me)

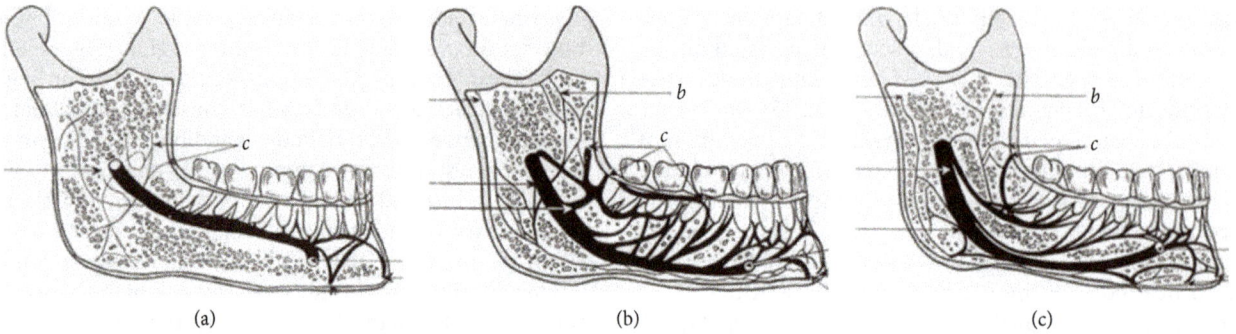

FIGURE 1: Schematic drawing of the intramandibular course of the inferior alveolar nerve, showing Types 1, 2, and 3 of the mandibular canal, as presented by Carter and Keen [8].

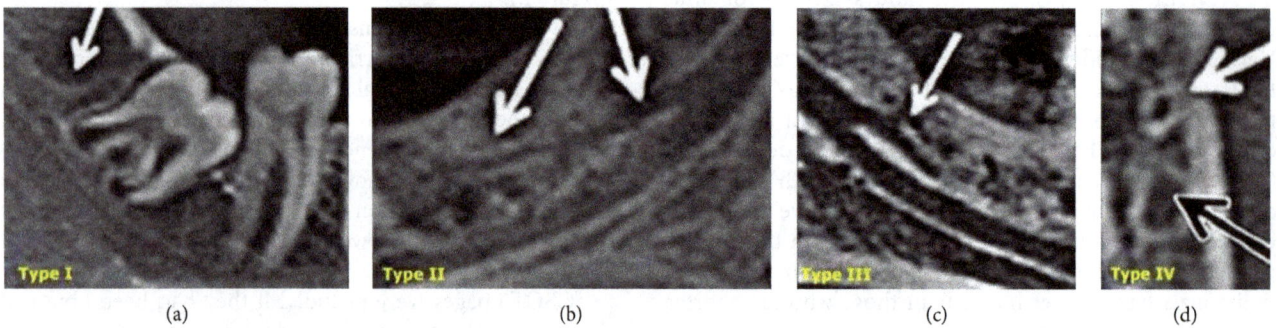

FIGURE 2: Images presented by Langlais et al. [9] showing different types of bifid mandibular canals. (a) Type I; (b) Type II; (c) Type III; (d) Type IV.

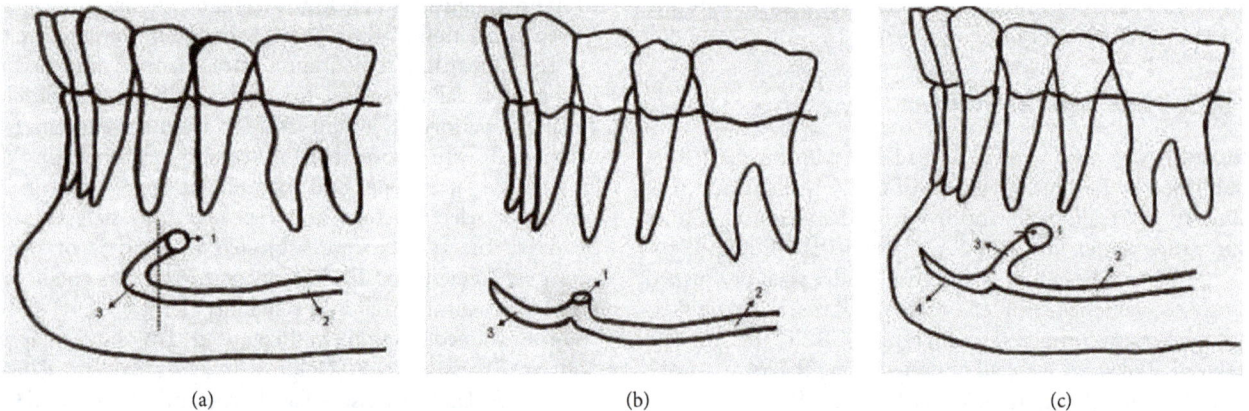

FIGURE 3: Schematic drawing presented by Greenstein and Tarnow [10]: Type A—schematic drawing illustration: 1, mental foramen outflow; 2, the course of the mandibular canal; 3, anterior loop. Type B—schematic drawing illustration: 1, mental foramen outflow; 2, the course of the mandibular canal; 3, incisive canal without anterior loop. Type C—schematic drawing illustration: 1, mental foramen outflow; 2, the course of the mandibular canal; 3, anterior loop; 4, incisive canal.

(Po-Or) is formed by the horizontal Frankfurt plane and the mandibular plane. (4) The height of the lower face angle (Xi-ENA) (X-Pm) is the angle formed by the Xi-ENA and Xi-PM planes. Its standard value is 47° with a standard deviation of +4°, and it remains constant with age. (5) The mandibular arch angle (DC-Xi) (X-Pm) is the angle formed by the body axis and the mandibular condylar axis. Its standard value is 26°, with a 0.5° increase with age for every year of life. This

system was used to establish three basic types of facial growth: mesofacial (balanced growth), dolichofacial (predominantly vertical growth), and brachyfacial (predominantly horizontal growth). The cephalometric points of this analysis were obtained using the Dolphin® Imaging program version 11.0 (Dolphin Imaging System). After marking the cephalometric points required for analysis, sagittal reconstruction was performed by overlapping the right and left sides to obtain a full cephalometric tracing. The program allows a close-up view of the area in question, and overlapping points were used to obtained linear and angular values automatically.

Images were processed using OnDemand3d® software. For analysis of CT images, anatomical planes were first corrected using multiplanar reconstruction. Axial images (thickness 0.25 mm) were used to establish a cutting plane along the alveolar ridge of each patient. This was used to obtain transverse slices from the panoramic images. Cross sections of 1.00 mm thickness, with an interslice distance of 1.00 mm, were used for standardization. In panoramic reconstructions, a slice thickness of 5.25 mm was used (Figure 4).

To improve the identification of the mandibular canal, minor changes were made to the bone edge in the cutting plane to correct brightness and contrast, and image filters were applied, as the anatomical structure of this path is not linear and needs to be individualized for each side of the patient. In cases in which bifid canals were detected, buccolingual oblique cuts were made to obtain suitable images.

2.1. Statistical Analyses. Data were arranged in absolute and relative frequency distribution tables. Chi-square and Fisher's exact tests were used to analyze the associations of facial type, age, sex, and anatomical variations of the mandibular canal. All analyses were performed using R program (R Core Team, 2015, a language and environment for statistical computing; R Foundation for Statistical Computing, Vienna, Austria (https://www.R-project.org/)). The statistical significance level was set at 5%.

3. Results

Of the patients assessed (174 CBCT scans and 348 hemimandibles), 52.9% were female and 47.1% male; 51.1% had a mesofacial type, 29.9% had a brachyfacial type, and 19.0% had a dolichofacial type. No significant associations of facial types with age and sex were observed ($p > 0.05$).

In the analyses of the right side of the face, the location of the mandibular canal was significantly associated ($p < 0.05$) with the facial type. In brachyfacial and mesofacial types, the mandibular canal mostly ran close to the root apexes (63.5% and 58.4% of cases, respectively). In dolichofacial types, the canal mostly ran closest to the base of the jaw, with branches to the root apexes (69.7%) and only 3.0% showed a main canal path running near the root apexes. In mesofacial types, we observed a lower prevalence of bifid mandibular canals than in the other facial types (Table 1).

The type of bifid canal on the right side was also significantly associated with the facial type ($p < 0.05$) (Figure 5). In the dolichofacial group, there was a higher prevalence of a bifid canal that joins into the base (Type II) than in the other two facial types. Type III bifid canals were only observed in the mesofacial group. Type IV bifid canals were observed only in dolichofacial types.

On the right side, the type of loop also showed a significant association with the facial type ($p < 0.05$) (Figure 6). In the dolichofacial group, there was a higher prevalence of

an anterior loop (Type A) and a lower prevalence of Type B canals than in the other facial types.

Table 2 presents the results for analysis of the left side of the mandible. The location of the mandibular canal on the left side was also significantly associated with facial type ($p < 0.05$). Again, brachyfacial and mesofacial types mostly presented with a canal running close to the root tips (67.3% and 52.3% of cases, respectively). In dolichofacial types, the main canal path ran closest to the base of the jaw, with branches extending to the root apexes (66.7%), and in only 6.1% did the main canal path run near the root apexes. In mesofacial types, we observed a lower prevalence of bifid mandibular canals than in the other facial types.

On the left side, there was no significant association of the type of bifid canal with the facial type ($p > 0.05$; Figure 7). The most prevalent type of bifurcation was the Type I bifurcation, accounting for 11.6%. The only case of two types of bifurcation occurring together was observed in a mesofacial individual. The only case of a bifurcated canal originating from separate foramens was observed in a mesofacial individual. The anterior loop types on the left side were not significantly associated with the facial type ($p < 0.05$; Figure 8), but the most common type encountered was Type A.

Table 3 shows the results of the study, regardless of side. The results of the data overall were similar to that for the sides individually; brachyfacial types and most mesofacial types presented with a canal path running next to the root apexes (65.4% and 55.4% of the studied canals, respectively). In dolichofacial types, canals mostly ran closest to the base of the jaw, with branches extending to the root apexes (68.2% of the canals), and only 4.5% of the canals presented with a course near the root tips. In the mesofacial types, there was a lower prevalence of bifid mandibular canals than in the other facial types.

The bifid canal type overall also showed a significant association with the facial type ($p < 0.05$; Figure 9). The dolichofacial group showed a higher prevalence of bifid canals where the bifurcations joined up within the base (Type II) than in the other two facial types. The only cases in which Type III canals were mesofacial types.

The anterior loop type overall was not significantly associated with the facial type ($p > 0.05$; Figure 10), and Type A was the most prevalent type overall.

4. Discussion

The present study demonstrated a significant association between the various facial types and anatomical variations of the mandibular canal. Brachyfacial and mesofacial types mostly had canal paths running close to the root apexes (65.4% ($n = 15$) and 55.4% ($n = 56$) of the studied canals, respectively). In dolichofacial types, the main canal mostly ran closest to the base of the jaw, with branches extending to the apexes (68.2% ($n = 45$) of the canals) and only 4.5% ($n = 3$) of cases showed a canal running near the root tips. Mesofacial types had a lower prevalence of bifid mandibular canals than the other facial types.

Our results contrast with those presented by Schmidt et al. [6], who found no significant association between

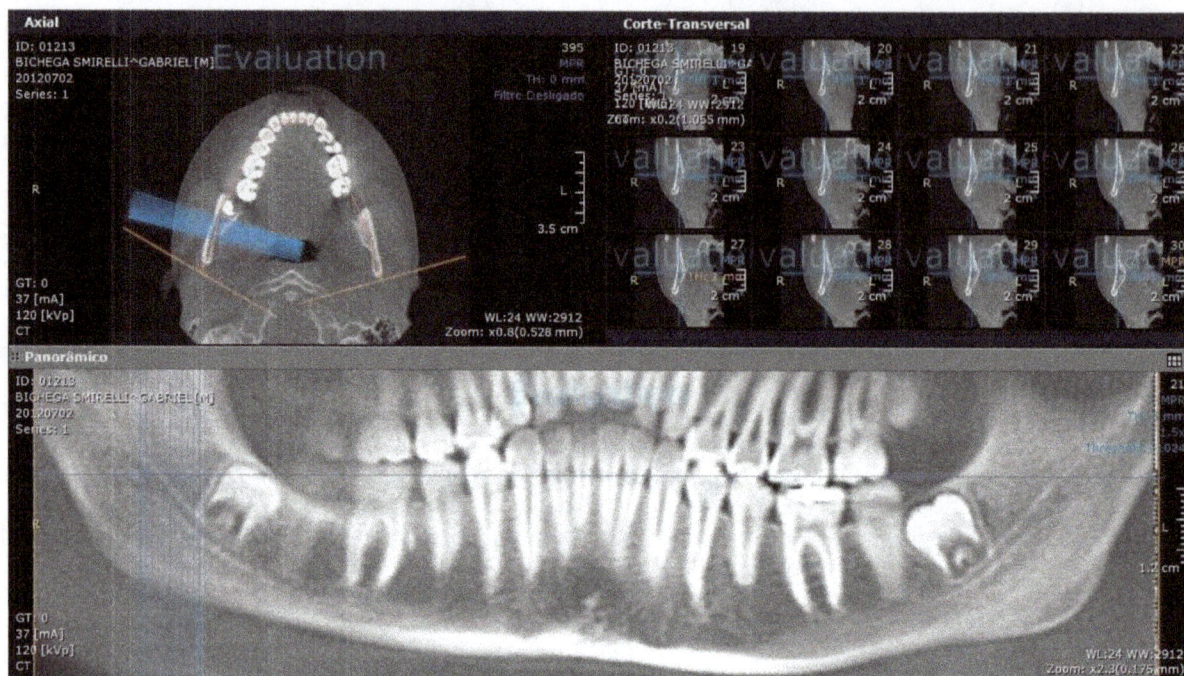

FIGURE 4: Image from OnDemand3D software, showing the axial slice planes, panoramic reconstruction, and transverse cuts.

TABLE 1: Absolute (*n*) and relative (%) frequency of the association between the prevalence of anatomical variations of the mandibular canal on the right side and facial type.

Variable		Total		Facial type						*p* value
				Brachyfacial		Mesofacial		Dolichofacial		
		n	%	*n*	%	*n*	%	*N*	%	
Location: right side	1	86	49.4	33	63.5	52	58.4	1	3.0	
	2	56	32.2	7	13.5	26	29.2	23	69.7	<0.0001
	3	32	18.4	12	23.1	11	12.4	9	27.3	
Bifid type, right side	I	18	10.3	10	19.2	4	4.5	4	12.1	
	II	11	6.3	2	3.8	5	5.6	4	12.1	
	III	2	1.1	0	0.0	2	2.2	0	0.0	0.0258
	IV	1	0.6	0	0.0	0	0.0	1	3.0	
	Absent	142	81.6	40	76.9	78	87.6	24	72.7	
Anterior loop, right side	A	77	44.3	22	42.3	34	38.2	21	63.6	
	B	53	30.5	14	26.9	36	40.4	3	9.1	
	C	43	24.7	15	28.8	19	21.3	9	27.3	0.0088
	Absent	1	0.6	1	1.9	0	0.0	0	0.0	

mandibular canal variants and facial types. This may be because they used panoramic radiographs for their examinations.

Rossi et al. [11] reported that genetic variation and ethnicity seemed to influence anatomical variations of the mandibular canal, with the prevalence of the types varying with geographic location. Although the current study did not set out to select samples by race and region, our sample contained a higher frequency of Caucasians, Africans and mulattos, and fewer Indian and Asian individuals; the current study results corroborated the finding of significant association between different facial types and different facial morphology of the mandibular canal.

CBCT has been shown to be a reliable tool to identify and measure the anterior loop [12]. Uchida et al. [13] found differences smaller than 0.1 mm between the anatomic measurements of the anterior loop in CBCT images, confirming the reliability of the CBCT for this purpose. Some studies have also used CBCT to measure the length and diameter of the anterior loop and incisor canal [13–15], while others have reported the prevalence of the incisive canal in certain populations [12, 16, 17]. Chen et al. [14] found racial influences when comparing the anterior loop measurement and reported that the anterior loop is longer in Taiwanese ($-1.81 + 7.61$ mm) than in American individuals (6.22 ± 1.81 mm).

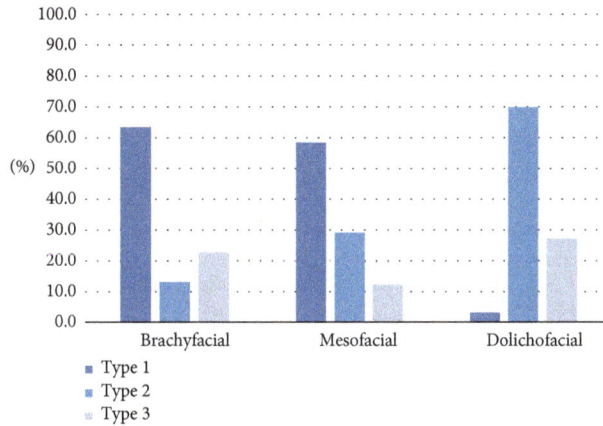

FIGURE 5: Association between the type of bifurcation in the mandibular canal on the right and the facial type.

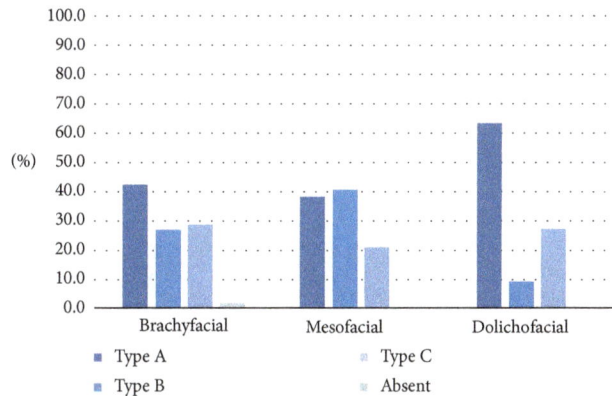

FIGURE 6: Association between the type of anterior loop on the right and the facial type.

TABLE 2: Analysis of the association between the prevalence of anatomical variations of the mandibular canal on the left side and facial type.

Variable		Total n (%)	Brachyfacial n (%)	Mesofacial n (%)	Dolichofacial n (%)	p value
Location: left side	1	83 (48.0)	35 (67.3)	46 (52.3)	2 (6.1)	
	2	60 (34.7)	8 (15.4)	30 (34.1)	22 (66.7)	<0.0001
	3	30 (17.3)	9 (17.3)	12 (13.6)	9 (27.3)	
Bifid type, left side	I	20 (11.6)	8 (15.4)	8 (9.1)	4 (12.1)	
	II	8 (4.6)	1 (1.9)	2 (2.3)	5 (15.2)	
	III	1 (0.6)	0 (0.0)	1 (1.1)	0 (0.0)	0.1009
	IV	1 (0.6)	0 (0.0)	1 (1.1)	0 (0.0)	
	Absent	143 (82.7)	43 (82.7)	76 (86.4)	24 (72.7)	
Anterior loop, left side	A	78 (45.1)	24 (46.2)	44 (50.0)	10 (30.3)	
	B	45 (26.0)	12 (23.1)	20 (22.7)	13 (39.4)	
	C	42 (24.3)	15 (28.8)	19 (21.6)	8 (24.2)	0.3295
	Absent	8 (4.6)	1 (1.9)	5 (5.7)	2 (6.1)	

In this study, we assessed anterior loop variants on CBCT images (Types A, B, and C), as previously described by Li et al. [17] and Do Nascimento et al. [18]. We found a higher prevalence of the anterior loop (Type A) and the lowest prevalence of Type B.

In terms of bifid canals, irrespective of the side studied, the Type 1 canal was the most frequent, accounting for about 12% of cases, and there was no significant difference in the prevalence between the sexes and with age, which is in agreement with results reported by Li et al. [17] in a Chinese population and differs from those of Fu et al. [19], who studied Taiwanese individuals, in which the prevalence of the bifid canal was higher in males.

This research is clinically relevant because knowledge about the correct location and anatomical variations of the mandibular canal is essential for the success of numerous

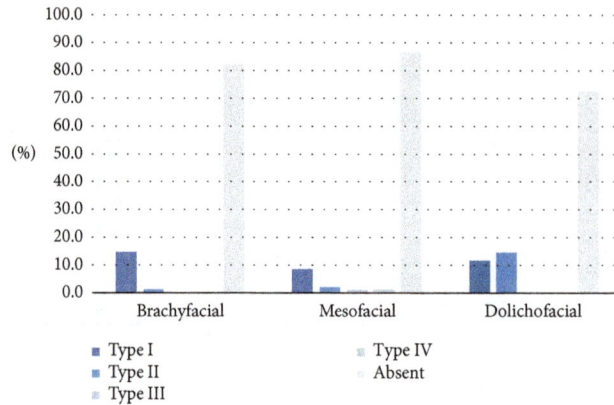

FIGURE 7: Association between the type of bifid mandibular canal on the left side and the facial type.

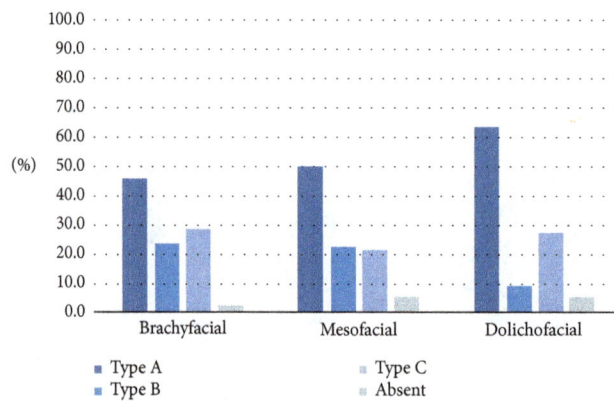

FIGURE 8: Association between the type of anterior loop on the left side and the facial type.

TABLE 3: Analysis of the association between the prevalence of anatomical variations of the mandibular canal and facial type (independent of side).

Variable		Total n (%)	Facial type			p value
			Brachyfacial n (%)	Mesofacial n (%)	Dolichofacial n (%)	
Location: independent of side	1	169 (48.7)	68 (65.4)	98 (55.4)	3 (4.5)	
	2	116 (33.4)	15 (14.4)	56 (31.6)	45 (68.2)	<0.0001
	3	62 (17.9)	21 (20.2)	23 (13.0)	18 (27.3)	
Bifid type: independent of side	I	38 (11.0)	18 (17.3)	12 (6.8)	8 (12.1)	
	II	19 (5.5)	3 (2.9)	7 (4.0)	9 (13.6)	
	III.	3 (0.9)	0 (0.0)	3 (1.7)	0 (0.0)	0.0032
	IV	2 (0.6)	0 (0.0)	1 (0.6)	1 (1.5)	
	Absent	285 (82.1)	83 (79.8)	154 (87.0)	48 (72.7)	
Anterior loop type: independent of side	A	155 (44.7)	46 (44.2)	78 (44.1)	31 (47.0)	
	B	98 (28.2)	26 (25.0)	56 (31.6)	16 (24.2)	
	C	85 (24.5)	30 (28.8)	38 (21.5)	17 (25.8)	0.7553
	Absent	9 (2.6)	2 (1.9)	5 (2.8)	2 (3.0)	

dental procedures involving the jaw, for instance, in anesthesia in routine dentistry practice, endodontics, periodontics, and pediatric dentistry, as well as for more invasive interventions, such as orthognathic surgery and implant installation [10, 20–23].

Stella and Tharanon [24] reported that mandibular canal anatomy may vary according to a number of factors, such as age, sex, race, and development of the alveolar bone. The results presented here contradicted their statement, as no significant associations of facial canal morphology and

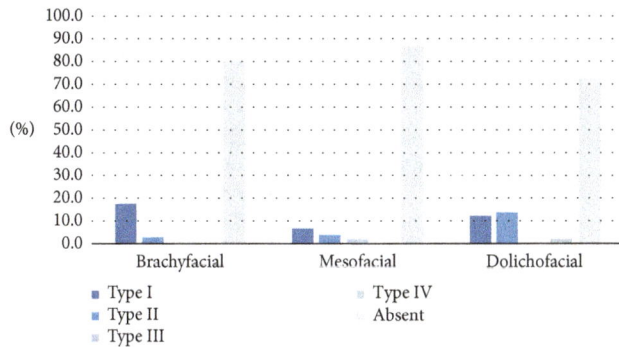

FIGURE 9: Association between the bifid canal type (regardless of side) and the facial type.

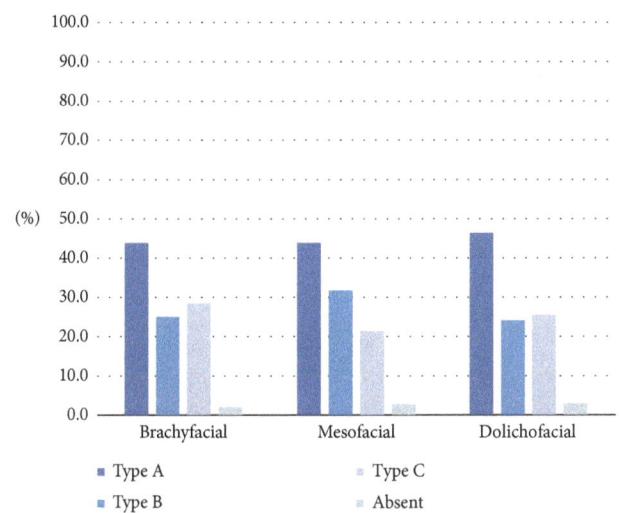

FIGURE 10: Association between the type of loop (regardless of side) and the facial type.

anatomical variations were found with age and sex. However, important factors identified in this study suggest that facial type may be considered an indicator of the location and morphology of the mandibular canal in clinical situations, which is important for planning surgical and dental procedures that require optimizing the quality of anesthesia.

Considering the importance of the issue and the lack of similar studies on the association between facial type and anatomical changes in the mandibular canal based on CBCT, further research is needed to verify the methodological approach used here to clarify the influence of facial types on the localization and morphology of the mandibular canal.

5. Conclusion

The morphology of the mandibular canal and its variations present significant association with different facial types, regardless of age, sex, or the side of the face studied.

Authors' Contributions

All authors have contributed significantly and are in agreement with the manuscript.

References

[1] J. H. Kang, K. S. Lee, M. G. Oh et al., "The incidence and configuration of the bifid mandibular canal in Koreans by using cone-beam computed tomography," *Imaging Science in Dentistry*, vol. 44, no. 1, pp. 53–60, 2014.

[2] K. Lew and G. Townser, "Failure to obtain adequate anesthesia associated with a bifid mandibular canal: a case report," *Australian Dental Journal*, vol. 51, no. 1, pp. 86–90, 2006.

[3] P. Rouas, J. Nancy, and D. Bar, "Identification of double bar mandibular canals: Literature review three case reports and CT scans and with cone beam CT," *Dentomaxillofacial Radiology*, vol. 36, no. 1, pp. 34–38, 2007.

[4] R. M. Ricketts, R. W. Bench, C. F. Gugino, J. J. Hilgers, and R. J. Schulho, *Bioprogresiva Technique Ricketts*, Panamericana, Buenos Aires, Argentina, 1982.

[5] C. J. Nortjé, A. G. Farman, and F. W. Grotepass, "Variations in the usual dental anatomy of the lower (mandibular) canal: a retrospective study of 3612 panoramic radiographs from routine dental patients," *British Journal of Oral Surgery*, vol. 15, no. 1, pp. 55–63, 1977.

[6] A. P. Schmidt, A. C. Rossi, R. A. Freire, F. C. Groppo, and F. B. Meadow, "Association between facial type and mandibular canal morphology—analysis in digital panoramic radiographs," *Brazilian Dental Journal*, vol. 27, no. 5, pp. 609–612, 2016.

[7] Z. J. Mellion, R. G. Behrents, and C. O. Johnston Jr., "The pattern of facial skeletal growth and its relationship to various common indexes of maturation," *American Journal of Orthodontics and Dentofacial Orthopedics*, vol. 143, no. 6, pp. 845–854, 2013.

[8] R. B. Carter and M. S. Keen, "The intramandibular course of the inferior alveolar nerve," *Journal of Anatomy*, vol. 108, no. 3, pp. 433–440, 1971.

[9] R. P. Langlais, R. Broadus, and B. J. Glass, "Bifid mandibular canals in panoramic radiographs," *Journal of the American Dental Association*, vol. 110, no. 6, pp. 923–926, 1985.

[10] G. Greenstein and D. Tarnow, "The foramen and mental nerve: clinical and Anatomical factors related to dental implant placement: a literature review," *Journal of Periodontology*, vol. 77, no. 12, pp. 1933–1943, 2006.

[11] P. Rossi, M. R. Bruker, and M. I. B. Rockenbach, "Forked jaw canals: analysis of panoramic radiographs," *Journal of Medical Sciences*, vol. 18, pp. 99–104, 2009.

[12] K. Filo, T. Schneider, M. C. Locher, A. L. Kruse, and H. T. Lübbers, "The inferior alveolar nerve's loop at the mental foramen and its implications for surgery," *Journal of the American Dental Association*, vol. 145, no. 3, pp. 260–269, 2014.

[13] Y. Uchida, N. Noguchi, M. Goto et al., "Measurement of anterior loop length for the mandibular canal and diameter of the mandibular incisive canal to avoid nerve damage when installing endosseous implants in the interforaminal region: a second attempt introducing cone beam computed tomography," *Journal of Oral and Maxillofacial Surgery*, vol. 67, no. 4, pp. 744–750, 2009.

[14] Z. Chen, D. Chen, L. Tang, and F. Wang, "Relationship between the position of the mental foramen and the previous loop of the inferior alveolar nerve determined by the cone beam computed tomography combined with mimics," *Journal of Computer Assisted Tomography*, vol. 39, no. 1, pp. 86–93, 2015.

[15] S. L. Kabak, N. V. Zhuravleva, Y. M. Melnichenko, and N. A. Savrasova, "Study of the mandibular incisive canal anatomy using cone beam computed tomography," *Surgical and Radiologic Anatomy*, vol. 39, no. 6, pp. 647–655, 2017.

[16] D. Apostolakis and J. E. Brown, "The anterior loop of the inferior alveolar nerve: Prevalence, measurement of its length and a recommendation for interforaminal implant installation based on cone beam CT imaging," *Clinical Oral Implants Research*, vol. 23, no. 9, pp. 1022–1030, 2012.

[17] X. Li, Z. K. Jin, H. Zhao, K. Yang, J. M. Duan, and W. J. Wang, "The prevalence, length and position of the anterior loop of the inferior alveolar nerve in Chinese, assessed by spiral computed tomography," *Surgical and Radiologic Anatomy*, vol. 35, no. 9, pp. 823–830, 2013.

[18] E. H. Do Nascimento, M. L. Dos Anjos Pontual, A. Dos Anjos Pontual et al., "Assessment of the anterior loop of the mandibular canal: a study using cone-beam computed tomography," *Imaging Science in Dentistry*, vol. 46, no. 2, pp. 69–75, 2016.

[19] E. Fu, M. Peng, C. Y. Chiang, H. P. Tu, Y. S. Lin, and E. C. Shen, "Bifid mandibular canals and the factors associated with their presence: a medical computed tomography evaluation in a Taiwanese population," *Clinical Oral Implants Research*, vol. 25, no. 2, pp. e64–e67, 2014.

[20] A. Chandra, A. Singh, M. Badni, R. Jaiswal, and A. Agnihotri, "Determination of sex by radiographic analysis of mental foramen in North Indian population," *Journal of Forensic Dental Sciences*, vol. 5, no. 1, pp. 52–55, 2013.

[21] T. von Arx, M. Fridli, P. Sendi, and S. Lozanoff, "Location and dimensions of the mental foramen: radiographic analysis by using cone-beam computed tomography," *Journal of Endodontics*, vol. 39, no. 12, pp. 1522–1528, 2013.

[22] Z. L. Zhang, J. G. Cheng, C. Li et al., "Detection accuracy of condylar bony defects in Promax 3D cone beam CT images scanned with different protocols," *Dentomaxillofacial Radiology*, vol. 42, no. 5, article 20120241, 2013.

[23] K. Saito, N. S. Araújo, M. T. Saito, J. J. V. Pine, and P. L. Oak, "Analysis of the mental foramen using cone beam computerized tomography," *Revista de Odontologia da UNESP*, vol. 44, no. 4, pp. 226–231, 2015.

[24] J. P. Stella and W. Tharanon, "The need radiographic method to determine the location of the inferior alveolar canal in the posterior edentulous mandible: implications for dental implants. Part 1: technique," *International Journal of Oral & Maxillofacial Implants*, vol. 5, pp. 15–22, 1990.

8

Analyzing Menton Deviation in Posteroanterior Cephalogram in Early Detection of Temporomandibular Disorder

Trelia Boel,[1] Ervina Sofyanti,[2] and Erliera Sufarnap[2]

[1]*Department of Dental Radiology, Faculty of Dentistry, University of Sumatera Utara, Medan, Indonesia*
[2]*Department of Orthodontics, Faculty of Dentistry, University of Sumatera Utara, Medan, Indonesia*

Correspondence should be addressed to Trelia Boel; trelia.boel@usu.ac.id

Academic Editor: Izzet Yavuz

Introduction. Some clinicians believed that mandibular deviation leads to facial asymmetry and it also had a correlation with temporomandibular disorders (TMDs). Posteroanterior (PA) cephalogram was widely reported as a regular record in treating facial asymmetry and craniofacial anomalies. The objective of this study was to analyze the relationship of menton deviation in PA cephalogram with temporomandibular disorders (TMDs) symptoms. *Materials and Methods.* TMJ function was initially screened based on TMD-DI questionnaire. PA cephalogram of volunteer subjects with TMDs ($n = 37$) and without TMDs ($n = 33$) with mean age of 21.61 ± 2.08 years was taken. The menton deviation was measured by the distance (mm) from menton point to midsagittal reference (MSR) horizontally, using software digitized measurement, and categorized as asymmetric if the value is greater than 3 mm. The prevalence and difference of menton deviation in both groups were evaluated by unpaired t-test. *Result.* The prevalence of symmetry group showed that 65.9% had no TMDs with mean of $1,815 \pm 0,71$ mm; in contrast, the prevalence of asymmetry group showed that 95.5% reported TMDs with mean of $3,159 \pm 1,053$ mm. There was a significant difference of menton deviation to TMDs ($p = 0.000$) in subjects with and without TMDs. *Conclusion.* There was a significant relationship of menton deviation in PA cephalogram with TMDs based on TMD-DI index.

1. Introduction

The relevance of temporomandibular disorders (TMDs) to malocclusion became a hot issue in recent years. TMDs are a collective complex term for a group of musculoskeletal and neuromuscular conditions which includes several clinical signs and symptoms involving the muscles of mastication, temporomandibular joint, and associated structures [1, 2]. The displacement of mandible can influence the modeling process of the TMJ, leading to asymmetry. Even though a small amount of asymmetry in the maxillofacial region is common, there is a critical threshold distance that is considered as asymmetric [3–6]. At the same time many authors have shown no or weak connection between orthodontics treatment and TMDs.

Malocclusion itself is a product of multiple factors that yields a significant influence on the patient's quality of life during craniomandibular growth and development even though, until aging, it can be treated by orthodontics or orthognathic surgery. The mandibular asymmetry is a major problem due to its effect on facial appearance directly, especially the chin area that represents the third lower facial part. There is an impact on the quality of life because functional problems that related to the role of temporomandibular joint are in the stomatognathic system and also affect the facial appearance, such as facial asymmetry [7, 8]. In daily practice, posteroanterior cephalogram is used widely in detection of asymmetry mandible that involved skeletal and dentoalveolar component [9]. Investigating the connection between morphologically anatomy landmarks with sign and symptom of TMDs has been a more interesting question than debating about malocclusion causes of TMDs or vice versa. Recent study reported sign and symptom of TMD as main risk factor in the occurrence of mandibulofacial asymmetry [10]. Asymmetry in mandibular usually results in a shift of the chin and 70% of patients with facial asymmetry and chin

TABLE 1: Temporomandibular disorder diagnostic index (TMD-DI).

Number	Question lists	Code	Filling instructions
1	Do you have symptom such as headache?		
2	Do you have symptom such as pain during closing and opening mouth?		
3	Do you have symptom of joint trismus when getting up in the morning?		Fill in code with
4	Do you have symptom of pain around neck?		0 = never
5	Do you have symptom of tinnitus?		1 = sometimes
6	Do you clench your teeth in worries?		2 = often
7	Do you clench your teeth when in anger?		3 = always
8	Do you clench your teeth when concentrating?		

Total score

Total score: 0–24

Total score ≤ 3: TMD symptom code = 0

Total score > 3: TMD code = 1

deviation presented structural and displacement asymmetry, while only 10% showed pure displacement asymmetry and facial askeletal asymmetry was reported to exist in patients with chin deviation [11, 12].

The aim of this study is to investigate the menton deviation that is presented at the chin position in a PA cephalogram. Early detection of TMDs symptom is performed by questionnaire, neglecting TMDs sign. Clarifying the relationship between menton deviation and TMDs symptoms is required to develop diagnosing and planning treatment of mandibular asymmetry.

2. Materials and Methods

All study volunteers who were female students of Dental Faculty of University of Sumatera Utara signed an informed consent form to participate in this study. This was a cross-sectional case-control study from March 2016 until August 2016 with 37 subjects with TMDs and 33 subjects without TMDs. An index as was showed in Table 1 was developed in Indonesia, called TMD diagnostic index (TMD-DI) as early detection of symptom was applied by the examiners in screening protocol of those volunteers [13].

The following inclusion criteria were used for volunteers participation in the study: (1) still being registered as active student in the Dental Faculty of University of Sumatera Utara; (2) no orthodontics treatment or occlusal adjustment history; (3) no facial traumatic injury or drug addiction history. These volunteers were from 18 years to 28 years (mean: 21.61 years ± 2.08 years) old.

The PA digital cephalogram of all the volunteers was taken under standard conditions and processed in the same X-ray machine OC 200 D 1-4-1 with digital sensor in Teaching Hospital Dental Faculty, University of Sumatera Utara, and measured digitally used Cliniview software version 10.1.2. Crista galli (Cg) is establishing in the midline of the skull and located on the midpart of the ethmoid bone which is common to be identified in the PA cephalogram. Menton as the lowest point on the symphyseal shadow of the mandible was

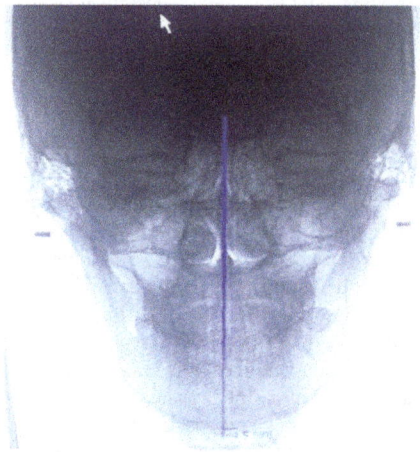

FIGURE 1: Menton deviation to MSR in PA cephalogram digital radiograph.

reported as one of landmarks that is common in frontal radiographs, such as panoramic and PA cephalogram in mandibular asymmetry [14]. The midsagittal reference (MSR) is constructed from crista galli (Cg) through the Anterior Nasal Spine (ANS) to the chin area. Then the menton deviation was done by measuring the distance of MSR to menton point [4, 15]. If the menton deviation is less than 3 mm, it was categorized as symmetrical group and vice versa if it is more than 3 mm, it was categorized as asymmetrical group (Figure 1).

Since both TMDs and symmetrical reference used categorize data, there was no normality distribution. The validity and reliability of intrarater digitized cephalometry measurements were obtained by measuring the mean of initial and second measurement and then calculated by using Bland-Altman analysis. The prevalence and amount of menton deviation in PA cephalogram in both groups were evaluated and compared by unpaired t-test (SPSS software, version 18.0 for Windows; SPSS, Chicago IL).

TABLE 2: Correlation of menton deviation horizontally to TMDs group (unpaired t-test).

Menton deviation	TMD-DI				Mean ± SD	p value
	(−)		(+)			
Symmetrical	29	65.9%	15	34.1%	1,815 ± 0,71 mm	0.000*
Asymmetrical	1	4.5%	21	95.5%	3,159 ± 1,053 mm	

*p < 0.05: significant correlation.

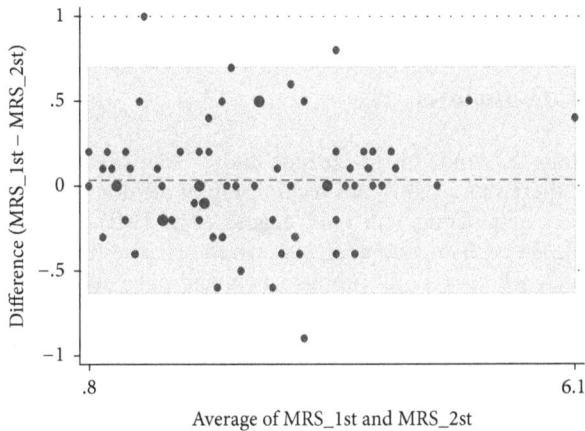

FIGURE 2: Bland-Altman analysis of combined group.

3. Results

This study is based on the tracings with intraexaminer reliability of the 70 PA cephalogram of volunteer subjects (mean: 21.61 years ± 2.08 years old) and performed by the same previously trained examiner (40 hours of training). In intraexaminer analysis, the validity and reliability of measurement by quantification of the agreement between two quantitative measurements had constructing limits of agreement of 95% as mean differences of first and second measurement showed no significant difference ($p = 0.057$). There were four measurement samples that showed out of 95% limits of agreement and were eliminated (Figure 2).

Analysis of unpaired t-test (sig. 2 tailed; $p < 0.05$) was used to compare the symmetrical mandible based on menton deviation to TMDs based on TMD-DI questionnaire.

The prevalence of symmetry group showed that 34.1% had TMDs; in contrast, the prevalence of asymmetry group showed that 95.5% reported TMDs in this group. There was a significant difference of menton deviation in both groups. The mean of non-TMDs showed menton deviation 1,815 ± 0,71 mm in non-TMDs and 3,159 ± 1,053 mm in TMDs group (Table 2).

4. Discussion

PA cephalogram, which has been reported to be widely used in orthodontics since 1990s, is an important radiodiagnostic in evaluating transverse skeletal and dentoalveolar asymmetry. Vertical and transverse measurement of skeletal and dentofacial structures were obtained relative to the reference lines by comparing the measurements of corresponding structures from the right and left sides. However, there were some limitations in difficulty when reproducing head posture and errors in identifying landmarks [16, 17]. Difficulty in reproducing good head posture might be related to confirming the postural changes of the head and body when taking the PA cephalogram. Adequate head position was required in taking PA cephalogram to avoid bias in measurement. Even though the PA cephalogram procedure was taken, tiny rotation head could affect the MSR analysis [18]. Nowadays, errors in identifying landmarks could be limited by computer-aided cephalometric analysis with digital radiography. Precise written definitions describing the landmarks and clinicians' training before intraexaminer measurement when digitizing landmarks are supposed to reduce the chance of interpretation error [16, 17].

There were several methods for constructing the vertical references lines using anatomic point at crista galli (Cg) to Nasion (Na), Anterior Nasal Spine (ANS), and menton [16]. Even though it was reported that Cg-ANS and Na-ANS had the lowest validity and should not be used in asymmetry cephalometric analysis, our study used an alternative way of constructing the MSR line, which is a line perpendicular to the line connecting the left and right intersection of the zygomaticofrontal suture and lateral orbital margin (ZF-ZF) through the Cg if anatomical variations in the upper and middle facial regions exist [15]. According to Broadbent, menton point is the most inferior point on the symphysis of the mandible in the median plane. There are several types of menton, such as concave type (the highest point between two mental protuberances); convex (the tip of the mandible in the prominent mandible); and flat type (the midpoint of the plat area).

The mandibular deviation resulting in chin deviation towards contralateral side should be considered in orthodontic treatment planning and evaluation of facial asymmetry patients. It means that the menton deviation, maxillomandibular midline angle, and the distance of lower incisor to the midsagittal reference might be compensated by leaning towards the deviated side of the menton during an orthodontic treatment, for example, using elastics [3]. This study used menton point because the chin deviation was easily identified in facial asymmetry patients and reported around 4% in mandibular asymmetry that required orthodontic treatment [19].

Some studies have shown that a small amount of asymmetry in the maxillofacial region is common in general populations and focused on deviation of menton, chin, or gonial angle. The facial asymmetry can be recognized if the menton is deviated by more than 4 mm [3, 15]. Other studies have reported more than 2 mm difference in these points to be recognized as asymmetry [6]. However, this study used 3 mm as the symmetrical guideline based on threshold of visual perception of facial asymmetry in a facial paralysis model that at least 3 mm of the oral commissure, brow, or both was assessed as facial asymmetry [4]. The other consideration in our study was that the subjects were female dental faculty students whose visual perception is more sensitive than layperson. Anamnestic data gathering was conducted according to the TMD-DI which should be considered different with layperson because the subjects of this study were dental faculty students where a person's appearance and self-esteem concern are probably higher than other subjects.

The impact of TMDs was found in some studies showing variation between activities and individuals. It was reported that 52.8% of 142 dental students at Dental school of Casablanca showed at least one sign of TMDs and 17.5% presented with pain [20]. Pain in TMDs has a significant negative impact on activities of daily living, especially to patients with malocclusion [21]. According to Olsson and Lindquist, orthodontic patients appear to be at greater risk of developing TMDs than individuals who only need minor treatment [21]. The presence of postural changes compared between women (mean age 18–45 years old) with migraine with or without TMDs showed clinically relevant postural changes [2]. In our study, the volunteer subjects were female dental student and early detection with TMD-DI questionnaire was performed as initial screening for TMD symptoms. Since we know that TMDs are multifactorial and have been demonstrated to induce mandibular asymmetry, any displacement of anatomical landmark of the mandible might induce skeletal change in the future. Our study was also similar with Purbiati's in adolescent population that reported TMDs as one of the main risk factors of mandibulofacial asymmetry [10]. Those studies indicated the possibility of early detection of TMDs through the presence of facial asymmetry.

Some studies reported that the prevalence of TMDs with various sign and symptoms was higher in older subjects. The prevalence of TMD increases by the age with a mean age of 32.7 ± 14.5 years, while the later comprised mean age of 54.2 ± 15.1 years. The homogenous subjects in age and sex related to the previous studies that reported at least two distinct age peaks are identifiable within this population of patients seeking for TMD treatment, one at about 30–35 years and the other one at about 50–55 years. The ratio of female patients who had sign and symptoms of TMDs was also reported to be higher than male patients. Even though sign and symptom of TMD showed no significant differences in age, sex, and race/ethnicity, the prevalence of female is higher than the male based on age distribution of group diagnoses [1]. There was a deviation of menton from the vertical plane in subjects with TMDs, highlighted by the significant differences of the angle from ANS-Me to the vertical plane among unilateral TMDs, bilateral TMDs, and no TMDs. The asymmetric index of the distances from the vertical plane to the chin or menton point ($p = 0.02$) was higher in subjects with unilateral TMDs [5]. In our study, the prevalence of symmetry group showed that 65.9% had no TMDs; in contrast, the prevalence of asymmetry group showed that 95.5% reported TMDs. There was a significant difference of menton deviation to TMDs ($p = 0.000$) in subjects with and without TMDs in this study. However, our hypothesis that the menton deviation might be useful as symmetrical guideline in early detection of TMDs required larger population sample and approved the clinical examination. The variation of morphological landmarks in PA cephalograms together with functional analysis might be considered as the sign of TMDs.

5. Conclusions

Within the limits of the current study, it can be concluded that there was a significant relationship of menton deviation in PA cephalogram with TMD diagnosed by TMD-DI index. Since PA cephalogram analyzes asymmetry cases in skeletal aspect, whereas TMD problem in mandibular asymmetry cases related to the difference of the skeletal measurement and shape of the condyle area, there is a close relationship between mandibular deviation and TMD. A further diagnostic study is needed to confirm PA analysis as an alternative tool for TMD diagnoses.

Ethical Approval

This study was approved by Research Ethics Committee of University of Sumatera Utara, under Protocol no. 322/2016.

Acknowledgments

The authors acknowledge the financial support received from Dana Hibah Fundamental Research University of Sumatera Utara that is granted by the Ministry of Education and Research Technology of Indonesia (no. 017/SP2H/LT/DRPM/II/2016). They thank all the volunteering subjects who were willing to participate in this study and also Purbiati M. for the discussion time.

References

[1] D. Manfredini, F. Piccotti, G. Ferronato, and L. Guarda-Nardini, "Age peaks of different RDC/TMD diagnoses in a patient population," *Journal of Dentistry*, vol. 38, no. 5, pp. 392–399, 2010.

[2] M. C. Ferreira, D. Bevilaqua-Grossi, F. É. Dach, J. G. Speciali, M. C. Gonçalves, and T. C. Chaves, "Body posture changes in women with migraine with or without temporomandibular disorders," *Brazilian Journal of Physical Therapy*, vol. 18, no. 1, pp. 19–29, 2014.

[3] N. Masuoka, A. Muramatsu, Y. Ariji, H. Nawa, S. Goto, and E. Ariji, "Discriminative thresholds of cephalometric indexes in the subjective evaluation of facial asymmetry," *American*

Journal of Orthodontics and Dentofacial Orthopedics, vol. 131, no. 5, pp. 609–613, 2007.

[4] E. A. Chu, T. Y. Farrag, L. E. Ishii, and P. J. Byrne, "Threshold of visual perception of facial asymmetry in a facial paralysis model," *Archives of Facial Plastic Surgery*, vol. 13, no. 1, pp. 14–19, 2011.

[5] O. C. Almasan, M. Baciut, M. Hedesiu, S. Bran, H. Almasan, and G. Baciut, "Posteroanterior cephalometric changes in subjects with temporomandibular joint disorders," *Dentomaxillofacial Radiology*, vol. 42, no. 1, Article ID 20120039, 2013.

[6] K. Y. Choi, "Analysis of Facial Asymmetry," *Archives of Craniofacial Surgery*, vol. 16, no. 1, pp. 1–10, 2015.

[7] O. S. Sezgin, P. Celenk, and S. Arici, "Mandibular asymmetry in different occlusion patterns," *Angle Orthodontist*, vol. 77, no. 5, pp. 803–807, 2007.

[8] M. T. Khan, S. K. Verma, S. Maheshwari, S. N. Zahid, and P. K. Chaudhary, "Neuromuscular dentistry: occlusal diseases and posture," *Journal of Oral Biology and Craniofacial Research*, vol. 3, no. 3, pp. 146–150, 2013.

[9] S. C. White and M. J. Pharoah, *Oral Radiology Principles and Interpretation*, vol. 7, Elsevier, 2014.

[10] M. Purbiati, M. K. Purwanegara, L. Kusdhany, and L. S. Himawan, "Prediction of mandibulofacial asymmetry using risk factor index and model of dentocraniofacial morphological pattern," *Journal of International Dental and Medical Research*, vol. 9, no. 3, pp. 195–201, 2016.

[11] W. Schmid, F. Mongini, and A. Felisio, "A computer-based assessment of structural and displacement asymmetries of the mandible," *AmericaN Journal of Orthodontics and Dentofacial Orthopedics*, vol. 100, no. 1, pp. 19–34, 1991.

[12] J Hwai, T. W. Ho, C. H. Ming et al., "Analysis of facial skeletal characteristics in patients with chin deviation," *Journal of the Chinese Medical Association*, vol. 73, no. 1, pp. 29–34, 2010.

[13] L. S. Himawan, L. Kusdhany, and I. Ismail, "iagnostic index for temporomandibular disorders in Indonesia," *Internal Journal of Clinical Preventif Dentistry*, vol. 10, no. 2, pp. 103–108, 2014.

[14] A. Agrawal, D. K. Bagga, P. Agrawal, and R. K. Bhutani, "An evaluation of panoramic radiograph to assess mandibular asymmetry as compared to posteroanterior cephalogram," *APOS Trends in Orthodontics*, vol. 5, no. 5, pp. 197–201, 2015.

[15] Q. Xie, C. Yang, D. He, X. Cai, and Z. Ma, "Is mandibular asymmetry more frequent and severe with unilateral disc displacement?" *Journal of Cranio-Maxillofacial Surgery*, vol. 43, no. 1, pp. 81–86, 2015.

[16] B. Trpkova, N. G. Prasad, E. W. N. Lam, D. Raboud, K. E. Glover, and P. W. Major, "Assessment of facial asymmetries from posteroanterior cephalograms: validity of reference lines," *American Journal of Orthodontics and Dentofacial Orthopedics*, vol. 123, no. 5, pp. 512–520, 2003.

[17] R. Leonardi, A. Annunziata, and M. Caltabiano, "Landmark identification error in posteroanterior cephalometric radiography," *Angle Orthodontist*, vol. 78, no. 4, pp. 761–765, 2008.

[18] K. Miyashita, "Contemporary cephalometric radiography," *Quintessence*, pp. 160–209, 1996.

[19] R. D. Sheats, S. P. McGorray, Q. Musmar, T. T. Wheeler, and G. J. King, "Prevalence of orthodontic asymmetries," *Seminars in Orthodontics*, vol. 4, no. 3, pp. 138–145, 1998.

[20] F. Bourzgui, H. Aghoutan, and S. Diouny, "Craniomandibular disorders and mandibular reference position in orthodontic treatment," *International Journal of Dentistry*, vol. 2013, Article ID 890942, 6 pages, 2013.

[21] E. Kaselo, T. Jagomagi, and U. Voog, "Malocclusion and the need for orthodontic treatment in patients with temporomandibular dysfunction," *Stomatologija Baltic Dental and Maxillofacial Journal*, vol. 9, no. 3, pp. 79–85, 2007.

9

Dentine Tubule Occlusion by Novel Bioactive Glass-Based Toothpastes

Luiza Pereira Dias da Cruz ⓘD, **Robert G. Hill, Xiaojing Chen, and David G. Gillam** ⓘD

Oral Bioengineering, Barts and the London School of Medicine and Dentistry, QMUL, London, UK

Correspondence should be addressed to David G. Gillam; d.g.gillam@qmul.ac.uk

Academic Editor: Ali I. Abdalla

There are numerous over-the-counter (OTC) and professionally applied (in-office) products and techniques currently available for the treatment of dentine hypersensitivity (DH), but more recently, the use of bioactive glasses in toothpaste formulations have been advocated as a possible solution to managing DH. *Aim.* The aim of the present study, therefore, was to compare several bioactive glass formulations to investigate their effectiveness in an established in vitro model. *Materials and Methods.* A 45S5 glass was synthesized in the laboratory together with several other glass formulations: (1) a mixed glass (fluoride and chloride), (2) BioMinF, (3) a chloride glass, and (4) an amorphous chloride glass. The glass powders were formulated into five different toothpaste formulations. Dentine discs were sectioned from extracted human teeth and prepared for the investigation by removing the cutting debris (smear layer) following sectioning using a 6% citric acid solution for 2 minutes. Each disc was halved to provide test and control halves for comparison following the brushing of the five toothpaste formulations onto the test halves for each toothpaste group. Following the toothpaste application, the test discs were immersed in either artificial saliva or exposed to an acid challenge. *Results.* The dentine samples were analyzed using scanning electron microscopy (SEM), and observation of the SEM images indicated that there was good surface coverage following artificial saliva immersion. Furthermore, although the acid challenge removed the hydroxyapatite layer on the dentine surface for most of the samples, except for the amorphous chloride glass, there was evidence of tubular occlusion in the dentine tubules. *Conclusions.* The conclusions from the study would suggest that the inclusion of bioactive glass into a toothpaste formulation may be an effective approach to treat DH.

1. Introduction

1.1. Overview. Dentine hypersensitivity (DH) affects approximately 10–30% of the adult population and may have a direct impact on the individual's quality of life [1]. There are numerous over-the-counter (OTC) and professionally applied (in-office) products and techniques available for the treatment of DH. Recently, the use of bioactive glasses in toothpaste formulations has been advocated as a possible long-term solution for managing DH [2]. Currently, most of the research activity focusses on the hydrodynamic theory as the basis for the therapeutic treatment of DH. The rationale being that, by blocking the dentinal tubules (tubular occlusion), there will a corresponding reduction of the fluid flow through dentine (dentine permeability) and a subsequent relief of pain [1, 3]. The mechanisms underpinning the hydrodynamic theory are generally investigated in several recognized models, for example, in vitro, in situ, in vivo human studies and animal studies (for nerve desensitizing mechanisms). The aim of the present in vitro study, therefore, was to investigate the effectiveness of experimental bioactive glasses designed for toothpaste formulations.

An ideal desensitizing agent should have a rapid action with long-term effects, be non-irritant to pulp, painless, easy to apply, and should not stain the tooth [4]. Toothpastes are considered the most economic method for using desensitizing in-home treatments and generally are classified by the regulatory authorities on the ingredients within the formulation (e.g., cosmetic and medicine/drug) [5, 6]. There are a plethora of products that are being developed for this condition, but currently, there does not appear to be one ideal product that can completely resolve the problem.

Bioactive materials have been considered for both medical and dental use particularly in bone defects. For example, in 1969, bioactive glasses were discovered as a second-generation alternative for the bonding of bone to an implant within the host's tissue through a chemical reaction. One of the advantages of these materials was that they have the capacity of producing hydroxyapatite and induce osteogenesis in physiological systems [7]. Since 1985, 45S5 Bioglass has been used clinically, as a third generation of biomaterials, for tissue reparation using gene activation properties. The first Bioglass-containing material established in the market was initially used to treat conductive hearing loss and also in several head and neck surgeries [7]. In dentistry, the application of bioactive glasses was related to bone replacement implants in edentulous patients, to provide a more stable ridge for denture construction. It was also used for periodontal diseases (PerioGlas®) and bone defects as a method of reconstruction of the bone. Dentine and bone have similarities in terms of tissue composition (e.g., hydroxyapatite); hence, biocompatible glasses may be an efficient material for incorporating into toothpaste formulations as a tubular occludent [8–10]. The composition of bioactive glasses is silicon, sodium, calcium, and phosphorus oxides with specific percentages. In addition, fluoride can be incorporated into the glass, and both fluoride and calcium ions are released in the presence of saliva [9, 10]. When in contact with a biological fluid such as saliva, Bioglass particles react and three processes occur: (1) leaching and formation of silanols, (2) dissolution of the glass network, and (3) precipitation. Precipitation is an important process for occluding dentine tubules. The formation of a layer composed of calcium and phosphate induced by the release of these ions from the glass can mechanically occlude dentinal tubules and lower fluid flow within the dentine. This layer is crystallized into hydroxyapatite, and the presence of silica can accelerate the maturation of hydroxyapatite. In the bone, bioactive glass triggers an osteoblast cell cycle leading to rapid cell proliferation and differentiation [7, 9, 11, 12].

Toothpaste formulations containing potassium designed to treat sensitive teeth can also have an analgesic effect. For example, potassium saline is responsible for maintaining high levels of potassium ion extracellularly, preventing repolarization of the nerve cell membrane and inhibiting the transmission of impulses. In brief, potassium nitrate has been postulated to act by blocking neural transmission to reduce DH symptoms. However, there are limited clinical data in humans to support the mode of action of potassium ions reducing DH. Several studies have reported that toothpastes containing calcium sodium phosphosilicate or NovaMin® (GSK) can occlude the dentinal tubules more effectively than potassium salts as evidenced in clinical studies and in vitro studies immersing the products in artificial saliva [6, 11, 12]. Usually toothpaste formulations are based on fluoride (to protect against caries), an abrasive component that provides the cleaning ability, substances that inhibit bacterial growth, and other ingredients [6, 12, 13]. Fluoride is a compound that may aid remineralization in enamel although evidence regarding its effect on DH is limited. It has been demonstrated, however, that fluoride in toothpastes can create a precipitation onto the dentine surface and block the dentine tubules,

increasing resistance against an acidic challenge [6]. The precipitation however may also contain silica particles that can occlude the dentinal tubules rather than the fluoride ion per se. The suggested actions of a bioactive glass toothpaste were through its chemical ability to occlude dentine tubules by the formation of calcium-phosphorous precipitates, calcium fluoride, and fluorapatite. Fluoride in toothpaste formulations however is important for its role in caries prevention by reducing the rate of demineralization, promoting remineralization of damaged tissue, and decreasing acid production by interfering with oral bacteria in the tooth biofilm, functioning as a biocide against S. mutans. Nevertheless, fluoride in combination with other ions may also enhance the effectiveness of any desensitizing effects [10, 14]. Toothpaste formulations may also induce the formation of calcium, phosphate, and fluoride and contribute to intratubular mineralization [6, 12, 13]. In addition, the use of calcium phosphate products has been considered promising for the treatment of DH. Calcium is also important for the remineralization in tooth restorations as it was the primary component of hydroxyapatite, with apatite as a form of calcium phosphate, which can be used in dental materials (e.g., hydroxyapatite and fluorapatite).

Precipitation of hydroxyapatite onto the exposed dentine surface can occlude dentine tubules, and it has been shown that calcium phosphate may occlude dentinal tubules without inhibiting the spontaneous remineralization of the tooth surface [10, 15]. Moreover, toothpaste formulations can also contain strontium, stannous, and calcium phosphate which can form physical barriers that may occlude the dentine tubules. These mechanisms occur by precipitating insoluble metal compounds on the dentine surface. Stannous chloride has also been reported to be effective in occluding dentine tubules although NovaMin® has been reported to be more effective than a strontium chloride and placebo toothpaste, particularly when exposed to citric acid and artificial saliva. [16] Stannous fluoride may also block the dentine tubules by forming SnF_2 and CaF_2. Additionally, strontium chloride has been reported to block the dentine tubules [6]. Tubule occlusion may, however, occur naturally through the normal remineralization processes by saliva and by dentine sclerosis through secondary dentine formation. Saliva also has a protective function against tooth wear. The biofilm layer has been reported to promote remineralization and reduce any mineral loss [14]. Therefore, using some of these dental products may help protect the dentine in order to enhance its resistance to both mechanical and chemical attack. One method of increasing the dentine surface resistance to wear by acid erosion and abrasion is to increase its mineral density; alternatively occluding the dentine tubules with a mineral substance, such as a calcium and phosphate toothpaste, would increase acid resistance of the dentine [13, 16].

1.2. Aim of the Project. The aim of the project, therefore, was to compare different bioactive glass formulations to investigate their effectiveness in the in vitro environment.

2. Materials and Methods

A 45S5 glass was synthesized in the laboratory together with several other glass formulations and subsequently formulated into five different toothpaste formulations (Section 2.4).

2.1. Preparation of Samples.
Caries-free extracted mandibular and maxillary molars were collected from the tooth bank with approval from the Queen Mary Research Ethics Committee QMREC 2011/99.

The teeth were cleaned with deionized water and stored in 70% ethanol. Each tooth was sliced into mid coronal sections by a diamond cut-off wheel machine. The teeth were embedded in an impression material to make blocks to stabilize them. The sections were required to be less than 1 mm thick; therefore, the machine was set to approximately 0.600 mm thickness. Subsequently, the dentine discs were polished using a carbide abrasive paper of P800, P2500, and P4000 consequently. A micrometre was used to measure the thickness after polishing, and it was established to be approximately 0.3 mm.

2.2. Glass Manufacture.
The 45S5 bioactive glass was manufactured in the laboratory within the University Department. The reagents including SiO_2 (45%), CaO (24.5%), P_2O_5 (6.0%), and Na_2O (24.5%) were mixed and placed in a crucible and melted at 1390°C for 1 hour in an electric furnace. The mixture was then quenched into cold water to prevent crystallization and ground in a Gyro Mill for two sets of 7 minutes. Finally, the particles were separated into two groups: (1) ≥38 microns and (2) ≤38 microns using a 38 μm sieve. The glass with a particle size ≤38 microns was used for further characterization.

2.3. Artificial Saliva and Toothpaste Application.
The artificial saliva was formulated using potassium chloride (2.236 g/L), potassium dihydrogen phosphate (1.361 g/L), sodium chloride (0.759 g/L), calcium chloride dihydrate (0.441 g/L), mucin (2.200 g), and sodium azide (0.2 g). These reagents were weighed in an electronic balance and dissolved in 8000 mL of deionized water; the pH was adjusted to 6.5 with KOH.

The paste was manufactured following the protocol by Mahmood et al. [12]. The components included glycerol, Carbopol (polyacrylic acid), PEG400 (polyethylene glycol), Syloid 63, synthetic amorphous silica, K acesulfame, titanium dioxide, and Na lauryl S (sodium dodecyl sulfate). The ingredients were weighed and mixed thoroughly in a plastic container. The pastes were divided into five portions with approximately 17 g each. Five batches of bioactive glass containing toothpastes (laboratory-manufactured 45S5, mixed glass, commercial BioMinF, CDL chloride glass, and amorphous chloride glass) were formulated by adding 1 g of bioactive glass into the paste and mixed thoroughly.

2.4. Experimental Design.
Five different types of bioactive glasses were investigated. The laboratory-manufactured 45S5, mixed glass containing fluoride and chloride, commercial BioMinF (BioMin Technologies Ltd., London, UK), chloride glass, and amorphous chloride glass (Table 1).

2.5. Scanning Electron Microscopy Study.
The discs were immersed in 6% citric acid for 30 seconds to remove the smear

TABLE 1: Five different types of bioactive glass formulations used for the study.

(1)	Laboratory-manufactured 45S5
(2)	Mixed glass containing fluoride and chloride
(3)	Commercially available BioMinF
(4)	Chloride glass
(5)	Amorphous chloride glass

TABLE 2: Test and control discs with the specific method of application of the toothpaste formulations.

Section 1	Control
Section 2	Brushed with toothpaste
Section 3	Brushed with toothpaste + artificial saliva
Section 4	Brushed with toothpaste + acid challenge

layer. The etched discs were then rinsed with deionized water and dried prior to the commencement of the experiment. For each glass-based toothpaste, one disc was cut into four halves. The first half was the control without brushing, and the other halves were brushed with a fixed amount of 50 mg toothpaste for 30 seconds. The second half was rinsed with deionized water, dried, and stored for SEM analysis. The third half was, subsequently to brushing, immersed in artificial saliva for 1 hour and then dried and stored for SEM. The fourth half was immersed in 6% citric acid for 2 minutes, rinsed with deionized water, dried, and stored for SEM (Table 2).

2.6. Quantification of Tubule Occlusion Based on SEM Observation.
The number of tubules was assumed to be constant between the control section of the etched dentine and the treated dentine section. This assumption was made because in many cases, the individual tubules were no longer visible after treatment. The number of tubules in each section of the control etched dentine varied between 56 and 72. However, for each sample, the control etched section was taken from the same mid coronal dentine slice and in close proximity to the etched dentine. Tubules were classified as fully open, partially occluded where particles were observed within the tubule or where materials were observed to have reduced the diameter significantly compared to the control section, or fully occluded. Since fully occluded tubules in many cases could not be observed, the number of fully occluded tubules was assumed to be the number of tubules in the control section minus the number of open tubules and partially occluded tubules. The results were converted to a percentage. Typically about 100 tubules were examined for each treatment representing a random statistical error of about 10%.

The dentine discs were mounted onto stubs with conducting carbon cement. Each part of the disc was mounted flat with the upper side exposed for brushing. The samples were subsequently sputter coated with gold/palladium for SEM analysis. The images were obtained from different fields of the disc at alternative magnifications such as 5000x and 10000x.

3. Results

It was evident from previous research in the department that the bioactive glasses have the capacity of occluding dentine

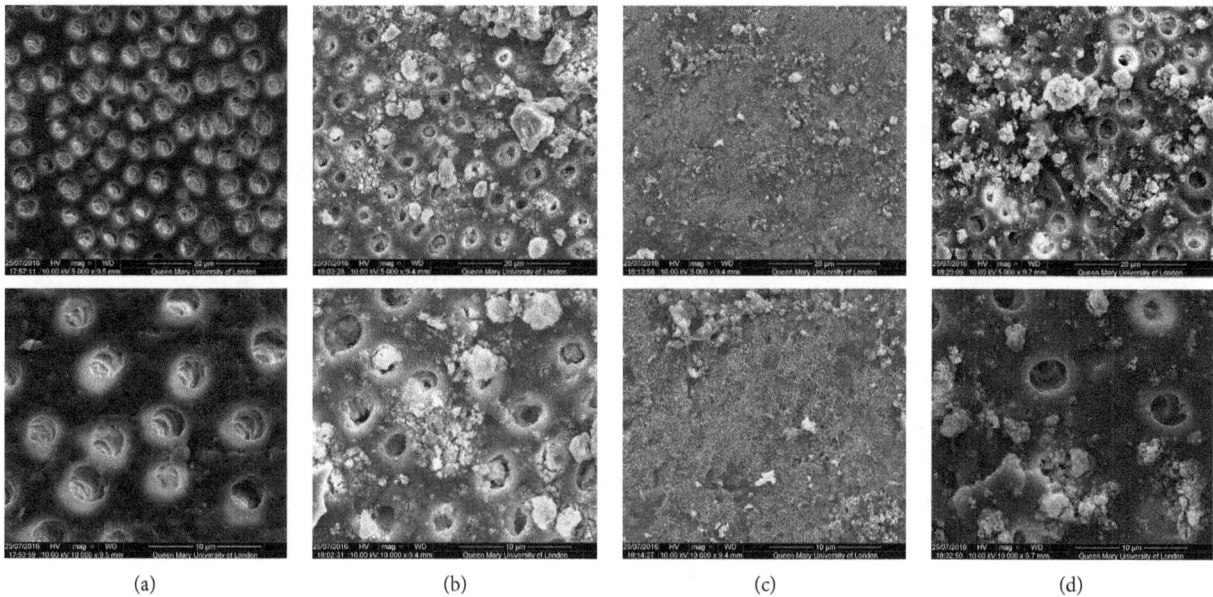

(a)	(b)	(c)	(d)

FIGURE 1: SEM images of the dentine surface morphology in disc 1 treated with a 45S5 glass-based toothpaste at 5000x (top) and 10000x (bottom) magnifications. (a) Control; (b) after brushing with a bioactive glass-based toothpaste; (c) after brushing with a bioactive glass-based toothpaste + artificial saliva immersion for 1 hour; (d) after brushing with a bioactive glass-based toothpaste + acid challenge with 6% citric acid.

tubules and as such may be an effective treatment for DH. In the present investigation, we used laboratory-made artificial saliva to mimic the in vivo environment following brushing of the discs. The results showed very good surface deposition with characteristic plate-like crystals or needle crystal-like formations in the various toothpaste samples. In the 45S5 sample, there was evidence that the Bioglass did not form apatite directly but may have formed a phase called octacalcium phosphate (OCP) which displays a plate-like morphology which may, then convert to a hydroxycarbonated apatite. The use of artificial saliva immersion following the toothpaste application was a useful addition to the methodology normally employed in in vitro studies in that it provided a similar environment to the oral cavity. For example, in the SEM images, there was clear evidence for hydroxyapatite formation with several hexagonal crystals observed following artificial saliva immersion. Apatite often has a hexagonal structure that can be recognized in the SEM images. Moreover, hydroxyapatite is a more stable crystal compared to other calcium phosphates, under physiological conditions. However, when exposed to an acid challenge, most of the hydroxyapatite layer formed with the artificial saliva dissolved although there was still a degree of tubule occlusion present.

SEM analysis of the test and control discs can be observed in the following figures (Figures 1–5); for example, an SEM image of a control etched dentine surface with visible open tubules can be observed in Figure 1. Please note that a residual smear layer deposit was present due to the samples not being cleaned ultrasonically before the commencement of the study in order to mimic real-life conditions.

The SEM images for the toothpaste containing 45S5 can be observed in Figure 1(a). In Figure 1(b), it may be noticed that, after brushing, some of the tubules were occluded by the particles. However, in Figure 1(c), when immersed in artificial saliva for 1 hour, all the tubules were occluded, as indicated by the clear formation of a layer covering the treated surface. This formation would lend some support to the fact that the effects of the product were improved when immersed in artificial saliva compared to when the discs were only brushed without immersion in saliva. After the acid challenge, in Figure 1(d), a significant part of that layer covering the tubules was removed, although it can be noted that some of the tubules were still occluded.

Figure 2(b) showed an improved coverage of the mixed glass product compared to 45S5. Nevertheless, the layer formed with the artificial saliva immersion was similar but with different formations of particles (Figure 2(c)). Following the acid challenge, as Figure 2(d) revealed, the layer was again rinsed away although some of the tubules remained occluded.

Figure 3(b) showed good coverage of the dentine surface with BioMinF. However, when immersed in artificial saliva, the layer formed was different to that formed with 45S5 and the mixed glass (Figure 3(c)). Particles of various sizes can be observed on the dentine surface and within the tubule lumen. Following the acid challenge, the results showed improvement compared to the other glasses. BioMinF was not totally washed away, and Figure 3(d) would suggest that almost the same amount of the dentine tubules maintained their occlusion (Figure 3(b)).

In Figure 4, the chloride glass sample showed basically the same coverage as with the other figures. This observation would suggest that although the layer covering the tubules was not formed with artificial saliva, the particles were not dissolved away with the acid challenge. Nevertheless, some of the tubules still remained open.

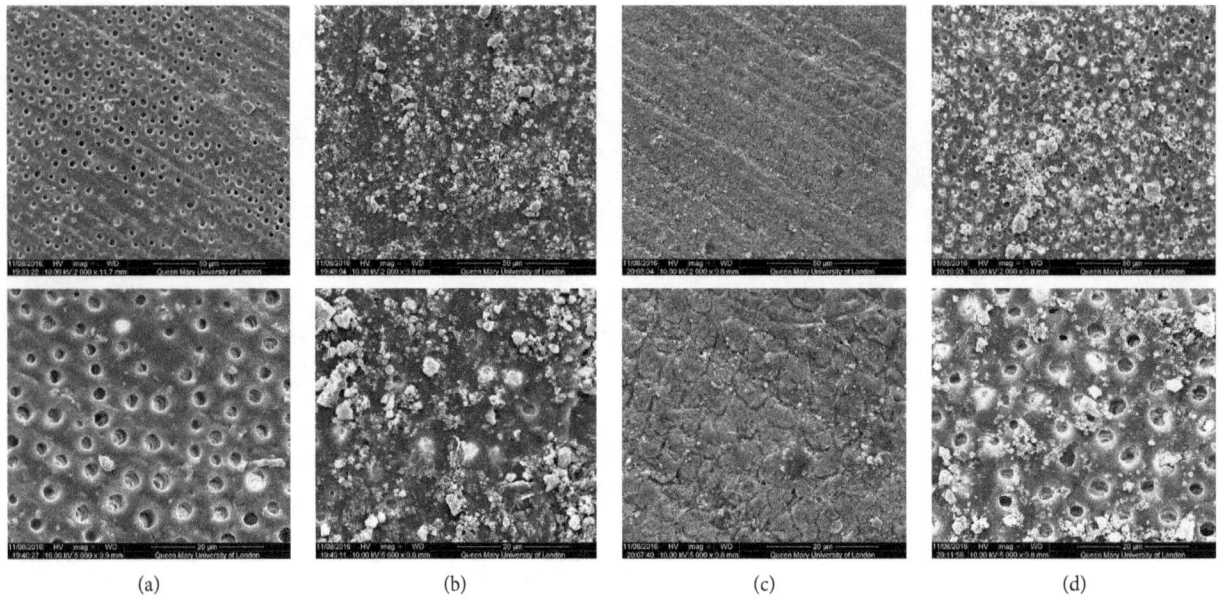

(a)   (b)   (c)   (d)

FIGURE 2: SEM images of the dentine surface morphology in disc 2 treated with a mixed glass-based toothpaste at 2000x (top) and 5000x (bottom) magnifications. (a) Control; (b) after brushing with a bioactive glass-based toothpaste; (c) after brushing with a bioactive glass-based toothpaste + artificial saliva immersion for 1 hour; (d) after brushing with a bioactive glass-based toothpaste + acid challenge with 6% citric acid.

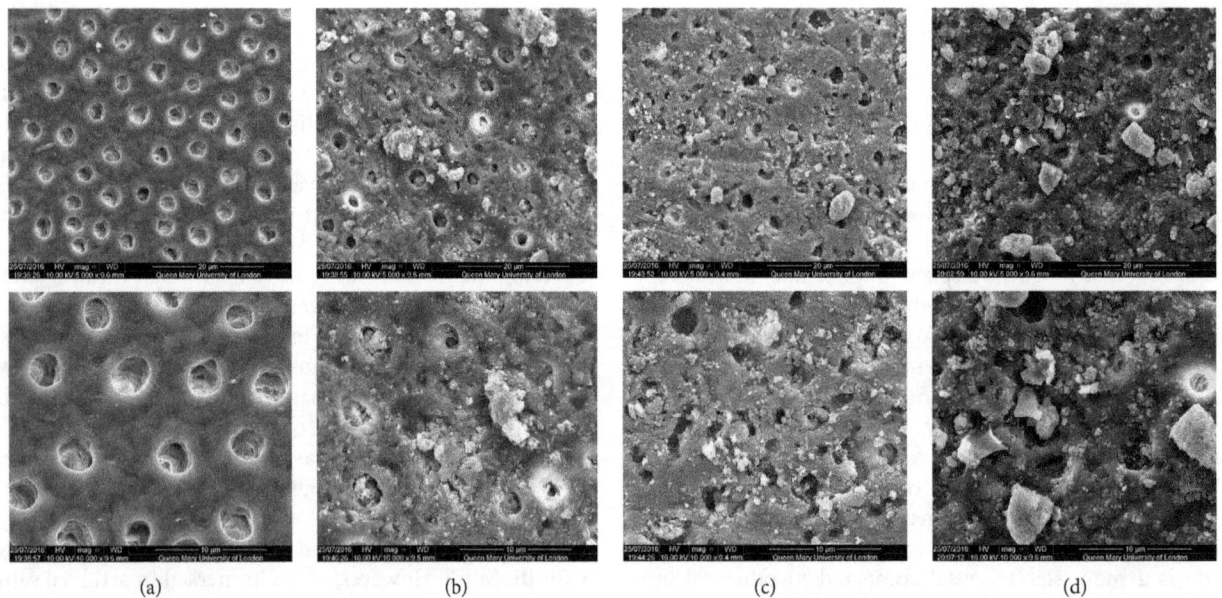

(a)   (b)   (c)   (d)

FIGURE 3: SEM images of the dentine surface morphology in disc 3 treated with a BioMinF glass-based toothpaste at 5000x (top) and 10000x (bottom) magnifications. (a) Control; (b) after brushing with a bioactive glass-based toothpaste; (c) after brushing with a bioactive glass-based toothpaste + artificial saliva immersion for 1 hour; (d) after brushing with a bioactive glass-based toothpaste + acid challenge with 6% citric acid.

Finally, Figure 5(b) showed an excellent surface coverage with the amorphous chloride glass-based toothpaste. Particles of various sizes occluded most of the tubules. In Figure 5(c), with artificial saliva immersion, the dentine surface appeared to be covered by the layer, and there were different formations covering the tubules. After an acid challenge, the results were also encouraging as many of the dentine tubules were still occluded, and although the surface layer was

dissolved away, there was evidence of tubular occlusion within the tubules (Figure 5(d)).

Figure 6 shows the percentages of open tubules, partially occluded tubules, and occluded tubules estimated from the SEM micrographs. It can be observed that all the toothpastes exhibited a significant increase in occlusion after brushing, with over >90% of all treatments resulting in complete and partially occluded tubules after brushing. Furthermore, the

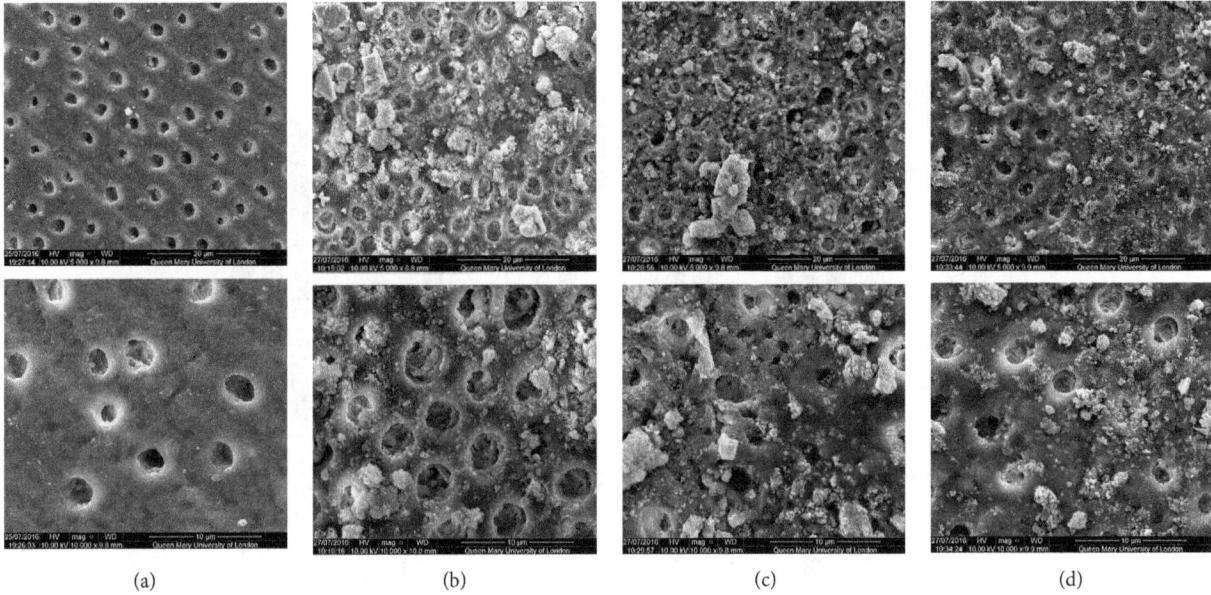

FIGURE 4: SEM images of the dentine surface morphology in disc 4 treated with a chloride glass-based toothpaste at 5000x (top) and 10000x (bottom) magnifications. (a) Control; (b) after brushing with a bioactive glass-based toothpaste; (c) after brushing with a bioactive glass-based toothpaste + artificial saliva immersion for 1 hour; (d) after brushing with a bioactive glass-based toothpaste + acid challenge with 6% citric acid.

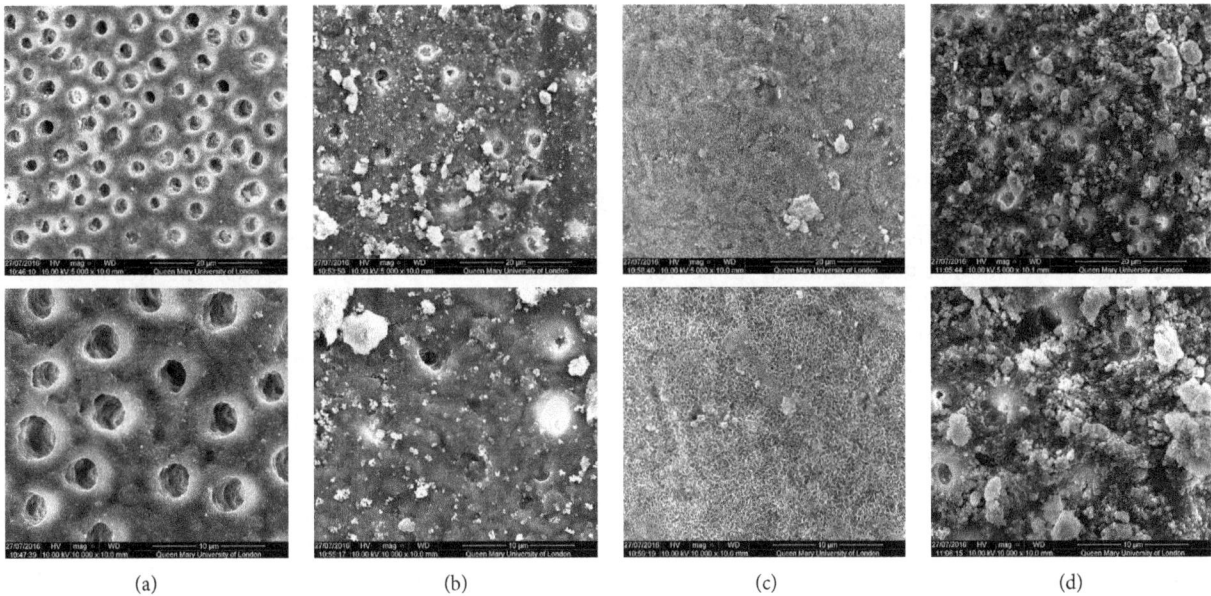

FIGURE 5: SEM images of the dentine surface morphology in disc 5 treated with an amorphous chloride glass-based toothpaste at 5000x (top) and 10000x (bottom) magnifications. (a) Control; (b) after brushing with a bioactive glass-based toothpaste; (c) after brushing with a bioactive glass-based toothpaste + artificial saliva immersion for 1 hour; (d) after brushing with a bioactive glass-based toothpaste + acid challenge with 6% citric acid.

tubule occlusion generally increased upon immersion in AS but generally declined after the acid challenge in citric acid. The exception here was the BioMinF which shows almost 100% tubule occlusion after the acid challenge.

When comparing the control images with those images following brushing with the bioactive glass-based toothpaste formulations, it may be concluded that all samples provided a degree of tubule occlusion following brushing with the respective toothpastes (Figures 1–5).

4. Discussion

It was evident from previous in vitro studies that bioactive glasses have the capacity for occluding dentine tubules and

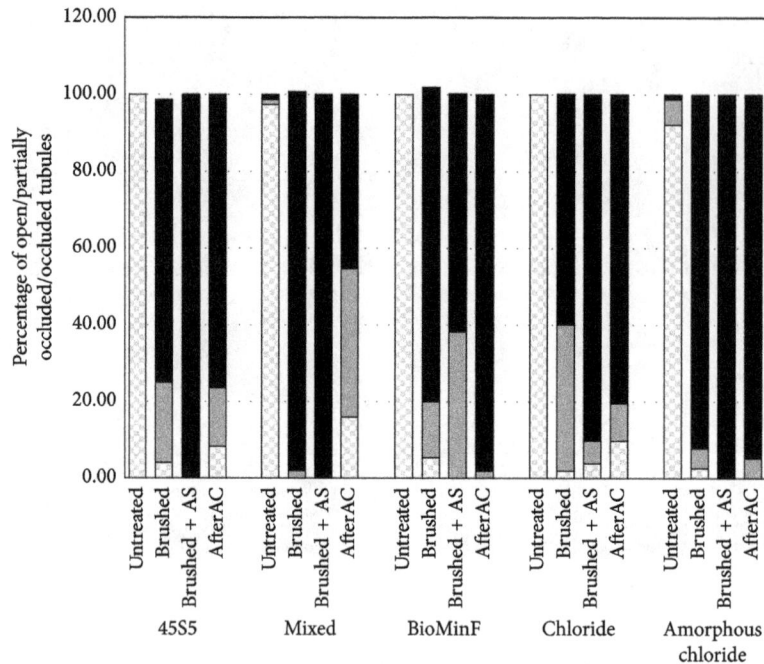

FIGURE 6: Percentage of open tubules (☐), partially occluded tubules (☐), and occluded tubules (■) present after different treatments.

as such incorporating these glasses into toothpaste formulations may be beneficial for those individuals who suffer from DH. In the present in vitro study, artificial saliva was formulated to simulate the in vivo environment following brushing the teeth. The results indicated that there was a good surface deposit with characteristic plate-like crystals and needle crystal formations in the different samples.

A study by Wang et al. [17] compared different types of bioactive glass-based toothpastes. Although these formulations were designed to deliver potassium ions to treat DH, the silica and calcium particles clearly occluded the tubules together with the smear layer produced by the application of the toothpaste. The SEM images of the toothpastes indicated that the toothpastes showed no resistance to an acid challenge, and the citric acid removed the particulate-coating layer from the tubule orifices. Furthermore, the precipitates formed were more resistant to an acid challenge when inside the dentine tubules. Another observation from this study which was of interest was that when a tooth was immersed in artificial saliva, there was an increase in fluid flow as measured in a hydraulic conductance model. This observation is somewhat contradictory as one would have expected a decrease in fluid flow following immersion.

In the 45S5 sample investigated in the present study, there was an indication that the Bioglass formulation does not form any apatite directly and may form an octacalcium phosphate (OCP) phase, which has a plate-like morphology. OCP is recognized to be a precursor for hydroxyapatite formation when the pH is ≤9 in the absence of fluoride. Moreover, the fluoride ions can either aid in the conversion of OCP to apatite or result in direct apatite formation. Therefore, OCP has an attractive potential for

remineralization since OCP can incorporate a source of fluoride for catalyzing the transformation of OCP to apatite and for the formation of a more acid-durable fluoridated apatite [18].

In a novel laboratory study [15], the investigators synthesized a varnish containing potassium chloride (KCl) and fluoridated hydroxyapatite (FHA). The SEM images obtained from this study indicated that the dentine tubules were occluded in the varnish FHA group. The KCl-FHA varnish could release potassium ions and reduce hydraulic conductance of the dentine discs and may therefore be a suitable option for the treatment of DH. FHA has the ability to occlude dentine tubules over time; however, the samples were not subjected to an acidic challenge or any other food and beverages that would have an impact in the clinical environment.

In the present study, the SEM images demonstrated evidence of hydroxyapatite formation as several hexagonal crystals were observed within the images following artificial saliva immersion. Apatite has a hexagonal structure that can be easily recognized. Moreover, hydroxyapatite is relatively stable when compared to many other calcium phosphates, under physiological conditions although it is not as stable as fluorapatite. When exposed to an acid challenge, most of the layer formed with the artificial saliva, which is thought to be hydroxyapatite, was dissolved, although there was still evidence of some tubule occlusion. The BioMinF treatment resulted in a layer consisting of fine highly elongated needle-like crystals in contrast to the more plate-like crystals or short stubby crystals formed with the fluoride-free toothpastes. Fluoride is known to promote the formation of fluorapatite, which generally forms as needle-like crystals and is much more acid durable. The BioMinF treatment resulted in the greatest tubule occlusion following the acid treatment, which probably reflects the formation of a more acid-resistant fluorapatite.

The needle-like formations, similar to those observed in the images, were also observed in both the chloride glass and amorphous chloride glass images. A study by Iijima et al. elucidated that the formation of needle-like structures after immersion in artificial saliva was enriched with both Ca and P, and as such the bioactive glass-coated alumina produced a crystal which may be calcium phosphate [19, 20].

Recent studies have made considerable progress in elucidating the effects of Bioglass particles on the tooth structure through the in vitro evaluation of different chemical composition(s) of Bioglass-containing toothpastes [21]. For example, several studies have reported different outcomes when evaluating chloride-containing toothpastes. Several in vitro studies have demonstrated that a small crystalline deposit was precipitated onto the dentine surface which can easily be rinsed away; however, other studies have reported positive effects of the chloride-containing products on the relief of DH [15, 22].

When comparing chlorine and fluoride toothpaste formulations, there were conflicting results reported in the published literature with several clinical studies indicating that there were no differences in efficacy between the two products and other studies indicating that there were differences in favour of chloride-containing toothpastes. This observation was also true when comparing in vitro studies alone as well as comparative studies using cross sections of dentine where no tubular occlusion was observed following treatment with an SnF_2-containing toothpaste [23].

A study published in 2013 [24] aimed at comparing the effectiveness of a one-minute application with a polishing prophylaxis paste containing 15% calcium sodium phosphosilicate with and without fluoride compared to a fluoride polishing control in reducing post-therapy DH following a dental scaling and root planning procedure. DH was assessed by both tactile and air blast stimuli at baseline, immediately following polishing and 28 days after the single application (subjects were provided with a non desensitizing toothpaste for the duration of the study). The results showed a significant reduction of sensitivity after 28 days of treatment for both groups with or without fluoride which would suggest that any improvement in DH was independent of the presence of fluoride (note that there are many confounding factors in running DH studies which could affect the results in this type of study) [25].

A further in vitro study [8] reported that the toothpaste formulations with different proportions of Bioglass replacing the silica compounds (2.5% and 7.5%) provided a greater surface coverage than the original Bioglass product. However, the study did not assess the composition of the particles deposited on the dentine surface or within the dentine tubules. Furthermore, there was no reported determination on whether the deposit was an abrasive component, for example, silica, or whether the deposit consisted of Bioglass particles or a precipitation of calcium phosphate following ion exchange on the surface of Bioglass.

Although the in vitro effectiveness of potassium-containing toothpastes was not the focus of the present study, a brief comparison of the effectiveness of products that occlude the dentine tubules (tubular occlusion) compared to the effect of potassium-containing toothpaste that claimed to work by blocking a pulp nerve response is worthy of some comment. For example, Acharya et al. compared the efficacy of toothpastes containing calcium sodium phosphosilicate and potassium nitrate and reported that calcium sodium phosphosilicate had a greater reduction in DH than potassium nitrate [11]. Moreover, this systematic review presented an overview on clinical trials of calcium sodium phosphosilicate (CSPS) to treat DH. CSPS was reported to provide superior results in reducing DH compared to potassium nitrate-containing toothpastes. Investigators have also suggested that when in contact with body fluids, CSPS reacts forming a layer of hydroxyapatite that can occlude dentine tubules. The results with CSPS were also reported to be more effective than the negative controls [26].

It is recognized, however, that the quantification of the number of occluded tubules is somewhat subjective, and perhaps, the limitation in the present study was the lack of fracture specimens to view the depth of penetration into the tubules. Nevertheless, the semi-quantification method used in the study does the support the observations from the SEMs that there was a degree of tubular occlusion which varied between the experimental toothpastes. Furthermore, evidence from an unpublished report that included this study indicated that the hydraulic conductance values of the BioMinF toothpaste supported the SEM observations indicating that the dentinal tubules were occluded [27].

One final review that may be relevant in this discussion on the effectiveness of CSPS is a systematic review by Talioti et al. [28]. These investigators compared the evidence of OTC desensitizing products (e.g., calcium sodium phosphosilicate, amorphous calcium phosphate, nanohydroxyapatite, and tooth mousse toothpaste/gels) in reducing DH. One of the problems reported by these investigators was that there was a lack of published studies directly comparing these four products. Furthermore, although there was evidence for the effectiveness of CSPS in occluding the dentine tubules from the in vitro studies, no conclusion could be made regarding the clinical efficacy of the various desensitizing toothpastes compared in the review. This was due in part to the different study designs and methodologies used in the various studies and the fact that there were relatively few randomized controlled trials (RCTs) available for analysis [28]. The systematic review and meta-analysis by Zhu et al. [26] also recognized the limitations of the published studies evaluating CSPS formulations in both toothpastes for DH and in prophylaxis polishing pastes for post periodontal therapy hypersensitivity. These investigators recommended that further non Industry (independent) supported clinical studies should be conducted prior to making any definitive recommendations regarding the efficacy of these formulations.

5. Conclusions

Of the various compositions of bioactive glasses assessed in the present in vitro study, all glass compositions demonstrated surface coverage after brushing with the formulated toothpaste. The formation of a hydroxyapatite layer occluding the dentine tubules following artificial saliva immersion may be considered an important stepping stone for further evaluation of these bioactive glass compositions. One of the innovative features of the study was the incorporation of an acid challenge to mimic the oral environment. Although the glass formulations, in particular Biomin, were resistant to an acid challenge, there was no doubt that further research was required to identify a different formulation or component that was not removed when immersed in a citric acid solution. In conclusion, the results from the present in vitro study would appear to support the growing evidence in the published literature that toothpaste formulations containing bioactive glasses occlude dentine tubules and therefore may be an effective approach treating DH.

Disclosure

Luiza Pereira Dias da Cruz is currently at the Departamento de Odontologia Social e Preventiva, Faculdade de Odontologia, Universidade Federal do Rio de Janeiro, Rio de Janeiro, RJ, Brazil.

References

[1] D. G. Gillam, "Management of dentin hypersensitivity," *Current Oral Health Reports*, vol. 2, no. 2, pp. 87–94, 2015.

[2] J. C. Pereira, S. H. Sales-Peres, L. F. Fran. sconi-dos-Rios et al., "Current and novel clinical approaches for the treatment of dentin hypersensitivity," in *Dentine Hypersensitivity*, D. Gillam, Ed., Springer, Cham, Switzerland, 2015.

[3] M. Brännström, "A hydrodynamic mechanism in the transmission of pain producing stimuli through the dentine," in *Sensory Mechanisms in Dentine*, D. J. Anderson, Ed., pp. 73–79, Pergamon Press, Oxford, UK, 1963.

[4] L. I. Grossman, "A systematic method for the treatment of hypersensitive dentine," *Journal of the American Dental Association*, vol. 22, no. 4, pp. 592–602, 1935.

[5] S. Miglani, V. Aggarwal, and B. Ahuja, "Dentin hypersensitivity: recent trends in management," *Journal of Conservative Dentistry*, vol. 13, no. 4, p. 218, 2010.

[6] I. Maldupa, A. Brinkmane, I. Rendeniece, and A. Mihailova, "Evidence based toothpaste classification, according to certain characteristics of their chemical composition," *Stomatologija*, vol. 14, no. 1, pp. 12–22, 2012.

[7] L. Hench, "The story of Bioglass®," *Journal of Materials Science: Materials in Medicine*, vol. 17, no. 11, pp. 967–978, 2006.

[8] D. Gillam, J. Tang, N. Mordan, and H. Newman, "The effects of a novel BioGlass dentifrice on dentine sensitivity: a scanning electron microscopy investigation," *Journal of Oral Rehabilitation*, vol. 29, no. 4, pp. 305–313, 2002.

[9] M. Khoroushi and F. Keshani, "A review of glass-ionomers: from conventional glass-ionomer to bioactive glass-ionomer," *Dental Research Journal*, vol. 10, no. 4, pp. 411–420, 2013.

[10] H. Davis, F. Gwinner, J. C. Mitchell, and J. L. Ferracane, "Ion release from, and fluoride recharge of a composite with a fluoride-containing bioactive glass," *Dental Materials* vol. 30, no. 10, pp. 1187–1194, 2014.

[11] A. Acharya, S. Surve, and S. Thakur, "A clinical study of the effect of calcium sodium phosphosilicate on dentin hypersensitivity," *Journal of Clinical and Experimental Dentistry* vol. 5, no. 1, pp. e18–e22, 2013.

[12] A. Mahmood, M. Mneimne, L. Zou, R. Hill, and D. Gillam, "Abrasive wear of enamel by bioactive glass-based toothpastes," *American Journal of Dentistry*, vol. 27, no. 5, 2014.

[13] K. Markowitz and D. Pashely, "Discovering new treatments for sensitive teeth: the long path from biology to therapy," *Journal of Oral Rehabilitation*, vol. 35, no. 4, pp. 300–315, 2008.

[14] L. Petersson, "The role of fluoride in the preventive management of dentin hypersensitivity and root caries," *Clinical Oral Investigations*, vol. 17, no. 1, pp. 63–71, 2012.

[15] Y. Lochaiwatana, S. Poolthong, I. Hirata, M. Okazaki, S. Swasdison, and N. Vongsavan, "The synthesis and characterization of a novel potassium chloride-fluoridated hydroxyapatite varnish for treating dentin hypersensitivity," *Dental Materials Journal*, vol. 34, no. 1, pp. 31–40, 2015.

[16] V. P. Pillai and P. Neelakantan, "Desensitizing toothpastes for treatment of dentin hypersensitivity," *International Journal of PharmTech Research*, vol. 5, no. 4, pp. 1769–1773, 2013.

[17] Z. Wang, Y. Sa, S. Sauro et al., "Effect of desensitising toothpastes on dentinal tubule occlusion: a dentine permeability measurement and SEM in vitro study," *Journal of Dentistry*, vol. 38, no. 5, pp. 400–410, 2010.

[18] R. Hill and D. G. Gillam, "Future strategies for the development of desensitising products," in *Dentine Hypersensitivity*, D. Gillam, Ed., Springer, Cham, Switzerland, 2015.

[19] M. Iijima, M. Hashimoto, N. Kohda et al., "Crystal growth on bioactive glass sputter-coated alumina in artificial saliva," *Dental Materials Journal*, vol. 32, no. 5, pp. 775–780, 2013.

[20] I. Farooq, I. Moheet, and E. AlShwaimi, "In vitro dentin tubule occlusion and remineralization competence of various toothpastes," *Archives of Oral Biology*, vol. 60, no. 9, pp. 1246–1253, 2015.

[21] A. F. Paes Leme, J. C. dos Santos, M. Giannini, and R. S. Wada, "Occlusion of dentin tubules by desensitizing agents," *American Journal of Dentistry*, vol. 17, no. 5, pp. 368–372, 2004.

[22] Z. Wang, T. Jiang, S. Sauro et al., "The dentine remineralization activity of a desensitizing bioactive glass-containing toothpaste: an in vitro study," *Australian Dental Journal*, vol. 56, no. 4, pp. 372–381, 2011.

[23] W. Arnold, M. Prange, and E. Naumova, "Effectiveness of various toothpastes on dentine tubule occlusion," *Journal of Dentistry*, vol. 43, no. 4, pp. 440–449, 2015.

[24] K. Neuhaus, J. Milleman, K. Milleman et al., "Effectiveness of a calcium sodium phosphosilicate containing prophylaxis paste in reducing dentine hypersensitivity immediately and 4 weeks after a single application: a double-blind randomized controlled trial," *Journal of Clinical Periodontology*, vol. 40, no. 4, pp. 349–357, 2013.

[25] F. A. Curro and D. G. Gillam, "Challenging the traditional approach for the conduct of dentine hypersensitivity studies: person-centric studies connecting the patient with their practitioner to optimise the clinical outcome," in *Dentine Hypersensitivity*, D. Gillam, Ed., Springer, Cham, Switzerland, 2015.

[26] M. Zhu, J. Li, B. Chen et al., "The effect of calcium sodium phosphosilicate on dentin hypersensitivity: a systematic review and meta-analysis," *PLoS One*, vol. 10, no. 11, article e0140176, 2015.

[27] L. P. D. da Cruz, *Unpublished Data: Dentine Tubule Occlusion by Novel Bioactive Glass Based Toothpastes, in Research Report for Science without Borders*, August 2016.

[28] E. Talioti, R. Hill, and D. G. Gillam, "The efficacy of selected desensitizing OTC products: a systematic review," *ISRN Dentistry*, vol. 2014, Article ID 865761, 14 pages, 2014.

10

Clinical Anxiety among Saudi Postgraduate Pediatric Dentistry Students in Jeddah City

Manal Almalik,[1] **Abeer Alnowaiser,**[2] **Omar El Meligy** ⓘ**,**[2,3] **Jamal Sallam,**[4] **and Yusra Balkheyour**[5]

[1]*Dental Department, King Fahd Armed Forces Hospital, Jeddah, Saudi Arabia*
[2]*Pediatric Dentistry Department, Faculty of Dentistry, King Abdulaziz University, Jeddah, Saudi Arabia*
[3]*Pediatric Dentistry and Dental Public Health Department, Faculty of Dentistry, Alexandria University, Alexandria, Egypt*
[4]*Ministry of Health, Jeddah, Saudi Arabia*
[5]*King Abdulaziz University, Jeddah, Saudi Arabia*

Correspondence should be addressed to Omar El Meligy; omeligy@kau.edu.sa

Academic Editor: Izzet Yavuz

Objective. To determine anxiety in relation to gender, Grade Point Average (GPA), level of education and academic and clinical situations in Jeddah, Saudi Arabia. Also, to identify academic and clinical anxiety levels among postgraduate pediatric dentistry students. *Methods.* A cross-sectional study at governmental training hospitals was conducted. All registered postgraduate students in pediatric dental programs during the year 2015-2016 were included in the study. A self-administered questionnaire was distributed electronically to 60 postgraduate pediatric dentistry students aged between 25 and 45 years old. The questionnaire is composed of 55 questions that investigated demographic data, academic and clinical related situations including investigations, diagnosis, treatment, and complications in treatment. *Results.* The study showed a higher anxiety level in younger age dental students (76.7% compared to 23.3%) and Saudi board residents (60%). Comparing gender differences in anxiety revealed that a significant difference (P 0.05) was found and anxiety seems to be more among female dental students (2% very anxious, 64% slightly anxious, and 34% not anxious) as compared to male dental students (8% very anxious, 69% slightly anxious, and 23% not anxious). *Conclusions.* There was increased awareness, detailed understanding, and handling of the patients by senior postgraduate pediatric dentistry students compared to junior students.

1. Introduction

Anxiety is a psychological and physiological state composed of feeling of worry, nervousness, or unease about something with an uncertain outcome [1].

Anxiety is potentially problematic for both patients and dentists. The origins of dentist anxiety in the dental clinic have a complex and multifactorial psychological and physiological etiology. Among dental students and practitioners, multiple researches were conducted to study the level of anxiety, stress, and their contributing factors [2–4].

The physical symptoms of anxiety may include one or more of the following: feelings of apprehension, trouble concentrating, anticipating the worst, irritability, restlessness, shortness of breath, heart palpitations, dry mouth, nausea, muscle tension, and cold or sweaty hands and feet as well as of numbness or tingling in the hands or feet. On the other hand, the psychological symptoms may also include one or more of the following: problems with concentration, difficulty with staying on task, memory difficulties, depressive symptoms like hopelessness, lethargy, and poor appetite, as well as becoming overly attached to a safety object or person, and finally avoiding crowded places [5–7].

An interesting finding in a cross-sectional study in 2009 by Al-Omari WM and Al-Omiri MK in Jordan on 600 medical, dental, and engineering undergraduate students showed that dental students had the lowest percentage of anxiety [8].

Another study was carried out in 2010 on 815 medical students in Nishtar Medical College and concluded that anxiety and depression were decreased with increasing student's age and with high anxiety levels in female students as compared to male students [9].

Furthermore, a study in 2011 in Plovdiv University, Bulgaria, revealed that dental students have a significantly higher level of dental anxiety at the beginning of their training than at its end [10].

Regarding postgraduate students, a study done in India on 50 postgraduate medical students showed that several factors such as age and type of the course contributed to raise the amount of stress and anxiety among these students [11].

Several studies were carried out to determine the anxiety provoking situations in medical and dental students [12–14]. To our knowledge, there were very few studies available that have investigated the association of anxiety among postgraduate pediatric dentistry students.

The objectives of this study were to determine anxiety in relation to gender, Grade Point Average (GPA), level of education and academic and clinical situations in the city of Jeddah, Saudi Arabia, and also to identify academic and clinical anxiety levels among postgraduate pediatric dentistry students.

2. Methods

This cross-sectional study was performed at governmental training hospitals in Jeddah, Kingdom of Saudi Arabia, and data were collected during the year 2015-2016.

Sixty postgraduate pediatric dentistry students (13 males and 47 females) aged between 25 and 45 years old, working in Saudi governmental training hospitals in Jeddah city, were included in the study. Thirty-six were Saudi board residents, 18 were master degree (MSc) students, and 6 were PhD students.

A structured questionnaire was used to gather the participants' data. The questionnaire was reviewed by three experts to ensure that the items were useful; there were agreements between the parts of the questionnaire, and the questions were relevant to the study. The experts rated each question, and their scores were analyzed to calculate the questionnaire's validity.

The self-administered questionnaire was distributed electronically to 60 postgraduate pediatric dentistry students. The questionnaire is composed of fifty-five questions that investigated demographic data, academic, and clinical-related situations including investigations, diagnosis, treatment, and complications in treatment.

Sixty respondents have completed the questionnaire successfully. Uncompleted questionnaires were excluded from the study.

2.1. Reliability Test. To determine the questionnaire reliability (intraexaminer), a test was done by distributing the questionnaire to 20 postgraduate pediatric dentistry students working at Saudi governmental hospitals. After 2 weeks, a retest was done by distributing the same questionnaire to the same 20 postgraduate pediatric dentistry students and comparing their responses (test-retest reliability).

2.2. Statistical Analysis. Data were fed to the computer using IBM Statistical Package for the Social Sciences (SPSS) software (version 20.0, SPSS Inc., Chicago, IL). The 0.05 level was used to indicate statistical significance.

2.3. Ethical Considerations. This study proposal has been approved by the Saudi governmental training hospitals, Jeddah, Saudi Arabia, and has therefore been performed in accordance with the ethical standards laid down in the 1964 Declaration of Helsinki and its later amendments (proposal number 096-01-17).

3. Results

Intraexaminer reliability was determined and was 0.95, representing excellent agreement. The overall response rate was 100%. All the 60 (13 males (21.7%) and 47 females (78.3%)) respondents have successfully completed the questionnaire. All the participants were postgraduate pediatric dentistry students aged between 25 and 45 years old. The study showed a higher anxiety level in younger age dental students (76.7% compared to 23.3%), females more than males (78.3% compared to 21.7%). For GPA, 3.3% of the respondents graduated with a GPA of 2.5–3; 76.6% graduated with a GPA of 3.1–4.4, while 20.1% had a GPA of 4.5–5. Regarding current study, 60% (36) of our respondents were Saudi board residents, 30% (18) were MSc students, and 10% (6) were PhD students. Seventeen (28.3%) students were first-year postgraduate dental students, 18 (30%) were second year, and 15 (25%) were third year, while 10 (16.7%) were final-year dental students (Table 1).

The level of clinical diagnosis, investigations, and treatment of the patients with respect to the postgraduate level and gender was the highest anxiety provoking situations for both male and female dental students. The senior postgraduate students in their final year were more likely to be anxious during clinical diagnosis and investigations than the first-year (junior) postgraduate students. There was a statistically significant difference ($P \leq 0.05$) between first-year and final-year students for the following questions: unable to diagnose patients, misdiagnosing patients, unable to answer the parents' questions as well as taking history and conducting patient examination, poor radiographic interpretation, prescribing medications and writing prescriptions, writing referral forms, referring patients for GA, or conscious sedation when needed (Figures 1 and 2).

Comparing gender differences in anxiety revealed that a significant difference ($P \leq 0.05$) was found, and anxiety seems to be more among female dental students (2% very anxious, 64% slightly anxious, and 34% not anxious) as compared to male dental students (8% very anxious, 69% slightly anxious, and 23% not anxious) (Figure 3).

Regarding the level of anxiety during academic situations, 23% were anxious regarding deadline for clinical case submission, 23% were anxious regarding studying for their exams, 23% were anxious regarding clinical case presentation, 16% were anxious regarding failure to interact with the child, 4% were anxious regarding application of

TABLE 1: The sociodemographic information of the participants.

Demographic data		Number (N)	Marginal percentage
Age (years)	25–35	46	76.7
	36–45	14	23.3
Grade Point Average (GPA)	2.5–3	2	3.3
	3.1–4.4	46	76.6
	4.5–5	12	20.1
Gender	Male	13	21.7
	Female	47	78.3
Postgraduate pediatric dentistry students	Saudi board	36	60
	MSc	18	30
	PhD	6	10
Current postgraduate year	1	17	28.3
	2	18	30
	3	15	25
	4	10	16.7
Total		60	100

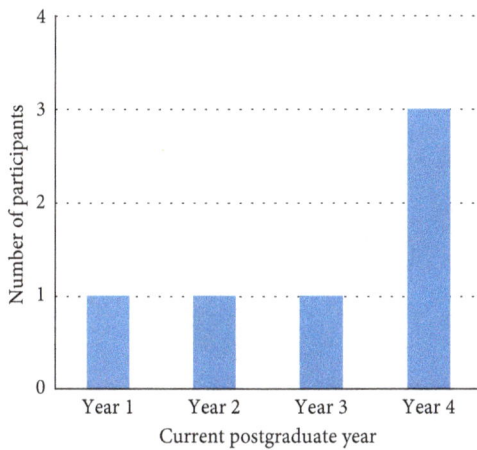

FIGURE 1: Level of anxiety during clinical investigations with respect to postgraduate current year.

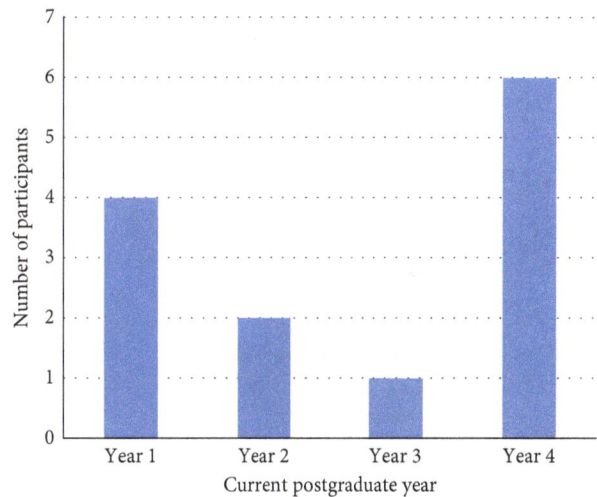

FIGURE 2: Level of anxiety during clinical diagnosis with respect to postgraduate current year.

behavior management methods with the child, 2% were anxious regarding communicating with parents, and 9% were anxious regarding communicating with other practitioners for consultation (Figure 4).

Concerning the level of anxiety during clinical complications, 7% were anxious regarding fracturing a tooth, 8% were anxious regarding extracting the wrong tooth, 9% were anxious being unsatisfied with fitting of space maintainers, 8% were anxious regarding iatrogenic gingival trauma, 8% were anxious regarding accidental pulp exposure, 10% were anxious regarding tooth perforation in bifurcation area, 10% were anxious regarding accidentally injuring the patient, 10% were anxious regarding getting infected by the patient, 10% were anxious regarding poor quality of restorations, 11% were anxious regarding patients got into deep sleep and being unable to wake them up during sedation, and 9% were anxious regarding failure to remove fractured roots (Figure 5).

With respect to the level of anxiety during various clinical treatments, 9% were anxious when treating a very

young child, 10% were anxious when treating psychiatric child, 9% were anxious when treating medically compromised patients, 10% were anxious when treating children with special health care needs, 9% were anxious when coping with uncooperative children, 11% were anxious when coping with difficult parents, 4% were anxious when administering local anesthesia, 2% were anxious during extraction of a tooth or a remaining root, 2% were anxious when controlling postoperative bleeding, 14% were anxious in dealing with emergency situations, 8% were anxious when treating patients under conscious sedation, 6% were anxious when treating patient under general anesthesia (GA), and 6% were anxious using restraints (Figure 6).

4. Discussion

Several studies were carried out to determine the anxiety provoking situations in medical and dental undergraduate

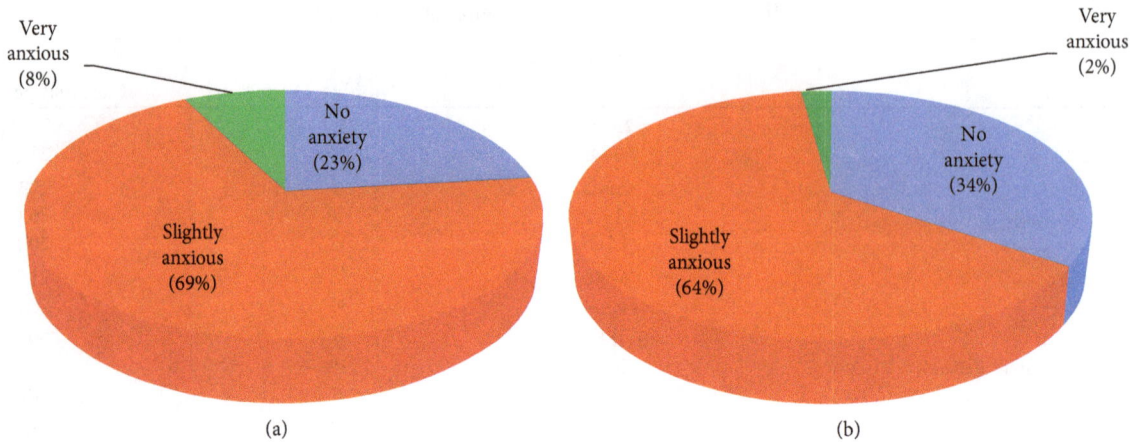

FIGURE 3: Level of total anxiety in relation to gender. (a) Percentage of total anxiety within males. (b) Percentage of total anxiety within females.

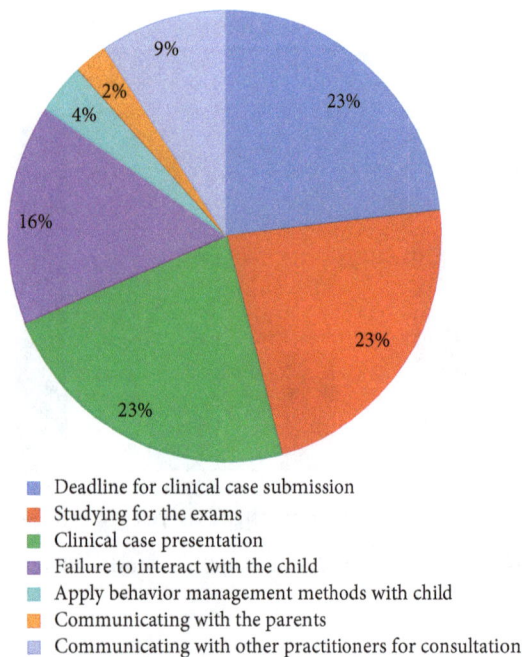

FIGURE 4: Level of anxiety during academic situations.

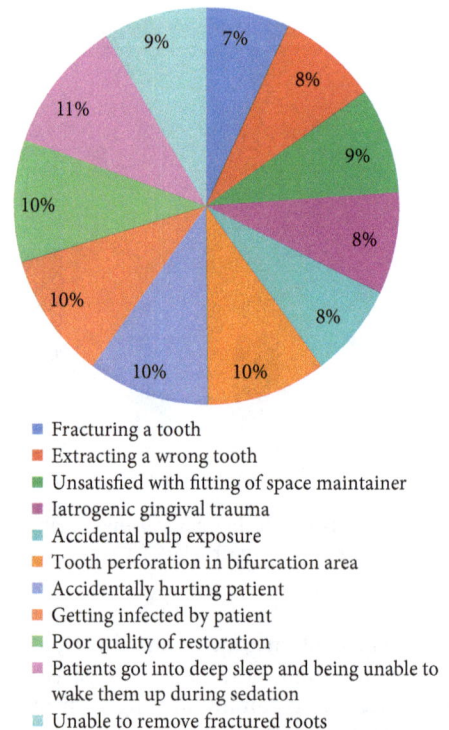

FIGURE 5: Level of anxiety during clinical complications.

students. Limited information is available about the association of anxiety among postgraduate pediatric dentistry students. The present study aimed to determine anxiety in relation to gender, GPA, and level of education and academic and clinical situations in the city of Jeddah, Saudi Arabia, and also to identify academic and clinical anxiety levels among postgraduate pediatric dentistry students.

The present study showed a higher anxiety level in younger age dental students (76.7% compared to 23.3%). This is in agreement with a study by Storjord et al. [13], who reported that dental anxiety was less in experienced dental students than new dental students. This strongly suggests that the dental program structure in universities may affect dental anxiety levels.

An explanation for variances in dental anxiety could be that the dental students in the first year are more susceptible to stress and anxiety because they are in an unacquainted study environment. Students just starting their studies can experience more stress due to the challenge of transitioning from high school to university, and a study from the United States showed that seniors and juniors have lower stress reactions than sophomores and freshmen [15]. The decrease in stress due to settling into university life might, therefore, be a generic process leading to lessening of particular anxiety (e.g., dental anxiety). Another explanation is that usually in later years of courses low failure rates make students less stressed and more self-confident [16].

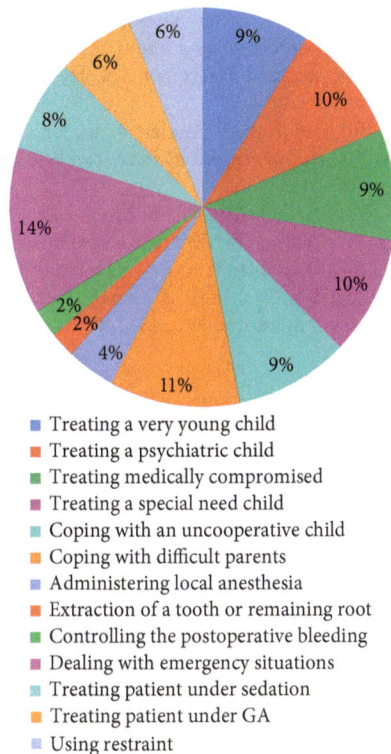

FIGURE 6: Level of anxiety during various clinical treatments.

- Treating a very young child
- Treating a psychiatric child
- Treating medically compromised
- Treating a special need child
- Coping with an uncooperative child
- Coping with difficult parents
- Administering local anesthesia
- Extraction of a tooth or remaining root
- Controlling the postoperative bleeding
- Dealing with emergency situations
- Treating patient under sedation
- Treating patient under GA
- Using restraint

Our study showed a higher anxiety level in females more than males (78.3% compared to 21.7%). In accordance with other studies, female students had reported higher scores of depression, anxiety, and stress compared with their male counterparts [17, 18]. This may be due to the fact that women articulate depressive symptoms, even minor ones, more easily [19]. Also, this dissimilarity may be described by women being better able to show their feelings of fear. Furthermore, physiological conditions such as fear, stress, depression, panic, and social phobia are more prevalent in females, and dental anxiety may be related with such feelings [20].

The current study showed an interesting finding, as senior postgraduate students in their final year were more likely to be anxious during clinical diagnosis and investigations than the first-year (junior) postgraduate students. Anxiety that have been reported during the final year may be due to nonsupportive and extremely perplexing environments as compared to the first year. This is in agreement with a study by Kulsoom and Afsar [21], who reported high stress and anxiety among first-year scholars, which climaxed in the fourth year, where the clerkship phase starts and students rotate through various disciplines of hospital as their chief training method. Also, they observed that the highest anxiety and depression results were reported in the fourth year.

Our study is in accordance with that of Alpert and Haber [22], where the level of anxiety during academic situations was the highest (23%) regarding deadline for clinical case submission, studying for their exams and clinical case presentation, while only 2% were anxious regarding communicating with parents.

Concerning the level of anxiety during clinical complications, the highest (11%) were anxious regarding patients got into deep sleep and being unable to wake them up during sedation, while the lowest (7%) were anxious regarding fracturing a tooth. This is in agreement with a study by Basudan et al. [14], who reported high occurrence of stress, anxiety, and depression among dental students.

Regarding the level of anxiety during various clinical treatments, the highest (14%) were anxious in dealing with emergency situations; however, 2% were anxious during extraction of a tooth or a remaining root and when controlling postoperative bleeding. This agrees with Ali et al. [23] who concluded that higher anxiety levels were reported by clinical and preclinical students during various clinical procedures.

Our results can point out that the dentistry program structure can be a major cause in decreasing dental anxiety.

The present study has several limitations. First, this study was a cross-sectional observational study using postgraduate pediatric dentistry students from only governmental training hospitals in Jeddah city, which means that findings may indicate institutional characteristics not representative of postgraduate pediatric dentistry students elsewhere in Saudi Arabia. Second, although all postgraduate pediatric dentistry students in governmental training hospitals in Jeddah city were included in this study, still the sample size is considered small to show significant differences in many areas in the study. Third limitation of this study was the lack of funding for the research project.

5. Conclusions

The study assists to understand the topic of anxiety among postgraduate dentists. There was increased awareness, detailed understanding, and handling of the patients by senior postgraduate pediatric dentistry students compared to junior students. The high anxiety levels seen in dental students indicate the need to provide support programs and to include stress management courses in their training programs.

6. Recommendations

Future research to further understand the topic of anxiety among postgraduate dentists is needed.

References

[1] T. Newton, K. Asimakopoulou, B. Daly, S. Scambler, and S. Scott, "The management of dental anxiety: time for a sense of proportion," *British Dental Journal*, vol. 213, no. 6, pp. 271–274, 2012.

[2] D. P. Appukuttan, "Strategies to manage patients with dental anxiety and dental phobia: literature review," *Clinical, Cosmetic and Investigation Dentistry*, vol. 8, pp. 35–50, 2016.

[3] V. B. Waghachavare, G. B. Dhumale, Y. R. Kadam, and A. D. Gore, "A study of stress among students of professional

colleges from an urban area in India," *Sultan Qaboos University Medical Journal*, vol. 13, no. 3, pp. 429–436, 2013.

[4] S. Gunjal, D. G. Pateel, and S. Parkar, "Dental anxiety among medical and paramedical undergraduate students of Malaysia," *International Journal of Dentistry*, vol. 2017, Article ID 4762576, 5 pages, 2017.

[5] R. E. Rada and C. Johnson-Leong, "Stress, burnout, anxiety and depression among dentists," *Journal of American Dental Association*, vol. 135, no. 6, pp. 788–794, 2004.

[6] L. N. Dyrbye, M. R. Thomas, and T. D. Shanafelt, "Systematic review of depression, anxiety, and other indicators of psychological distress among U.S. and Canadian medical students," *Academia Medicine*, vol. 81, no. 4, pp. 354–373, 2006.

[7] P. Singh, D. S. Aulak, S. S. Mangat, and M. S. Aulak, "Systematic review: factors contributing to burnout in dentistry," *Occupational Medicine*, vol. 66, no. 1, pp. 27–31, 2016.

[8] W. M. Al-Omari and M. K. Al-Omiri, "Dental anxiety among university students and its correlation with their field of study," *Journal of Applied Oral Science*, vol. 17, no. 3, pp. 199–203, 2009.

[9] N. A. Jadoon, R. Yaqoob, A. Raza, M. A. Shehzad, and S. C. Zeshan, "Anxiety and depression among medical students: a cross-sectional study," *Journal of Pakistan Medical Association*, vol. 60, no. 8, pp. 699–702, 2010.

[10] D. G. Kirova, "Dental anxiety among dental students," *Journal of IMAB-Annual Proceeding*, vol. 17, no. 2, pp. 137–139, 2011.

[11] A. N. Shete and K. D. Garkal, "A study of stress, anxiety, and depression among postgraduate medical students," *CHRISMED Journal of Health and Research*, vol. 2, no. 2, pp. 119–123, 2015.

[12] N. Ibrahim, D. Al-Kharboush, L. El-Khatib, A. Al-Habib, and D. Asali, "Prevalence and predictors of anxiety and depression among female medical students in King Abdulaziz University, Jeddah, Saudi Arabia," *Iranian Journal of Public Health*, vol. 42, no. 7, pp. 726–736, 2013.

[13] H. P. Storjord, M. M. Teodorsen, J. Bergdahl, R. Wynn, and J. A. Johnsen, "Dental anxiety: a comparison of students of dentistry, biology, and psychology," *Journal of Multidisciplinary Healthcare*, vol. 7, pp. 413–418, 2014.

[14] S. Basudan, N. Binanzan, and A. Alhassan, "Depression, anxiety and stress in dental students," *International Journal of Medical Education*, vol. 8, pp. 179–186, 2017.

[15] R. Misra and M. McKean, "College students' academic stress and its relation to their anxiety, time management, and leisure satisfaction," *American Journal of Health Studies*, vol. 16, no. 1, pp. 41–51, 2000.

[16] H. M. Abdulghani, A. A. AlKanhal, E. S. Mahmoud, G. G. Ponnamperuma, and E. A. Alfaris, "Stress and its effects on medical students: a cross-sectional study at a college of medicine in Saudi Arabia," *Journal of Health, Population and Nutrition*, vol. 29, no. 5, pp. 516–522, 2011.

[17] A. N. Supe, "A study of stress in medical students at Seth G.S. Medical College," *Journal of Postgraduate Medicine*, vol. 44, pp. 1–6, 1998.

[18] A. Singh, A. Lal, and C. Shekhar, "Prevalence of depression among medical students of a private medical college in India," *Online Journal of Health Allied Sciences*, vol. 9, no. 4, pp. 1–3, 2010.

[19] R. E. Noble, "Depression in women," *Metabolism*, vol. 54, no. 5, pp. 49–52, 2005.

[20] S. Arslan, E. Erta, and M. Ulker, "The relationship between dental fear and sociodemographic variables," *Erciyes Medical Journal*, vol. 33, pp. 295–300, 2011.

[21] B. Kulsoom and N. A. Afsar, "Stress, anxiety, and depression among medical students in a multiethnic setting," *Neuropsychiatric Disease and Treatment*, vol. 16, no. 11, pp. 1713–1722, 2015.

[22] R. Alpert and R. N. Haber, "Anxiety in academic achievement situations," *Journal of Abnormal and Social Psychology*, vol. 61, no. 2, pp. 207–215, 1960.

[23] S. Ali, I. Farooq, S. Q. Khan, I. A. Moheet, B. A. Al-Jandan, and K. S. Al-Khalifa, "Self-reported anxiety of dental procedures among dental students and its relation to gender and level of education," *Journal of Taibah University Medical Sciences*, vol. 10, no. 4, pp. 449–453, 2015.

11

Shaping Ability of Superelastic and Controlled Memory Nickel-Titanium File Systems: An In Vitro Study

Raidan A. Ba-Hattab ⓘ[1] **and Dieter Pahncke**[2]

[1]Department of Clinical Dental Sciences, College of Dentistry, Princess Nourah Bint Abdulrahman University, Riyadh, Saudi Arabia
[2]Department of Operative Dentistry and Periodontology, Dental School, University of Rostock, Rostock, Germany

Correspondence should be addressed to Raidan A. Ba-Hattab; rabahattab@pnu.edu.sa

Academic Editor: Carlos A. Munoz-Viveros

Improvements in the thermomechanical processing procedures of NiTi wires have led to the development of new NiTi instruments that compose mainly of martensite crystals, making the wire stable at clinical condition. This study aimed at comparing the shaping ability of two rotary nickel-titanium systems manufactured from different NiTi wires. Twenty simulated root canals each with a curvature of 35° in resin blocks were divided into two groups of 10 canals each. Canals in the first group were prepared with superelastic F360 instruments (Gebr. Brasseler, Germany) while canals in the second group were prepared using controlled memory HyFlex®CM™ instruments (Coltène Whaledent, Switzerland). Images were taken before canal preparation and after the use of each instrument. The assessment of the canal shapes was accomplished with a computer image analysis program. Data were statistically analyzed using SPSS program. Within the limitation of this in vitro study, HyFlex®CM™ instruments remained better centered in the apical third of the canals. In most canal segments, no significant differences were observed between either system in the amount of material removed. Both systems were comparable to each other in regards to their ability to enlarge root canal in the same way without procedural errors.

1. Introduction

During the last decade, many dental companies have been directed for manufacturing of different NiTi rotary instruments with different designs including noncutting tips, radial lands, different cross sections, different helical angle, and varying tapers with the aim to improve their performance and to simplify the preparation procedure [1]. Recently, thermal treatment of NiTi alloy is frequently used [2, 3] to further increase flexibility and fatigue resistance of rotary NiTi instruments rather than changes in instrument geometry [4].

HyFlex®CM™ NiTi files (Coltène Whaledent, Switzerland) are made from an innovative thermomechanical process of NiTi alloy with the property of "Controlled Memory" rather than "Superelastic property" of other conventional NiTi files [4]. These instruments are in the martensite condition at body temperature [5]. Instruments with sizes 20/0.02, 20/0.06, 30/0.04, and 40/0.04 have triangular cross section with three blades and three flutes, other instruments with sizes 20/0.04 and 25/0.04 have quadrangular cross section with four blades and four flutes [6].

The recent F360 system (Komet Dental, Lemgo, Germany) is a 2-file system. The instruments have a 4% taper and are available in sizes 25, 35, 45, and 55. They have a modified double S-shaped cross section and are made of conventional, superelastic NiTi alloy [7].

The null hypothesis was that there would be no difference between superelastic, conventional NiTi instruments (F360) and controlled memory NiTi instruments (HyFlex®CM™) regarding their shaping ability in simulated root canals.

2. Materials and Methods

2.1. Resin Blocks and Experiment Design. A total of twenty transparent canals made of clear polyester resin (Endo Training Block 02 taper, REFA 0177; Dentsply Maillefer,

CH-1338 Ballaigues, Switzerland) were used in this study. All canals had an apical foramen of 0.15 mm, a taper of 0.02, and an angle of curvature of 35°. Canal length was 17 mm with a straight section of 12 mm and a curved section of 5 mm. The samples were randomly divided into two experimental groups ($n = 10$). Using a diamond bur, a small hole was drilled on one side of the preinstrumented block to ensure superimposition accuracy of pre- and post-instrumentation canal pictures during subsequent image analysis. Then, red solution (Caries Marker, coloured caries indicator, VOCO, Cuxhaven, Germany) was injected into the canals to recognize them easily from the post-instrumented canal.

To secure a stable position of the resin blocks, a metal holder was made in which the resin blocks could be placed and repositioned in exactly the same position. A digital camera EOS 400 Digital (Canon Inc., Tokyo, Japan) with a macro-objective "Tamron SP AF 60 mm F/2 Dill Macro 1 : 1" (Tamron Co., Ltd., Saitama, Japan) was used in a fixed position to capture pictures before and after canal instrumentation, and the pictures are saved directly as JPEG format files in a computer. A black background was placed behind the blocks, and the simulated canals were prepared with any of the two systems: F360 and HyFlex®CM™.

2.2. Preparation of the Simulated Canals. The instruments were set into CanalPro CL cordless motor handpiece (Coltène Whaledent, Switzerland) with contra-angle head of 16 : 1. Torque limits and the rotational speeds of each file which recommended by the manufacturers were entered and stored manually by the operator. The instrumentation of all blocks was carried out by one experienced operator.

2.2.1. Group 1: Superelastic Group. Root canals were prepared using F360 instruments (Gebr. Brasseler, Germany). File sizes 25/0.04 and 35/0.04 were used in a single-length technique at a constant rotational speed of 300 rpm and a torque-control level of 1.8 N·cm as recommended by the manufacturer. The instruments were placed in the canals sequentially with a gentle picking motion.

2.2.2. Group 2: Controlled Memory Group. Root canals were prepared using HyFlex®CM™ System (Coltène Whaledent, Switzerland). The instruments were used in a single-length technique at a constant rotational speed of 500 rpm and a torque-control level of 2.5 N·cm as the suggested settings by the manufacturer. To standardize the apical preparation, two files of HyFlex®CM™ (25/0.04 and 35/0.04) were used to prepare the canals instead of conventional full sequence. The files were also placed sequentially in the canals with a gentle picking motion.

Each instrument was coated with FileCare (EDTA, VDW, München, Germany) to lubricate the canals during instrumentation, and a total of 5 ml water was used repeatedly after the use of each instrument. Each instrument was used to shape one canal only. Once the instrument had reached the full working length and rotated freely, it was removed.

2.3. Assessment of Canal Preparation. Image analysis software (GSA Image Analyser Software development and Analytics Bansemer and Scheel GbR, Germany) was used for the assessment of canal curvature modification. The pictures of the simulated canals before and after instrumentation were superimposed using the software, producing a composite image for each canal (Figure 1). The area between canal walls before and after instrumentation was determined both for the inner and outer canal curvature using the same image software. The composite image was sectioned by ten concentric circles spaced 1 mm apart. The centers of the circles were targeted over the tip of the preinstrumented canal, i. e., the first circle radius was 1 mm from the canal tip, and the last circle radius was 10 mm from the canal tip, resulting in 10 measuring segments on the outer and inner sides of the canal, for a total of 20 measuring segments (Figure 2). These segments (material removed) were measured as a surface area (mm^2) automatically using the GSA Image Analyser program.

Moreover, procedural errors occurred during instrumentation described by Thompson and Dummer [8] were also assessed based on the composite images.

2.4. Data Analysis. All data were recorded and statistically analyzed using SPSS (version 19.0, IBM Corporation, USA). The significance level was set at $P \leq 0.05$. The Wilcoxon test was used to compare the area removed from the inner and outer canal walls of one group. The Kruskal–Wallis test was used to compare canal transportation between the groups.

3. Results

The mean values and standard deviations of the area removed from the inner and outer curvature of the canals are detailed in Table 1. The two systems removed significantly ($p \leq 0.05$) more material on the outer wall than the inner wall in the coronal part of the canal (segments 8–10). In the middle part of the canal (segments 5–7), more material was removed on the inner wall than the outer wall; the difference was statistically significant ($p < 0.05$) except in segments 5 and 7 of F360 and HyFlex®CM™ groups, respectively. Apically (segments 1–4), the difference between the material removed from the inner and outer canal walls was not statistically significant in segment 2 of F360 group and in segments 1 and 2 of HyFlex®CM™ group.

There was no statistically significant difference between the F360 and HyFlex®CM™ groups in the mean material removed from the inner and outer wall of the canals (Table 2), except in two segments (8 and 9) on the inner wall and only one segment (8) on the outer wall ($p \leq 0.05$).

Regarding procedural errors, no loss of working length or canal aberration was recorded during canal instrumentation in any of the groups.

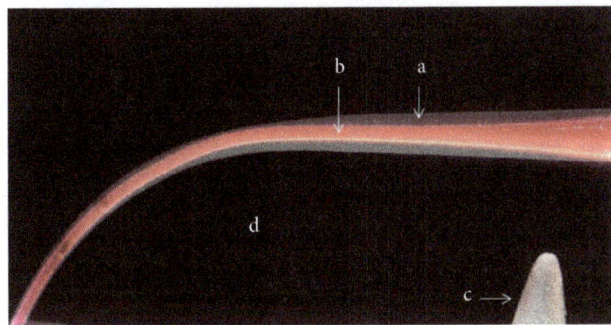

FIGURE 1: A composite image of the simulated canal from the HyFlex CM group (a) after instrumentation (white area) and (b) before preparation (red area) with (c) black background and (d) a drilled hole to secure superimposition of the canals.

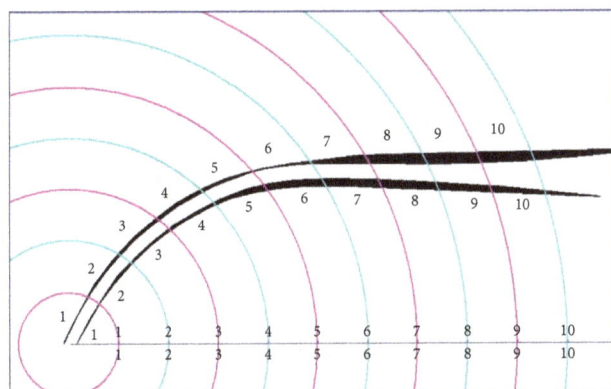

FIGURE 2: 20 segments (10 segments in the inner wall and 10 segments in the outer wall) are created by the ten concentric circles (F360 group).

4. Discussion

The purpose of this study was to compare the shaping ability of two NiTi endodontic instruments manufactured from different NiTi wires: superelastic NiTi instruments (F360) and controlled memory NiTi instruments (HyFlex®CM™) in simulated root canals in resin blocks. HyFlex®CM™ instruments are manufactured from a special NiTi alloy that has been claimed to have a lower percent in weight of nickel **52%** [9] and subjected to thermomechanical processing that creates a mixture of martensite and austenite structures [5].

In this study, simulated canals in resin blocks had been used as an experimental model for assessment of shaping ability of the instruments. These simulated canals are an alternative to the real human extracted teeth and have been used in several studies to test the shaping ability of files [10, 11]. Although the major advantage of using extracted human teeth is the reproduction of the clinical situation, the variations in three-dimensional root canal morphology makes standardization difficult [12]. Resin blocks provide standardized experimental conditions but may not fully represent the clinical settings as they have several limitations related to their mechanical properties which differ from human dentin and heat generation during instrumentation which might lead to instrument separation [13].

Standardization of the apical end preparation is essential to compare the shaping ability of different root canal instruments [14]. In this investigation, the apical end of the canals was prepared using instruments.

According to the results of this study, HyFlex®CM™ and F360 systems did not remain perfectly within the center of the root canal and showed canal straightening toward the inner wall in the middle third and toward the outer wall apically and coronally. Centering ability of the instruments is influenced by several parameters such as instrument design and alloy from which the instrument is manufactured. Instruments with small cross-sectional designs proved better centering ability [15] as the minimal amount of the residual core improves instrument flexibility [16]. Although HyFlex®CM™ instruments have a larger cross-sectional design (quadrangular and triangular cross section for size 25/0.04 and 35/0.04, respectively) in comparison with the small, modified S-shaped cross section of F360 instruments, the instruments remained better centered apically than F360, where nearly the same amount of resin material was removed from the first and second segments of the canal. This might be explained by the good flexibility of the unique, controlled memory (CM) wire of HyFlex®CM™ instruments. Furthermore, the elongation of their spirals during canal preparation allows better removal of debris from the canal [17]. F360 instruments are manufactured from conventional, superelastic NiTi alloy, and this means that the instrument straighten itself while preparing curved canal and attempts to regain its original shape which result in uneven stress on canal walls and consequently uneven material removal from the canal [18].

Recently, Gu et al. [19] stated that the alloy type of the instruments influenced canal transportation more than their cross-sectional designs ($p < 0.05$), and the CM-wire based instruments created the most favorable preparations amongst the thermally treated NiTi instruments in resin canals.

The results of the present study are in agreement with those reported by Bürklein et al. [20], who used the same way as in this study to compare five systems: WaveOne (Dentsply Maillefer, Ballaigues, Switzerland), Reciproc (VDW), OneShape (Micro-Mega), HyFlex®CM™, and F360. They found less transportation in canals prepared with F360, OneShape, and HyFlex®CM™ when compared with instruments of reciprocating motion. Similar conclusions were reached by Rashid and Saleh [21], who compared WaveOne, Reciproc, OneShape, and F360. They concluded that all systems maintained root canal curvature well and were safe to use, and canals prepared with the F360 and OneShape systems were better centered compared with the Reciproc and WaveOne systems.

James et al. [22] stated that HyFlex®CM™ files produce less canal transportation when compared with other thermally treated NiTi Files. A study by Łęski and Radwański [23] showed that HyFlex®CM™ files are more flexible than ProTaper Next® (Dentsply Maillefer, Ballaigues, Switzerland). Another study showed that Hyflex CM instruments resulted in significantly less canal straightening as compared to the use of ProTaper Universal [24].

TABLE 1: Area removed[1] (mm^2) for each instrument.

Segments	1	2	3	4	5	6	7	8	9	10
F360										
Outer wall	0.03 ± 0.01	0.04 ± 0.02	0.06 ± 0.02	0.07 ± 0.02	0.07 ± 0.02	0.05 ± 0.02	0.08 ± 0.03	0.13 ± 0.02	0.16 ± 0.03	0.16 ± 03
Inner wall	0.02 ± 0.01	0.03 ± 0.01	0.03 ± 0.01	0.04 ± 0.02	0.09 ± 0.03	0.13 ± 0.03	0.12 ± 0.02	0.10 ± 0.01	0.10 ± 0.01	0.09 ± 02
P values	**0.047***	0.396	**0.007***	**0.011***	0.128	**0.005***	**0.005***	**0.005***	**0.005***	**0.005***
HyFlex®CM™										
Outer wall	0.03 ± 0.01	0.03 ± 0.02	0.06 ± 0.02	0.07 ± 0.02	0.05 ± 0.02	0.04 ± 0.01	0.08 ± 0.01	0.11 ± 0.02	0.14 ± 0.02	0.15 ± 0.02
Inner wall	0.03 ± 0.01	0.04 ± 0.02	0.03 ± 0.01	0.05 ± 0.02	0.10 ± 0.02	0.13 ± 0.02	0.10 ± 0.02	0.08 ± 0.01	0.08 ± 0.02	0.07 ± 0.02
P values	0.096	0.726	**0.008***	**0.015***	**0.009***	**0.005***	0.076	**0.009***	**0.007***	**0.005***

[1]Mean ± standard deviation; *values are statistically significant.

TABLE 2: Comparison between the instruments of the area removed[2] (mm^2) from canal walls.

Segments	1	2	3	4	5	6	7	8	9	10
Outer wall										
F360	0.03 ± 0.01	0.04 ± 0.02	0.06 ± 0.02	0.07 ± 0.01	0.07 ± 0.02	0.05 ± 0.02	0.08 ± 0.03	0.13 ± 0.02	0.16 ± 0.03	0.16 ± 0.03
HyFlex®CM™	0.03 ± 0.01	0.03 ± 0.02	0.06 ± 0.02	0.07 ± 0.02	0.05 ± 0.02	0.04 ± 0.01	0.08 ± 0.01	0.11 ± 0.02	0.14 ± 0.02	0.15 ± 0.02
P values	0.812	0.439	0.592	0.585	0.301	0.133	0.319	**0.017***	0.055	0.135
Inner wall										
F360	0.02 ± 0.01	0.03 ± 0.01	0.03 ± 0.01	0.04 ± 0.02	0.09 ± 0.03	0.13 ± 0.03	0.12 ± 0.02	0.10 ± 0.01	0.10 ± 0.01	0.09 ± 0.02
HyFlex®CM™	0.03 ± 0.01	0.04 ± 0.02	0.03 ± 0.01	0.05 ± 0.02	0.10 ± 0.02	0.13 ± 0.02	$0.10 \pm .002$	0.08 ± 0.01	0.08 ± 0.02	0.07 ± 0.02
P values	0.218	0.908	0.540	0.966	0.254	0.909	0.086	**0.021***	**0.019***	0.066

[2]Mean ± standard deviation; *values are statistically significant.

In summary, the current study showed that both HyFlex®CM™ and F360 instruments prepared canals without significant shaping errors and there was no significant difference between them. Therefore, the null hypothesis was accepted.

5. Conclusions

Within the experimental limitation and the results of the present study, it could be concluded that both systems were comparable to each other in regard to their ability to enlarge root canal in the same way without procedural errors.

Acknowledgments

The authors thank Gebr. Brasseler (Germany) and Coltène Whaledent (Switzerland) for providing the root canal instruments used in this study.

References

[1] S. B. R. Cohen, *Pathways of the Pulp*, Mosby-Year Book, Louis, MO, USA, 6th edition, 1994.

[2] S. Miyazaki, Y. Ohmi, K. Otsuka, and Y. Suzuki, "Characteristic of deformation and transformation pseudoelasticity in Ti-Ni alloys," *Le Journal de Physique Colloques*, vol. 43, no. C4, pp. C4-255–C4-260, 1982.

[3] C. P. Frick, A. M. Ortega, J. Tyber et al., "Thermal processing of polycrystalline NiTi shape memory alloys," *Materials Science and Engineering: A*, vol. 405, no. 1-2, pp. 34–49, 2004.

[4] S. Zinelis, T. Eliades, and G. Eliades, "A metallurgical characterization of ten endodontic Ni-Ti instruments: assessing the clinical relevance of shape memory and superelastic properties of Ni-Ti endodontic instruments," *International Endodontic Journal*, vol. 43, no. 2, pp. 125–134, 2010.

[5] Y. Shen, H. Zhou, Y. Zheng, L. Campbell, B. Peng, and M. Haapasalo, "Metallurgical characterization of controlled memory wire nickel-titanium rotary instruments," *Journal of Endodontics*, vol. 37, no. 11, pp. 1566–1571, 2011.

[6] C. Poggio, A. Dagna, M. Chiesa, R. Beltrami, and S. Bianchi, "Cleaning effectiveness of three NiTi rotary instruments: a focus on biomaterial properties," *Journal of Functional Biomaterials*, vol. 6, no. 1, pp. 66–76, 2015.

[7] A. Dagna, "F360 and F6 skytaper: SEM evaluation of cleaning efficiency," *Annali di Stomatologia*, vol. 6, p. 69, 2015.

[8] S. A. Thompson and P. M. H. Dummer, "Shaping ability of proFile.04 taper series 29 rotary nickel-titanium instruments in simulated root canals. part 1," *International Endodontic Journal*, vol. 30, no. 1, pp. 1–7, 1997.

[9] L. Testarelli, G. Plotino, D. Al-Sudani et al., "Bending properties of a new nickel-titanium alloy with a lower percent by weight of nickel," *Journal of Endodontics*, vol. 37, no. 9, pp. 1293–1295, 2011.

[10] K. T. Ceyhanli, A. Kamaci, M. Taner, N. Erdilek, and D. Celik, "Shaping ability of two M-wire and two traditional nickel-titanium instrumentation systems in S-shaped resin canals," *Nigerian Journal of Clinical Practice*, vol. 18, no. 6, pp. 713–717, 2015.

[11] H. Wu, C. Peng, Y. Bai, X. Hu, L. Wang, and C. Li, "Shaping ability of ProTaper Universal, WaveOne and ProTaper Next in simulated L-shaped and S-shaped root canals," *BMC Oral Health*, vol. 15, no. 1, p. 27, 2015.

[12] M. Hülsmann, O. Peters, and P. M. H. Dummer, "Mechanical preparation of root canals: shaping goals, techniques and means," *Endodontic Topics*, vol. 10, no. 1, pp. 30–76, 2005.

[13] L. Zhang, H. X. Luo, X. D. Zhou, H. Tan, and D. M. Huang, "The shaping effect of the combination of two rotary nickel-titanium instruments in simulated S-shaped canals," *Journal of Endodontics*, vol. 34, no. 4, pp. 456–458, 2008.

[14] F. Paque, U. Musch, and M. Hulsmann, "Comparison of root canal preparation using RaCe and ProTaper rotary Ni-Ti instruments," *International Endodontic Journal*, vol. 38, no. 1, pp. 8–16, 2005.

[15] D. Kandaswamy, N. Venkateshbabu, and I P. G. Porkodi, "Canal-centering ability: an endodontic challenge," *Journal of Conservative Dentistry*, vol. 12, p. 3, 2009.

[16] C. J. Ruddle, "The ProTaper technique," *Endodontic Topics*, vol. 10, no. 1, pp. 187–190, 2005.

[17] COLTENE, *HyFlex™ CM NiTi Files*, 2018, https://www.coltene.com/products/endodontics/rotary-files/hyflex-rotary-files/hyflexTM-cm-niti-files/#description.

[18] J. Vaudt, K. Bitter, K. Neumann, and A. M. Kielbassa, "Ex vivo study on root canal instrumentation of two rotary nickel–titanium systems in comparison to stainless steel hand instruments," *International Endodontic Journal*, vol. 42, no. 1, pp. 22–33, 2009.

[19] Y. Gu, K-Y Kum, H Perinpanayagam et al., "Various heat-treated nickel–titanium rotary instruments evaluated in S-shaped simulated resin canals," *Journal of Dental Sciences*, vol. 12, no. 1, pp. 14–20, 2017.

[20] S. Bürklein, T. Poschmann, and E. Schäfer, "Shaping ability of different nickel-titanium systems in simulated S-shaped canals with and without glide path," *Journal of Endodontics*, vol. 40, no. 8, pp. 1231–1234, 2014.

[21] A. Rashid and A. R. Saleh, "Shaping ability of different endodontic single-file systems using simulated resin blocks," *Indian Journal of Multidisciplinary Dentistry*, vol. 6, p. 61, 2016.

[22] A. James, A. Shetty, and M. M. C. Hegde, "Evaluation of apical transportation using 3 different rotary systems: Hyflex Files, Twisted Files, Protaper next by morphometric analysis," *IOSR-Journal of Dental and Medical Sciences*, vol. 15, pp. 21–24, 2016.

[23] M. Łęski and M. P. H. Radwański, "Comparison of the shaping ability of Hyflex® CM™ files with ProTaper Next® in simulated L-curved canals," *Dental and Medical Problems*, vol. 52, pp. 54–56, 2015.

[24] Y. Liu, Q. Ning, X. Ming, C. Wang, X. Yu et al., "Comparison of shaping ability of five nickel-titanium rotary instruments in simulated curved canals," *Journal of Dentistry and Oral Health*, vol. 3, pp. 1–5, 2017.

12

Incidence of Tooth Loss in Adults: A 4-Year Population-Based Prospective Cohort Study

Manoelito Ferreira Silva-Junior,[1] **Marília Jesus Batista,**[2] **and Maria da Luz Rosário de Sousa**[1]

[1]*Department of Community Dentistry, Piracicaba Dental School, University of Campinas, Avenue Limeira 901, 13414-903 Piracicaba, SP, Brazil*
[2]*Department of Community Health, Faculty of Medicine Jundiaí, R. Francisco Telles, No. 250, Vila Arens II, 13202-550 Jundiaí, SP, Brazil*

Correspondence should be addressed to Maria da Luz Rosário de Sousa; luzsousa@fop.unicamp.br

Academic Editor: Gilberto Sammartino

Objective. To verify the incidence of tooth loss in extended age group of adults in 4 years. *Materials and Methods.* The prospective cohort study assessed adults (20–64 years old) between 2011 and 2015, from Piracicaba, São Paulo, Brazil. The dependent variable was cumulative incidence of tooth loss, assessed by difference between missing teeth (M) of decayed, missing, and filled tooth index (DMFT) in 2011 and 2015. Participants were stratified into young (20–44 years old) and older (45–64 years old) adults. Mann–Whitney U test ($p < 0.05$) was used to compare the means of incidence of tooth loss between age groups. *Results.* After four years, 57.7% ($n = 143$) of adults were followed up and the mean incidence of tooth loss was 0.91 (SD = 1.65); among these, 51 adults (35.7%) who lost their teeth showed mean tooth loss of 2.55 (SD = 1.86). In older adults, incidence of tooth loss was higher ($p = 0.008$), but no difference between age groups was found when only adults with incidence of tooth loss were assessed ($p = 0.844$). *Conclusion.* There was higher incidence of tooth loss in older adults after four years, however, without difference between age groups when only those who lost teeth were evaluated.

1. Introduction

Tooth loss, still ranked among the hundred health conditions that most affect the world's population [1], is an oral condition that leads to functional, aesthetic, and social damage with impact on people's quality of life [2, 3] and is responsible for causing 7.6 million DALY (disability-adjusted life years) [1].

In spite of the more conservative philosophy within professional dental practice, where tooth extraction is treated as the last treatment option, there are cases in which this is the only choice [4, 5]. This is because time is a determinant factor in the progression and severity of oral diseases, such as caries and periodontal disease, and due to its cohort effect, the incidence of tooth loss during adulthood is higher [6, 7].

A review of 15 longitudinal studies from seven countries regarding tooth loss showed an annual incidence of the loss of one or more teeth ranging from 1.3% to 13.7% and the number of teeth lost varied from 3 to 38 per 100 subjects/year [8]. Although tooth loss can be prevented, its incidence has not declined in recent decades [1, 6] and it is still considered a public health care issue [1, 6, 9, 10]. In Brazil, the mean number of teeth lost in adults (35–44 years) is almost four times higher than that in adolescents (15–19 years) and half of mean number in older persons (65–74 years) [11]; therefore, it is important to investigate the distribution of tooth loss in the age range between the age groups of adolescents, adults, and older persons. This justified the use of an extended age group of adults in the present study.

The clinical aspects of tooth loss, such as most affected teeth, their distribution [12, 13], and condition before tooth extraction, have been more exploited in clinical studies [4, 14, 15] and may not correspond to the reality of the population.

Observational studies with adults are rarely found in the literature and may present more detailed data on clinical conditions of tooth loss [16]. Tooth loss studies are usually cross-sectional [9, 11, 12, 14, 17–20] and assess factors associated with this condition, mainly socioeconomic and oral health service utilization [8–12, 14, 15, 17–20].

The data on the distribution of tooth loss in a population-based cohort, mainly in an extended age group of adults, would be able to infer more reliable data for the planning of actions in public health and may also serve as a basis for verifying the impact of the public health policies implemented. To this end, the objective of this study was to verify the incidence of tooth loss in an extended age group of adults (20–64 years) in a period of 4 years.

2. Material and Methods

2.1. Study Design and Location. This prospective cohort study conducted in Piracicaba, São Paulo, Brazil, was part of a dissertation entitled "Longitudinal tooth loss study in adults and associated factors" [5].

2.2. Ethical Aspects. This research was approved by the Research Ethics Committee of the Piracicaba Dental School (CEP-FOP/Unicamp) (177/2009).

2.3. Population and Sample

2.3.1. Baseline. To calculate the representative sample of adults (20–64 years) living in Piracicaba, São Paulo, oral health conditions were assessed in different age groups and two different calculations were estimated for the sample size of young adults (20–44 years) and older adults (45–64 years). We adopted a design effect of 1.5; margin of error of 10.0%; and 95.0% confidence interval, data concerning the prevalence of caries for each age group (70.2% and 90.9%, resp. [18]), and added 20% to the total to compensate occasional losses. The sample size for adults aged 20–44 years was 172, and for those aged 45–64 years, 68, totaling 240 adults. We added 30% to the final sample size for selecting adults, foreseeing the possibility of losses and refusals, resulting in 342 households, 11.4 households for each census tract [3].

The sample selection was planned based on the Brazilian Demographic Census (2000) [21], the latest data compiled at the time when the study was conducted. The Piracicaba population of adults from 20 to 64 years old was 202, 131; 30 census tracts were randomly selected using probability sampling; 11 households were randomly selected in each sector, according to a varying fraction determined by the number of households. One adult per house was examined [3].

2.3.2. Follow-Up. For the purpose of following up the same subjects, the home census tracts related to their current residences were not considered [5].

2.4. Data Collection

2.4.1. Baseline. Data collection took place between June and September 2011. The research consisted of one clinical oral examination and one interview. Clinical oral examinations were measured by the number of decayed, missing, and filled teeth index (DMFT) and need for dental caries treatment was performed in the households, under artificial lighting without prior prophylaxis or drying, using CPI-probes and front surface mouth mirrors, as recommended by the World Health Organization [22]. In addition, each volunteer answered a questionnaire on demographic (sex, age, race, and marital status) and socioeconomic (family income and education) factors.

Inclusion criteria were living in one of the residences drawn in Piracicaba, São Paulo, and to be between 20 and 64 years of age in 2011. Exclusion criteria were those with physical and psychological conditions that would interfere in the clinical procedures or in the understanding of the questionnaire [3].

At baseline, one examiner conducted the study, after being trained by a benchmark examiner, through theoretical and practical discussions, lasting for a total of 16 hours, obtaining agreement equal to or greater than 90.0% for coronal caries and treatment needs for dental caries. Intraexaminer agreement was from 96.5% to 100.0% and the Kappa coefficient ranged from 0.89 to 1.00, within reliability standards [3].

At this stage, there was a loss of 24.0% ($n = 82$) adults because they did not agree to participate in the study or were not found during one of the three visits; however, a minimum number of 240 adults was obtained, or representativeness of adults of the studied municipality. At baseline, the sample was composed of 248 adults, representing the 149,635 adults (20–64 years old) living in Piracicaba, São Paulo, Brazil.

2.4.2. Follow-Up. Data collection was made between June and September 2015. Inclusion criterion was to have participated in the independent baseline of the current census tract of residences in 2015. Exclusion criterion was physical and psychological conditions that would interfere with the clinical procedures [5].

During follow-up, two examiners participated in this stage of data collection; they were trained by benchmark examiner (baseline examiner) with theoretical and practical discussions, calibrated in a total of 20 hours, and obtained at least 90.0% agreement relative to coronal caries and treatment needs for dental caries. Intraexaminer and interexaminer agreement was from 96.5% to 100.0% and the Kappa coefficient ranged from 0.89 to 1.00, within reliability standards [5].

The same individuals were sought at their addresses and invited to participate in the study. If the individual was not found, at least three more attempts were made. Participants signed the Term of Free and Informed Consent to participate in the study. The same oral clinical conditions were assessed, using the same criteria and examination protocol as that used at baseline [3]. At the time of data collection, each individual kept the same baseline identification.

At this stage, the sample was composed of 143 (follow-up rate = 57.7%) adults. The reasons for not participating were 64 (25.8%) could not be found, 33 (13.3%) refused to participate, and 8 (3.2%) died [5].

2.5. Variables. The dependent variable was cumulative incidence of tooth loss, assessed by the difference between missing teeth (M) of decayed, missing, and filled teeth index (DMFT) in 2011 and 2015. Missing teeth (M) were considered the teeth with codes 4 (tooth loss due to dental caries experience) and 5 (tooth loss due to other causes) of the DMFT index. Treatment needs for dental caries were determined as restorative (in one or more surfaces and a single crown) and endodontic treatment and extraction. For calculating the clinical variables, the 32 teeth were considered.

As reference for the sample characterization, we used the socioeconomic and demographic data collected at baseline. Age was stratified into two groups: young (20–44 years) and older (45–64 years) adults at baseline (2011), so that there would be no transition among the studied groups. Racial groups were defined by self-declaration, and these were categorized as white and non-white (black, brown, yellow, or indigenous). Marital status was categorized as stable relationship (married or cohabitation) and nonstable relationship (single, divorced, or widowed). Family income was categorized as low (less than 1 minimum wage (MW)), average (1-2 MW), and high (greater than 2 MW). Educational level was categorized according to the number of years of completed education (≤4 years, between 5–10 years, and ≥11 years).

2.6. Data Analysis. The data were tabulated with Statistical Package for the Social Sciences version 20.0 (SPSS) and Microsoft Excel®. A descriptive analysis was performed, thus obtaining the absolute and percentage distribution, mean, and standard deviation (SD) of the studied variables. The Mann–Whitney U test ($p < 0.05$) was used to compare the mean values of incidence of tooth loss between age groups.

3. Results

The majority of the participants were women (72.0%), older (51.0%), in stable relationship (78.3%), and with a mean family income (63.6%) and had studied for more than 11 years (53.1%) (Table 1).

After the 4-year follow-up, 12.6% ($n = 18$) adults still had no tooth loss, 1.4% ($n = 2$) presented their first tooth loss and one 0.7% ($n = 1$) adult became edentulous.

A total of 51 adults (35.7%) had lost at least one tooth, among these 24.3% ($n = 17$) of the young adults and 46.6% ($n = 34$) of the older adults. There was a higher incidence of 35.0% ($n = 18$) of one tooth loss per individual (Figure 1).

Table 2 shows the mean incidence of tooth loss was 0.91 (SD = 1.65); among these, 51 adults (35.7%) showed the loss of 2.55 (SD = 1.86) teeth. The incidence of tooth loss in older adults ($p = 0.008$) was higher, but there was no difference between age groups when only adults with incidence of tooth loss were assessed ($p = 0.844$) (Table 2).

At baseline, the prevalence of tooth loss was higher in the maxilla (53.7%), with the maxillary molars being the most affected (29.1%) and the front teeth the least affected (8.1%). In the follow-up, the incidence was similar in the maxilla (50.8%) and mandible (49.2%); the mandibular molars

TABLE 1: Demographic and socioeconomic characteristics of sample of adults living in Piracicaba, São Paulo, Brazil.

Characteristics	n (%)
Demographics	
Sex	
Male	40 (28.0)
Female	103 (72.0)
Age	
Young adults	70 (49.0)
Older adults	73 (51.0)
Race	
White	122 (85.3)
No white	21 (14.7)
Marital status	
Stable relationship	112 (78.3)
No stable relationship	31 (21.7)
Socioeconomics	
Family income	
Low	23 (16.1)
Average	91 (63.6)
High	25 (17.5)
Missing	4 (2.8)
Education	
≤4 years	30 (21.0)
5–10 years	37 (25.9)
≥11 years	76 (53.1)

Note. *Reference data (2011).

(22.3%) were the most affected teeth, and maxillary premolars (11.5%) the least affected (Figure 2).

For the adults who had incidence of tooth loss, in total 130 teeth were lost in the last four years; and at baseline, the majority had treatment needs for caries, which was restorative treatment (64.9%) (Table 3).

4. Discussion

The findings of this population-based prospective cohort study with a sample of adults in expanded age group are of great relevance for understanding tooth loss. While data were compiled on tooth loss and treatment needs for dental caries at baseline, in the follow-up it was possible to check clinical changes in the teeth over the course of time. Over one-third of the sample had incidence of tooth loss in 4 years, and the incidence increased according to the age group studied. The incidence of tooth loss among young adults was, however, equal to that of older adults, considering only individuals who had lost teeth.

The present study presented some limitations, such as the higher number of women participating, a fact also verified in other reports of home collection [3, 9, 11–13]. The sample loss expected in cohort studies also occurred in this study [8, 15, 16, 23]. However, the sample retained the characteristic of being mostly composed of women. Among the treatment needs identified relative to the lost teeth, in the present

TABLE 2: Number of teeth lost by age group of adults for simple total and adults with incidence of tooth loss in 4 years of follow-up. Piracicaba, São Paulo, Brazil, 2011–2015.

Incidence of tooth loss	Total Mean (SD)	Young adults Mean (SD)	Older adults Mean (SD)	p value[*]
Simple total ($n = 143$)	0.91 (1.65)	0.67 (1.64)	1.14 (1.64)	0.008
Among adults with incidence ($n = 51$)	2.55 (1.86)	2.76 (2.33)	2.44 (1.60)	0.844

[*]Mann–Whitney U test ($p < 0.05$).

TABLE 3: Absolute frequency of treatment needs for dental caries at baseline (2011) and incidence of tooth loss (2015) according to the number of teeth in the arch. Piracicaba, São Paulo, Brazil, 2011–2015.

Tooth number in arch	Treatment needs for dental caries (2011)				Incidence of tooth loss (2011–2015)
	Restorative	Endodontics	Extraction	Total	Total
	n	n	n	n	n
18	4	0	3	7	4
17	1	2	2	5	6
16	4	0	0	4	0
15	3	1	1	5	4
14	1	1	1	3	3
13	3	0	2	5	1
12	2	0	0	2	3
11	6	0	0	6	5
21	7	0	0	7	5
22	2	2	0	4	2
23	4	0	1	5	6
24	1	2	0	3	3
25	2	1	0	3	5
26	3	4	0	7	3
27	2	0	2	4	7
28	1	0	0	1	7
38	4	0	2	6	9
37	1	3	1	5	6
36	6	2	1	9	2
35	1	0	0	1	2
34	1	0	0	1	3
33	3	0	0	3	4
32	2	0	0	2	4
31	1	0	0	1	3
41	2	0	0	2	5
42	3	0	0	3	2
43	1	0	0	1	3
44	4	2	1	7	7
45	2	1	0	3	4
46	3	2	1	6	3
47	3	1	0	4	2
48	2	1	3	6	7
Total	85 (64.9%)	25 (19.1%)	21 (16.0%)	131 (100.0)	130 (100.0)

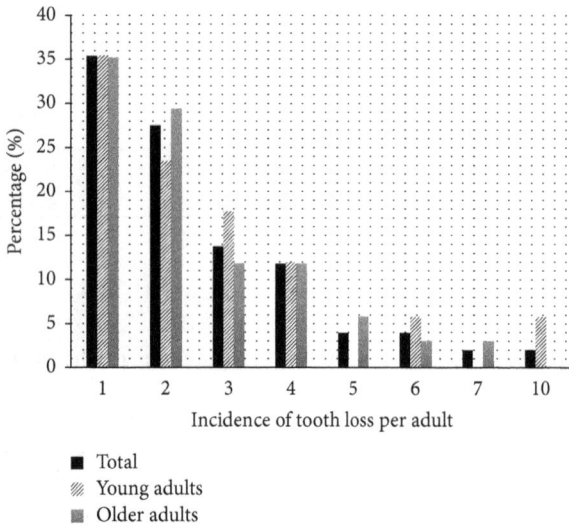

FIGURE 1: Frequency of total incidence and by age group of the number of teeth lost by adults in the 4-year follow-up. Piracicaba, São Paulo, Brazil, 2011–2015.

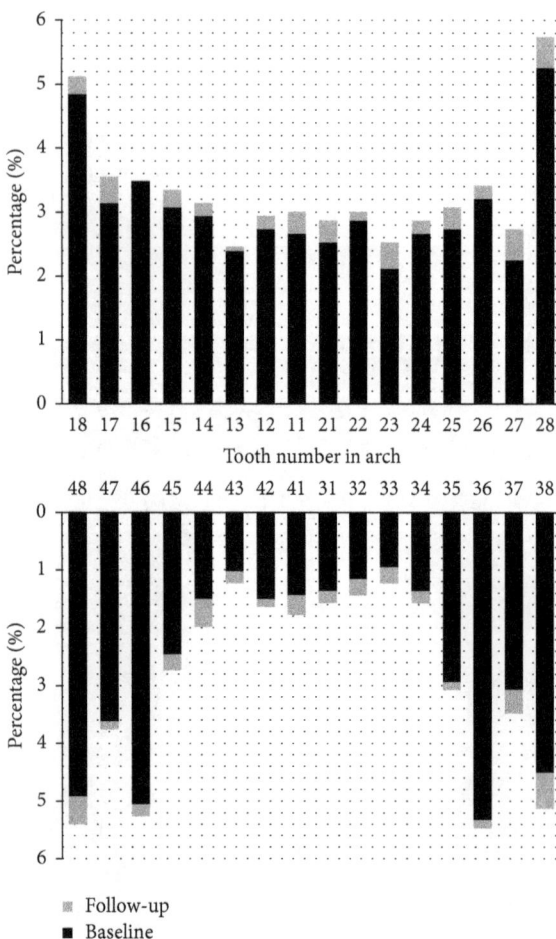

FIGURE 2: Percentage of tooth loss according to affected teeth in adults at the baseline and follow-up. Piracicaba, São Paulo, Brazil, 2011–2015.

study, only caries requirements were considered; and other previous conditions of the teeth, such as previous restorations or periodontal conditions were not verified. Thus, the authors recommend that future cohort studies should include other oral health care needs with the purpose of preventing future tooth loss.

In this study, expanded age groups and stratification into the two age groups of our study allowed us to verify important differences between the distribution of tooth loss in young adults and older adults. In spite of differences in the methodology of longitudinal tooth loss studies, such as the exclusion of third molars from analysis [11, 12], use of a restricted age group, between 35 and 44 years [22], as recommended by WHO, and number of years of follow-up, it was possible for the authors of the present study to verify a methodological pattern of higher incidence of tooth loss as the period of the follow-up increased [15, 16, 20] and the age group studied was older [24]. Moreover, even if most studies considered age an associated or risk factor of tooth loss [5, 18, 19, 25], this association is questionable, because there is no established evidence between tooth loss and the physiology of aging [24].

In present study, the number of adults with incidence of tooth loss was almost twice as high among older adults. The mean number of teeth lost was higher in older adults when compared with the total sample, whereas there was no difference between the mean number of teeth lost when the age groups studied were compared between adults with incidence of tooth loss. This result denotes a polarization of tooth loss in young adults, as happens with dental caries in children, because the highest burden of the condition is concentrated in a small portion of individuals [26]. Although the incidence of tooth loss was restricted to a small number of young adults, it was equal to the mean incidence in older adults.

The highest incidence of one tooth lost per individual was in agreement with values in the literature [15, 16, 25]. In present study, only one individual became edentulous. In the past decades, studies have verified a reduction in the prevalence of edentulism [27], which may denote less invasive oral health care practices today, as tooth extraction is considered the last treatment option.

We also found that the incidence of tooth loss per group of teeth was similar to the data found for prevalence of tooth loss [18]. When prevalence of tooth loss at baseline and follow-up was assessed, distribution was similar to that found in the literature [15, 18]; the mandibular molars were the first teeth lost and the mandibular front teeth are those that remained longest. Examination of the incidence of tooth loss showed a different pattern: premolars and teeth in the mandibular dental arch were least frequently missing. This may be explained by the fact that this study was conducted with expanded age groups and included individuals in different stages of life, but it should be noted that the molars continued to be the most frequently missing teeth. Another aspect that could justify why the mandibular teeth are kept, mainly the mandibular anterior teeth, is the professional choice of these teeth as prosthetic abutments for greater retention of prosthesis in the mandibular ridge [5].

In the evaluation of each tooth that was lost at follow-up and the treatment needs for dental caries at baseline, the majority of participants needed restorative treatment. From this, we inferred a greater need for low complexity treatments that could have been made by primary oral health care in the initial stages of dental caries [17]. Most studies have, however, demonstrated the need for more dental services in secondary care for adults [9, 19], mostly due to the high accumulated demand [28]. This result becomes important since tooth loss is a direct consequence of lack of dental caries treatment. Therefore, it is difficult to think of reducing tooth loss without thinking of reducing tooth decay. This restates the necessity of providing proper knowledge on oral hygiene and diet, for example, rational consumption of sugar, regular use of the dental services, and healthy choices to maintain and keep teeth functional throughout their entire life time.

From this perspective, to meet the oral health care needs of the Brazilian people and to achieve integrality in health care, oral health care was included in the Unified Health System (SUS), with the creation of the National Oral Health Policy in 2003 and deployment of Dental Specialties Centers (DSC). DSC provides users with specialized oral health treatments capable of rehabilitating teeth with severe damage and tissue loss [9].

Although Brazil has developed oral health policies, for example, increase in the number of Oral Health Teams (OHT) in the Family Health Strategy, other aspects should be discussed. As verified in our study, although large investments have been made to expand OHT, in Piracicaba as well, where 14-OHT modality type I, and two DSC have been implemented up to now, this is still not enough to reduce dental caries and its main threat to the adult population: tooth loss. Nevertheless, in Brazil these changes and investments in public oral health are usually made over time; therefore, longitudinal studies are necessary to measure these aspects.

Outcomes from this study may assist with planning adult oral health policies, because they demonstrated the eminent need for promoting basic oral health care. This restates the necessity to focus on oral health care promotion regardless of the age group of adults studied, as a continuous approach, and as early as possible, in order to prevent oral health diseases and their worsening, because they may have an impact on the other life cycles of individuals, and lead to tooth loss.

Access of the economically active population, the greater part of the adult population, to health care services becomes difficult where opening hours are concerned. Alternative opening hours, at night or weekends, would facilitate access to public dental services. Another important aspect of the discussion on tooth loss is related to professional practice, often still centered on the biomedical model, strengthened by repetitive restorative cycles and without prioritizing risk factors, preventing oral health diseases, and promoting oral health care. Further aspects concern personal motivation, both relative to the late demand for treatment, that is, motivated by pain or beliefs that make individuals choose tooth extraction [5, 26], and the low value they assign to their teeth. These hypotheses, however, require further research, in order to provide more subjective explanations of factors that cause tooth loss in the long-term.

5. Conclusion

After four years, it was possible to verify a higher incidence of tooth loss in older adults, however, without difference between age groups when only those who lost teeth were evaluated.

Acknowledgments

The authors thank *Fundação de Amparo à Pesquisa do Estado de São Paulo*, FAPESP (2009/16560-0, 2011/00545-1, and 2017/11771-9), and cooperation agreement with FAPESP and *Coordenação de Aperfeiçoamento de Pessoal de Nível Superior*, CAPES (2014/15184-2), for supporting this research. The authors also thank *Espaço da Escrita, Coordenadoria Geral da Universidade, UNICAMP*, for the language services provided.

References

[1] N. J. Kassebaum, A. G. C. Smith, E. Bernabé et al. et al., "Global, regional, and national prevalence, incidence, and disability-adjusted life years for oral conditions for 195 countries, 1990–2015: A systematic analysis for the global burden of diseases, injuries, and risk factors," *Journal of Dental Research*, vol. 96, no. 4, pp. 380–387, 2017.

[2] A. E. Gerritsen, P. F. Allen, D. J. Witter, E. M. Bronkhorst, and N. H. J. Creugers, "Tooth loss and oral health-related quality of life: a systematic review and meta-analysis," *Health and Quality of Life Outcomes*, vol. 8, article 126, p. 552, 2010.

[3] M. J. Batista, H. P. Lawrence, and M. D. L. R. de Sousa, "Impact of tooth loss related to number and position on oral health quality of life among adults," *Health and Quality of Life Outcomes*, vol. 12, no. 1, article no. 165, 2014.

[4] M. Jafarian and A. Etebarian, "Reasons for extraction of permanent teeth in general dental practices in Tehran, Iran," *Medical Principles and Practice*, vol. 22, no. 3, pp. 239–244, 2013.

[5] M. F. Silva-Junior, *Tooth loss longitudinal study in adults and associated factors. Piracicaba-SP. Thesis [Master in Dentistry]*, University of Campinas, Piracicaba Dental School, 2016.

[6] N. J. Kassebaum, E. Bernabé, M. Dahiya, B. Bhandari, C. J. L. Murray, and W. Marcenes, "Global Burden of Severe Tooth Loss: A Systematic Review and Meta-analysis," *Journal of Dental Research*, vol. 93, pp. 20–28, 2014.

[7] F. Müller, M. Naharro, and G. E. Carlsson, "What are the prevalence and incidence of tooth loss in the adult and elderly population in Europe?" *Clinical Oral Implants Research*, vol. 18, no. 3, pp. 2–14, 2007.

[8] O. Haugejorden, K. S. Klock, and T. A. Trovik, "Incidence and predictors of self-reported tooth loss in a representative sample of Norwegian adults," *Community Dentistry and Oral Epidemiology*, vol. 31, no. 4, pp. 261–268, 2003.

[9] P. R. Barbato, H. C. M. Nagano, F. N. Zanchet, A. F. Boing, and M. A. Peres, "Tooth loss and associated socioeconomic, demographic, and dental-care factors in Brazilian adults: an analysis of the Brazilian Oral Health Survey, 2002-2003," *Cadernos de Saúde Pública*, vol. 23, no. 8, pp. 1803–1814, 2007.

[10] B. F. Jaleel, R. Nagarajappa, A. K. Mohapatra, and G. Ramesh, "Risk indicators associated with tooth loss among Indian adults," *Oral Health and Dental Management*, vol. 13, no. 2, pp. 170–178, 2014.

[11] M. A. Peres, P. R. Barbato, S. C. G. B. Reis, C. H. S. D. M. Freitas, and J. L. F. Antunes, "Tooth loss in Brazil: Analysis of the 2010 Brazilian oral health survey," *Revista de Saude Publica*, vol. 47, no. 3, pp. 78–89, 2014.

[12] S. Nascimento, P. Frazao, A. Bousquat, and J. L. F. Antunes, "Dental health in Brazilian adults between 1986 and 2010," *Revista de Saúde Pública*, vol. 47, no. suppl 3, pp. 69–77, 2013.

[13] M. J. Batista, D. D. Silva, and M. L. R. Sousa, "Oral health in an adult population in a municipality of Paulínia, São Paulo," *Revista de Odontologia da UNESP*, vol. 39, no. 4, pp. 185-91, 2010.

[14] S. Khazaei, A. H. Keshteli, A. Feizi, O. Savabi, and P. Adibi, "Epidemiology and risk factors of tooth loss among Iranian adults: Findings from a large community-based study," *BioMed Research International*, vol. 2013, Article ID 786462, 2013.

[15] U. Van Der Velden, A. Amaliya, B. G. Loos et al., "Java project on periodontal diseases: Causes of tooth loss in a cohort of untreated individuals," *Journal of Clinical Periodontology*, vol. 42, no. 9, pp. 824–831, 2015.

[16] S. Fure, "Ten-Year Incidence of Tooth Loss and Dental Caries in Elderly Swedish Individuals," *Caries Research*, vol. 37, no. 6, pp. 462–469, 2003.

[17] M. J. Batista, L. B. Rihs, and M. da Luz Rosário de Sousa, "Workers oral health: A cross-sectional study," *Brazilian Journal of Oral Sciences*, vol. 12, no. 3, pp. 178–183, 2013.

[18] M. J. Batista, L. B. Rihs, and M. D. L. R. de Sousa, "Risk indicators for tooth loss in adult workers," *Brazilian Oral Research*, vol. 26, no. 5, pp. 390–396, 2012.

[19] M. J. Batista, H. P. Lawrence, and M. D. L. R. de Sousa, "Tooth loss classification: Factors associated with a new classification in an adult population group," *Ciencia e Saude Coletiva*, vol. 20, no. 9, pp. 2825–2835, 2015.

[20] G. H. Gilbert, R. P. Duncan, and B. J. Shelton, "Social Determinants of Tooth Loss," *Health Services Research*, vol. 38, no. 6, pp. 1843–1862, 2003.

[21] Brazilian Institute of Geography and Statistics (IBGE), "2010, Brazilian Demographic Census – 2000," http://www.ibge.gov .br/home/.

[22] World Health Organization, *Oral Heath Surveys: Basic Methods*, World Heath Organization, Geneva, Switzerland, 4th edition, 1997.

[23] A. N. Haas, E. J. Gaio, R. V. Oppermann, C. K. Rösing, J. M. Albandar, and C. Susin, "Pattern and rate of progression of periodontal attachment loss in an urban population of South Brazil: A 5-years population-based prospective study," *Journal of Clinical Periodontology*, vol. 39, no. 1, pp. 1–9, 2012.

[24] P. C. Narvai and P. Frazão, "Oral health in Brazil far beyond the palate," Rio de Janeiro: Editora Fiocruz; 2008.

[25] R. J. De Marchi, J. B. Hilgert, F. N. Hugo, C. M. D. Santos, A. B. Martins, and D. M. Padilha, "Four-year incidence and predictors of tooth loss among older adults in a southern Brazilian city," *Community Dentistry and Oral Epidemiology*, vol. 40, no. 5, pp. 396–405, 2012.

[26] P. C. Narvai, P. Frazão, A. G. Roncalli, and J. L. F. Antunes, "Dental caries in Brazil: decline, polarization, inequality and social exclusion," *Revista Panamericana de Salud Pública*, vol. 19, no. 6, pp. 385–393, 2006.

[27] E. Bernabé and A. Sheiham, "Tooth loss in the United Kingdom - Trends in social inequalities: An age-period-and-cohort analysis," *PLoS ONE*, vol. 9, no. 8, Article ID e104808, 2014.

[28] M. H. Baldani, W. H. Brito, J. A. C. Lawder, Y. B. E. Mendes, F. F. M. Silva, and J. L. F. Antunes, "Individual determinants of dental care utilization among low-income adult and elderly individuals," *Revista Brasileira de Epidemiologia*, vol. 13, no. 1, pp. 150–162, 2010.

13

A Therapeutic Educational Program in Oral Health for Persons with Schizophrenia

Audrey Peteuil,[1] Corinne Rat,[2] Sahar Moussa-Badran,[3] Maud Carpentier,[4] Jean-François Pelletier,[5] and Frederic Denis ⓘ[2,3,6]

[1]Instance Régionale d'Éducation et de Promotion de la Santé, 21000 Dijon, France
[2]Clinical Research Unit, La Chartreuse Psychiatric Centre, 21033 Dijon, France
[3]UFR Odontology and Public Health Department, 1 Avenue du Maréchal Juin, F-51095 Reims, France
[4]Direction de la Recherche Clinique, University Hospital of Dijon, 21079 Dijon, France
[5]Department of Psychiatry, Montreal University, Yale Program for Recovery and Community Health, Montreal, Canada
[6]EA 75-05 Education, Ethique, Santé, Université François-Rabelais Tours, Faculté de Médecine, 37032 Tours, France

Correspondence should be addressed to Frederic Denis; f.f.denis@orange.fr

Academic Editor: Maha El Tantawi

Objective. The aim of this study was to test the feasibility of a therapeutic educational program in oral health (TEPOH) for persons with schizophrenia (PWS). *Design.* In a qualitative study, we explored the representation of oral health before and after a TEPOH. *Clinical Setting*: PWS are at greater risk of decayed and missing teeth and periodontal diseases. In a previous publication, we described the different steps in building a TEPOH by taking into account the experiences of PWS concerning oral health quality of life. This TEPOH aimed at promoting a global health approach. *Participants*: Voluntary PWS and their caregivers were recruited during face-to-face interviews at "Les Boisseaux" (a psychiatric outpatient centre) in Auxerre (France) and were included in the study between November and December 2016. *Intervention*: We explored the experiences of participants and their perceptions of oral health before and after the TEPOH with focus group meetings. *Results.* Four females and three males participated in the study, and the mean age was 29.4 ± 5. Before the TEPOH, the PWS produced 28 ideas about oral health perception and 37 after the TEPOH. After the TEPOH, elements relating to the determinants of oral health (smoking and poor diet) emerged. *Conclusions.* These results show an evolution in oral health representation, and after some adjustments to the TEPOH, the second step will be to test this program in a large sample to generate a high level of evidence of the impact of TEPOH in the long term.

1. Background

Analysis of the literature shows a gap in health between persons with severe mental illnesses, such as schizophrenia, and the general population. The life expectancy of people with severe mental illnesses is 15 to 20 years shorter than that of the general population, and they are more prone to excess morbidity [1]. In oral health, descriptive studies indicated that this population is also at a greater risk of developing tooth decay, missing teeth, and periodontal diseases [2]. Oral health as part of the general health of persons with schizophrenia (PWS) involves complex interactions between their mental illness, the social and medical support systems

in which these people live, and the health care they receive [3]. PWS frequently do not recognize their health need along with the adverse effects of the different psychiatric treatments, like hyposalivation induced by antipsychotics [4] or hypersalivation with clozapine [5]. Other side effects do occur. First-generation antipsychotics can induce neurological effects (e.g., dystonia and dyskinesia), especially shaking, which prevents effective tooth brushing and impairs chewing and swallowing [6]. Second-generation antipsychotics tend to induce metabolic side effects, such as obesity or diabetes, rather than neurological effects [7]. Periodontal disease is associated with metabolic side effects [8], and it is now generally accepted that poor oral health is associated with chronic medical conditions such as myocardial infarction and stroke.

Evidence suggested that mental health risk factors may be associated with oral symptoms [9]. PWS are recognized as a priority group in need of support to improve oral health. However, Khokhar et al. noted that there are currently no studies supporting the need for routine clinical practices in this field [10].

A report by the Kings Fund (2016) in Australia "Bringing together physical and mental health: A new frontier for integrated care" argues that there needs to be a stronger focus on the integration of physical and mental health and that this aspect of integration should lead to the development of new models of care for all nurses and other health care professionals to address existing health inequalities [11].

In a previous publication, we described a study protocol to assess the effectiveness of a therapeutic educational programme in oral health (TEPOH) for PWS in France, with a cluster randomized controlled trial. We also explained the different steps necessary for building a TEPOH while accounting for the experiences of PWS in oral health quality of life and their active participation in the building process of the TEPOH. This TEPOH was aimed at promoting a global health approach and developing appropriate strategies to encourage multidisciplinary treatment of dental disorders, prospective support for PWS, and the development of training in oral health or mental health caregivers [12]. The TEPOH consisted of three workshops: an introductory session and a debriefing session each lasting 90 min and 2 weeks apart. The different themes of the workshops were mobilization of motivational approaches by improving self-esteem and well-being, called "Yes we can". The second was demystifying dental surgery and was called "Even more afraid". The third theme was improvement of oral health by a transverse approach to quality of life (cessation of smoking, controlling diabetes, management of good diet, etc.) and was called "Take care of myself" [12].

However, before assessing the effectiveness of this programme in a large sample, it was necessary to test the programme in real conditions with a cluster of PWS.

Therefore, the aim of this study was to test in a qualitative study the feasibility of the TEPOH through the evaluation of oral health in a sample of PWS.

2. Methods and Materials

2.1. Patients. Voluntary PWS (7) and their caregivers were recruited following face-to-face interviews at "Les Boisseaux" (a psychiatric outpatient centre) in Auxerre (France) and were included in the study between November and December 2016. The inclusion criteria were patients over 18 years of age with a diagnosis of schizophrenia, according to the Diagnostic and Statistical Manual of Mental Disorder-Fifth edition: DSM-5 [13]. Informed consent was obtained for participation in this study. The exclusion criteria were diagnosis other than schizophrenia, persons not stabilized from a psychiatric viewpoint, and patients with a decompensated organic disease and mental retardation. This decision was made by the psychiatrist of the patient. PWS who could not understand or had a poor understanding of French were excluded from the study. We confirm that participation was voluntary, that the participants could not be identified from the material presented, and that no plausible harm to participating individuals could result from the study. After providing participants with a complete description of the study, a written informed consent was obtained from each participant (or from their legal guardians for persons under guardianship).

The trial received ethical approval from the Committee for the Protection of Persons Number II of Eastern France (Approval reference: 2015-A00407-42).

2.2. Method

2.2.1. Design. We used a focus group (FG) meeting to explore the evolution of the markers of oral health before and after the TEPOH.

First, we explained the TEPOH to the PWS and their caregivers. Second, we explored the experiences of the participants and the meaning of oral health for approximately 90 min using the following questions:

(i) What do you think about your oral health?

(ii) Why you don't take care of your oral health?

(iii) Are you afraid of the dentist?

(iv) Do you think there is a link between oral health and dental health?

These open questions served to guide the interview and were selected from the qualitative study we conducted to build the TEPOH content with an expert group made up of health professionals, PWS, and PWS caregivers [12].

The post-it meeting technique was used to collect information and was classified into three categories on a paper board: positives, negatives, or neutral experiences about oral health (Figure 1(a)).

According to researchers, positive assertions were assertions made by the PWS indicating ways to improve oral health. Negative assertions were assertions made by the PWS indicating a lack of proper oral hygiene. Neutral assertions involved other topics that emerged during the FG meeting. Group interactions encouraged respondents to provide insights that would not have surfaced during individual interviews. Participants were free to talk to other group members. The FG meeting covered personal data and insights that would have been less accessible without interactions in a group setting. The FG meeting was conducted by a specialist in therapeutic education. The caregiver did not participate in the FG meeting but was solely an observer. He assisted in creating a favourable environment during the study and participated in the debriefing process with the researchers.

Third, the same specialist in therapeutic education conducted the TEPOH sessions for two weeks. Full details of this specific TEPOH for PWS are published elsewhere [12].

Fourth, at the end of the TEPOH, the same methodology as that used in the first step was used to access the evolution of markers of oral health (Figure 1(b)).

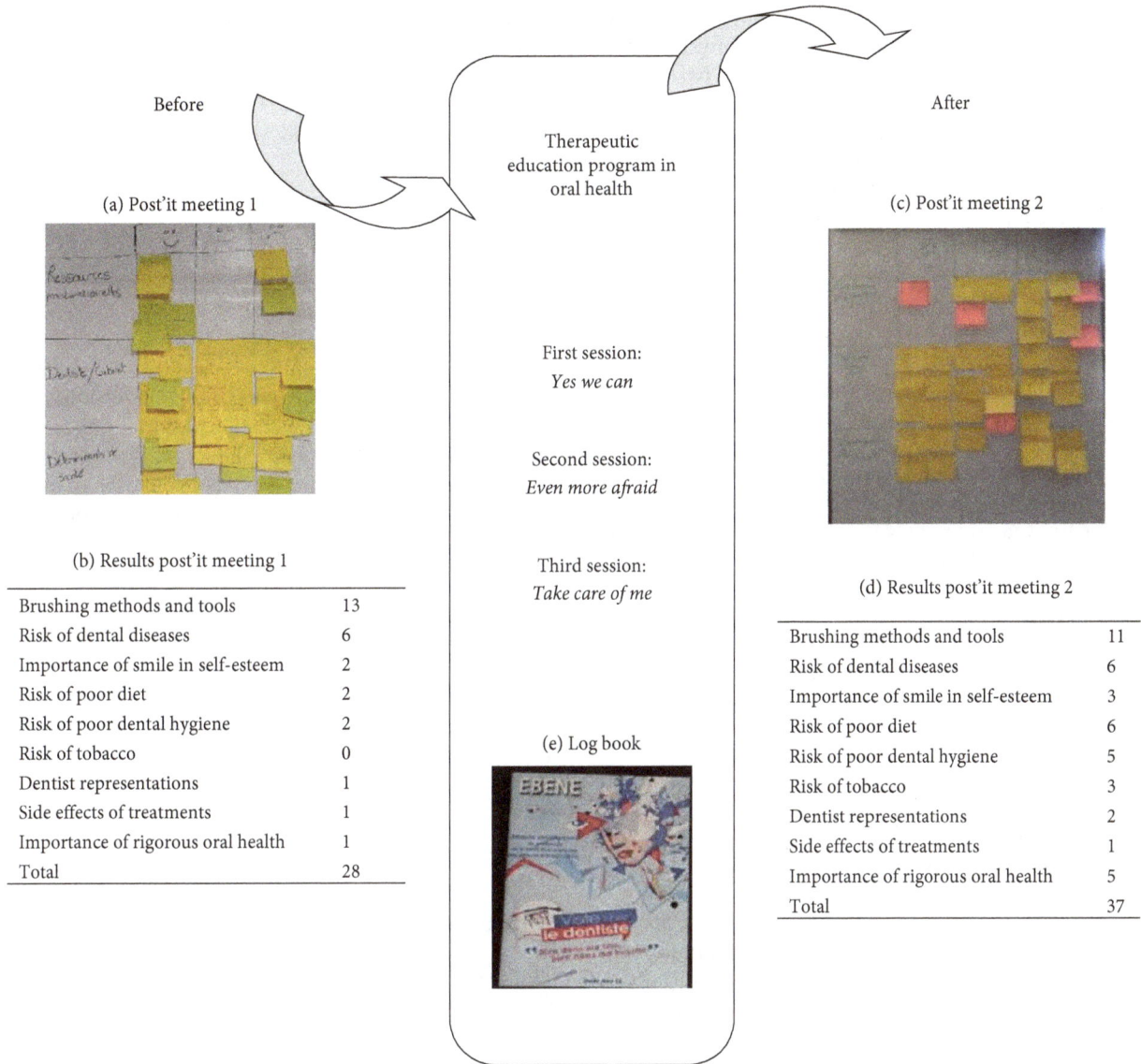

FIGURE 1: Evolution of the representations in oral health in a sample of PWS.

The audio recordings of all the FGs were analysed by a working group of researchers composed of a specialist in therapeutic education, a dentist, and a nurse specializing in mental health.

During this feasibility study, we tested the tools of the TEPOH, especially the log book for helping patients in their daily life to take care of their own oral health and the movie used to demystify dental consultations.

2.2.2. Sample Size. In total, 7 PWS participated in the two FG meetings. Generally, FGs are composed of groups of 4 to 12 people. In this case, the sample size of the FG meetings was sufficient [14]. Guest et al. [15] suggested that a sample size of two to three FGs will likely capture at least 80% of the themes. Thus, 7 individuals were sufficient to assess the feasibility of the TEPOH and to offer complimentary data for some adjustments if necessary [16].

3. Results

Four females and three males participated in this study, and the mean age was 29.4 ± 5. Before the TEPOH, the PWS produced 28 ideas regarding oral health perception (Figure 1(b)) and 37 after the TEPOH (Figure 1(d)).

One caregiver from "Les Boisseaux" (a psychiatric outpatient centre) in Auxerre (France) was present during the course of the study. This ensured proper organization of the sessions (paper board, room meeting, etc.), and the caregiver also contributed to the creation of a friendly atmosphere, thus allowing the good progress of the FG meetings. The caregiver suggested the organization of two sessions in the future in order to encourage more PWS to use the log book.

Before the TEPOH, the most frequently cited positive elements were related to the methods and tools used for tooth brushing along with the risks of dental diseases (pain, infections, etc.). We have not identified any negative assertions. All participants were motivated to improve their oral health. At this step, the determinants of oral health were not spontaneously addressed.

After the TEPOH, the elements related to the methodology of tooth brushing were less cited (13 to 11) than at the inaugural session. Conversely, the determinants of oral health (tobacco and poor diet) emerged.

These results emphasize an evolution in oral health representation, which translates, as indicated by the content and the number of words produced, into an enlargement of the general knowledge concerning the subject.

Other topics emerged (neutral) such as the cost of dental treatment and the different payment methods, which was an emergent problem for PWS.

The log book was of little use in noting the patients' efforts to improve their oral health (Figure 1(e)). Generally, the patients declared "I forgot to make it". On the contrary, the movie was a good resource to help patients demystify the process of the dental consultation.

4. Discussion

This TEPOH aimed at supporting caregivers to help patients in improving their oral health and promoting a global approach to health, not only with regard to dental care-centred approach.

We found that PWS understand that oral health can be improved by reducing tobacco consumption, with a good diet, or a good dental hygiene and that oral health can contribute to the improvement of self-esteem and oral health-related quality of life.

In this study, we noticed the motivation of the PWS to improve this health problem. The caregiver of the "Les Boisseaux" psychiatric outpatient centre was implicated in this study and helped to create a good environment to promote the programme. A key component of this TEPOH will be the long-term participation and involvement of the different health teams in introducing TEPOH in their practices to support the current practices in oral health for PWS.

This pilot study confirmed that PWS have significant knowledge of oral health, as observed during the building stage of the TEPOH [12].

It is important to take into account the cost of dental care and to introduce in the TEPOH an explanation for the different possible dental services and financial resources for PWS. In France, medical and dental care costs are partly covered in cases of conservative and surgical dental care (70%) and prosthetics and orthodontics treatment (30 to 50%) by national health insurance and complementary health insurance or by PUMa (Protection Universelle Maladie) for people with low income levels (below 8723€ per year in 2017). PUMa is free [17]. An additional module will be introduced in the TEPOH.

Although the log book has been of little use in noting the efforts to improve oral health, the chapter of the log book with guidelines for accessing a dental office gave them the confidence to engage themselves and consult a dentist more frequently. The movie helped them to further demystify this process. In a previous study conducted by our group, we confirmed the importance of an integrative guide to improve access to primary care for the management of chronic diseases and health promotion among patients with severe mental illnesses [18].

5. Limitation

Regardless of the procedure used to obtain seven patients in this qualitative study, the cohorts were composed of volunteers who differed from a representative population of PWS. Indeed, their cognitive level and oral health status may probably be higher than those observed in a representative sample of PWS. Furthermore, taking into account the small sample size of the PWS and the implementation of only two FGs, we can assume that our results are probably not exhaustive.

6. Conclusions

The TEPOH showed the capacity to improve patient knowledge and patient questioning about oral health. After some adjustments, the second step will be to test this programme in a larger sample and over a longer period of time.

Abbreviations

TEPOH: Therapeutic educational program in oral health
PWS:　　 Persons with schizophrenia
FG:　　　 Focus group
PUMa:　　 Protection Universelle Maladie.

Acknowledgments

The authors would like to thank Philip Bastable for his help with English language correction and are grateful to the French Ministry of Health (Direction Générale de l'Offre de Soins) and the University Hospital of Dijon for the support given to the study. The authors would like to especially thank the schizophrenic persons for their contribution to the study. This trial was funded by the French Ministry of Health (Direction Générale de l'Offre de Soins).

References

[1] S. Saha, D. Chant, and J. McGrath, "A systematic review of mortality in schizophrenia: is the differential mortality gap worsening over time?," *Archives of General Psychiatry*, vol. 64, no. 10, pp. 1123–1131, 2007.

[2] M. C. Wey, S. Loh, J. G. Doss et al., "The oral health of people with chronic schizophrenia: a neglected public health burden," *Australian and New Zealand Journal of Psychiatry*, vol. 50, no. 7, pp. 685–694, 2016.

[3] S. Brown, H. Inskip, and B. Barraclough, "Causes of the excess mortality of schizophrenia," *British Journal of Psychiatry*, vol. 177, no. 3, pp. 212–217, 2000.

[4] A. Bardow, B. Nyvad, and B. Nauntofte, "Relationships between medication intake, complaints of dry mouth, salivary flow rate and composition, and the rate of tooth demineralization in situ," *Archives of Oral Biology*, vol. 46, no. 5, pp. 413–423, 2001.

[5] T. E. Matos Santana, N. A. Capurso, M. Ranganathan, and G. Yoon, "Sublingual atropine in the treatment of clozapine-induced sialorrhea," *Schizophrenia Research*, vol. 182, pp. 144-145, 2017.

[6] J. Nielsen, P. Munk-Jørgensen, S. Skadhede, and C. U. Correll, "Determinants of poor dental care in patients with schizophrenia: a historical, prospective database study," *Journal of Clinical Psychiatry*, vol. 72, no. 2, pp. 140–143, 2011.

[7] D. Vancampfort, B. Stubbs, A. J. Michell et al., "Risk of metabolic syndrome and its components in people with schizophrenia and related psychotic disorders, bipolar disorder and major depressive disorder: a systematic review and meta-analysis," *World Psychiatry*, vol. 14, no. 3, pp. 339–347, 2015.

[8] E. K. Kaye, N. Chen, H. J. Cabral, P. Vokonas, and R. I. Garcia, "Metabolic syndrome and periodontal disease progression in men," *Journal of Dental Research*, vol. 95, no. 7, pp. 822–828, 2016.

[9] K. Y. Do and K. S. Lee, "Relationship between mental health risk factors and oral symptoms in adolescents: Korea Youth Risk Behavior Web-based Survey," *Community Dental Health*, vol. 4, pp. 88–92, 2013.

[10] W. A. Khokhar, A. Clifton, H. Jones, and G. Tosh, "Oral health advice for people with serious mental illness," *Cochrane Database of Systematic Reviews*, vol. 11, article 008802, 2011.

[11] P. Das, C. Naylor, and A. Majeed, "Bringing together physical and mental health within primary care: a new frontier for integrated care," *Journal of the Royal Society of Medicine*, vol. 109, pp. 364–366, 2016.

[12] F. Denis, I. Millot, N. Abello et al., "Study protocol: a cluster randomized controlled trial to assess the effectiveness of a therapeutic educational program in oral health for persons with schizophrenia," *Journal of Mental Health Systems*, vol. 10, no. 1, p. 65, 2016.

[13] American Psychiatric Association, *Desk Reference to the Diagnostic Criteria from DSM*, Vol. 5, American Psychiatric Association, Philadelphia, VA, USA, 2013.

[14] R. A. Krueger and M. A. Casey, *Focus Groups. A Practical Guide for Applied Research*, Sage Publications, Thousand Oaks, CA, USA, 2000.

[15] G. Guest, E. Namey, and K. McKenna, "How many focus groups are enough? Building an evidence base for non-probability sample sizes," *Field Methods*, vol. 29, pp. 3–22, 2017.

[16] M. Q. Patton, *Qualitative Research & Evaluation Methods*, Sage Publications, Inc, 3rd, 2002.

[17] *La-mise-en-place-de-la-Protection-Universelle-Maladie-PUMA-au-1er-janvier*, Le portail du service public de la Securite social, France, 2016, http://www.securite-social.fr/.

[18] J. F. Pelletier, A. Lesage, C. Boisvert, F. Denis, J. P. Bonin, and S. Kisely, "Feasibility and acceptability of patient partnership to improve access to primary care for the physical health of patients with severe mental illnesses: an interactive guide," *International Journal for Equity in Health*, vol. 14, no. 1, p. 78, 2015.

14

Secondary Bleedings in Oral Surgery Emergency Service

Sebastian Igelbrink,[1] Stefan Burghardt,[2] Barbara Michel,[3] Norbert R. Kübler,[2] and Henrik Holtmann ⓘ[2]

[1]Clinic for Oral and Maxillofacial Surgery, University of Münster, Albert-Schweitzer-Campus 1, 48149 Münster, Germany
[2]Clinic for Oral and Maxillofacial Surgery, University Clinic of Duesseldorf, Moorenstr 5, 40225 Duesseldorf, Germany
[3]Doctor's Practice for Oral and Maxillofacial Surgery, Uhlstraße 97, 50321 Brühl, Germany

Correspondence should be addressed to Henrik Holtmann; henrik.holtmann@med.uni-duesseldorf.de

Academic Editor: Izzet Yavuz

Introduction. Bleeding after dental surgery is still a common cause for emergency presentation in patients using anticoagulants. Our aim was to analyze pertinent characteristic features on the one hand and to bare existing problems in handling on the other. *Materials and Methods.* The study included 76 patients. We documented basic data, anticoagulant medication, type of surgery, and tooth socket sutures in respective patients. *Results.* The vast majority of patients took a coumarin derivative (41) and acetylsalicylic acid (27). Nine (12%) of the patients had to be hospitalized due to ongoing bleeding despite local haemostyptic steps and/or circulatory dysregulation. Most patients could be successfully treated in outpatient settings. No statistically significant correlation between bleeding, level of INR value, number of extracted teeth, and sewed alveoli could be shown. Sixty-five percent of cases with tooth extractions did not have suture of tooth sockets. Eighty-seven percent of the patients denied being informed about possible self-treatment options by their surgeon/dentist, and none of the patients got presurgical-fabricated bandage plate(s). *Conclusions.* Patients taking coumarin derivative currently, furthermore, represent the biggest anticoagulant after-bleeding group in dentoalveolar surgery. The major part of after-bleedings (90%) can be handled in an outpatient setting with simplest surgical interventions. Unfortunately, the biggest part of the patient collective got no suture, no prefabricated dental bandage plate(s), and no explanation by their dentist how to handle in case of after-bleeding. Therefore, dental practitioners should furthermore get enlightenment on how to prevent after-bleeding situations.

1. Introduction

Secondary bleedings after dental surgeries can lead to emergency presentation. Influencing factors include medication, the performed surgery, and patient factors. With regard to the management of perioperative coagulation, for example, the guidelines of the European Society of Cardiology (ESC) and the European Society of Anaesthesiology (ESA) state that noncardiac operations can be carried out safely at an INR of <1.5 [1]. According to the German Cardiac Society, for dentoalveolar surgery, an INR of 1.8–2.0 may be acceptable should a patient's thromboembolic risk require it [2].

Numerous papers on the issue of secondary bleeding after oral surgery [3–13] can be found in the literature. Recommendations for perioperative bleeding management especially advocate for suture of the tooth sockets following exodontia [14, 15].

However, all these works have some limitations. Some do not break down, for which surgeries were performed [11, 16]. Others focus largely or exclusively on tooth extractions [3, 5, 7–10, 13, 17]. Also, some papers do not mention their surgical management of secondary bleedings [12]. Some works mainly included patients operated on in university settings, thus reducing their validity for the nonacademic sector considerably [5, 13]. One study concludes that there is heterogeneity and poor comparability within the present literature [6].

Therefore, our study aimed to answer the following questions in particular:

(i) Which is the mean INR value in patients using phenprocoumon medication/vitamin K antagonists? (In Germany, physicians typically prescribe phenprocoumon rather than warfarin as a coumarin derivative.) In after-bleeding, is there a statistically significant difference of the INR value between cases with single- versus multiple-teeth extractions?

(ii) Do tooth-extracted patients whose alveoli were sewed over have higher INR values than patients whose alveoli were not? Are all anticoagulant patients regularly sewed over? Do they possess prefabricated bandage plates?

(iii) Does an ongoing medication with acetylsalicylic acid play numerous roles concerning anticoagulant patients and bleeding after dentoalveolar surgery?

(iv) What is the actual role in dentoalveolar secondary hemorrhage of the new direct oral anticoagulants (DOACs) in comparison to the classical ones?

(v) How extensive is the needed therapy in after-bleeding cases, and what is the percentage of patients with an inpatient treatment? What is the reason for inpatient treatment in dentoalveolar after-bleeding patients?

(vi) Are patients well informed about easy and appropriate measures which they can do on their own against bleeding by their medical practitioner who did dentoalveolar surgical intervention?

2. Materials and Methods

2.1. Study Aim, Design, and Setting. The aim was to analyze characteristic features in patients with emergency presentation due to bleedings following dental surgery. We designed a cross-sectional study at the University Clinic of Duesseldorf. The study was conducted after registration with the Ethics Committee of the Medical Faculty of the Heinrich Heine University of Duesseldorf.

2.2. Patients. All patients who presented to the Department of Oral and Maxillofacial Surgery, University Clinic of Duesseldorf, with secondary bleedings following dental surgery and use of anticoagulants were eligible. We comprised patients into the study over a period of 12 month (April 2015–March 2016).

We excluded patients with concomitant haemostaseologic or hematological diseases and those presenting with (intraoral) bleedings from tumor arrosion.

2.3. Data and Statistical Analysis. Following informed consent, we recorded demographics, surgical history (type of oral surgery performed, setting, and technique of anesthesia), anticoagulant medication, and its last intake. In cases

with phenprocoumon medication, we also recorded the initial INR value in patients' presentation. We noted the number of extracted teeth and whether the pretreating surgeon had sewed over the alveoli. In addition, we asked the patients by questionnaire and recorded whether they were informed about actions they can do on their own in case of bleeding, the reason for dentoalveolar surgery, and whether the patients were in possession of/wore presurgical dentist-fabricated bandage plate(s). Finally, we documented the ensuing surgical procedures performed in our clinic, the duration and reason of/for any inpatient stay (if necessary), and whether erythrocyte concentrates had to be given.

Statistical analysis was done using Excel 2013 (Microsoft Corporation, Redmond, Washington, USA). We calculated t-tests and selected the appropriate subtype after performing an F-test to evaluate the variance of the compared groups. Confidence intervals were calculated at 95% level. Student's t-test was chosen in case of a group size < 30. In case of a group size > 30, we assumed a normal distribution and calculated the confidence intervals accordingly. We also calculated odds ratios to compare groups. Finally, Cohen's d or Cramer's V for groups of different sizes are given to describe strengths of association between characteristics [18].

3. Results

3.1. Participants. Seventy-six patients, 51 men (67%) and 25 (33%) women, were included. The mean age of these patients was 67.5 years.

3.2. Anticoagulation. Forty-one patients stated to be taking phenprocoumon, 27 acetylsalicylic acid, 4 acetylsalicylic acid combined with clopidogrel, 2 rivaroxaban, and 2 dabigatran (Figure 1). For the indications for intake of anticoagulation, see Table 1. The mean duration of drug holiday in patients with phenprocoumon medication was 2.6 days before surgery; however, 19 patients had continued to take phenprocoumon.

3.3. Surgical History. Sixty-eight of the patients had undergone tooth extraction. Eighteen patients got their extraction(s) isolated due to caries, 43 due to a combination of caries and chronic parodontitis, and 7 due to isolated acute/chronic parodontitis (latter data: patient's self-assessment). In 2 of the remaining patients, scaling and root planing was performed, and apicoectomy was performed in 6 patients.

In the phenprocoumon patients, 8 patients had a single tooth extracted, 31 patients had multiple teeth, and 2 patients had undergone apicoectomy (Table 2). 66 (87%) of the operations had been performed in a practice, 10 (13%) of the operations in a clinic. An average of 2.9 teeth had been extracted in the exodontia patients. In only 24 (35%) of the patients after tooth extraction, the pretreating surgeons/dentists had sewed over the alveoli. In the subgroups of patients with phenprocoumon, the extraction sockets had been sewed over in 15 cases (38%) and in those with ASA medication in 6 cases (27%) (Table 3).

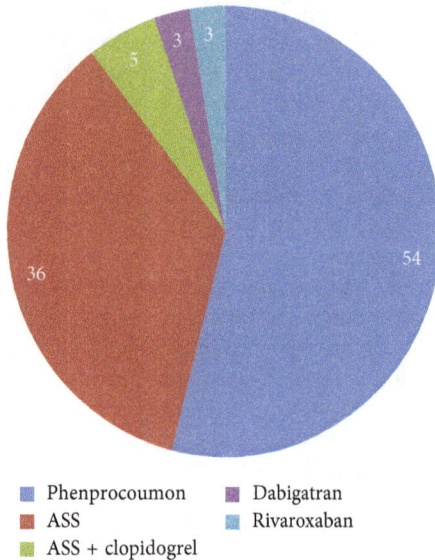

FIGURE 1: Percentages of primary anticoagulant substances taken.

Legend:
- Phenprocoumon
- ASS
- ASS + clopidogrel
- Dabigatran
- Rivaroxaban

TABLE 1: Reasons for anticoagulation (multiple entries were possible).

Stent:	10
Stroke:	5
Atrial fibrillation:	17
Valve replacement:	22
Myocardial infarction:	18
Thrombosis:	12
Others:	2

TABLE 2: Performed surgeries

Surgery	Number
Tooth extraction	68
Apicoectomy	6
Periodontal	2
Total	76

Concerning our question if patients were well informed about easy and appropriate measures which they can do on their own against bleeding by their medical practitioner who did dentoalveolar surgical intervention, 87% of the patients negated this. Furthermore, none of the presented patients declared the possession of or wore (a) presurgical-fabricated bandage plate(s).

3.4. INR. In the 41 patients of the phenprocoumon group, the mean INR was 1.9 (1.78, 2.02). The lowest INR was 1.3 and the highest INR was 3.0.

In the phenprocoumon bleeding group, the INR did not differ statistically significantly with regard to the presence of sutures of the alveoli as well as extraction of one versus multiple teeth ($p = 0.31$) (Table 4).

3.5. Further Treatment. Local ambulant treatment was sufficient in 67 (88 (81, 95) %) patients (bite swab with or

TABLE 3: Number (percentage) of extraction sockets with and without sutures in patients with respective anticoagulation.

	Suture	No suture
All	24 (35%)	44 (65%)
Phenprocoumon	15 (38%)	24 (62%)
ASA	6 (27%)	16 (73%)
ASA + clopidogrel	0 (0 %)	3 (100 %)
Dabigatran	1 (50%)	1 (50%)
Rivaroxaban	2 (100%)	0 (0%)

without tranexamic acid, suture, and haemostyptic agent). Only 9 (12 (5, 19) %) of the patients had to be hospitalized due to isolated ongoing bleeding despite local haemostyptic steps ($n = 5$) and/or circulatory dysregulation ($n = 3/n = 1$). 6 of these patients had taken phenprocoumon, 2 patients had taken acetylsalicylic acid, and 1 patient had taken clopidogrel + acetylsalicylic acid. The mean age of patients who had to be hospitalized was 68 (53.5, 82.8) years. The duration of the inpatient stay was 2.8 (2.3, 3.3) days on average. No case required the transfusion of erythrocyte concentrates.

3.6. Comparison of Patients with Consecutive Inpatient Admission with Outpatients. Patients after tooth extraction had to be admitted significantly less frequently (9% versus 38%, $\chi2$ test = 0.02, and odds ratio = 0.16), but with very weak association (Cramer's V = 0.02). Patients who were hospitalized after tooth extraction showed no statistically significantly higher extraction number (4.2 versus 2.7. $p = 0.14$). Similarly, phenprocoumon patients whose INR were not statistically significant were more likely to be hospitalized than other patients ($p = 0.49$). Patients after periodontal surgery, on the other hand, had to be admitted statistically significantly more frequently ($p < 0.001$); however, as mentioned, there were totally only 2 periodontal cases (Table 5).

In all 9 patients who were admitted, we took impressions for wound covers. Those patients following exodontia and apicoectomy also received additional sutures. In the two periodontal cases, we applied periodontal dressing (Peri-pac®, Dentsply). For residual minor bleedings, tranexamic acid gauze was used as needed (4 cases).

4. Discussion

The mean INR of phenprocoumon patients was only 1.9 (1.78, 2.02). In particular, there was no statistically significant difference in INR values between patients with single-tooth extractions and those with multiple-tooth extractions. The statistical significance was closely missed ($p = 0.08$); however, even if it had been met, the result would have had little effect as a $\chi2$ test of 0.08 was shown. An explanation for this could be that lower values rarely lead to secondary bleeding, and higher values are rare due to bridging to heparine. There was also no statistically significant difference with respect to the INR (1.94 versus 1.88, $p = 0.31$) concerning extraction patients whose alveoli were sewed and patients whose alveoli were not.

TABLE 4: INR values (phenprocoumon patients) with regard to sutures to the alveoli and extent of exodontia.

	Number	INR (mean)	Statistical test	Results
Sutures	15	1.94 (1.73, 2.15)[1]	One-sided t-test, equal variances/d_{Cohen}	0.31/0.15
No sutures	24	1.88 (1.71, 2.04)		
Single-tooth extraction	8	2.08 (1.68, 2.47)	One-sided t-test, unequal variances/d_{Cohen}	0.08/0.08
Multiple-teeth extraction	31	1.85 (1.72, 1.99)		

[1]95% confidence interval each.

TABLE 5: Statistical comparisons of patients who were admitted/were not admitted to the hospital.

	Admitted	Not admitted	Statistical test	Results
Total	9 (12 (5, 19)[1]%)	67 (88 (81, 95) %)	—	—
Mean age (years)	68	66	One-sided t-test, unequal variances/d_{Cohen}	0.46/0.05
Surgical history				
Exodontia	6 (9%)	62 (91%)	Odds ratio/$\chi2$ test/Cramer's V	0.16/0.02[2]
Number of extracted teeth (mean)	4.2	2.7	One-sided t-test, unequal variances/d_{Cohen}	0.14/0.88
Periodontal surgery	2 (100%)	0 (0%)	$\chi2$ test/Cramer's V	<0.001[2]/0.001
Apicoectomy	1 (17%)	5 (83%)	Odds ratio/$\chi2$ test/Cramer's V	1.55/0.70[2]/0.10
Anticoagulation				
Phenprocoumon	6 (15%)	35 (85%)	Odds ratio/$\chi2$ test/Cramer's V	1.83/0.41/0.07
INR (mean)	1.80	1.92	One-sided t-test, unequal variances/d_{Cohen}/d_{Cohen}	0.25/0.31
ASA	2 (7%)	25 (93%)	Odds ratio/$\chi2$ test/Cramer's V	0.48/0.37/0.07
ASA + clopidogrel[3]	1 (33%)	3 (67%)		
Dabigatran	0 (0%)	2 (100%)		
Rivaroxaban	0 (0%)	2 (100%)		

[1]95% confidence interval each; [2]expected values of the $\chi2$ test too low → limited accuracy; [3]due to very small number of cases, no further statistical testing was carried out.

At the first sight, this result seems to suggest that neither single-tooth extractions nor sutures of the alveoli allow for higher tolerable perioperative INRs. However, this conclusion would be premature: the average INR in the basic population was not known, and the same was true for the proportions of patients with sutures of the alveoli and single-tooth extractions.

The percentage of patients who had to be admitted to the hospital was 12% [5, 19] (9 patients) with no indication to blood transfusion. This correlates to the current literature which shows that in most cases of bleeding, secondary to oral surgery easy measures are enough to stop the bleeding [16, 20]. On the other hand, the small proportion of patients needing inpatient stay shows that the recommendations for the ongoing use of anticoagulants during oral surgery seems to be appropriate [16, 21, 22].

The mean age of patients (68 years) probably represents the age group affected in industrialized countries with considerably ageing populations well. This is especially true when compared to the work of Pereira et al. from Brazil [9]. In his study, the mean age of patients with phenprocoumon was 49 years.

The gender ratio of 67 : 33% men to women is consistent with the data by Koertke (approx. 70% share of men) and Maegerlein (74%) regarding phenprocoumon medication after mechanical heart valve replacement [19, 23]. The patient sample is likely to be representative for the ambulatory sector as well because of the large catchment area of a university emergency department.

A Hawthorne effect on the part of pretreating surgeons and patients can be excluded because both groups were not aware of the study before a participant's presentation to our emergency room. Furthermore, the cross-sectional design makes this effect unlikely.

Considering the study collective at all, one could find further interesting facts: first thing was that patients using DOAC up to now do not play a numerous important roles in dentoalveolar after-bleeding up to now. We could only identify four patients using them in our collective. None of them had an inpatient stay. Contrary to this fact, coumarin-intake patients took the vast majority of all after-bleeding patients (41 patients). Additionally, as mentioned before, the highest percentage of patients reported that they were not informed properly about easy measures they could do on their own against after-bleeding (87%), and none of them possessed prophylactica bandage plates. Unfortunately, 2/3 of the after-bleeding patients had no suture. The fact that 1/3 had after-bleedings despite suture may have special reasons one could speculate for: ease of the suture material perhaps due to solid food, misleading preparation and mobilization of sore rand, increase of blood pressure due to postoperative pain, inadequate sewed wounds, and basic need for more protective measures than only suture (additional need for hemostytic agents and bandage plates) in cases of extended dentoalveolar surgery. Unfortunately, these data could not be obtained in this study. Further studies could pursue these conjectures.

For inpatient treatment, phenprocoumon also numerously played the most important role. For inpatient care, no blood transfusion or antagonization of anticoagulation was necessary, which fits to the literature published before [16].

Due to the study setting with patients who had had surgery alio loco in most cases and presented in an emergency, reliable bridging protocols could not be obtained. However, such data would have had to rely solely on possibly incomplete patient information in many cases.

The vast majority of our patients had undergone extractions due to a combination of caries and parodontitis or isolated parodontitis (50/68) with a presumable higher amount of granulation tissue before extraction. Additionally, patients after periodontal surgery had to be statistically more often treated inpatient. This could present a correlation between higher amounts of infection/granulation tissue and dentoalveolar bleeding risk. Nevertheless, these findings have to be interpreted with care due to the fact that the number of inpatient treatments was small, and the statements to the reason of initial surgical intervention was made by the patients themselves and not by the primary surgeon.

5. Conclusions

Bleeding secondarily to oral surgical interventions is still an important topic to talk about although numerous papers as well as national and international guidelines are written about that.

Our data reveal that about 90% of dentoalveolar after-bleedings could be handled in an outpatient setting with simplest surgical interventions (bite swab with or without tranexamic acid, suture, hemostyptic agent, and prefabricated bandage plate by a dentist/surgeon). Furthermore, all anticoagulant patients should always be given information about easy measures against after-bleeding before surgical intervention (antiseptic mouth rinse, soft costume, external cool packs, and bite swabs) and all patients should be sewed over within surgical intervention.

The possibility to handle mostly all patients in outpatient settings by simple measures underlines current literature findings which recommend no interruption of classical or direct oral anticoagulants. An interruption could lead to strong side effects like myocardial infarction or a stroke instead. Medication should be in its therapeutic range, and patients should closely be monitored. Furthermore, a precise time planning for dentoalveolar surgery is the most important thing for patients using DOAC [16, 21].

In addition, special attention should be put on vitamin K antagonist patients as they are the most numerous populations in secondary bleeding after dental surgery in our study collective and furthermore the biggest proportion of a small population needing inpatient treatment. One should handle therefore these patients with care and discuss any surgical step with their general practitioner.

Summarizing the data of the presented study, there is an ongoing need for more clarification for dental practitioners doing dental surgery for anticoagulant patients.

Abbreviations

DOAC: Direct (new) oral anticoagulant
ESC: European Society of Cardiology
INR: International normalized ratio.

Ethical Approval

This study has been approved by the Ethics Committee of the Medical Faculty of the University of Duesseldorf (Study no. 4925R, year 2016).

Authors' Contributions

Stefan Burghardt, Sebastian Igelbrink, Henrik Holtmann, and Barbara Michel performed the literature research. Stefan Burghardt, Sebastian Igelbrink, and Henrik Holtmann conceived and designed the study. Sebastian Igelbrink collected the data. Stefan Burghardt and Sebastian Igelbrink performed statistical analysis. Sebastian Igelbrink aims to do his doctoral thesis out of the data. Henrik Holtmann wrote the draft of the manuscript. All authors read and approved the final manuscript.

References

[1] S. D. Kristensen and J. Knuuti, "ESC/ESA guidelines on non-cardiac surgery: cardiovascular assessment and management," European Heart Journal, vol. 35, no. 35, pp. 2383–2431, 2014.

[2] H. M. Hoffmeister, C. Bode, H. A. Darius, K. Huber, K. Rybak, and S. Silber, "Unterbrechung antithrombotischer Behandlung (Bridging) bei kardialen Erkrankungen," Kardiologe, vol. 4, no. 5, pp. 365–374, 2010.

[3] S. Salam, H. Yusuf, and A. Milosevic, "Bleeding after dental extractions in patients taking warfarin," British Journal of Oral and Maxillofacial Surgery, vol. 45, no. 6, pp. 463–466, 2007.

[4] C. Bacci, M. Maglione, L. Favero et al., "Management of patients undergoing anticoagulant treatment. Results from a large, multicentre, prospective, case-control study," Thrombosis and Haemostasis, vol. 104, no. 11, pp. 972–975, 2010.

[5] J. Handschel, C. Willamowski, R. Smeets et al., "Complications after oral surgery in patients with congenital or drug-induced bleeding disorders," In Vivo, vol. 25, pp. 283–286, 2011.

[6] P. Kosyfaki, W. Att, and J. R. Strub, "The dental patient on oral anticoagulant medication: a literature review," Journal of Oral Rehabilitation, vol. 38, no. 8, pp. 615–633, 2011.

[7] E. D. Karslı, Ö. Erdogan, E. Esen, and E. Acartürk, "Comparison of the effects of warfarin and heparin on bleeding caused by dental extraction: a clinical study," Journal of Oral and Maxillofacial Surgery, vol. 69, no. 10, pp. 2500–2507, 2011.

[8] Y. Morimoto, H. Niwa, and K. Minem, "Risk factors affecting postoperative hemorrhage after tooth extraction in patients receiving oral antithrombotic therapy," Journal of Oral and Maxillofacial Surgery, vol. 69, no. 6, pp. 1550–1556, 2011.

[9] C. M. Pereira, P. F. Gasparetto, D. S. Carneiro, M. E. Corrêa, and C. A. Souza, "Tooth extraction in patients on oral anticoagulants: prospective study conducted in 108 brazilian patients," ISRN Dentistry, vol. 2011, Article ID 203619, 4 pages, 2011.

[10] Y. Morimoto, H. Niwa, and K. Minem, "Risk factors affecting hemorrhage after tooth extraction in patients undergoing continuous infusion with unfractionated heparin," Journal of Oral and Maxillofacial Surgery, vol. 70, no. 3, pp. 521–526, 2012.

[11] C. Hong, J. J. Napenas, M. Brennan, S. Furney, and P. Lockhart, "Risk of postoperative bleeding after dental procedures in patients on warfarin: a retrospective study," *Oral Surgery, Oral Medicine, Oral Pathology and Oral Radiology*, vol. 114, no. 4, pp. 464–468, 2012.

[12] F. I. Broekema, B. van Minnen, J. Jansma, and R. R. Bos, "Risk of bleeding after dentoalveolar surgery in patients taking anticoagulants," *British Journal of Oral and Maxillofacial Surgery*, vol. 52, no. 3, pp. e15–e19, 2014.

[13] M. E. Prokopidi, *Postoperative Bleeding after Oral Surgeries: Causes, Risk Profile of Patients and Therapy Approaches*, Dissertation, Universität Regensburg, Regensburg, Germany, 2012.

[14] W. Reich, M. S. Kriwalsky, H. H. Wolf, and J. Schubert, "Bleeding complications after oral surgery in outpatients with compromised haemostasis: incidence and management," *Oral and Maxillofacial Surgery*, vol. 13, no. 2, pp. 73–77, 2009.

[15] C. H. Hong, J. J. Napeñas, M. T. Brennan, S. L. Furney, and P. B. Lockhart, "Frequency of bleeding following invasive dental procedures in patients on low-molecular-weight heparin therapy," *Journal of Oral and Maxillofacial Surgery*, vol. 68, no. 5, pp. 975–979, 2010.

[16] P. W. Kämmerer, B. Frerich, J. Liese, E. Schiegnitz, and B. Al-Nawas, "Oral surgery during therapy with anticoagulants-a systematic review," *Clinical Oral Investigations*, vol. 19, no. 2, pp. 171–180, 2015.

[17] D. Blinder, Y. Manor, U. Martinowitz, and S. Taicher, "Dental extractions in patients maintained on oral anticoagulant therapy: comparison of INR value with occurrence of postoperative bleeding," *International Journal of Oral and Maxillofacial Surgery*, vol. 30, no. 6, pp. 518–521, 2011.

[18] Psychometrica, *Berechnung von Effektstärken*, December 2016, https://www.psychometrica.de/effektstaerke.html.

[19] H. Koertke, A. Zittermann, G. Tenderich et al., "Low-dose oral anticoagulation in patients with mechanical heart valve prostheses: final report from the early self-management anticoagulation trial II," *European Heart Journal*, vol. 28, no. 20, pp. 2479–2484, 2007.

[20] S. Sindet-Pedersen, G. Ramström, S. Bernvil, and M. Blombäck, "Hemostatic effect of tranexamic acid mouthwash in anticoagulant-treated patients undergoing oral surgery," *New England Journal of Medicine*, vol. 320, no. 13, pp. 840–843, 1989.

[21] J. P. Patel, S. A. Woolcombe, R. K. Patel et al., "Managing direct oral anticoagulants in patients undergoing dentoalveolar surgery," *British Dental Journal*, vol. 222, no. 4, pp. 245–249, 2017.

[22] F. Fialka and F. J. Kramer, "Dental Surgery in patients receiving oral anticoagulatory drugs–guidlines and their consequences for the cooperation of general practioners and dentists," *Zeitschrift für Allgemeinmedizin*, vol. 82, no. 12, pp. 562–566, 2006.

[23] C. Maegerlein, *Blutgerinnungsmanagement nach mechanischem Herzklappenersatz*, Dissertation, Ludwig-Maximilians-Universität, München, Germany, 2009.

15

Relative Efficacy of Quercetin Compared with Benzydamine Hydrochloride in Minor Aphthae: A Prospective, Parallel, Double Blind, Active Control, Preliminary Study

Maitreyi Pandya,[1] **Anupama N. Kalappanavar,**[2]
Rajeshwari G. Annigeri,[2] **and Dhanya S. Rao**[3]

[1]*Oral Medicine and Radiology, Private Practice, New Delhi, India*
[2]*Oral Medicine and Radiology, College of Dental Sciences, Davangere, India*
[3]*Oral Medicine and Radiology, A. J. Institute of Dental Sciences, Mangalore, India*

Correspondence should be addressed to Dhanya S. Rao; dhanyarao21@gmail.com

Academic Editor: Manal Awad

Background and Objectives. Recurrent aphthous stomatitis is an inflammatory condition present since ancient era wherein numerous treatment modalities have been tried. But complete eradication of the disease has not been possible and hence newer agents are being introduced. One such agent is a flavonoid named quercetin with proven antioxidant, anti-inflammatory, and ulcer healing properties. *Methods.* 40 patients with minor aphthous ulcers were divided equally into two groups: A and B. Group A patients were advised to apply quercetin gel and Group B patients were advised to take benzydamine hydrochloride mouth wash. Clinical evaluation including assessment of ulcer size and pain score and questionnaire about the acceptability of both the drugs in terms of taste and ease of application was carried out. Each criterion was compared and statistically analyzed. *Results.* There was statistically significant reduction in the mean score of pain sensation and ulcer area in both the groups. Quercetin showed statistically highly significant ulcer size reduction as compared to benzydamine hydrochloride. *Conclusion.* From the present study, it is evident that quercetin is safe, well tolerated, and effective therapy which promotes complete ulcer healing in a short duration of time.

1. Introduction

"Medicine Is a Science of Uncertainty and an Art of Probability" *(Louis Pasteur).* Recurrent aphthous stomatitis (RAS) is one of the most common oral mucosal disorders affecting 5–25% of the general population. When specific ethnic, high socioeconomic groups or selected populations were studied, the prevalence could be as high as 50–60% [1, 2]. Patients with recurrent aphthous stomatitis experience oral pain causing discomfort, ranging from simple annoyance to an intensely painful period that interferes with normal oral activities at some time in their lives [3]. Despite extensive investigations, the exact etiology of RAS remains elusive though various factors such as local trauma, familial tendency, nutritional deficiencies, immune disturbances,

hormonal imbalance, microbial factors (both bacterial and viral), underlying systemic diseases, medications, stress, and allergy may contribute to the pathogenesis of this clinical entity [1, 2].

Treatment for oral aphthous ulcers includes antibacterial, anti-inflammatory, and analgesic mouth rinses, immunomodulators, hormones, and lasers. In patients with frequent exacerbations or more severe forms of aphthae that are unresponsive to topical treatments, systemic agents such as corticosteroids, colchicines, dapsone, or antibacterials are indicated [4]. However, the treatment of aphthous ulcers remains unsatisfactory, since both topical and systemic therapies provide only palliative care, thereby reducing only the severity of symptoms. Thus, substantial need exists for an effective and well tolerated agent that can promote complete ulcer healing within a short period of time without any side effects.

Quercetin is a naturally occurring flavonoid that has a long history of consumption as part of the normal human diet [5]. Several biological and pharmacological functions have been ascribed to quercetin, including strong antioxidant and anti-inflammatory properties [5]. Quercetin being one of the most powerful flavonoids protects the body against reactive oxygen species, by direct scavenging of free radicals. It also chelates ions of transition metals such as iron which can initiate the formation of oxygen free radicals [6] and inhibits xanthine oxidase activity and nitric oxide induced radical damage, all of which have been implicated in the etiopathogenesis of RAS [6, 7]. Tumor necrosis factor-alpha (TNF-α), an important inflammatory mediator and a critical cytokine for adequate host defense which is increased in RAU, is significantly inhibited by quercetin [8], indicating that it has the capacity to modulate the immune response and has potential anti-inflammatory activity [6, 7].

Quercetin also exerts an enzyme inhibitory action on phospholipases which catalyses the release of arachidonic acid from phospholipids stored in cell membranes thereby decreasing synthesis of thromboxane, prostaglandins, and leukotrienes [4, 5]. In addition, quercetin also inhibits the enzymes cyclooxygenase and lipooxygenase which catalyses the conversion of arachidonic acid to its metabolites suggesting it to be a potent anti-inflammatory agent [6]. Also quercetin seems to exert antimicrobial activity against many strains of bacteria, thereby removing the bacterial contamination [6]. The healing properties of quercetin include enhancement of myofibroblast and epithelial cell growth, which are vital to the tissue repair process, as suggested in a number of animal studies conducted for the management of gastric and colon ulcers [4].

Benzydamine HCL is a nonsteroidal anti-inflammatory drug which is devoid of activity on arachidonic acid metabolism [8, 9]. The anti-inflammatory activity of benzydamine has been recently related to its capacity to inhibit the production of proinflammatory cytokines (TNFa, IL-1b), without significantly affecting other inflammatory cytokines (IL-6, IL-8) and, importantly, anti-inflammatory cytokines (IL-10, IL-1ra). It has also been seen that benzydamine inhibits the migration of inflammatory leukocytes and that this effect is associated with inhibition of the mitogen-activated protein kinase (MAPK) pathway. Inhibition of MAPK activation and cell migration in response to chemotactic agents is also likely to contribute to the anti-inflammatory activity of this compound [9]. Studies have proved that benzydamine has general antimicrobial properties with a rapid biocidal activity against a variety of organisms at concentrations less than those advocated for treatment of inflammatory conditions [10]. It has been hypothesized that benzydamine produces local analgesia by stabilisation of the cellular membrane and inhibition of prostaglandin synthesis [11].

Given the adverse effects and limited efficacy of the current treatment modalities, the present study was undertaken to unearth a newer treatment modality by determining the potential healing properties of quercetin as compared to an active control drug benzydamine hydrochloride in otherwise healthy patients presenting with minor aphthous ulcers.

2. Materials and Methods

The present randomized, prospective, parallel-group, active controlled clinical study was conducted in the Department of Oral Medicine and Radiology, College of Dental Sciences, Davangere, from 2012 to 2014, wherein 40 patients with characteristic clinical features of minor aphthous ulcers and willing to undertake the treatment until complete healing of the ulcer were included. Patients with major or herpetiform aphthous ulcers, any other associated oral mucosal diseases, systemic diseases affecting healing of ulcers, and deleterious habit history of tobacco in any form and patients on other medications for minor aphthous ulcers were excluded from the study. Institutional ethical clearance was obtained and informed consent was procured from the participants of the study after explaining the entire procedure of the study. Two observers conducted the study, with one dispensing the drug and the other measuring the parameters, thereby preventing bias.

2.1. Data Collection. Patients in generally good health, irrespective of the site and gender with RAS, were selected. A diagnosis of aphthous ulcer was made if it occurred in the nonkeratinized mucosa as a shallow crateriform ulcer covered by a whitish yellow pseudomembrane and presented with a round, regular border with a surrounding erythematous halo [12].following data were recorded.

Number of Ulcers and Duration. Subjects with <3 ulcers were included for ease of assessment. Diagrammatic representation of each ulcer was done in the proforma.

Pain Intensity. It was measured using VAS consisting of a 10 cm line [13], with 0 being no pain and 10 being severe pain.

Aggravating factors like menstruation and stress were also recorded. In addition to this, patients were also questioned about the presence of any joint pain, eye or skin lesions, and gastrointestinal disturbances [1] and general physical examination was carried out to rule out the same.

Size of Each Ulcer. A transparent plastic sheet was directly applied on the ulcer and using a permanent water proof marker pen the circumference of the ulcer was traced and then placed on a graph paper and the number of mm^2 units included inside the area drawn was counted [4]. Pretreatment photographs were taken and the treatment was commenced on the same day with strict infection control measures.

2.2. Quercetin Gel: (Table 1). Hydroxyethyl cellulose and distilled water required for the gel preparation were continuously stirred by mechanical stirrer, till the polymer dissolves, and then the appropriate quantity of quercetin dissolved in small quantity of water was added, followed by methyl paraben which served as preservative, glycerine as a humectant, and peppermint oil as a flavoring agent. The prepared gel

TABLE 1: Ingredient list.

Ingredient	Quantity
Quercetin	2 g
Methyl paraben	0.01 g
Glycerine	4 g
Peppermint oil	0.02 ml
Polymer (hydroxyethyl cellulose)	100 g qs
Water	75 ml approx.

was packed in sterile 10 ml aluminum collapsible tubes and the tubes were sealed and labeled.

2.3. Drug Administration. 40 patients were randomly assigned to 2 groups, A and B. Group A patients received a gel containing approximately 2% quercetin to be applied topically on the ulcers TID for total of 7 days and were restrained from eating, drinking, or rinsing the mouth for 30 minutes after each application [14]. Group B patients received 0.15% benzydamine hydrochloride mouthwash (Tantum oral rinse) to be rinsed for 30 seconds and then expelled out, approximately 15 minutes before meals TID for 7 days [15].

Patients were recalled on 2nd, 4th, and 7th day of the treatment. Ulcer size and pain assessment was done on each visit. Allergic reaction was also monitored. At day 7 a questionnaire about the acceptability of the quercetin and benzydamine hydrochloride in terms of taste and ease of application was provided to the subject. The demographic and clinical examination data so gathered was sorted and tabulated into a master chart which was subjected to appropriate statistical analysis.

2.4. Statistical Analysis. Statistical analysis was carried out using SPSS package (version 19). Results were expressed as mean ± SD. One-way ANOVA and post hoc Tukey's test were used for groupwise comparisons. Pairwise comparison was made by paired t-test. For all the tests, a p value of 0.05 or less was considered as statistically significant.

3. Results

An age range of 9–58 years was seen, with the mean age of patients in group A being 25.1 ± 13.79 years and group B being 27 ± 13.29 years. Group A had 14 males and 6 females whereas group B had 12 males and 8 females. The mean duration of occurrence of ulcers in group A was 2.1±0.85 days and group B was 2.1 ± 0.71 days. No statistical significance with respect to gender, age, and duration of the ulcers was seen between both the groups. In group A, 12 (60%) patients showed complete ulcer healing and 8 (40%) patients showed partial ulcer healing on day 7 whereas in group B they were 7 (35%) and 13 (65%), respectively.

The mean pain score of ulcers at the baseline (1st visit) was 5.35 ± 1.84 for group A and 4.95 ± 1.7 for group B. During the treatment period, the mean pain score at day 2 (2nd visit), day 4 (3rd visit), and day 7 (4th visit) was 2.9±1.71, 0.75±1.29, and 0.1±0.44 and 3.25±1.91, 1.6±2.13, and 0.45±1.19 for groups A

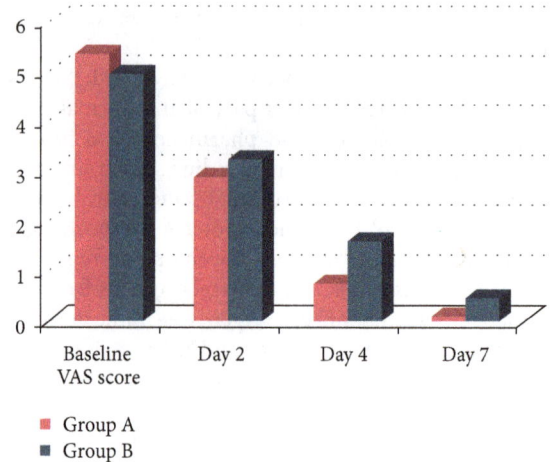

FIGURE 1: Intergroup comparison of VAS score for pain assessment.

and B, respectively. Hence, the mean reduction in pain score from baseline to day 2 was 2.45, from baseline to day 4 was 4.6, and from baseline to day 7 was 5.25 for group A and 1.7, 3.35, and 4.50 for group B. Also, the mean reduction in pain score from day 2 to day 4 was 1.65 and from day 2 to day 7 was 2.8 for group A and 1.65 and 2.8 for group B. The mean reduction in pain score from day 4 to day 7 was 0.65 for group A and 1.15 for group B. All these mean reductions were statistically highly significant ($p < 0.001$) (Figure 1). At the baseline (1st visit) the mean pain scores difference for groups A and B was 0.40. At day 2, the difference was 0.35, at day 4 difference was 0.85, and at day 7 the difference was 0.35. All these were statistically nonsignificant. The mean difference for the pain score from baseline to day 7 was 5.25 in group A and 4.5 for group B which were both statistically highly significant ($p < 0.001$). But, the mean difference for the pain score between groups A and B on day 7 was 0.35 which was not statistically significant ($p = 0.246$).

The mean score of ulcer area at the baseline for group A was 28.25 ± 6.71 whereas for group B it was 29.7 ± 8.4. During the treatment period, the mean score of ulcer area at day 2, day 4, and day 7 was 15.75 ± 4.5, 6.95 ± 2.91, and 1.3 ± 1.94, respectively, for group A and 23.1 ± 7.6, 13.8 ± 6.7, and 5.9± 6.5, respectively, for group B (Figures 2 and 3). Hence, the mean reduction in ulcer area from baseline to day 2 was 12.5, from baseline to day 4 was 21.3, and from baseline to day 7 was 26.9 for group A and 6.5, 15.9, and 23.8 for group B. Also, the mean reduction in ulcer area from day 2 to day 4 was 8.8 and from day 2 to day 7 was 14.45 for group A and 9.3 and 17.2 for group B. The mean reduction in ulcer area from day 4 to day 7 was 5.65 and 7.9 for groups A and B, respectively. All these mean reductions were statistically highly significant ($p < 0.001$). At the baseline, groups A and B had a mean difference in their ulcer area of 1.45 and it was statistically nonsignificant ($p = 0.55$). At day 2 mean difference was 7.4, at day 4 the difference was 6.85, and at day 7 the difference was 4.6. These were statistically highly significant ($p < 0.001$).

The mean difference for the ulcer size in group A from baseline to day 7 was 26.95 and in group B was 23.8. On intergroup comparison, the mean difference for the ulcer

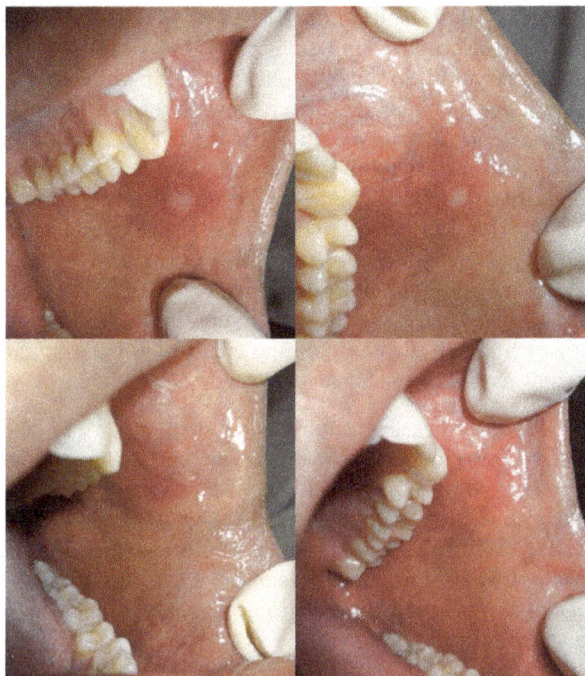

FIGURE 2: Ulcer healing seen in group A.

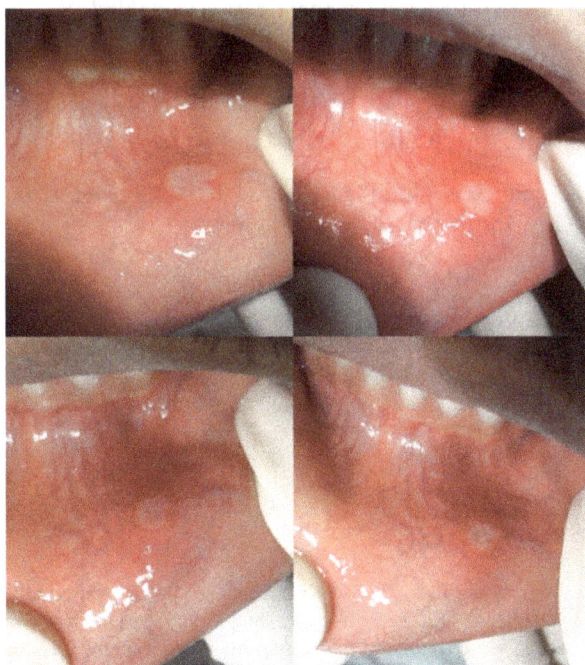

FIGURE 3: Ulcer healing seen in group B.

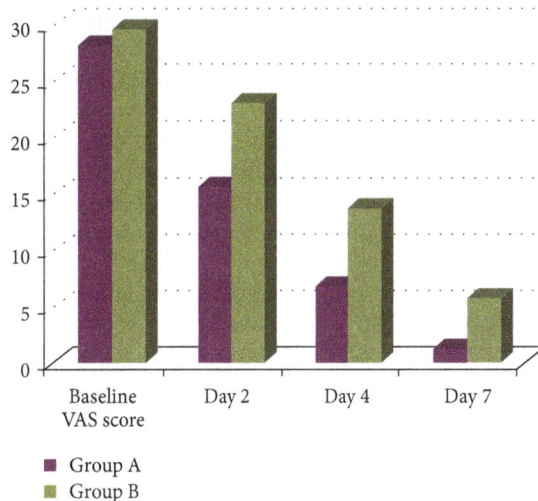

FIGURE 4: Intergroup comparison of ulcer areas (in mm^2).

4. Discussion

Aphthous stomatitis has been studied for many years by numerous investigators. Recently, oxidant-antioxidant imbalance has been given prime importance in the etiology of recurrent aphthous stomatitis [16]. Several biological and pharmacological functions have been ascribed to quercetin, including strong antioxidant and anti-inflammatory properties.

60% of patients in group A and 35% patients in group B showed complete ulcer healing on day 7. These results were similar to the study conducted by Mostafa and Ibrahem [4]. The rapid ulcer healing in the quercetin group can be attributable to the anti-inflammatory and antioxidative properties of the drug. Benzydamine, on the other hand, provides only pain relief and does not accelerate ulcer healing [17].

Pain reduction is the cornerstone in the management of RAS patients. In the present study, the study drug quercetin successfully achieved this goal by producing highly statistically significant reduction in pain scores from baseline to day 2, day 4, and day 7 during the treatment period. Similarly the active control drug benzydamine hydrochloride also showed significant pain reduction over the 7-day period, but, on intergroup comparison, there was no statistically significant difference between the two groups with regard to pain reduction. These findings were in contrast to the study conducted by Mostafa and Ibrahem [4] wherein a moderately significant difference (<0.01) was noted between the two groups. The significant pain reduction in group A could be attributable to the fact that quercetin induces an antinociceptive effect primarily by modulating the adrenergic pathways [18]. Quercetin also has a powerful anti-inflammatory action which could be responsible for the analgesia [19, 20]. Also, the rapid healing of the ulcers in this group could account for the significant decrease in the symptoms associated with it. Likewise, in case of the active control group, benzydamine hydrochloride has anti-inflammatory, analgesic, and local anaesthetic properties when applied topically [9, 11]. In a

size between groups A and B on day 7 was 4.6 which was statistically highly significant ($p < 0.001$) (Figure 4).

With regard to the taste of the gel, 80% reported good taste and with respect to the ease of application 75% found it easy to apply. With regard to the taste of the mouthwash, 74% found the taste acceptable and, with respect to the ease of application, 80% found it easy to apply.

study conducted by Matthews et al. [21], comparing the efficacy of benzydamine HCL to that of chlorhexidine and placebo groups, no statistically significant differences were noted between any of the treatments tested. Similarly in the present study too, no statistically significant difference was noted between the two groups with respect to pain reduction.

In the present study, the study drug quercetin produced highly statistically significant reduction in ulcer area from baseline to day 2, day 4, and day 7 during the treatment period. Similarly benzydamine hydrochloride also showed highly statistically significant reduction in ulcer area over the 7-day period. On intergroup comparison, the mean score of ulcer area at the baseline was statistically nonsignificant ($p = 0.55$). However, statistically highly significant difference was noted between the two groups during the subsequent visits. These findings were consistent with the study conducted by Mostafa and Ibrahem [4] wherein a highly significant difference ($p = 0.004$) was noted between the two groups for ulcer size. This clinical improvement could be due to antiulcerative action of quercetin wherein it enhances myofibroblast and epithelial cell growth, which are vital to the tissue repair process [4]. Accelerated ulcer healing also requires removal of bacterial contamination from the wound to provide favourable grounds for mucosal cell growth and repair [4]. Various studies have shown quercetin has antibacterial property as well [6]. On the other hand, benzydamine hydrochloride provides only palliative care whereby it reduces the pain perception but does not aid in the ulcer healing [16]. Furthermore, quercetin was given in the form of a gel which provided a thick encompassing coat over the ulcer area preventing it from bacterial contamination and mechanical trauma; also the retention period of a gel over the ulcer surface is more than that of a mouth rinse, thus providing prolonged therapeutic benefits.

The ease of application of benzydamine hydrochloride was better than that of the quercetin gel. This could be ascribed to the fact that benzydamine hydrochloride given in the form of a mouth rinse was more accessible to the various areas in the oral cavity as compared to quercetin which was given in a gel form. These results were found to be similar to those of Mostafa and Ibrahem [4] and Roopashri et al. [15] studies.

None of the patients in our study reported any serious side effects due to the study drugs. In the benzydamine hydrochloride group, 8 patients experienced a transient stinging sensation shortly following the rinsing with the drug. In a study conducted by Matthews et al. [21], it was noted that eight patients stated a personal preference for benzydamine because of the local anaesthetic effect of benzydamine, which gave pain relief in spite of the transient stinging sensation associated with its usage. Topical use of high potency glucocorticoids may cause oral pseudomembranous candidiasis and suppression of the HPA axis. In 2.1% of 991 patients treated with topical amlexanox, adverse effects like stinging, dryness, bumps on the lips, and mucositis were noted. Chlorhexidine mouthwash has a bitter taste and causes brown staining of the teeth and tongue. On the contrary, no adverse effects were seen in the study drug quercetin and this was consistent with the study conducted by Mostafa and Ibrahem [4].

Although the results of the study are highly encouraging, there were also a few limitations that were encountered in the present study. So far only one study using quercetin in RAS management has been documented in the literature. The sample size in the present study was small. The application of the medicament to the remote areas of the oral cavity was relatively difficult due to inaccessibility of quercetin in the gel form. The patients with multiple ulcers and major aphthous ulcers could not be included in the study for ease of assessment of the clinical parameters. Furthermore the study involved the comparison of a mouth rinse to that of a gel, which added the confounding factor of comparing two different modes of local drug delivery systems.

Further studies are recommended on a larger sample of patients, over a longer follow-up period, in a larger multicentric setup, and with the evaluation of immunological markers to maximize the sensitivity for detecting subtle changes of the mucosa during the course of the treatment. Quercetin gel is not available commercially as of now; it is recommended that commercial preparation of topical quercetin gel be made available in the near future.

In conclusion, the results from our study are highly encouraging; the use of topically applied quercetin gel has shown salutary results compared to benzydamine hydrochloride in minor RAS patients and further research with this drug entity might prove beneficial.

Ethical Approval

This study was ethically approved by College of Dental Sciences' Institutional Ethical Committee.

Acknowledgments

The authors acknowledge Department of Pharmacology, Bapuji Pharmacy College, for their timely help for gel preparation.

References

[1] G. S. Vijayabala, A. N. Kalappanavar, R. G. Annigeri, R. Sudarshan, and S. S. Shettar, "Single application of topical doxycycline hyclate in the management of recurrent aphthous stomatitis," *Oral Surgery, Oral Medicine, Oral Pathology, Oral Radiology, and Endodontology*, vol. 116, no. 4, pp. 440–446, 2013.

[2] J. A. Ship, E. M. Chavez, P. A. Doerr, B. S. Henson, and M. Sarmadi, "Recurrent aphthous stomatitis," *Quintessence International*, vol. 31, no. 2, pp. 95–112, 2000.

[3] S. Yunus, K. Basal, and O. Perihan, "Assessment of salivary serum antioxidant vitamins lipid peroxidation in patients with recurrent aphthous ulceration," *The Tohoku Journal of Experimental Medicine*, vol. 206, pp. 305–312, 2005.

[4] M. A. Mostafa and M. A. Ibrahem, "Management of aphthous ulceration with topical quercetin," *Cairo Dental Journal*, vol. 25, no. 1, p. 15, 2009.

[5] M. Harwood, B. Danielewska-Nikiel, J. F. Borzelleca, G. W. Flamm, G. M. Williams, and T. C. Lines, "A critical review of the data related to the safety of quercetin and lack of evidence of in vivo toxicity, including lack of genotoxic/carcinogenic properties," *Food and Chemical Toxicology*, vol. 45, no. 11, pp. 2179–2205, 2007.

[6] P. Lakhanpal and D. K. Rai, "Quercetin: a versatile flavonoid," *Internet Journal of Medical Update*, vol. 2, no. 2, pp. 22–37, 2007.

[7] A. Gurel, H. C. Altinyazar, M. Unalacak, F. Armutcu, and R. Koca, "Purine catabolic enzymes and nitric oxide in patients with recurrent aphthous ulceration," *Oral Diseases*, vol. 13, no. 6, pp. 570–574, 2007.

[8] M. Dogan, C. Yilmaz, H. Caksen, and A. S. Guven, "A case of benzydamine HCL intoxication," *Eastern Journal of Medicine*, vol. 11, pp. 26–28, 2006.

[9] E. Riboldi, G. Frascaroli, P. Transidico et al., "Benzydamine inhibits monocyte migration and MAPK activation induced by chemotactic agonists," *British Journal of Pharmacology*, vol. 140, no. 2, pp. 377–383, 2003.

[10] N. H. Fanaki and M. A. El-Nakeeb, "Antimicrobial activity of benzydamine, a non-steroid anti-inflammatory agent," *Journal of Chemotherapy*, vol. 4, no. 6, pp. 347–352, 1992.

[11] A. Valijan, "Pain relief after tonsillectomy Effect of benzydamine hydrochloride spray on postoperative pain relief after tonsillectomy," *Anaesthesia*, vol. 44, no. 12, pp. 990-991, 1989.

[12] T. F. Meiller, M. J. Kutcher, C. D. Overholser, C. Niehaus, L. G. DePaola, and M. A. Siegel, "Effect of an antimicrobial mouthrinse on recurrent aphthous ulcerations," *Oral Surgery, Oral Medicine, Oral Pathology, Oral Radiology, and Endodontology*, vol. 72, no. 4, pp. 425–429, 1991.

[13] A. Khandwala, R. G. Van Inwegen, and M. C. Alfano, "5% amlexanox oral paste, a new treatment for recurrent minor aphthous ulcers: I. Clinical demonstration of acceleration of healing and resolution of pain," *Oral Surgery, Oral Medicine, Oral Pathology, Oral Radiology, and Endodontology*, vol. 83, no. 2, pp. 222–230, 1997.

[14] S. S. Natah, Y. T. Konttinen, N. S. Enattah, N. Ashammakhi, K. A. Sharkey, and R. Häyrinen-Immonen, "Recurrent aphthous ulcers today: a review of the growing knowledge," *International Journal of Oral and Maxillofacial Surgery*, vol. 33, no. 3, pp. 221–234, 2004.

[15] G. Roopashri, K. Jayanthi, and R. Guruprasad, "Efficacy of benzydamine hydrochloride, chlorhexidine, and povidone iodine in the treatment of oral mucositis among patients undergoing radiotherapy in head and neck malignancies: A drug trail," *Contemporary Clinical Dentistry*, vol. 2, no. 1, pp. 8–12, 2011.

[16] S. Saxena, "Assessment of plasma and salivary antioxidant status in patients with recurrent aphthous stomatitis," *RSBO*, vol. 8, no. 3, pp. 261–265, 2011.

[17] C. Scully and S. Porter, "Oral mucosal disease: recurrent aphthous stomatitis," *British Journal of Oral and Maxillofacial Surgery*, vol. 46, no. 3, pp. 198–206, 2008.

[18] R. Kaur, D. Singh, and K. Chopra, "Participation of $\alpha2$ receptors in the antinociceptive activity of quercetin," *Journal of Medicinal Food*, vol. 8, no. 4, pp. 529–532, 2005.

[19] M. Hämäläinen, R. Nieminen, P. Vuorela, M. Heinonen, and E. Moilanen, "Anti-inflammatory effects of flavonoids: Genistein, kaempferol, quercetin, and daidzein inhibit STAT-1 and NF-κB activations, whereas flavone, isorhamnetin, naringenin, and pelargonidin inhibit only NF-κB activation along with their inhibitory effect on iNOS expression and NO production in activated macrophages," *Mediators of Inflammation*, vol. 2007, Article ID 45673, 10 pages, 2007.

[20] http://examine.com/supplements/Quercetin/#thingstoknow.

[21] R. W. Matthews, C. M. Scully, B. G. H. Levers, and W. S. Hislop, "Clinical evaluation of benzydamine, chlorhexidine, and placebo mouthwashes in the management of recurrent aphthous stomatitis," *Oral Surgery, Oral Medicine, Oral Pathology, Oral Radiology, and Endodontology*, vol. 63, no. 2, pp. 189–191, 1987.

16

Teeth and Covariates: Association with Risk of Falls

Shivani Kohli[iD],[1] **Aaron Lam Wui Vun,**[2] **Christopher Daryl Philip**[iD],[2]
Cassamally Muhammad Aadil[iD],[2] **and Mahenthiran Ramalingam**[iD][2]

[1]*Department of Prosthodontics, Faculty of Dentistry, MAHSA University, Selangor, Malaysia*
[2]*Faculty of Dentistry,MAHSA University, Selangor, Malaysia*

Correspondence should be addressed to Shivani Kohli; shivani@mahsa.edu.my

Academic Editor: Manal Awad

Purpose. Falls occur commonly in geriatric populations and undesirably influence their life, morbidity, and mortality. The aim of this study was to analyze the association between the number of teeth present among the elderly population and covariates in relation to the risk of falls. *Materials and Methods.* This study was conducted at various old age homes in the Klang Valley region of Malaysia involving the geriatric population aged 60 years and above. A detailed questionnaire consisting of sociodemographic data including sex, age, household income, and dental variables such as the number of teeth and chewing difficulty was obtained. The Tinetti test (TT) was used to evaluate the patients' ability to walk, to maintain postural balance, and to determine their risk of falling. The short version of the Geriatric Depression Scale was used to assess depression among the participants, and the Barthel Scale was used to analyze the subject's ability to perform the activities of daily living (ADL). *Results.* Statistically significant association was observed in relation to the number of teeth present and risk of falls ($p < 0.05$). Subjects who had 19 teeth or less in total had moderate to highest risk of falls ($p = 0.001$) in comparison with subjects who had 20 teeth or more. Those aged 70 years and above showed the highest risk of falls ($p = 0.001$) in comparison with the subjects aged between 60 and 69 years. Subjects with depression ($p = 0.03$) and presence of illness related to fall showed statistically significant difference ($p = 0.001$) in comparison with those who did not suffer from the same. Compromised ADL ($p = 0.001$) (which included ability to perform several tasks like indoor mobility, climbing stairs, toilet use, and feeding) and low monthly income ($p = 0.03$) was also observed among subjects who had higher risk of falls. *Conclusion.* According to the results achieved, there was a high statistically significant association observed between the number of teeth present, age, depression, ADL, and presence of illness in relation to the risk of falling among the geriatric population. Henceforth, oral rehabilitation of elderly patients with less number of teeth may reduce their risk of falls.

1. Introduction

According to the World Health Organization (WHO), falls are defined as "inadvertently coming to rest on the ground, floor or other lower level, excluding intentional change in position to rest in furniture, wall or other objects" [1]. Falls have been reported to be a common problem among older people and can be the cause of morbidity and mortality among the later [2]. Incidence of falls of older people is increasing with increasing age and with increasing frailty and dependency. Elderly residents staying in the old age home are approximately three times more prone to falling in comparison with those staying in the community; such falls might even result in bone fracture or hospital admission [3].

Fall incidents may result in hip fracture, joint dislocations, brain injury, facial fracture (head injuries), lower extremity fracture, forearm/wrist fracture, humeral fracture, rib/scapular fracture, severe lacerations, and other soft tissue injuries [4, 5]. Subsequently, falls may restrict daily activities such as bathing, feeding, or dressing and increase the risk of admission to a nursing home [6]. Falls also increase the use of long-term medical services and account for significant care costs [4].

Risk factors for fall injuries have been identified by a number of studies which include older age, white race, arthritis, cerebrovascular disease depression, history of falls, and mainly impairment of muscle strength and balance [7–9]. In view of these risk factors, fall prevention programs have been carried out in the past; however, as they were ineffective, additional risk factors must be investigated [10].

The number of elderly people within a population has been reported to be rising in developing countries including Malaysia [11]. Demographers have estimated that, by the year 2020, almost 10% of Malaysian population will be 60 years and above [12] and aging may also have a detrimental effect on the oral tissues and functions [13]. The elderly are at higher risk of chronic diseases such as dental infections, benign mucosal lesions, xerostomia, and oral candidiasis wherein tooth loss due to caries or periodontal disease has been generally reported as the most common oral condition [14].

Gangloff has investigated the relationship of dental occlusion on gaze and posture stabilization in order to maintain balance and proprioception [15]. Proprioception of the mandible includes the masticatory muscular system and dentoalveolar ligaments (innervation from the trigeminal nerve) which provide sensory afferent input to the central nervous system via vestibular and visual receptors [16]. Alteration in chewing due to lesions in the masticatory muscles or dentoalveolar ligaments could also result in postural imbalances [15]. The effect of different mandibular positions (altered by occlusal collapse) on body equilibrium has also been investigated in the past [17]. Urbanowicz stated that the changes in vertical dimension of occlusion could cause change in head and neck posture [18]. Okuyama et al. associated the loss of dental occlusion with balance function and decline in lower extremities dynamic strength which was the prerequisite for neuromuscular capacity to prevent fall [19]. Several studies have reported the influence of occlusal condition on motor performances and muscle strength of the extremities [20]. However, whether or not the loss of teeth actually predicts the risk of falls is largely unknown. Therefore, the aim of this study was to investigate the influence of the number of teeth present and its covariates in relation to the risk of falls among the elderly aged 60 years and above within Klang Valley region, Malaysia.

2. Materials and Methods

This cross-sectional study was conducted over a period of 6 months involving the elderly aged 60 years and above residing in the various cities and towns of the Klang Valley region which was densely populated with a population of approximately 6 million people. The Klang Valley region consists of Wilayah Persekutuan Kuala Lumpur, Wilayah Putrajaya, and subdistricts of Selangor state (Gombak, Hulu Langat, Sepang, Petaling, and Klang).

The study was conducted through one-on-one interview technique, and different tests were performed by the participants which were assessed by the evaluator. Informed consent forms were provided to the participants (either verbal or written) prior to interviews. Subjects aged 60 years and older, both genders, and from any racial background in the Klang Valley region were included. Subjects suffering from physical or cognitive disabilities and those who could not verbally communicate or refused to participate were excluded from the study. The time taken for the interview was based on how fast the participants could respond to the specific question and

their capability to perform the physical test; it took approximately 30 minutes per participant to conduct the study. Ethical clearance was obtained from the MAHSA Research Review Committee prior to the commencement of this research.

2.1. Study Sample and Recruitment. The sample size was calculated using sample size formula for finite population. The present geriatric population aged 60 and above within the Klang Valley was estimated to be 395276 people according to the latest reports of the Department of Statistics, Malaysia Official Website updated in 2011. The prevalence of home injuries among the elderly in Malaysia was reported as $p = 5.8\%$ and 95% confidence intervals (CI) in accordance with the study conducted among the elderly people in Malaysia by Lim et al. in 2013 [21].

Normal deviation corresponding to 95% CI [t] was set as 1.96, and the absolute error [d] was set to 5%. q is $[1 - p]$. The total geriatric sample size was estimated to be 77, which was reconfirmed with RAOSOFT calculator, an online calculator used to calculate sample size estimation:

$$\frac{Nt^2 pq}{d^2 [N-1] + t^2 pq}. \tag{1}$$

Convenience sampling technique was used for data collection. Old age homes in the Klang Valley regions were identified; potential participants were initially screened according to eligibility criteria. The interview was conducted using the English, Malay, or Chinese version of the study information based on the participant's language preference.

2.2. Study Variables and Questionnaire. A detailed questionnaire consisting of sociodemographic data including sex, age, household income, and dental variables such as the number of teeth present were obtained from the participants by the interviewer. The number of teeth present were observed by the interviewer and categorized into 4 groups: subjects having 20 natural teeth or more, 19 natural teeth or fewer with dentures, 19 natural teeth or fewer without dentures, and absence of teeth as missing.

The participants' ability to masticate was ascertained by asking questions such as "Can eat everything?", "Can eat most food?", "Cannot eat most food?", or "Cannot eat at all?" Their responses were received and evaluated accordingly.

There are studies in the past showing association of falls with sex [7, 21], age [4, 7], activities of daily living [1, 21, 22], depression [4], personal health [21], and movement and socioeconomic factors [23]. Hence, all these parameters were also analyzed in this study. Self-reported current medical conditions such as stroke, osteoporosis, joint disease, neuralgia, and fracture were also recorded as conditions responsible for presence of illness related to fall.

The Tinetti test (TT) was used to evaluate patients' ability to walk, maintain postural balance, and determine their risk of fall [24]. Firstly, the participants were asked to perform the gait component of the test wherein the evaluator walked closely behind the subject to evaluate any abnormality in the gait (steppage) and drift, following which the balance

TABLE 1: Master chart of number of teeth present and covariates in relation to the risk of fall.

Master chart	Total	Tinetti test (TT)		
		Lowest risk of falls	Moderate risk of falls	Highest risk of falls
Total number of teeth present				
≥20 natural teeth	28	17 (60.7)	5 (17.9)	6 (21.4)
≤19 natural teeth with dentures	34	25 (73.5)	3 (8.8)	6 (17.6)
≤19 natural teeth without dentures	42	13 (31.0)	7 (16.7)	22 (52.4)
Missing	6	4 (66.7)	0	2 (33.3)
Chewing difficulty				
Can eat everything	41	25 (61.0)	10 (24.4)	6 (14.6)
Can eat most foods	39	21 (53.8)	0	18 (46.2)
Cannot eat most foods	28	12 (42.9)	4 (14.3)	12 (42.9)
Cannot eat at all	2	1 (50)	0	1 (50)
Sex				
Male	48	26 (54.2)	6 (12.5)	16 (33.3)
Female	62	33 (53.2)	8 (12.9)	21 (33.9)
Presence of illness related to fall				
Yes	21	4 (19.1)	4 (19.1)	13 (61.9)
No	89	55 (61.8)	10 (11.2)	24 (27.0)
Activity of daily living				
Dependent	29	6 (20.7)	5 (17.2)	18 (62.1)
Independent	81	53 (65.4)	9 (11.1)	19 (23.5)
Use of drugs				
Yes	73	35 (47.9)	11 (15.1)	27 (37.0)
No	37	24 (64.9)	3 (8.1)	10 (27.0)
Self-evaluated health				
Excellent	8	2 (25)	2 (25)	4 (50)
Good	62	39 (62.9)	9 (14.5)	14 (22.6)
Fair	39	17 (43.6)	3 (7.7)	19 (48.7)
Poor	1	1 (100)	0	0
Monthly household income (Malaysian ringgit)				
<500	93	46 (49.5)	13 (14)	34 (36.6)
500–999	4	4 (100)	0	0
1000–1999	5	3 (60)	1 (20)	1 (20)
>2000	8	6 (75)	0	2 (25)

component was executed wherein they performed standing, sitting, and other different actions. Scores of both the components were totaled to determine the level of dependence and risk of falls. The subjects with the highest risk of falls obtained the lowest scores (≤18); moderate risk consisted of people with scores of 19–23 points, which reflected moderate dependence and falling risk; and the group with minimal risk had scores of ≥24 points. To assess depression among the participants, the short version of the Geriatric Depression Scale with fifteen questions constructed for simple answering by means of a straightforward yes/no format was used. It was classified into three groups: 0–4 (no depression), 5–9 (mild depression), and 10–15 (moderate to severe depression). The Barthel Scale was used to analyze subjects' ability to perform the activities of daily living (ADL) which included several tasks like indoor mobility, climbing stairs, toilet use, and feeding [24]. Accordingly, the subjects were categorized as "dependent" or "independent" based on their performances.

2.3. Statistical Analysis. Data obtained were tabulated and analyzed using Statistical Package of Social Science version 22, with significance level of 0.05 and 95% confidence intervals. To test the association between the variables and risk of falls, Pearson's chi-square test and Fisher's exact test were employed. Additionally, all covariates were analyzed individually with the risk of falls. Univariate analysis was done to study the relationship between all the variables and risk of fall.

3. Results

Out of the 154 participants encountered, 110 were eligible to participate in the study, while others were disqualified according to the exclusion criteria. In order to calculate the p value together with the odds ratio and 95% confidence interval for univariate analysis, the total number of teeth present were grouped into subjects having 20 natural teeth or more with or without dentures and 19 natural teeth or less with or without dentures, while the age was grouped into 70 years and above and 60 to 69 years.

Table 1 shows the master chart of the number of teeth present and covariates in relation to the risk of fall wherein 36 (32.73%) out of 110 respondents reported having high risk of fall. It also showed that subjects with less number of teeth, chewing difficulty, older age, females, presence of

TABLE 2: Univariate associations of the number of teeth present and covariates with risk of falls.

Covariates	Total	Risk of falls (TT)		p value	OR	95% CI
		Lowest risk of falls	Moderate to highest risk of falls			
Total number of teeth present						
20 teeth or more with/without denture	62	42	20	0.001	0.26	0.12–0.58
19 teeth or less with/without denture	48	17	31			
Age						
70 years old and above	53	17	36	<0.001	5.92	2.59–13.52
60 to 69 years old	57	42	15			
Sex						
Male	48	26	22	0.92	0.9629	0.45–2.05
Female	62	33	29			
Depression						
No	98	56	42	0.03*	0.25	0.06–0.98
Mild to severe	12	3	9			
Presence of illness related to fall						
Yes	21	4	17	0.001	6.87	2.13–22.15
No	89	55	34			
Activity of daily living (ADL)						
Dependent	29	6	23	<0.001	7.25	2.64–19.89
Independent	81	53	28			
Use of drugs						
Yes	73	35	38	0.09	2.00	0.88–4.53
No	37	24	13			
Self-evaluated health						
Healthy	70	41	29	0.16	0.57	0.26–1.26
Not very healthy	40	18	22			
Monthly household income (Malaysian ringgit)						
500 or less	93	46	47	0.03	3.32	1.00–10.93
501 or more	17	13	4			

*Calculated using Fisher's exact test.

illness, compromised daily activity, and low monthly income were associated with the risk of falling.

Table 2 shows univariate associations of the number of teeth present and covariates with risk of falls. Subjects having 19 natural teeth or less with or without using dentures have moderate to highest risk of falls (OR 0.27, 95% CI 0.12 to 0.58, $p = 0.001$) compared with those having 20 natural teeth or more with or without dentures. Those aged 70 years and above showed a significant result (OR 5.92, 95% CI 2.59 to 13.52, $p = 0.001$). Participants with depression showed positive association with risk of falls compared to those without depression (OR 0.25, 95% CI 0.06 to 0.98, $p = 0.03$). Subjects with presence of illness related to fall also showed statistically notable relationship (OR 6.87, 95% CI 2.13 to 22.15, $p = 0.001$). Activity of daily living also had a significant relation to risk of fall (OR 7.25, 95% CI 2.64 to 19.89, $p < 0.001$). The monthly household income was also recorded to be a crucial factor in relation to the risk of fall (OR 3.32, 95% CI 1.00 to 10.93, $p = 0.03$). There is no significant association observed between risk of fall and chewing difficulty, sex, use of drugs, and self-evaluated health.

4. Discussion

This was a pilot study to evaluate relationship between remaining teeth and risk of falling among Malaysian elderly population. The present study showed that there was an association between the total number of teeth present and risk of falls. Subjects with 19 or fewer teeth (teeth include both natural and artificial) had a considerably high risk of falls compared to those with more than 20 teeth along with other various extraneous variables such as age, physical health, and household income.

These findings were compatible with the longitudinal cohort study conducted by Yamamoto et al. among Japanese population aged 65 years and above which showed that participants with 19 or lesser number of teeth who were not using partial or complete dental prosthesis (dentures) had more chances of falling compared to people having 20 or more number of teeth [25]. Another longitudinal study by Yoshida et al. [26] conducted among 146 elderly with dementia showed that subjects with functionally inadequate dental status had higher significance of frequent falls compared to those with functionally adequate occlusion composed of natural teeth, denture, or both. They also discovered that falling risk among the geriatric population having 19 remaining teeth or less in total will not increase even if they wear dentures. Such outcomes propose that poor occlusion due to the loss of teeth and without replacing will increase the risk of falling among the elderly subjects with 19 or lesser number of teeth.

There are several possible pathways that relate dentition and incidence of falls, as it is known that falls occur due to loss of balance [22, 27, 28]. Balance is gained through various types of sensory information emanating from proprioceptive systems. The stomatognathic system (maxilla and mandible, dental arches, salivary glands, nervous and vascular supplies, temporomandibular joint, and masticatory muscles) may affect muscular function in other parts of the body, range of movement, and balance control [15, 23, 29–31]. Dental occlusion does influence postural stabilization through sensory afferent input from the ligaments around the teeth and the masticatory system. Consequently, improper occlusion may reduce the proprioception and interfere with the head stabilization [19]. Miyaura et al. in 2000 also showed that denture use improves postural balance [32].

In the present study, self-reported chewing difficulty was not associated with the risk of falls. This result was similar to the study conducted by Yamamoto et al. in 2012 [25] but was in contrast with another study conducted by Takata et al. [31] in 2004 which showed significant association between chewing ability and balance, as self-reported chewing ability can be very subjectively answered based on the type of food intake (soft food or solid food).

Brito et al. in 2014 reported the occurrence of falls was accompanied with depressive symptoms and disturbances in balance as recorded in the present study [33]. Fall happens more often to people with lower functional status which was similar to the results obtained in this study [34]. For the other covariates discussed in this present study, the gender was not the risk factors for fall which is in accordance with existing scientific guidelines for prevention of falls [22, 35]. Self-reported finding such as general health was the limitation of the present study. Future study with a larger sample size would be more helpful to confirm the impact of different variables in relation to the risk of fall among the elderly.

5. Conclusion

The purpose of this study was to evaluate the importance of the presence of teeth among the geriatric population, and care should be taken to preserve them in order to reduce their risk of falls. Highly statistically significant association was observed between the number of teeth present and the risk of fall; hence, dental health education including taking care of own teeth, yearly dental checkup, and proper use of denture may help in preventing falls. Among the covariates, statistically significant association was seen between age, depression, presence of illness related to fall, ADL, and household income in relation to the risk of fall. Retrospectively, people with high risk of falling may be identified through dental checkup, and oral rehabilitation can be done to reduce their risk of falls. Further studies testing the influence of maintaining oral health and denture usage on prevention of falls should be carried out.

References

[1] World Health Organization, *WHO Global Report on Falls Prevention in Older Age*, World Health Organization, Geneva, Switzerland, 2007.

[2] K. E. Ensrud, "Epidemiology of fracture risk with advancing age," *Journals of Gerontology Series A: Biological Sciences and Medical Sciences*, vol. 68, no. 10, pp. 1236–1242, 2013.

[3] M. Q. Vu, N. Weintraub, and L. Z. Rubenstein, "Falls in the nursing home: are they preventable?," *Journal of the American Medical Directors Association*, vol. 5, no. 6, pp. 401–406, 2004.

[4] R. Gelbard, K. Inaba, O. T. Okoye et al., "Falls in the elderly: a modern look at an old problem," *American Journal of Surgery*, vol. 208, no. 2, pp. 249–253, 2014.

[5] M. E. Tinetti, M. Speechley, and S. F. Ginter, "Risk factors for falls among elderly persons living in the community," *New England Journal of Medicine*, vol. 319, no. 26, pp. 1701–1707, 1988.

[6] M. Tinetti and C. S. William, "Falls, injuries due to falls, and the risk of admission to a nursing home," *New England Journal of Medicine*, vol. 337, no. 18, pp. 1279–1284, 1997.

[7] M. Ueno, S. Kawai, T. Mino et al., "Systematic review of fall-related factors among the house-dwelling elderly in Japan," *Nippon Ronen Igakkai Zasshi*, vol. 43, no. 1, pp. 92–101, 2006.

[8] J. C. L. Neyens, B. P. J. Dijcks, J. C. M. van Haastregt et al., "The development of a multidisciplinary fall risk evaluation tool for demented nursing home patients in the Netherlands," *BMC Public Health*, vol. 6, no. 1, p. 74, 2006.

[9] M. R. de Jong, M. van der Elst, and A. Hartholt, "Drug-related falls in older patients: implicated drugs, consequences, and possible prevention strategies," *Therapeutic Advances in Drug Safety*, vol. 4, no. 4, pp. 147–154, 2013.

[10] F. E. Shaw, J. Bond, D. A. Richardson et al., "Multifactorial intervention after a fall in older people with cognitive impairment and dementia presenting to the accident and emergency department: randomised controlled trial," *BMJ*, vol. 326, no. 7380, pp. 73–75, 2003.

[11] T. Aizan, *Population Ageing in Malaysia, 2015. Department of Statistics, Malaysia (DSM) 2011. Population Distribution and Basic Demographic Characteristics 2010*, Population and Housing Census of Malaysia, Putrajaya, Malaysia, 2010.

[12] M. Mafauzy, "The problems and challenges of the aging population of Malaysia," *Malaysian Journal of Medical Sciences*, vol. 7, no. 1, pp. 1–3, 2000.

[13] R. Guiglia, A. Musciotto, D. Compilato et al., "Effects in hard and soft tissues," *Current Pharmaceutical Design*, vol. 16, no. 6, pp. 619–630, 2010.

[14] W. C. Gonsalves, A. S. Wrightson, and R. G. Henry, "Common oral conditions in older persons," *American Family Physician*, vol. 78, no. 7, pp. 845–852, 2008.

[15] P. Gangloff, J. P. Louis, and P. P. Perrin, "Dental occlusion modifies gaze and posture stabilization in human subjects," *Neuroscience Letters*, vol. 293, no. 3, pp. 203–206, 2000.

[16] H. Rouviere and A. Delmas, *Anatomie Humaine Descriptive, Topographique et Fonctionnelle*, vol. 1, Masson, Paris, France, 1974.

[17] M. A. Salonen, A. M. Raustia, and J. Huggare, "Head and cervical spine postures in complete denture wearers," *Journal of Craniomandibular Practice*, vol. 11, no. 1, pp. 30–33, 1993.

[18] M. Urbanowicz, "Alteration of vertical dimension and its effect on head and neck posture," *Cranio*, vol. 9, no. 2, pp. 174–179, 1991.

[19] N. Okuyama, T. Yamaga, A. Yoshihara et al., "Influence of dental occlusion on physical fitness decline in a healthy Japanese elderly population," *Archives of Gerontology and Geriatrics*, vol. 52, no. 2, pp. 172–176, 2011.

[20] M. O. Williams, S. J. Chaconas, and P. Bader, "The effect of mandibular position on appendage muscle strength," *Journal of Prosthetic Dentistry*, vol. 49, no. 4, pp. 560–567, 1983.

[21] K. H. Lim, K. Jasvindar, I. Normala et al., "Risk factors of home injury among elderly people in Malaysia," *Asian Journal of Gerontology and Geriatrics*, vol. 9, pp. 16–20, 2014.

[22] A. C. Grundstrom, C. E. Guse, and P. M. Layde, "Risk factors for falls and fall related injuries in adults 85 years of age and older," *Archives of Gerontology and Geriatrics*, vol. 54, no. 3, pp. 421–428, 2012.

[23] American Geriatrics Society, British Geriatrics Society, and American Academy of Orthopaedic Surgeons Panel on Falls Prevention, "Guideline for the prevention of falls in older persons," *Journal of the American Geriatrics Society*, vol. 49, no. 5, pp. 664–672, 2001.

[24] M. S. Kamińska, J. Brodowski, and B. Karakiewicz, "Fall risk factors in community-dwelling elderly depending on their physical function, cognitive status and symptoms of depression," *International Journal of Environmental Research and Public Health*, vol. 12, no. 4, pp. 3406–3416, 2015.

[25] T. Yamamoto, K. Kondo, J. Misawa et al., "Dental status and incident falls among older Japanese: a prospective cohort study," *BMJ Open*, vol. 2, no. 4, pp. 1–7, 2012.

[26] M. Yoshida, H. Morikawa, Y. Kanehisa, T. Taji, K. Tsuga, and Y. Akagawa, "Functional dental occlusion may prevent falls in elderly individuals with dementia," *Journal of the American Geriatrics Society*, vol. 53, no. 9, pp. 1631-1632, 2005.

[27] A. F. Kayser, "Shortened dental arches and oral function," *Journal of Oral Rehabilitation*, vol. 8, no. 5, pp. 457–462, 1981.

[28] A. Yoshihara, R. Watanabe, M. Nishimuta, N. Hanada, and H. Miyazaki, "The relationship between dietary intake and the number of teeth in elderly Japanese subjects," *Gerodontology*, vol. 22, no. 4, pp. 211–218, 2005.

[29] C. Fernandez-de-las-Penas, M. Carratala-Tejada, L. Luna-Oliva, and J. C. Miangolarra-Page, "The immediate effect of hamstring muscle stretching in subjects' triggers points in the masseter muscle," *Journal of Musculoskeletal Pain*, vol. 14, no. 3, pp. 27–35, 2006.

[30] M. Maruya, K. Shimizu, T. Ohnuma et al., "The effect of wearing denture and changes of occlusal position on body sway in edentulous patient," *Journal of Japan Prosthodontic Society*, vol. 44, no. 6, pp. 781–785, 2000.

[31] Y. Takata, T. Ansai, S. Awano, T. Hamasaki, Y. Yoshitake, and Y. Kimura, "Relationship of physical fitness to chewing in an 80-year-old population," *Oral Diseases*, vol. 10, no. 1, pp. 44–49, 2004.

[32] K. Miyaura, M. Morita, Y. Matsuka, A. Yamashita, and T. Watanabe, "Rehabilitation of biting abilities in patients with different types of dental prostheses," *Journal of Oral Rehabilitation*, vol. 27, no. 12, pp. 1073–1076, 2000.

[33] T. A. Brito, R. S. Coqueiro, M. H. Fernandes, and C. S. de Jesus, "Determinants of falls in community-dwelling elderly: hierarchical analysis," *Public Health Nursing*, vol. 31, no. 4, pp. 290–297, 2014.

[34] I. Melzer and I. Kurz, "Self-reported function and disability in late life: a comparison between recurrent fallers and non-fallers," *Disability and Rehabilitation*, vol. 31, no. 10, pp. 791–798, 2009.

[35] J. Moreland, J. Richardson, D. Chan, J. O'Neill, A. Bellissimo, and R. Grum, "Evidence-based guidelines for the secondary prevention of falls in older adults," *Gerontology*, vol. 49, no. 2, pp. 93–116, 2003.

17

Vitamin D Deficiency as it Relates to Oral Immunity and Chronic Periodontitis

R. A. G. Khammissa⑩, R. Ballyram, Y. Jadwat, J. Fourie, J. Lemmer, and L. Feller⑩

Department of Periodontology and Oral Medicine, Sefako Makgatho Health Sciences University, Medunsa 0204, South Africa

Correspondence should be addressed to R. A. G. Khammissa; razia.khammissa@smu.ac.za

Academic Editor: Wael Sabbah

The biologically active form of vitamin D, 1,25 dihydroxyvitamin D ($1,25(OH)_2D$) and its receptor, the vitamin D receptor (VDR), play roles in maintaining oral immunity and the integrity of the periodontium. Results of observational cross-sectional clinical studies investigating the association between vitamin D serum level and the incidence and severity of chronic periodontitis indicate that, perhaps owing to the immunomodulatory, anti-inflammatory, and antibacterial properties of $1,25(OH)_2$ D/VDR signalling, a sufficient serum level of vitamin D is necessary for the maintenance of periodontal health. In cases of established chronic periodontitis, vitamin D supplementation is associated with reduction in the severity of periodontitis. As cross-sectional studies provide only weak evidence for any causal association and therefore are of questionable value, either longitudinal cohort studies, case controlled studies, or randomized control trials are needed to determine whether or not deficiency of vitamin D is a risk factor for chronic periodontitis, and whether or not vitamin D supplementation adjunctive to standard periodontal treatment is in any way beneficial. In this article, we discuss the relationship between vitamin D, oral immunity and periodontal disease and review the rationale for using vitamin D supplementation to help maintain periodontal health and as an adjunct to standard periodontal treatment.

1. Introduction

Chronic periodontitis is an inflammatory disease caused by dentogingival bacterial plaques and if left untreated, it causes progressive destruction of periodontal tissues, ultimately leading to tooth loss. In a subset of subjects with chronic periodontitis, there may be an increased risk of cardiovascular disease, diabetes mellitus, and complications of pregnancy [1–4]. Periodontitis affects up to 50% of the adult population [5–7].

Vitamin D plays a role in maintaining the homeostasis of various biological systems including the neuromuscular, skeletal, cutaneous, cardiovascular, and immune systems. In addition, vitamin D has tumour suppressing, anti-inflammatory, and antibacterial properties [8–12] (Figure 1). While there is no doubt about the essential role of vitamin D in maintaining bone and calcium homeostasis, its role in other biological systems is less well-defined [13].

Cross-sectional observational studies show that vitamin D deficiency may be associated with increased risk of chronic periodontitis [1, 6, 14–17], and that supplementation with vitamin D alone, or with vitamin D together with calcium may help to maintain periodontal health, may increase mineral density of the jaws, and may inhibit inflammatory alveolar bone resorption [15, 18–21]. Furthermore, in subjects with adequate vitamin D, surgical treatment for chronic periodontitis appears to be more successful than in subjects with vitamin D deficiency [22]. However, results of some longitudinal studies show that vitamin D deficiency is a poor predictor of progressive tissue destruction in subjects with chronic periodontitis [7] and conversely, vitamin D sufficiency does not protect against progression of chronic periodontitis [23]. These longitudinal studies do not provide any information regarding the association between vitamin D levels and chronic periodontitis in the general population. The two studies deal only with

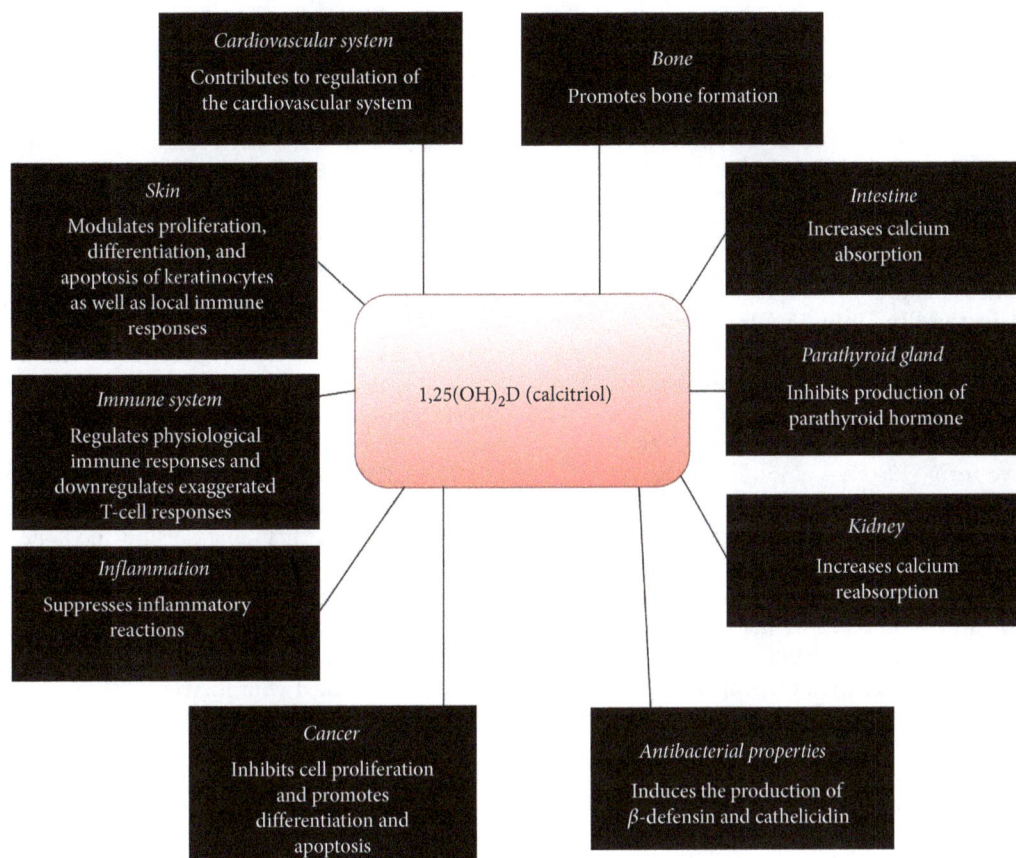

FIGURE 1: The functions of vitamin D.

a selected population of men over the age of 65 recruited for a study of "Osteoporotic Fractures in Men" [7], and with a selected population of postmenopausal women enrolled in the "Buffalo OsteoPerio Study" [23].

Cross-sectional observational studies also show that vitamin D deficiency, independently of chronic periodontitis, is associated with increased risk of cardiovascular disease [9, 10, 24], but it is not known if concurrence of periodontal disease and vitamin D deficiency poses a cumulative cardiovascular risk. In any case, there are no strong evidence-based data to show that supplementation with vitamin D reduces the incidence or the severity of cardiovascular or of any immunoinflammatory diseases [9, 24, 25]. Nevertheless, vitamin D has been used in prevention or treatment of a number of infections including respiratory infections [26], gingivitis [27], and influenza [28] and in the management of asthma [29]. Owing to climatic variations and variations in skin pigmentation, according to generally accepted norms of serum levels of vitamin D, deficiency of vitamin D is very common. In fact, if vitamin D deficiency is defined as a serum level of 25(OH)D below 50 nmol/L, then up to 40% of Europeans can be considered to be deficient [30].

Standard treatment of periodontal disease focuses on reducing the dentogingival bacterial load through personal and professional mechanical disruption of the biofilm, by the use of local or systemic antibacterial agents, or by downregulating the immunoinflammatory response with drugs in order to reduce the bacteria-induced inflammation and to arrest the progression of periodontal tissue damage [31]. If indeed vitamin D were to be found to be effective in the prevention and treatment of periodontitis, then it should be added to the arsenal of biologically active therapeutic agents.

In this narrative review, we describe the possible mechanisms by which vitamin D deficiency may play roles in the pathogenesis of chronic periodontitis and in maintaining the homeostasis of the oral epithelium and the integrity of oral immunity.

2. Vitamin D and Vitamin D Receptor (VDR)

About 80% of vitamin D in the body is derived from ultraviolet B (UVB)-induced photoconversion in the skin of 7-dehydrocholesterol to vitamin D_3 (cholecalciferol) and the remainder from animal dietary sources in the form of vitamin D_3 or of vitamin D_2 (ergocalciferol). In a modern diet, food supplements substantially augment the natural sources. The term vitamin D refers either to vitamin D_2 or to vitamin D_3 or to both, and either can be used for correcting vitamin D deficiency [25, 32].

Exposure to sunlight is essential for achieving a sufficient level of vitamin D [25, 29, 33], but as the available evidence suggests that excessive exposure to sunlight raises the risk of skin cancer, it is common practice to avoid exposure to sunlight or to wear protective clothing and to use sunscreen with high protection factors when outdoors [34, 35]. Under these circumstances, it is difficult without supplementation to attain sufficient levels of vitamin D for vitamin D-related physiological activities [25]. Because melanin reduces the penetration of UVB into the skin, diminishing the photoproduction of vitamin D, black people are more frequently vitamin D deficient than white people [5, 30]. This may contribute minimally to the greater severity of chronic periodontitis in blacks than in whites [5].

Both vitamin D_2 and D_3 are biologically inactive and are converted in the liver into 25(OH)D which then is converted mainly by the proximal tubular cells of the renal nephrons into $1,25(OH)_2D$. This is the biologically active vitamin D (Figure 2). However, other tissues can also to a lesser extent convert vitamin D2 and D3 to the biologically active form [13, 25, 32, 36].

As the $1,25(OH)_2D$ has a half-life of only about 4 hours, 25(OH)D with a half-life of 2-3 weeks is used to determine serum levels of vitamin D. Metabolites of vitamin D are transported in the circulation by the vitamin D binding protein, and upon reaching their target cells, they dissociate from the binding protein and enter the cells [8, 19, 25, 32, 37, 38]. The biochemical properties of vitamin binding protein which is the principle transporter of vitamin D and its metabolites, determine the free levels of free vitamin D available to the tissues [33].

Regulation of the concentration of circulating 25(OH)D and $1,25(OH)_2D$ is a complex process which is modulated by multiple factors including age, sunlight exposure (duration and intensity), diet (oily fish such as tuna, salmon, sardines; cod liver oil; yeast and fungi), plasma calcium, parathyroid hormone, direct feedback by $1,25(OH)_2D$, fibroblast growth factor 23, diseases (i.e., malabsorption syndromes, sarcoidosis, and impaired calcium metabolism), systemic inflammatory reactions, and medications (i.e., glucocorticoids, anticonvulsants, and barbiturates) [13, 25, 36, 38, 39]. As older adults are often less exposed to sunlight and have reduced capacity to produce biologically active vitamin D metabolites and to absorb vitamin D from the intestine and may be suffering from chronic diseases requiring multiple-drug treatment, they are at particular risk of vitamin D deficiency [12].

According to the Endocrine Society Clinical Practice Guideline [25], Vitamin D deficiency is defined as levels of 25 (OH)D below 50 nmol/L and insufficiency as 25(OH)D levels of 52.5–72.5 nmol/L. For people with vitamin D deficiency, in order to attain blood levels of 25(OH)D above 75 nmol/L, they should be treated daily with 6000 IU of either vitamin D_2 or vitamin D_3, followed by a maintenance dose of 1500–2000 IU/day [25, 29]. Although about 70 nmol/L of vitamin D enhances both calcium and phosphorus absorption from the intestine and enhances bone health and muscle function, the adequate levels of 25(OH)D for nonskeletal tissue health are unknown [25]. For the best clinical outcomes of vitamin D supplementation, daily doses are better than higher weekly or monthly doses [12] because daily doses result in a more stable serum and tissue concentration [38].

$1,25(OH)_2D$ exerts most of its activities through the widespread vitamin D nuclear receptor (VDR) which functions as a transcription factor. VDR forms a heterodimer with the retinoid X receptor (RXR), and this VDR/RXR binds to vitamin D response elements in target genes, regulating gene expression either by activation or by repression of gene transcription [8, 10, 40].

$1,25(OH)_2D/VDR/RXR$-induced transcription of target genes is modulated by other transcriptional coactivators and corepressors which are recruited to the vitamin D response elements. However, VDR may mediate cellular functions in a ligand-independent manner [13]. $1,25(OH)_2D/VDR$ and glucocorticoid receptor intracellular signalling pathways cross-talk so that increased levels of vitamin D may upregulate responsiveness of certain target cells to glucocorticoids; and as VDR and glucocorticoid receptor share some transcriptional coactivators, VDR may promote transcription of certain genes induced by glucocorticoids [13].

The $1,25(OH)_2D/VDR$ signalling pathway interacts with other signalling pathways in the regulation of many biological processes, including calcium and bone homeostasis, inflammation, cell mediated immunity, cell-cycle progression, and apoptosis [8]. The $1,25(OH)_2D/VDR$ signalling pathway has the capacity to mediate antibacterial, antiviral, and anti-inflammatory activity [29]. VDR polymorphism has been associated with increased risk of several diseases, with some of the genetic variants being less responsive than others to $1,25(OH)_2D$ in suppressing inflammatory processes, thus favouring the development of cutaneous inflammatory conditions [41] and possibly of chronic periodontitis [5, 42].

$1,25(OH)_2D/VDR$ signalling in osteoblasts may crosstalk with the transforming growth factor β, insulin growth factor 1, interferon, parathyroid hormone, and Wnt/β catenin signalling pathways to mediate physiological activities of osteoblasts [13]. $1,25(OH)_2D/VDR$ pathways directly or indirectly can mediate differentiation and maturation of osteoblasts and osteoclasts, thus influencing bone remodelling. $1,25(OH)_2D/VDR$ pathways in osteoblasts enhance the expression of osteogenic genes such as those encoding type I collagen, alkaline phosphatase, osteocalcin, and osteopontin which drive bone formation and upregulate the expression by osteoblasts of RANKL which subsequently promotes differentiation and activity of osteoclasts [13]. Vitamin D deficiency has the potential to interfere with bone homeostasis, but as long as calcium serum levels are normal, bone metabolism appears not to be affected by vitamin D deficiency [13].

3. Oral Mucosal Immunity

The oral mucosal epithelium separates a microorganism-ridden environment from the underlying connective tissue. It acts as the physical barrier that protects the deeper tissues from penetration of water and a wide range of water-soluble molecules, from invasion by microorganisms with their associated antigens and toxins, and from minor mechanical damage [43]. $1,25(OH)_2D$ is produced, and VDR is expressed by keratinocytes of the basal and spinous layers of the oral epithelium, and $1,25(OH)_2D/VDR$ signalling influences proliferation, differentiation, and apoptosis of keratinocytes, and local immune responses [8, 44]. In fact,

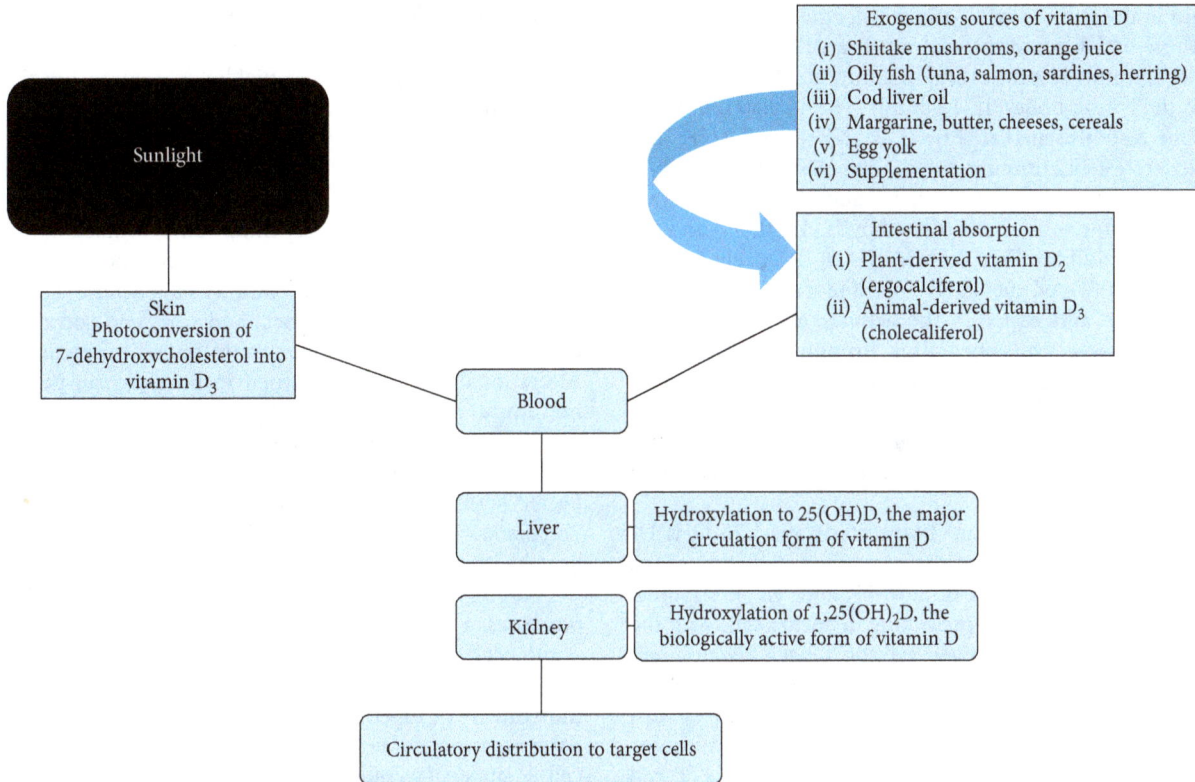

FIGURE 2: Synthesis of vitamin D precursors and metabolites.

$1,25(OH)_2D$/VDR signalling in oral keratinocytes mediates antiproliferative and prodifferentiation effects, and vitamin D-deficient laboratory animals show increased proliferation of oral epithelium without any morphological or histological abnormalities [45].

The epithelium and the underlying lamina propria of the oral mucosa are populated by innate immune cells including macrophages, natural killer (NK) cells, NKT cells, polymorphonuclear leukocytes, and dedicated antigen-presenting cells, with all their related cytokines and chemokines [43]. In response to antigenic stimulation, activated keratinocytes produce antimicrobial agents such as β-defensins and cathelicidins and can mediate immunoinflammatory reactions [46]. Salivary flow, salivary secretory immunoglobulin A, and gingival crevicular fluid are additional physical and biological elements of oral mucosal immunity [43].

Oral mucosal immunity has many functions including control of colonization of the oral mucosa by pathogenic microorganisms, generation of protective immunoinflammatory responses against invading pathogens, mediation of immune tolerance to commensal microorganisms and foreign antigens derived from exogenous sources, and neutralization of harmful exogenous antigens [47].

Oral keratinocytes and innate immune cells in the lamina propria of the oral mucosa express molecular pattern-recognition receptors that can detect microorganisms and harmful endogenous molecules derived from tissue damage. There are several families of molecular pattern-recognition receptors including the Toll-like receptor (TLR)

family, the c-type lectin receptor family, and the mannose receptor family [46, 47]. Stimulation of TLR receptors by periodontopathic bacteria breaching the crevicular epithelium triggers the production of antibacterial and chemotactic agents, inflammatory mediators, and cytokines. All of these induce a nonspecific inflammatory reaction and mobilize dedicated antigen-presenting cells to the infected gingival site. In turn, these biological reactions initiate and drive adaptive immunoinflammatory reactions [43, 46, 47].

Invasion of the gingival epithelium by periodontopathic bacteria brings about activation of keratinocytes, myeloid dendritic cells, and macrophages. After having recognized molecular patterns of periodontopathic bacteria through TLRs, local immature myeloid dendritic cells process the pathogenic antigen and undergo maturation, with upregulation of expression of major histocompatibility complex (MHC) and costimulatory surface molecules. In the presence of MHC surface molecules, the mature dendritic cells can effectively present antigens to the naïve T cells in draining lymph nodes, initiating cross-priming and mediating the generation of T cell immune responses [43].

The primed T cells in the lymph nodes then differentiate into antigen-specific memory effector CD4+ and CD8+ T cells and into regulatory T (Treg) cells. The subtype and the magnitude of the antigen-specific T cell response in the lymph nodes is determined by the nature of the infective agent, by the cytokine profile in the microenvironment, by the specific T cell receptor repertoire, and by the profile of the cell surface molecules expressed by antigen-presenting dendritic cells [43, 47]. Some of the effector T cells will remain in the lymph nodes, others will enter the circulation, and those which reach the oral mucosa will engage in local effector immune responses and in immune surveillance [43].

In the lymph nodes, IL-12 and IL-18 will generate a Th1 immune response mediated by IL-2, INF-Y, and TNF; IL-4 will generate a Th2 immune response mediated by IL-4, IL-5, IL-6, and IL-13; and TNF-β, IL-1β, and IL-6 will generate a Th17 immune response mediated by IL-17, IL-21, and IL-22 [46]. In addition, Treg cells *via* IL-10 downregulate the induction of T-cell-mediated immune responses in the lymph nodes and suppress the activity of T-cells in the peripheral tissue, thus mediating immune tolerance and preventing upregulation of immunoinflammatory reactions [43, 47]. Despite this process of T cell polarization, the polarized T cells retain some functional versatility, having the capacity to produce cytokines which are not considered lineage-specific [43].

In the context of immune homeostasis, the 1,25(OH)$_2$D/VDR signalling pathway can modulate the production of the proinflammatory cytokines IL-2, IL-17, and INF-α; suppress the maturation of antigen-presenting dendritic cells with the consequent decrease in antigen-specific T cell activation and proliferation; and promote the activity of Treg cells. Together, these fine-tuned physiological immune responses can downregulate hyperactive T cell mediated immunoinflammatory reactions and moderate autoimmune T cell responses [9, 11, 48–50].

However, despite all this, the evidence for a causal association between vitamin D deficiency and the incidence and severity of immunoinflammatory diseases is weak, and augmenting standard treatment with vitamin D supplementation or its biologically active analogues does not seem to improve the efficacy of the treatment of any autoimmune or immunoinflammatory diseases [9, 51].

In addition, it has been shown that VDR polymorphism, in the presence of exogenous aetiological factors (i.e., tobacco smoke and alcohol), is associated with increased risk of chronic periodontitis and other inflammatory conditions. Some genetic variants may be less responsive to 1,25(OH)$_2$D in suppressing inflammation, thus favouring bacteria-induced tissue damage, while other variants are associated with low bone-mineral density, thus making alveolar bone vulnerable to bacterial plaque-induced inflammatory bone resorption [5, 41, 42, 52, 53].

4. Periodontitis

Periodontitis is a bacterial plaque-induced inflammatory disease characterized by exudation of cervicular fluid, increased periodontal probing depths, bleeding on probing, and loss of alveolar crestal bone. The pathogenesis is multifactorial with complex interaction between bacterial agents and bacteria-induced immunoinflammatory responses, on a background of inherent genetic predisposition. Risk factors such as smoking, uncontrolled diabetes, vitamin D deficiency, and deep periodontal pockets that favour proliferation of periodontopathic bacteria, all have the capacity to aggravate the course of the disease (Figure 3) [52–54].

The metabolic products of early, mainly aerobic bacterial colonisers, together with environmental organic and inorganic compounds form a biofilm in which the pioneer bacteria multiply. The chemical and physical properties of this biofilm within the ecological niche favour proliferation of late bacterial colonisers, including anaerobic periodontopathic bacteria. The biofilm is retained *in-situ* by its adhesive and cohesive properties and provides some protection to the bacterial flora against penetration of antibiotics [54].

In gingival health, the commensal bacteria including Gram-positive facultative cocci and rods and some anaerobes and the gingival tissues are in biological equilibrium. Alterations in the local microenvironment or in the host's immunity may favour multiplication of Gram-negative anaerobic bacterial species, including the periodontopathic bacteria *Porphyromonas gingivalis*, *Aggregatibacter actinomycetemcomitans*, *Prevotella intermedia*, and *Treponema denticolo*, bringing about a disturbance in the host-bacterial biological equilibrium [54].

P. gingivalis, the main periodontopathic bacterium, possesses a number of virulence factors and micromorphological structures including gingipain, lipopolysaccharides (LPS), fimbriae, and outer membrane vesicles which individually or together can cause direct tissue damage [55]. After having become attached to a gingival sulcular epithelial cell, *P. gingivalis* enters the cell inducing remodelling of the actin and tubulin cytoskeleton, and after intracellular multiplication, it spreads *via* actin bridges to neighbouring cells, thus infecting a field of epithelial cells. Within the infected cell, *P. gingivalis* can survive, ultimately inducing apoptosis, lysis of the infected cell [31, 55, 56], and thence invading connective tissue cells and osteoblasts of the alveolar bone. *P. gingivalis* can then inhibit differentiation and ultimately induce apoptosis of infected osteoblasts, thus inhibiting bone turnover [57, 58].

In subjects with chronic periodontitis, the expression of TLR2 and TLR4 by cells of the periodontium is upregulated in response to the preponderance of periodontopathic bacteria [55]. Lipopolysaccharides of *P. gingivalis*, via TLR 2/4, trigger the activation of the transcription factors NF-κB, AP-1 (activator protein 1), and the STAT-3 (nuclear signal transducers and activators of transcription-3). These upregulate the expression of genes encoding inflammatory mediators including cytokines, chemokines, prostaglandins, and proteinases [31, 55, 59], generating an initial inflammatory reaction. This reaction will be amplified and propagated by activated immunoinflammatory cells of the adaptive arm of the immune system recruited to the infected periodontal site [31], causing marginal alveolar bone loss with increased periodontal pocket depths, raised pH, and decreased local redox potential. All these together favour proliferation of anaerobic bacteria, and unless interrupted by treatment, a vicious cycle of bacterial multiplication, inflammation, and progressive alveolar bone destruction will occur, ultimately resulting in tooth loss [54]. Thus, while bacteria do cause some direct tissue damage, most of the damage of chronic periodontitis is mediated by immunoinflammatory reactions in response to the challenge of the periodontopathic bacteria [59].

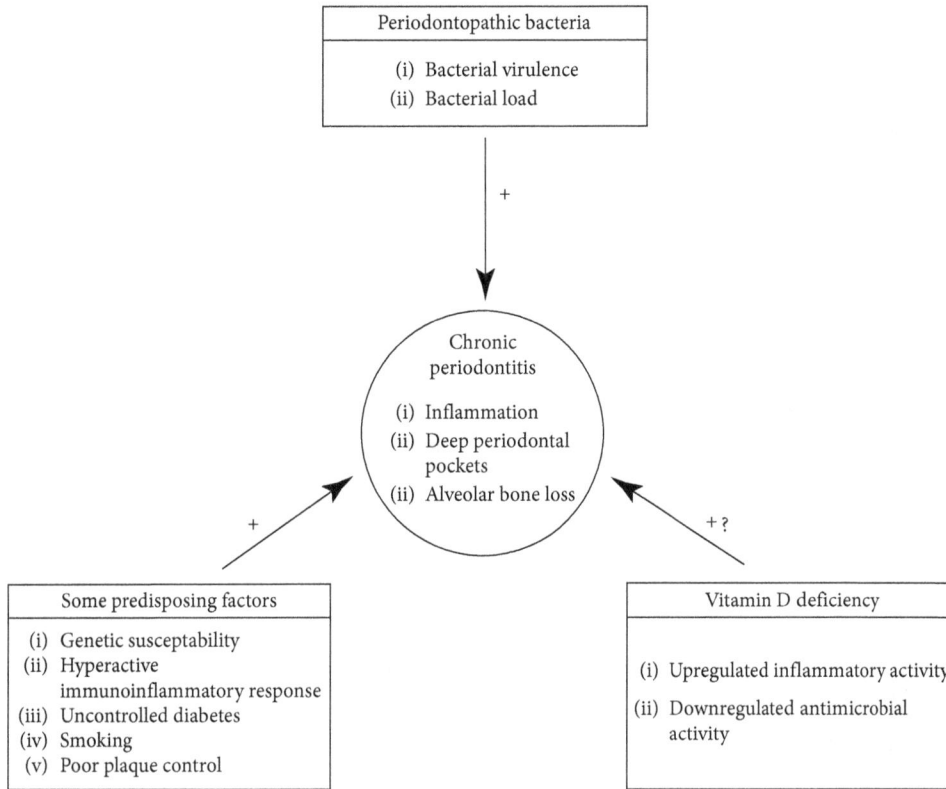

FIGURE 3: Pathogenesis of periodontal disease.

The interaction between molecular patterns of certain periodontopathic bacteria and TLR1/2 of innate oral immunocytes including monocytes/macrophages and keratinocytes may also induce the expression of VDR and the production of $1,25(OH)_2D$ by these cells. In turn, the $1,25(OH)_2D$/VDR signalling induces the expression of genes encoding the antibacterial agents cathelicidin and β defencin [1, 10, 51] which may provide some protection against the development of bacterial plaque-induced chronic periodontitis [13].

Alveolar bone loss in chronic periodontitis is brought about by increased expression of receptor activator of nuclear factor kappa-B ligand (RANKL), by Th17-derived IL-17 and by TNF-α all of which have the capacity directly or indirectly to promote osteoclastogenesis. Lipopolysaccharides of anaerobic bacteria, *via* stimulation of TLRs, upregulate the expression of RANKL by fibroblasts, osteoblasts, and/or by T and B lymphocytes, resulting in differentiation and activation of osteoclasts; Th17-derived IL-17 can also upregulate the expression of RANKL by osteoblasts and CD4+ T cells; and TNF-α produced by neutrophils, macrophages, and Th1 cells directly promotes osteoclastogenesis. All these bring about the resorption of supporting alveolar bone characteristic of chronic periodontitis [31].

In progressive chronic periodontitis, dissemination of periodontopathic bacteria and of inflammatory mediators from the inflamed periodontal tissues is not uncommon. As a result, in a subset of genetically predisposed persons with upregulated immunoinflammatory responses, active chronic periodontitis can increase the risk of cardiovascular disease, stroke, inadequate glycaemic control in diabetes mellitus, and complications of pregnancy [1, 4]. Indeed, it has been reported that after adjustment for confounding variables, compared to those with minimal periodontal disease, subjects with advanced periodontitis have a 25% increased risk of coronary heart disease [4].

The statistical association between vitamin D status represented by 25(OH)D levels and resistance to periodontal disease observed in cross-sectional studies might be explained in terms of several biological mechanisms. Firstly, $1,25(OH)_2D$, the biologically active form of vitamin D, through its positive role in maintaining calcium and bone homeostasis can increase the mineral density of alveolar bone, and thus may reduce alveolar bone resorption, with a consequent decrease in the severity of chronic periodontitis and may help to maintain periodontal health [5, 11, 49, 60].

Secondly, $1,25(OH)_2D$/VDR signalling can downregulate transcription of genes encoding proinflammatory cytokines, can suppress cyclo-oxygenase-2 (COX-2) and prostaglandin pathways, and can inhibit production of matrix metalloproteinases. Taken together, all these effects of 1,25 dihydroxyvitamin D/VDR signalling may reduce the bacteria-induced inflammatory process of periodontal disease [49, 55, 60].

Thirdly, $1,25(OH)_2D$/VDR signalling plays some supportive role in wound healing. It mediates proliferation and differentiation of keratinocytes and recruitment of monocytes/macrophages during the inflammatory phase of tissue repair, and VDR-deficient laboratory animals show impairment in the formation of granulation tissue characterized by low vascularization and extracellular matrix content [61]. Thus, vitamin D deficiency may inhibit periodontal tissue healing.

Lastly, in response to bacterial stimulation, 1,25 $(OH)_2D/VDR$ signalling in activated keratinocytes, monocytes, and macrophages of the periodontium, may induce the production of the antibacterial agents cathelicin and β-defensin [5, 9, 11, 49], thus playing a role in reducing the bacterial burden; and supplementation with vitamin D may amplify the local antimicrobial effector response against periodontopathic bacteria [5, 49].

5. Comments

It is difficult to interpret the information from observational cross-sectional clinical studies of the association between the incidence and severity of chronic periodontitis and vitamin D serum levels [6, 14–17, 62]. Follow-up periods have been short, study populations often heterogeneous, and risk factors such as ethnicity, old age, and smoking are common to both subjects with low-levels serum vitamin D and subjects with chronic periodontitis [6, 13–15, 17, 62]. Furthermore, the effects of supplementation of calcium together with vitamin D was investigated in some of the studies, thus ruling out any conclusion as to the effect of vitamin D alone [63].

Epidemiologically, the extent, severity, and rate of progression of chronic periodontitis are extremely variable [63, 64], and as the tissue destruction in chronic periodontitis is known to be episodic with short periods of disease activity and longer periods of disease quiescence, follow-up periods of several years would be necessary to detect whether vitamin D supplementation could reduce the risk and the severity of chronic periodontitis [63].

In general, observational cross-sectional studies, like most of those investigating the link between vitamin D and chronic periodontitis, provide only weak evidence of any causal association, and as such are of questionable value in determining whether or not vitamin D deficiency increases the risk of chronic periodontitis [5, 65]. Either longitudinal cohort studies, case controlled studies, or randomized controlled trials would be needed to demonstrate any causal associations or to determine the value of vitamin D in the maintenance of periodontal health or in periodontal treatment [65].

In any case, as medicine is not a precise science, treatment modalities which according to evidence-based research have not been found to be completely effective for an observed group may still be beneficial for a subset of the general population [66]. Therefore, the use of vitamin D supplementation as an adjunct to standard periodontal treatment should be considered in subjects with vitamin D deficiency.

6. Conclusion

Studies investigating the link between vitamin D and chronic periodontitis do not provide direct experimental evidence of any causal association between vitamin D deficiency and chronic periodontitis, or that vitamin D supplementation has any beneficial role in the treatment of chronic periodontitis; these studies do provide coherent and consistent evidence of the potential role of vitamin D in maintaining oral health. However, there appears to be no justification for vitamin D screening for persons with chronic periodontitis who are not at risk of vitamin D deficiency.

References

[1] J. do Amaral Bastos, L. C. Ferreira de Andrade, F. de Andrade et al., "Serum levels of vitamin D and chronic periodontitis in patients with chronic kidney disease," *Jornal Brasileiro de Nefrologia*, vol. 35, no. 1, pp. 20–26, 2013.

[2] R. I. Garcia, M. M. Henshaw, and E. A. Krall, "Relationship between periodontal disease and systemic health," *Periodontology 2000*, vol. 25, no. 1, pp. 21–36, 2001.

[3] G. R. Persson and R. E. Persson, "Cardiovascular disease and periodontitis: an update on the associations and risk," *Journal of Clinical Periodontology*, vol. 35, no. 8S, pp. 362–379, 2008.

[4] J. D. Beck, G. Slade, and S. Offenbacher, "Oral disease, cardiovascular disease and systemic inflammation," *Periodontology 2000*, vol. 23, no. 1, pp. 110–120, 2000.

[5] W. B. Grant and B. J. Boucher, "Are Hill's criteria for causality satisfied for vitamin D and periodontal disease?," *Dermato-Endocrinology*, vol. 2, no. 1, pp. 30–36, 2010.

[6] K. A. Boggess, J. A. Espinola, K. Moss, J. Beck, S. Offenbacher, and C. A. Camargo Jr., "Vitamin D status and periodontal disease among pregnant women," *Journal of Periodontology*, vol. 82, no. 2, pp. 195–200, 2011.

[7] U. Schulze-Spate, R. Turner, Y. Wang et al., "Relationship of bone metabolism biomarkers and periodontal disease: the osteoporotic fractures in men (MrOS) study," *Journal of Clinical Endocrinology & Metabolism*, vol. 100, no. 6, pp. 2425–2433, 2015.

[8] C. J. Rosen, J. S. Adams, D. D. Bikle et al., "The nonskeletal effects of vitamin D: an Endocrine Society scientific statement," *Endocrine Reviews*, vol. 33, no. 3, pp. 456–492, 2012.

[9] S. Christakos, P. Dhawan, A. Verstuyf, L. Verlinden, and G. Carmeliet, "Vitamin D: metabolism, molecular mechanism of action, and pleiotropic effects," *Physiological Reviews*, vol. 96, no. 1, pp. 365–408, 2016.

[10] S. Christakos, M. Hewison, D. G. Gardner et al., "Vitamin D: beyond bone," *Annals of the New York Academy of Sciences*, vol. 1287, no. 1, pp. 45–58, 2013.

[11] S. H. Stein, R. Livada, and D. A. Tipton, "Re-evaluating the role of vitamin D in the periodontium," *Journal of Periodontal Research*, vol. 49, no. 5, pp. 545–553, 2014.

[12] S. W. Muir and M. Montero-Odasso, "Effect of vitamin D supplementation on muscle strength, gait and balance in older adults: a systematic review and meta-analysis," *Journal of the American Geriatrics Society*, vol. 59, no. 12, pp. 2291–2300, 2011.

[13] R. A. G. Khammissa, J. Fourie, M. H. Motswaledi, R. Ballyram, J. Lemmer, and L. Feller, "The biological activities of vitamin D and its receptor in relation to calcium and bone homeostasis, cancer, immune and cardiovascular systems, skin

biology, and oral health," *BioMed Research International*, vol. 2018, Article ID 9276380, 9 pages, 2018.

[14] T. Dietrich and R. I. Garcia, "Associations between periodontal disease and systemic disease: evaluating the strength of the evidence," *Journal of Periodontology*, vol. 76, no. 11S, pp. 2175–2184, 2005.

[15] D. D. Miley, M. N. Garcia, C. F. Hildebolt et al., "Cross-sectional study of vitamin D and calcium supplementation effects on chronic periodontitis," *Journal of Periodontology*, vol. 80, no. 9, pp. 1433–1439, 2009.

[16] T. Dietrich, K. J. Joshipura, B. Dawson-Hughes, and H. A. Bischoff-Ferrari, "Association between serum concentrations of 25-hydroxyvitamin D3 and periodontal disease in the US population," *American Journal of Clinical Nutrition*, vol. 80, no. 1, pp. 108–113, 2004.

[17] A. E. Millen, K. M. Hovey, M. J. LaMonte et al., "Plasma 25-hydroxyvitamin D concentrations and periodontal disease in postmenopausal women," *Journal of Periodontology*, vol. 84, no. 9, pp. 1243–1256, 2013.

[18] M. N. Garcia, C. F. Hildebolt, D. D. Miley et al., "One-year effects of vitamin D and calcium supplementation on chronic periodontitis," *Journal of Periodontology*, vol. 82, no. 1, pp. 25–32, 2011.

[19] C. F. Hildebolt, "Effect of vitamin D and calcium on periodontitis," *Journal of Periodontology*, vol. 76, no. 9, pp. 1576–1587, 2005.

[20] D. Dixon, C. F. Hildebolt, D. D. Miley et al., "Calcium and vitamin D use among adults in periodontal disease maintenance programmes," *British Dental Journal*, vol. 206, no. 12, pp. 627–631, 2009.

[21] E. N. Alshouibi, E. K. Kaye, H. J. Cabral, C. W. Leone, and R. I. Garcia, "Vitamin D and periodontal health in older men," *Journal of Dental Research*, vol. 92, no. 8, pp. 689–693, 2013.

[22] J. D. Bashutski, R. M. Eber, J. S. Kinney et al., "The impact of vitamin D status on periodontal surgery outcomes," *Journal of Dental Research*, vol. 90, no. 8, pp. 1007–1012, 2011.

[23] A. E. Millen, C. A. Andrews, M. J. LaMonte et al., "Vitamin D status and 5-year changes in periodontal disease measures among postmenopausal women: the Buffalo OsteoPerio Study," *Journal of Periodontology*, vol. 85, no. 10, pp. 1321–1332, 2014.

[24] K. Kienreich, M. Grubler, A. Tomaschitz et al., "Vitamin D, arterial hypertension and cerebrovascular disease," *Indian Journal of Medical Research*, vol. 137, no. 4, pp. 669–679, 2013.

[25] M. F. Holick, N. C. Binkley, H. A. Bischoff-Ferrari et al., "Evaluation, treatment, and prevention of vitamin D deficiency: an Endocrine Society clinical practice guideline," *Journal of Clinical Endocrinology & Metabolism*, vol. 96, no. 7, pp. 1911–1930, 2011.

[26] G. Iacobucci, "Vitamin D supplementation does cut respiratory infections, new study suggests," *BMJ*, vol. 356, p. j847, 2017.

[27] V. P. Hiremath, C. B. Rao, V. Naik, and K. V. Prasad, "Anti-inflammatory effect of vitamin D on gingivitis: a dose-response randomised control trial," *Oral Health & Preventive Dentistry*, vol. 11, no. 1, pp. 61–69, 2013.

[28] M. Urashima, T. Segawa, M. Okazaki, M. Kurihara, Y. Wada, and H. Ida, "Randomized trial of vitamin D supplementation to prevent seasonal influenza A in schoolchildren," *American Journal of Clinical Nutrition*, vol. 91, no. 5, pp. 1255–1260, 2010.

[29] A. R. Martineau, C. J. Cates, M. Urashima et al., "Vitamin D for the management of asthma," *Cochrane Database of Systematic Reviews*, vol. 9, article CD011511, 2016.

[30] K. D. Cashman, "Vitamin D: dietary requirements and food fortification as a means of helping achieve adequate vitamin D status," *Journal of Steroid Biochemistry and Molecular Biology*, vol. 148, pp. 19–26, 2015.

[31] A. Di Benedetto, I. Gigante, S. Colucci, and M. Grano, "Periodontal disease: linking the primary inflammation to bone loss," *Clinical and Developmental Immunology*, vol. 2013, Article ID 503754, 7 pages, 2013.

[32] M. F. Holick, "Vitamin D deficiency," *New England Journal of Medicine*, vol. 357, no. 3, pp. 266–281, 2007.

[33] R. F. Chun, "New perspectives on the vitamin D binding protein," *Cell Biochemistry and Function*, vol. 30, no. 6, pp. 445–456, 2012.

[34] N. H. Wood, R. Khammissa, R. Meyerov, J. Lemmer, and L. Feller, "Actinic cheilitis: a case report and a review of the literature," *European Journal of Dentistry*, vol. 5, no. 1, pp. 101–106, 2011.

[35] L. Feller, N. H. Wood, M. H. Motswaledi, R. A. Khammissa, M. Meyer, and J. Lemmer, "Xeroderma pigmentosum: a case report and review of the literature," *Journal of Preventive Medicine and Hygiene*, vol. 51, no. 2, pp. 87–91, 2010.

[36] R. Vieth, "How to optimize vitamin D supplementation to prevent cancer, based on cellular adaptation and hydroxylase enzymology," *Anticancer Research*, vol. 29, no. 9, pp. 3675–3684, 2009.

[37] D. A. Searing and D. Y. Leung, "Vitamin D in atopic dermatitis, asthma and allergic diseases," *Immunology and Allergy Clinics of North America*, vol. 30, no. 3, pp. 397–409, 2010.

[38] B. W. Hollis and C. L. Wagner, "Clinical review: the role of the parent compound vitamin D with respect to metabolism and function: why clinical dose intervals can affect clinical outcomes," *Journal of Clinical Endocrinology & Metabolism*, vol. 98, no. 12, pp. 4619–4628, 2013.

[39] D. Reid, B. J. Toole, S. Knox et al., "The relation between acute changes in the systemic inflammatory response and plasma 25-hydroxyvitamin D concentrations after elective knee arthroplasty," *American Journal of Clinical Nutrition*, vol. 93, no. 5, pp. 1006–1011, 2011.

[40] V. Dimitrov, R. Salehi-Tabar, B. S. An, and J. H. White, "Non-classical mechanisms of transcriptional regulation by the vitamin D receptor: insights into calcium homeostasis, immune system regulation and cancer chemoprevention," *Journal of Steroid Biochemistry and Molecular Biology*, vol. 144, pp. 74–80, 2014.

[41] A. Piotrowska, J. Wierzbicka, and M. A. Zmijewski, "Vitamin D in the skin physiology and pathology," *Acta Biochimica Polonica*, vol. 63, no. 1, pp. 89–95, 2016.

[42] L. L. Chen, H. Li, P. P. Zhang, and S. M. Wang, "Association between vitamin D receptor polymorphisms and periodontitis: a meta-analysis," *Journal of Periodontology*, vol. 83, no. 9, pp. 1095–1103, 2012.

[43] L. Feller, N. H. Wood, R. A. Khammissa, and J. Lemmer, "Review: allergic contact stomatitis," *Oral Surgery, Oral Medicine, Oral Pathology and Oral Radiology*, vol. 123, no. 5, pp. 559–565, 2017.

[44] L. Barrea, M. C. Savanelli, C. Di Somma et al., "Vitamin D and its role in psoriasis: an overview of the dermatologist and nutritionist," *Reviews in Endocrine and Metabolic Disorders*, vol. 18, no. 2, pp. 195–205, 2017.

[45] F. N. Yuan, J. Valiyaparambil, M. C. Woods et al., "Vitamin D signaling regulates oral keratinocyte proliferation in vitro and in vivo," *International Journal of Oncology*, vol. 44, no. 5, pp. 1625–1633, 2014.

[46] L. Feller, R. A. Khammissa, R. Chandran, M. Altini, and J. Lemmer, "Oral candidosis in relation to oral immunity," *Journal of Oral Pathology & Medicine*, vol. 43, no. 8, pp. 563–569, 2014.

[47] L. Feller, M. Altini, R. A. Khammissa, R. Chandran, M. Bouckaert, and J. Lemmer, "Oral mucosal immunity," *Oral Surgery, Oral Medicine, Oral Pathology and Oral Radiology*, vol. 116, no. 5, pp. 576–583, 2013.

[48] M. T. Cantorna, L. Snyder, Y. D. Lin, and L. Yang, "Vitamin D and 1,25(OH)2D regulation of T cells," *Nutrients*, vol. 7, no. 4, pp. 3011–3021, 2015.

[49] Y. Amano, K. Komiyama, and M. Makishima, "Vitamin D and periodontal disease," *Journal of Oral Science*, vol. 51, no. 1, pp. 11–20, 2009.

[50] H. D. Hendrik and E. J. Raubenheimer, "Vitamin D nuclear receptor and periodontal disease: a review," *JBR Journal of Interdisciplinary Medicine and Dental Science*, vol. 3, no. 1, article 1000157, 2015.

[51] R. Wei and S. Christakos, "Mechanisms underlying the regulation of innate and adaptive immunity by vitamin D," *Nutrients*, vol. 7, no. 10, pp. 8251–8260, 2015.

[52] R. B. de Brito Junior, R. M. Scarel-Caminaga, P. C. Trevilatto, A. P. de Souza, and S. P. Barros, "Polymorphisms in the vitamin D receptor gene are associated with periodontal disease," *Journal of Periodontology*, vol. 75, no. 8, pp. 1090–1095, 2004.

[53] B. J. Hennig, J. M. Parkhill, I. L. Chapple, P. A. Heasman, and J. J. Taylor, "Association of a vitamin D receptor gene polymorphism with localized early-onset periodontal diseases," *Journal of Periodontology*, vol. 70, no. 9, pp. 1032–1038, 1999.

[54] R. A. Khammissa, L. Feller, R. Meyerov, and J. Lemmer, "Peri-implant mucositis and peri-implantitis: bacterial infection," *SADJ*, vol. 67, no. 2, pp. 70–74, 2012.

[55] X. Tang, Y. Pan, and Y. Zhao, "Vitamin D inhibits the expression of interleukin-8 in human periodontal ligament cells stimulated with Porphyromonas gingivalis," *Archives of Oral Biology*, vol. 58, no. 4, pp. 397–407, 2013.

[56] J. Lane, "Investigation into toll like receptor mechanisms of action, in relation to *Porphyromonas gingivalis* in periodontitis," *The Plymouth Student Scientist*, vol. 6, no. 2, pp. 355–367, 2013.

[57] W. Zhang, E. B. Swearingen, J. Ju, T. Rigney, and G. D. Tribble, "Porphyromonas gingivalis invades osteoblasts and inhibits bone formation," *Microbes and Infection*, vol. 12, no. 11, pp. 838–845, 2010.

[58] P. Zhang, Y. Wu, Z. Jiang, L. Jiang, and B. Fang, "Osteogenic response of mesenchymal stem cells to continuous mechanical strain is dependent on ERK1/2-Runx2 signaling," *International Journal of Molecular Medicine*, vol. 29, no. 6, pp. 1083–1089, 2012.

[59] L. Feller, M. Altini, and J. Lemmer, "Inflammation in the context of oral cancer," *Oral Oncology*, vol. 49, no. 9, pp. 887–892, 2013.

[60] Y. Zhan, S. Samietz, B. Holtfreter et al., "Prospective study of serum 25-hydroxy vitamin D and tooth loss," *Journal of Dental Research*, vol. 93, no. 7, pp. 639–644, 2014.

[61] S. Rieger, H. Zhao, P. Martin, K. Abe, and T. S. Lisse, "The role of nuclear hormone receptors in cutaneous wound repair," *Cell Biochemistry and Function*, vol. 33, no. 1, pp. 1–13, 2015.

[62] S. Jabbar, J. Drury, J. Fordham, H. K. Datta, R. M. Francis, and S. P. Tuck, "Plasma vitamin D and cytokines in periodontal disease and postmenopausal osteoporosis," *Journal of Periodontal Research*, vol. 46, no. 1, pp. 97–104, 2011.

[63] E. A. Krall, C. Wehler, R. I. Garcia, S. S. Harris, and B. Dawson-Hughes, "Calcium and vitamin D supplements reduce tooth loss in the elderly," *American Journal of Medicine*, vol. 111, no. 6, pp. 452–456, 2001.

[64] M. Jimenez, E. Giovannucci, E. Krall Kaye, K. J. Joshipura, and T. Dietrich, "Predicted vitamin D status and incidence of tooth loss and periodontitis," *Public Health Nutrition*, vol. 17, no. 4, pp. 844–852, 2014.

[65] G. J. van der Putten, J. Vanobbergen, L. De Visschere, J. Schols, and C. de Baat, "Association of some specific nutrient deficiencies with periodontal disease in elderly people: a systematic literature review," *Nutrition*, vol. 25, no. 7-8, pp. 717–722, 2009.

[66] G. Klein, "Evidence-based medicine," in *This Idea Must Die*, J. Brockman, Ed., pp. 220–222, HarperCollins, New York, NY, USA, 2015.

18

Detection of Bone Defects using CBCT Exam in an Italian Population

Gianluca Gambarini,[1] **Gabriele Miccoli,**[1] **Gianfranco Gaimari,**[1] **Deborah Pompei,**[1] **Andrea Pilloni,**[1] **Lucila Piasecki,**[2] **Dina Al-Sudani,**[3] **Dario Di Nardo,**[1] **and Luca Testarelli**[1]

[1]*Department of Oral and Maxillofacial Sciences, Sapienza University of Rome, Rome, Italy*
[2]*Department of Periodontics and Endodontics, University at Buffalo, Buffalo, NY, USA*
[3]*Department of Restorative Dental Sciences, College of Dentistry, King Saud University, Riyadh, Saudi Arabia*

Correspondence should be addressed to Gabriele Miccoli; miccoligabriele@gmail.com

Academic Editor: Manal Awad

Background. The aim of this study was to evaluate the *in vivo* incidence and the location of fenestrations in a young Italian population by using CBCT. *Materials and Methods*. Fifty patients who had previously performed CBCT for planning third molar extraction or orthodontic therapy were selected for the study. No previous dental treatment had been performed on these patients. Overall, 1,395 teeth were evaluated. Root fenestrations were identified according to the definition of Davies and the American Association of Endodontists. Data was collected and statistically analyzed. *Results*. Fenestrations were observed in 159 teeth out of 1,395 (11% of teeth). In the lower jaw, we found 68 fenestrations (5%) and 91 in the maxilla (6,5%). Incisors were the teeth with the highest incidence of fenestrations. *Conclusion*. The relative common finding (11%) of fenestration supports the need for CBCT exams before any surgical/implant treatment to avoid complications related to the initial presence of fenestrations. CBCT was found to be an effective and convenient tool for diagnosing fenestration.

1. Background

Bone defects like dehiscence and fenestrations are common findings in natural dentition, being more frequent on the facial bone than on the lingual bone, and in the anterior teeth [1]. Fenestrations are isolated areas in which roots are denuded of bone and root surfaces are covered only by periosteum and overlying gingiva, but marginal bone is intact. Therefore, the marginal bone in fenestrations is intact [2].

Clinical diagnosis of fenestration is a challenge. Information derived from probing the gingival tissues in association with traditional radiographic diagnostic imaging provides guidelines for assessing the alveolar bone height and checking for the presence of bone defects, but they can very rarely detect fenestrations [3].

Moreover, fenestrations can also occur as an iatrogenic error in implant dentistry. In such cases, a fenestration is defined as a "vestibular or linguopalatal defect" or as an expression of a bone thickness deficiency that creates partial exposure of an implant that is completely surrounded by bone. This means that when buccal fenestrations occur, the implant partially protrudes through an opening in the intact bone plate, mostly on the buccal side. There fenestrations that occur in implant dentistry are divided into two cases [1]. A Class 1 fenestration is a minor penetration of the implant through the intact bone plate. A Class 2 fenestration is the formation of a convexity enclosing a "significant portion of the implant exposed." The distinction between these two classes of fenestrations is important because they call for different repair measures.

Diagnosis of such fenestrations can be accomplished at two stages: (a) as early as implant placement during the surgery or (b) delayed during recall appointments of the implant patient. Since fenestrations can be a result of implant placement but can be also naturally present in the dentition; it is important to determine why and when the fenestration occurred and to differentiate between a natural finding and an iatrogenic error. A limited number of researches were

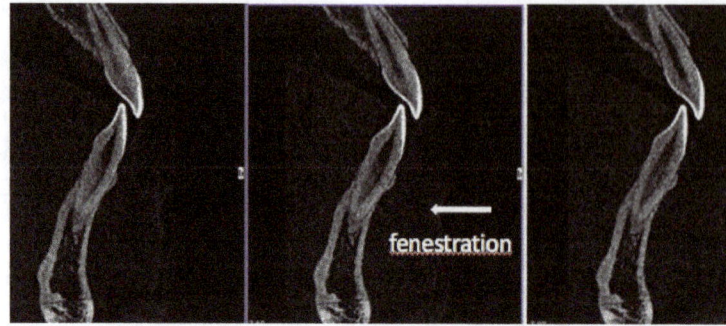

FIGURE 1: Cone-beam computed tomography (CBCT) images showing fenestrations in the area of the incisors.

conducted specifically on fenestrations, and most of them were conducted on skulls, with no relation to previous dental treatment, including extractions, periodontal surgery, and orthodontic therapy [3, 4]. Therefore, the aim of the present study was to evaluate the incidence and the location of fenestrations by using a CBCT exam in a young population, who had no previous dental treatment performed.

2. Materials and Methods

CBCT examinations were selected from Italian (Caucasian) patients between 18 and 30 years old, who had already performed the CBCT exams for third molar extraction or orthodontic purposes but had no dental treatment previously done. Criteria of inclusion were age lower than 30 years old, teeth present in both dental arches, without any previous orthodontic, restorative, surgical (extraction), or prosthodontic treatment.

Fifty CBCT exams were examined, for a total of 1,395 teeth (five agenesia were recorded). Images were obtained by using a CBCT exam (iCAT, Imaging Sciences International, Hatfield, PA, USA), with a single 360-degree rotation and 0,3 mm voxel dimension (exposition of 5,0 mA, 120 kV, 9,6 s for time exposition, and 0,3 of axial section). The sections used were 1 mm (FOV, $4 \times 4 \times 6$ cm) and 1,28 mm thickness. This passes through the center of the root perpendicular to the alveolar crest. The long axis of the root has dictated the vertical orientation of the section. The measurements were performed with the maximum possible zoom.

Root fenestration (RF) was identified according to the definition of Davies et al. [5] and the American Association of Endodontists [6] as a tooth root protruding from a window-like opening or a defect in the alveolar bone without involvement of the alveolar margin. Three points should be emphasized in this definition. (1) A window-like opening or defect of the alveolar bone means that both the cortical bone and the cancellous bone are penetrated simultaneously, and the root either is in direct contact with the overlying mucosa or exposed to the oral environment. (2) The exposed root protrudes beyond the bone. (3) The exclusion of the alveolar margin emphasized to differentiate fenestration from dehiscence, which is the crest of buccal and/or lingual bone that lies at least 4 mm apical to the crest of the interproximal bone [5, 7, 8]. Figure 1 shows an example.

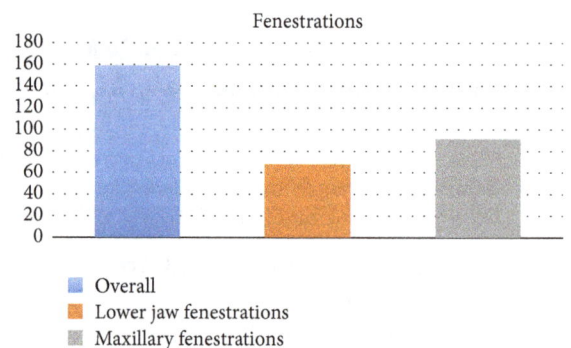

FIGURE 2: Incidence of fenestrations in maxilla and in mandible.

Data was analyzed using a Pearson chi-square test, performed using the Statistical Package for the Social Sciences (version 18.0; SPSS, Inc., Chicago, IL). The age, gender, number of fenestrations, and their location were displayed by frequency and percentage. The relations between the groups were analyzed by using the Pearson chi-square test. The level of significance was 5% ($P < 0.05$) and data was presented with 95% confidence intervals where applicable. All assessment was done by a double examiner to eliminate the interexaminer errors. All data regarding patient identification was kept confidential.

3. Results

The average age of patients was 24.5 years old, with 24 males (48%) and 26 females (52%).

In 588 teeth (42%), dehiscence, fenestrations, or both bone defects, were found. Fenestrations were present in 159 teeth out of 1,395, corresponding to the 11%.

A significant difference was found ($P = 0.0311$) between the lower jaw presenting 68 fenestrations (5%) and the maxilla with 91 fenestrations (6,5%), as shown in Figure 2.

Incisors were teeth with the highest incidence of fenestrations: 90 fenestrations (56%) were found in incisors, 50 in the maxilla (31%) and 40 in the lower jaw (25%); 36 cases (22%) were found in canines, 22 in the maxilla (13%) and 14 for the lower jaw (0.8%). Thirty-one (19%) fenestrations were found on premolars, 18 in the maxilla (11%) and 13 on the lower jaw (0.8%). The smallest incidence was found on molars in only 2

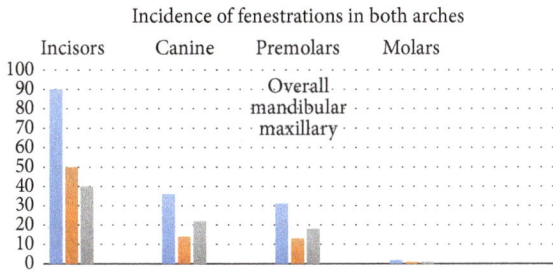

FIGURE 3: Incidence of fenestrations by tooth type.

cases, 1 in the maxilla (0.1%) and 1 in the lower jaw (0,06%). Significant differences were found amongst these groups, with the exception of the canines compared to premolars (P = 0.068), as shown in Figure 3.

A significant difference was found (P = 0.0001) between 157 (99%) fenestrations observed in the labial-buccal side, compared with the two observed in the plagal-lingual side (1%). Multiple defects were significantly (P = 0,119) found more often (9.6%), when compared to patients showing only one defect (4%).

4. Discussion

Results of the present study showed that 11% of teeth have fenestrations as a natural finding, without any relation to previous dental treatments. This data confirms some, but not all, results from previous studies which had been performed on skulls, and consequently not in a young and healthy population. An in vivo study was performed to achieve more precise and detailed information. In cadavers skulls, due to differences in the composition of teeth and alveolar bone, the extent of degradation and damage differs between these two hard tissues. The alveolar plates in dried skulls, especially on the labial or buccal side, may be physically damaged more easily after exposure to air and soil, which may explain the higher prevalence of fenestration in skulls.

Fenestrations were present in 9.32% of teeth in skulls in the study conducted by Jorgic-Srdjak et al. in 1998 [9]; on the contrary, in the Nimigean et al. study [7], fenestrations were found in 69,56% of skulls. The latter results could have been influenced by surgical extractions, periodontal or other diseases [9–11].

In the present study, fenestrations were more common in the maxilla than in the mandible, which is consistent with previous reports [5, 7, 9–14]. However, differences can be found in the prevalence in some teeth. Previous studies reported the relative frequency of tooth type with fenestrations as follows: maxillary first molar, mandibular first molar, maxillary and mandibular canines, and mandibular lateral incisors [5, 7, 9, 11]. On the contrary, in the present study, fenestrations were found more common in incisors and rare in molars, probably due to the lack of any dental treatment, including extractions, in the molar area.

The present study confirmed that fenestrations were more frequent on the labial-buccal side than on the palatal-lingual. Elliot and Bower [15] reported only one unspecified lingual

fenestration in a mandibular third molar. Edel [13] reported two lingual fenestrations in mandibular incisors because of inclined roots. Nimigean et al. [7] examined 3,646 teeth but reported no palatal or lingual fenestrations. A clear explanation of this phenomenon has not been reported, but it can be hypothesized that since most fenestrations occur in maxillary teeth, this might be a potential contributing factor, as many teeth in this arch have root tips inclined to the labial-buccal [7].

The traditional method of investigating the prevalence and morphology of fenestrations has been on dry human skulls. Visual examination and direct measurement make this method highly accurate and reliable; however, disadvantages are that studies of dried skulls offer no clinical information and no dental history, and the method can never be applied to clinical surgical diagnosis [16]. On the contrary, both in vivo and ex vivo studies have indicated that CBCT may be a useful and more practical clinical tool to detect these defects. The low dose of radiation and excellent image quality of CBCT compared with conventional CT makes CBCT the ideal means for the diagnosis of fenestration defects [17]. The use of CBCT allows clinicians to examine the form and the size of the alveolar bone without the disadvantages of common radiography. These images are not subject to distortions or overlaps. In the present study, CBCT scans were used to evaluate alveolar bone defects with axial and transverse sections. Fenestration was easily detected, confirming the conclusions of the Bayat et al. study [18]. CBCT currently represents the gold standard to evaluate fenestrations and dehiscences furcation lesions, instead of the common radiology.

To date, only few investigations have taken advantage of CBCT to study fenestration. The studies of Leung et al. [19], Ising et al. [20], and Patcas et al. [2] indicated that CBCT is a reliable, accurate, and noninvasive method for diagnosing fenestrations in the clinical setting and for investigating its prevalence. Visualizing dehiscences and fenestrations is not possible with traditional two-dimensional (2D) radiographs because of superimposition. CBCT allows the visualization of these defects with more accurate three-dimensional (3D) images [21–24].

Of course, unpredictable occurrences, such as iatrogenic errors during implant placement, cannot be eliminated by any precautionary measures, but a preoperative CBCT can help to ensure proper placement in implant angulation and to ensure a proper distance from the adjacent tooth and the external bone surface.

Other studies [25] used CBCT to compare the correlations between the presence of fenestrations and malocclusions. Significant differences in the presence of fenestration were found among subjects with skeletal Class I, Class II, and Class III malocclusions. Fenestrations had greater prevalence in the maxilla and were more common in Class II. A study on Chinese population [26] found a higher presence of fenestrations (31,93% of teeth) in Class III patients. The tooth site which was most commonly affected was lower canine, while the least was upper central incisor. All these studies indicated that malocclusions are potential factors for bone defects and fenestrations. In the present study, it was not possible to check this correlation in an Italian population because half of the patients had been previously scanned for surgical purposes and no orthodontic parameters had been registered.

5. Conclusion

Fenestrations of the buccal bone are unpredictable anatomical findings, difficult to diagnose by traditional clinical and radiographic technique. It is important to diagnose these defects before any surgical, implant, or orthodontic therapy, since undetected fenestrations may adversely affect the clinical outcome of these treatments. The relative common finding of fenestrations in an Italian population supports the need of a preoperative CBCT exam to accurately diagnose the initial presence of fenestrations, for a more precise and reliable surgical approach and implant placement.

References

[1] L. Steier and G. Steier, "Successful dental implant placement surgeries with buccal bone fenestrations," *Journal of Oral Implantology*, vol. 41, no. 1, pp. 112–118, 2015.

[2] R. Patcas, L. Müller, O. Ullrich, and T. Peltomäki, "Accuracy of cone-beam computed tomography at different resolutions assessed on the bony covering of the mandibular anterior teeth," *American Journal of Orthodontics and Dentofacial Orthopedics*, vol. 141, no. 1, pp. 41–50, 2012.

[3] N. Bagis, M. E. Kolsuz, S. Kursun, and K. Orhan, "Comparison of intraoral radiography and cone-beam computed tomography for the detection of periodontal defects: An in vitro study," *BMC Oral Health*, vol. 15, no. 1, article no. 64, 2015.

[4] M. Trottini, M. Bossù, D. Corridore et al., "Assessing risk factors for dental caries: A statistical modeling approach," *Caries Research*, vol. 49, no. 3, pp. 226–235, 2015.

[5] R. M. Davies, M. C. Downer, P. S. Hull, and M. A. Lennon, "Alveolar defects in human skulls," *Journal of Clinical Periodontology*, vol. 1, no. 2, pp. 107–111, 1974.

[6] American Association of Endodontists (2012) Glossary of endodontic terms, http://www.aae.org/Publications/Content.aspx.

[7] V. R. Nimigean, V. Nimigean, M. A. Bencze, N. Dimcevici-Poesina, R. Cergan, and S. Moraru, "Alveolar bone dehiscence and fenestration: an anathomical study and review," *Romanian Journal of Morphology and Embryology*, vol. 50, no. 3, pp. 391–397, 2009.

[8] T. Yoshioka, I. Kikuchi, C. G. Adorno, and H. Suda, "Periapical bone defects of root filled teeth with persistent lesions evaluated by cone-beam computed tomography," *International Endodontic Journal*, vol. 44, no. 3, pp. 245–252, 2011.

[9] K. Jorgic-Srdjak, D. Plancak, A. Bosnjak, and Z. Azinovic, "Incidence and distribution of dehiscence and fenestrations in human skulls," *Collegium Antropologicum*, pp. 111–116, 1998.

[10] G. Urbani, G. Lomardo, P. Filippini, and FP. Nocini, "Dehiscences and fenestrations: study of distribution and incidence in a homogeneous population model," *Stomatologia Mediterranea*, vol. 11, no. 2, pp. 113–118, 1991.

[11] R. D. Rupprecht, G. M. Horning, B. K. Nicoll, and M. E. Cohen, "Prevalence of dehiscences and fenestrations in modern American skulls," *Journal of Periodontology*, vol. 72, no. 6, pp. 722–729, 2001.

[12] H. Tal, "Alveolar dehiscences and fenestrae in dried south African Negro mandibles," *American Journal of Physical Anthropology*, vol. 61, no. 2, pp. 173–179, 1983.

[13] A. Edel, "Alveolar bone fenestrations and dehiscences in dry Bedouin jaws," *Journal of Clinical Periodontology*, vol. 8, no. 6, pp. 491–499, 1981.

[14] D. C. Larato, "Alveolar plate fenestrations and dehiscences of the human skull," *Oral Surgery, Oral Medicine, Oral Pathology, Oral Radiology, and Endodontology*, vol. 29, no. 6, pp. 816–819, 1970.

[15] J. R. Elliot and G. M. Bower, "Alveolar dehiscence and fenestration," *Periodontics*, vol. 1, pp. 245–248, 1963.

[16] H. Y. Pan, H. Yang, R. Zhang et al., "Use of cone-beam computed tomography to evaluate the prevalence of root fenestration in a Chinese subpopulation," *International Endodontic Journal*, vol. 47, no. 1, pp. 10–19, 2014.

[17] A. Kasaj and B. Willershausen, "Digital volume tomography for diagnostics in periodontology," *International Journal of Computerized Dentistry*, vol. 10, no. 2, pp. 155–168, 2007.

[18] S. Bayat, A. R. Talaeipour, and F. Sarlati, "Detection of simulated periodontal defects using cone-beam CT and digital intraoral radiography," *Dentomaxillofacial Radiology*, vol. 45, no. 6, Article ID 20160030, 2016.

[19] C. C. Leung, L. Palomo, R. Griffith, and M. G. Hans, "Accuracy and reliability of cone-beam computed tomography for measuring alveolar bone height and detecting bony dehiscences and fenestrations," *American Journal of Orthodontics and Dentofacial Orthopedics*, vol. 137, no. 4, pp. S109–S119, 2010.

[20] N. Ising, K. B. Kim, E. Araujo, and P. Buschang, "Evaluation of dehiscences using cone beam computed tomography," *The Angle Orthodontist*, vol. 82, no. 1, pp. 122–130, 2012.

[21] A. Baysal, T. Uysal, I. Veli et al., "Evaluation of alveolar bone loss following rapid maxillary expansion using cone-beam computed tomography," *Korean Journal of Orthodontics*, vol. 43, pp. 83–95, 2013.

[22] F. A. Quereshy, T. A. Savell, and J. M. Palomo, "Applications of Cone Beam Computed Tomography in the Practice of Oral and Maxillofacial Surgery," *Journal of Oral and Maxillofacial Surgery*, vol. 66, no. 4, pp. 791–796, 2008.

[23] S. Enhos, T. Uysal, A. Yagci, I. Velid, F. I. Ucare, and T. Ozerf, "Dehiscence and fenestration in patients with different vertical growth patterns assessed with cone-beam computed tomography," *The Angle Orthodontist*, vol. 82, no. 5, pp. 868–874, 2012.

[24] S. Q. Buyuk, E. Ercan, M. Celikoglu, A. S. Ercan, and Hatipoglu M., "Evaluation of dehiscence and fenestration in adolescent patients affected by unilateral cleft lip and palate: a retrospective cone beam computed tomography study," *The Angle Orthodontist*, vol. 86, no. 3, pp. 431–436, 2016.

[25] A. Yagci, I. Veli, T. Uysal, F. I. Ucar, T. Ozer, and S. Enhos, "Dehiscence and fenestration in skeletal Class I, II, and III malocclusions assessed with cone-beam computed tomography," *The Angle Orthodontist*, vol. 82, no. 1, pp. 67–74, 2012.

[26] L.-Y. Sun, B. Wang, and B. Fang, "The prevalence of dehiscence and fenestration on, anterior region of skeletal Class III malocclusions: a cone-beam CT study," *Shanghai Kou Qiang Yi Xue*, vol. 22, no. 4, pp. 418–422, 2013.

19

Investigation of Clinical Characteristics and Etiological Factors in Children with Molar Incisor Hypomineralization

Maria Rita Giuca, Maria Cappè, Elisabetta Carli, Lisa Lardani, and Marco Pasini ⓘ

Department of Surgical, Medical, Molecular Pathology and Critical Area, Dental and Oral Surgery Clinic, Unit of Pediatric Dentistry, University of Pisa, Via Savi 10, 56126 Pisa, Italy

Correspondence should be addressed to Marco Pasini; dr.marcopasini@yahoo.it

Academic Editor: Louis M. Lin

Aim. The purpose of the present study was to evaluate the clinical defects and etiological factors potentially involved in the onset of MIH in a pediatric sample. *Methods.* 120 children, selected from the university dental clinic, were included: 60 children (25 boys and 35 girls; average age: 9.8 ± 1.8 years) with MIH formed the test group and 60 children (27 boys and 33 girls; average age: 10.1 ± 2 years) without MIH constituted the control group. Distribution and severity of MIH defects were evaluated, and a questionnaire was used to investigate the etiological variables; chi-square, univariate, and multivariate statistical tests were performed (significance level set at $p < 0.05$). *Results.* A total of 186 molars and 98 incisors exhibited MIH defects: 55 molars and 75 incisors showed mild defects, 91 molars and 20 incisors had moderate lesions, and 40 molars and 3 incisors showed severe lesions. Univariate and multivariate statistical analysis showed a significant association ($p < 0.05$) between MIH and ear, nose, and throat (ENT) disorders and the antibiotics used during pregnancy (0.019). *Conclusions.* Moderate defects were more frequent in the molars, while mild lesions were more frequent in the incisors. Antibiotics used during pregnancy and ENT may be directly involved in the etiology of MIH in children.

1. Background

The term "molar incisor hypomineralization (MIH)" is a definition introduced by Weerheijm et al. to describe enamel defects affecting the first permanent molars and, frequently, permanent incisors; furthermore, the second permanent molars and permanent canines can also be involved [1].

MIH is a relatively common condition with a world prevalence range from 2.8% to 44% [2]. Mulic et al. observed that females exhibit a higher prevalence of mineralization than males of the same age and that the maxillary first molars and incisors were more often affected in comparison to mandibular teeth [3].

Clinical features of MIH include white-to-yellow/brown large demarcated porous opacities caused by changes in mineral and protein enamel composition, anomaly in the tissue translucency, tooth hypersensitivity that is due to the exposure of dentin, posteruption enamel breakdown, and rapid dental caries progression.

In a systematic review of Americano et al., a positive association between dental caries and MIH was found as the enamel breakdown predisposes for higher dental biofilm accumulation. The authors concluded that children with MIH were 2 to 4 times more likely to show caries than young patients of the control group [4].

Bozal et al. [5] evaluated the ultrastructural aspects of the surface of the teeth with MIH and found a loss of prismatic pattern, a porous ultrastructure with cracks, decreased levels of calcium and phosphate, and alterations in ionic composition. These enamel alterations may interfere with the dental restorative procedures.

MIH lesions can be classified into three categories: mild (isolated enamel opacities without enamel sensitivity), moderate (occlusal or incisal third involvement with no or slight sensitivity), and severe (presence of posteruptive

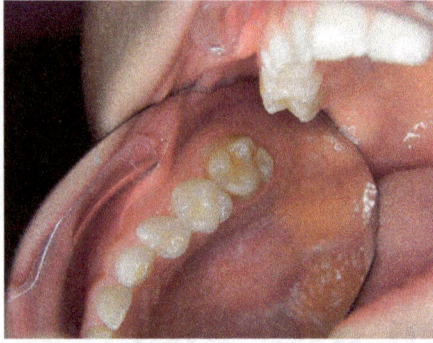

FIGURE 1: Mild molar hypomineralization.

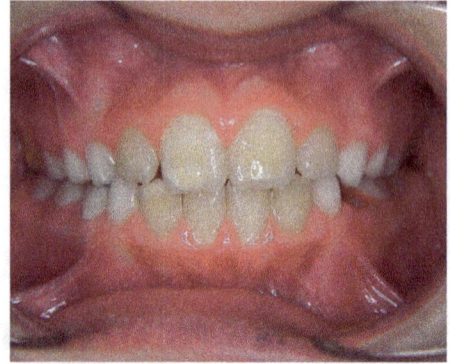

FIGURE 3: Mild incisor hypomineralization.

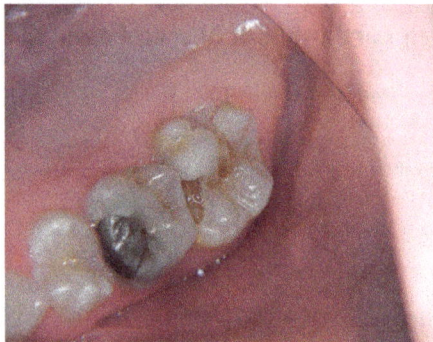

FIGURE 2: Severe molar hypomineralization.

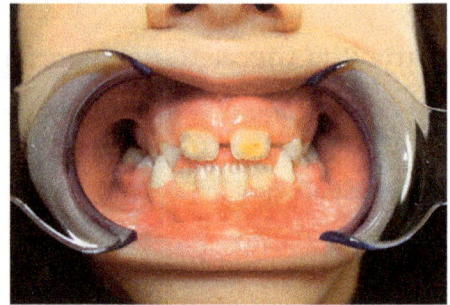

FIGURE 4: Severe incisor hypomineralization.

enamel breakdown and widespread caries that determine both functional and esthetic complications) (Figures 1–4) [6].

Early detection, intervention, and appropriate therapy can prevent severe complications and improve both masticatory function and esthetic. It was stated that the age of 8 years is the best age for a correct diagnosis, as at this stage, all upper and lower permanent incisors and mandibular and maxillary permanent first molars are fully erupted [7]. Differential diagnosis includes amelogenesis imperfecta, hypoplasia, and fluorosis.

Although the etiology of MIH is still not clear, a combination of different factors that may affect the ameloblasts during the enamel formation has been proposed. There is not often a family history of enamel hypomineralization such as in cases of amelogenesis imperfecta.

Mineralization of the first permanent molars usually starts at birth (just before or shortly after birth), and it is fully completed at 4-5 years of age [8]; anomalies that occur during the enamel matrix secretion cause enamel hypoplasia, while enamel anomalies during the maturation stage can determine the onset of hypomineralization.

In a recent systematic review [9], a possible link between MIH lesions and both systemic and environmental factors that may play a role during the enamel maturation stage was suggested.

Health problems that occurred during pregnancy and early childhood illness (i.e., asthma and pneumonia) were selected as the main possible etiological factors.

However, as the authors stated, the validity of several previous reports was impaired by poor protocol design.

As regards pathogenesis, it was hypothesized that the lesions are linked to an alteration in the oxygen supply of ameloblasts with a consequent decrease of enamel mineralization [10]. In particular, every systemic physiological stress may influence the ameloblasts' activity before or at birth and in the first years of life [11].

Several prenatal (i.e., diabetes and hypocalcemia), perinatal (i.e., premature birth and prolonged delivery), and postnatal (i.e., antibiotics and nutrition problems) etiological factors were proposed; however, to date, there is no conclusive evidence on MIH etiology [12].

For this reason, further studies are needed in order to individuate the etiology of MIH.

Therefore, the purpose of the present study was to investigate the possible etiological factors potentially involved in the onset of MIH.

2. Materials and Methods

In the present study, 60 children (25 boys and 35 girls; average age: 9.8 ± 1.8 years) with MIH (test group) and 60 children (27 boys and 33 girls; average age: 10.1 ± 2 years) without MIH (control group) were included. Patients were selected at the unit of pediatric dentistry of the university hospital. The control group consisted of patients in general good health and without MIH, that were comparable to the test group for age and sex.

A written consent (signed by parents or legal guardians) to participate in the study was obtained for each child, and all procedures were conducted in accordance with the Declaration of Helsinki. Moreover, this study was approved by the Ethics Committee.

The inclusion criteria were as follows: age from 6 to 13 years, Caucasian, presence of at least one permanent molar with a MIH with or without the incisors involved (for the test group).

The exclusion criteria were as follows: the presence of hypoplastic lesions or hypomineralization, fluorosis, amelogenesis imperfecta, tetracycline stains, and history of dental trauma for the incisors.

The clinical dental examination was performed by the same operator, who is an expert in pediatric dentistry and who had received extensive training on clinical pictures of MIH lesions; each tooth affected by MIH was cleaned with a rotating brush, and tartar deposits were removed with ultrasound. Clinical examination of MIH was performed on wet teeth after cleaning. The criteria used to diagnose MIH were those indicated by Weerheijm et al., and for each tooth involved, the severity was assessed: mild (color change of the smooth surface without enamel defects), moderate (loss of enamel without dentine involvement), or severe degree (dentine involvement, atypical restorations, and teeth extracted because of severe lesions) [13].

All patients of the test group were reevaluated by a second operator in order to confirm the diagnosis and the score of MIH.

A questionnaire was distributed to parents in order to investigate the possible etiological factors of MIH which were divided into prenatal, perinatal, and postnatal parameters.

Each variable was linked to the child or parental history, especially the mothers.

2.1. Statistical Analysis. The chi-square test was used for the clinical parameters (severity and distribution).

Univariate and multivariate statistical analyses, based on the general linear model procedures, were used to investigate the relationship between MIH and etiological factors. The variables were included in multivariate analysis when they were found to be significant in statistical univariate analysis.

We calculated the odds ratios and 95% confidence intervals for each parameter included in the questionnaire, and the Wald test was used to test all standard hypotheses in the univariate and multivariate model; the level of significance was set at $p < 0.05$.

The statistical analysis was performed using the SPSS (Statistical Package for Social Sciences, Chicago, USA) 22.0 program.

3. Results

It was observed that 32 (53.3%) children of the test group exhibited both molar and incisor involvement, while 28 (46.7%) patients had only molars affected. No statistically significant difference was found between the two percentages (chi-square test $p = 0.47$; relative risk 1.14; confidence interval 0.8–1.64).

The severity of MIH is reported in Table 1.

TABLE 1: Severity score.

	Mild	Moderate	Severe
Molars	55 (29.6%)	91 (48.9%)	40 (21.5%)
Incisors	75 (76.5%)	20 (20.4%)	3 (3.1%)

TABLE 2: Prenatal, perinatal, and postnatal variables (percentages) in the test group (with MIH) and in the controls (without MIH).

Possible etiological factors	Test group (%)	Control group (%)
Fluoride supplements in pregnancy	8	6
Gestational diabetes	27	13
Drug use in pregnancy	22	13
Full-term baby delivery	82	73
Smoking during pregnancy or breastfeeding	11	13
Natural vaginal birth	60	73
Childbirth complications	9	7
Breastfeeding	58	40
Allergies	24	13
Penicillin	84	27
Vitamin D	53	27
Infectious diseases	55	13
Ear, nose, and throat (ENT) disorders	60	7
Respiratory disorders	31	7
Physiological weaning for breastfeeding	75	87

As regards molars, moderate lesions were significantly ($p < 0.05$) more frequent in comparison to both mild defects (chi-square test $p = 0.001$; relative risk 1.48; confidence interval 1.22–1.81) and severe lesions (chi-square test $p = 0.001$; relative risk 1.76; confidence interval 1.45–2.14). No significant difference was detected between mild molar defects and severe lesions frequencies (chi-square test $p = 0.07$; relative risk 0.8; confidence interval 0.62–1.04).

As regards incisors, mild defects were significantly more frequent in comparison to moderate (chi-square test $p = 0.001$; relative risk 3.12; confidence interval 2.16–4.51) and severe lesions (chi-square test $p = 0.001$; relative risk 4.93; confidence interval 3.41–7.14).

Furthermore, moderate incisor lesions were significantly higher than severe lesions (chi-square test $p = 0.002$; relative risk 1.93; confidence interval 1.54–2.42).

Table 2 provides the prevalence of prenatal, perinatal, and postnatal etiological variables associated with MIH in the two groups.

Univariate analysis showed a statistically significant correlation ($p < 0.05$) between MIH and antibiotics, infectious diseases, and respiratory and ear, nose, and throat (ENT) disorders.

However, with multivariate analysis, a statistical association ($p < 0.05$) was found only between MIH and antibiotics and ENT disorders (Table 3).

4. Discussion

MIH diagnosis might be difficult to outpoint, and a standardized protocol is necessary for the dentists and for the reports in epidemiological studies of MIH [14].

TABLE 3: Univariate and multivariate analysis for etiological factors of MIH.

Variable	Univariate analysis			Multivariate analysis		
	p	OR	95% CI	p	OR	95% CI
Breastfeeding	0.236	0.487	0.148–1.602			
Allergies	0.373	0.476	0.093–2.443			
Antibiotics	0.001*	0.067	0.017–0.272	0.019*	0.138	0.026–0.717
Vitamin D	0.081	0.318	0.088–1.151			
Childbirth complications	0.788	0.732	0.075–7.113			
Gestational diabetes	0.301	0.423	0.083–2.157			
Drug use in pregnancy	0.461	0.538	0.104–2.793			
Fluoride supplements in pregnancy	0.623	0.571	0.061–5.323			
Smoking during pregnancy or breastfeeding	0.817	1.231	0.213–7.119			
Full-term baby delivery	0.459	0.595	0.150–2.354			
Infectious diseases	0.044*	0.192	0.039–0.953	0.644	0.628	0.087–4.535
Ear, nose, and throat (ENT) disorders	0.005*	0.048	0.006–0.395	0.038*	0.093	0.010–0.880
Respiratory disorders	0.058*	0.158	0.019–1.324	0.755	0.678	0.059–7.837
Natural vaginal birth	0.357	1.833	0.504–6.663			
Physiological weaning	0.373	2.103	0.409–10.80			

*$p < 0.05$

As regards the lesion distribution, a slight higher prevalence of both molar and incisor involvement was observed, while the percentage of children showing only molar involvement were slightly lower. The results in the literature are partially contradictory: Jasulaityte et al. found that 77.4% of schoolchildren exhibited MIH defects only in molars, while a lower percentage (22.6%) showed both molar and incisor enamel lesions [15].

However, in the Dutch National Epidemiological Survey of 2003, a higher percentage (57.1%) of both molar and incisor involvement was recorded [16].

Also in a study conducted on 360 Greek children aged 8–12 years, it was observed that a lower percentage of patients (28.4%) showed only molars affected, while more than 70% of the children exhibited both incisor and molar lesions [17].

The results of our study showed that mild defects were more frequent in molars. In the literature, it was observed by Buchgraber et al. [18] that demarcated enamel opacities were the most frequent lesions in Austrian children aged 6–12 years.

Jasulaityte et al. [16] found that children with MIH exhibited only demarcated opacities in high percentage (55.6%), while 20.6% of the patients showed at least one tooth with occlusal breakdown. These data are partially in agreement with the results of our study as we found a 21.5% of severe lesions in molars.

In our research, it was noticed that incisors showed milder enamel defects in comparison to molars, and this result was in line with a previous study, conducted on 277 children aged 8–12 years, showing that the severity of MIH defects was significantly more in molars compared to incisors [19].

Moreover, also in a recent study conducted on 154 Malaysian children aged 7–12 years, it was found that incisor involvement was less frequent than molar involvement (58%) and mild lesions exhibited a very high percentage (96.6%) [20].

Our results are also in agreement with those recorded by Lygidakis et al. [17] that observed a higher percentage (37.9%) of molars with moderate or severe lesions in

comparison with incisors (4.9%); in both incisors and molars, mild defects were detected in highest prevalence (62.1% in molars and 95.1% in incisors).

In the present study, a positive association was observed between MIH and antibiotics (penicillin use) and ENT disorders even if, in the literature, this association is still uncertain.

Mulic et al. [3] examined 103 children with MIH and found that the use of penicillin due to adenoid infections in the first five years was associated with a higher prevalence of enamel lesions.

Furthermore, Laisi et al. [21] stated that an altered pattern of amelogenesis may interfere with the process of enamel mineralization and that the early use of amoxicillin is one of the main causative factors of MIH. However, these results should be interpreted with caution as it is not possible to determine if it is the antibiotic use or the disease or a combination of both that can lead to the enamel lesions.

In the literature, other possible etiological factors of MIH were also found; in fact, in a recent systematic review, a positive association was observed between maternal alcohol consumption, infantile fever, and ethnicity; however, as the authors stated, the validity of these results was impaired by poor study design and other methodological errors [9]. In the present study, no association between MIH and prenatal and perinatal variables was found, and these results are in accordance with those reported by Basak et al. [22].

A limitation of this study, in addition to the small number of patients included, is that, using a questionnaire, there is a lack of validity, as the respondent may be forgetful or not be thinking within the full context of the situation. Furthermore, the present study was limited only in our region, and the results of this study may not accurately reflect a larger international sample.

5. Conclusion

In the present study, similar percentages of only molar involvement and molar/incisor involvement were detected.

Furthermore, it was observed that molars exhibited higher severity scores in comparison to incisors.

The results of this study show that, among the possible etiological factors of MIH, antibiotics and ear, nose, and throat diseases, during the first years of life, seem to be the predominant factors, while no positive association between prenatal/perinatal factors and MIH lesions was found.

References

[1] K. L. Weerheijm, B. Jälevik, and S. Alaluusua, "Molar-incisor hypomineralisation," *Caries Research*, vol. 35, no. 5, pp. 390-391, 2001.

[2] M. Hernandez, J. R. Boj, and E. Espasa, "Do we really know the prevalence of MIH?," *Journal of Clinical Pediatric Dentistry*, vol. 40, no. 4, pp. 259-263, 2016.

[3] A. Mulic, E. Cehajic, A. B. Tveit, and K. R. Stenhagen, "How serious is molar incisor hypomineralisation (MIH) among 8- and 9-year-old children in Bosnia-Herzegovina? A clinical study," *European Journal of Paediatric Dentistry*, vol. 18, no. 2, pp. 153-157, 2017.

[4] G. C. Americano, P. E. Jacobsen, V. M. Soviero, and D. Haubek, "A systematic review on the association between molar incisor hypomineralization and dental caries," *International Journal of Paediatic Dentistry*, vol. 27, no. 1, pp. 11-21, 2017.

[5] C. B. Bozal, A. Kaplan, A. Ortolani, S. G. Cortese, and A. M. Biondi, "Ultrastructure of the surface of dental enamel with molar incisor hypomineralization (MIH) with and without acid etching," *Acta Odontologica Latinoamericana*, vol. 29, no. 2, pp. 192-198, 2015.

[6] M. Pasini, M. R. Giuca, M. Scatena, R. Gatto, and S. Caruso, "Molar incisor hypomineralization treatment with casein phosphopeptide and amorphous calcium phosphate in children," *Minerva Stomatologica*, vol. 67, no. 1, pp. 20-25, 2018.

[7] N. Garg, A. K. Jain, S. Saha, and J. Singh, "Essential of early diagnosis of molar incisor hypomineralization in children and review of its clinical presentation, etiology and management," *International Journal of Clinical Pediatric Dentstry*, vol. 5, no. 3, pp. 190-196, 2012.

[8] S. Caruso, S. Bernardi, M. Pasini et al., "The process of mineralisation in the development of human tooth," *European Journal of Paediatric Dentistry*, vol. 17, no. 4, pp. 322-326, 2016.

[9] M. J. Silva, K. J. Scurrah, J. M. Craig, D. J. Manton, and N. Kilpatrick, "Etiology of molar incisor hypomineralization- a systematic review," *Community Dentistry and Oral Eidemiology*, vol. 44, no. 4, pp. 342-353, 2016.

[10] W. E. Amerongen and C. M. Kreulen, "Cheese molars: a pilot study of the etiology of hypocalcifications in first permanent molars," *ASDC Journal Dentistry for Children*, vol. 62, no. 2, pp. 266-269, 1995.

[11] R. Ahmadi, N. Ramazani, and R. Nourinasab, "Molar incisor hypomineralization: a study of prevalence and etiology in a group of Iranian children," *Iranian Journal of Pediatrics*, vol. 22, no. 2, pp. 245-251, 2012.

[12] A. R. Vieira and E. Kup, "On the etiology of molar-incisor hypomineralization," *Caries Research*, vol. 50, no. 2, pp. 166-169, 2016.

[13] K. L. Weerheijm, M. Duggal, I. Mejàre et al., "Judgement criteria for molar incisor hypomineralisation (MIH) in epidemiological studies: a summary of the European meeting on MIH held in Athens," *European Journal of Paediatic Dentistry*, vol. 4, no. 3, pp. 110-113, 2003.

[14] A. Ghanim, M. J. Silva, M. E. C. Elfrink et al., "Molar incisor hypomineralisation (MIH) training manual for clinical field surveys and practice," *European Archives of Paediatric Dentistry*, vol. 18, no. 4, pp. 225-242, 2017.

[15] L. Jasulaityte, J. S. Veerkamp, and K. L. Weerheijm, "Molar incisor hypomineralization: review and prevalence data from the study of primary school children in Kaunas/Lithuania," *European Archives of Paediatric Dentistry*, vol. 8, no. 2, pp. 87-94, 2007.

[16] L. Jasulaityte, K. L. Weerheijm, and J. S. Veerkamp, "Prevalence of molar-incisor-hypomineralisation among children participating in the Dutch National Epidemiological Survey (2003)," *European Archives of Paediatric Dentistry*, vol. 9, no. 4, pp. 218-223, 2008.

[17] N. A. Lygidakis, G. Dimou, and E. Briseniou, "Molar-incisor-hypomineralisation (MIH). Retrospective clinical study in Greek children. I. Prevalence and defect characteristics," *European Archives of Paediatric Dentistry*, vol. 9, no. 4, pp. 200-208, 2008.

[18] B. Buchgraber, L. Kqiku, and K. A. Ebeleseder, "Molar incisor hypomineralization: proportion and severity in primary public school children in Graz, Austria," *Clinical Oral Investigations*, vol. 22, no. 2, pp. 757-762, 2017.

[19] S. D. Yannam, D. Amarlal, and C. V. Rekha, "Prevalence of molar incisor hypomineralization in school children aged 8-12 years in Chennai," *Journal of Indian Society of Pedodontics and Preventive Dentistry*, vol. 34, no. 2, pp. 134-138, 2016.

[20] A. S. Hussein, M. Faisal, M. Haron, A. M. Ghanim, and M. I. Abu-Hassan, "Distribution of molar incisor hypomineralization in Malaysian children attending university dental clinic," *Journal of Clinical Pediatric Dentirsty*, vol. 39, no. 3, pp. 219-223, 2015.

[21] S. Laisi, A. Ess, C. Sahlberg, P. Arvio, P. L. Lukinmaa, and S. Alaluusua, "Amoxicillin may cause molar incisor hypomineralization," *Journal of Dental Research*, vol. 88, no. 2, pp. 132-136, 2009.

[22] D. Basak, A. Zerrin, P. Sertac, and K. Betul, "Possible medical aetiological factors and characteristics of molar incisor hypomineralization in a group of Turkish children," *Acta Stomatologica Croatica*, vol. 47, no. 4, pp. 297-305, 2013.

20

Missing Teeth and Prosthetic Treatment in Patients Treated at College of Dentistry, University of Dammam

Shaimaa M. Fouda,[1] Fahad A. Al-Harbi,[1] Soban Q. Khan,[2] Jorma I. Virtanen,[3,4] and Aune Raustia[4,5]

[1]*Department of Substitutive Dental Sciences, College of Dentistry, University of Dammam, P.O. Box 1982, Dammam 31411, Saudi Arabia*

[2]*Department of Clinical Affairs, College of Dentistry, University of Dammam, P.O. Box 1982, Dammam 31411, Saudi Arabia*

[3]*Research Unit of Oral Health Sciences, Department of Community Dentistry, Faculty of Medicine, University of Oulu, P.O. Box 5281, 90014 Oulu, Finland*

[4]*Medical Research Center Oulu, Oulu University Hospital and University of Oulu, Oulu, Finland*

[5]*Research Unit of Oral Health Sciences, Department of Prosthetic Dentistry and Stomatognathic Physiology, Faculty of Medicine, University of Oulu, P.O. Box 5281, 90014 Oulu, Finland*

Correspondence should be addressed to Shaimaa M. Fouda; shaimaa.fouda@hotmail.com

Academic Editor: Manal Awad

The percentage of completely and partially edentulous patients and their prosthetic treatment at the Department of Substitutive Dental Sciences (SDS), College of Dentistry, University of Dammam, were investigated. Panoramic radiographs and medical records of adult patients ($n = 479$, mean age 45.9 years, and range 25–96 years) treated in 2011–2014 were examined. 6% of the patients were completely edentulous, 8% had single jaw edentulousness, and 74% were partially edentulous. Edentulousness was significantly correlated with age and the number of missing teeth was significantly higher among males ($p < 0.026$). Diabetes was significantly associated with complete edentulousness, single edentulous jaw (p value 0.015), and partial edentulousness (p value 0.023). Kennedy class III was the most frequent class of partial edentulousness in single and/or both jaws ($p = 0.000$). Patients having class I and/or class II were treated most often with removable partial dentures (RPD) ($p = 0.000$), while patients having class III were treated with fixed partial dentures (FPD). It was found that complete edentulousness increases in older age and the number of missing teeth was significantly higher among males. Kennedy class III was most common in both upper and lower jaw and was treated more often with FPD than with RPD.

1. Introduction

Tooth loss considerably reduces quality of life [1]. It causes impairment of speech, aesthetics, and mastication, as well as social impairment [1, 2]. It also has a negative impact on the patient's psychological status. It may cause depression and reduced self-esteem due to the loss of an important part of the body and an impaired self-image [1, 2].

Many factors lead to edentulousness, for example, caries and periodontal diseases, which are considered the main causes of tooth loss [3]. Other factors such as the quality of oral health services, socioeconomic status, educational level, smoking, area of residence, and pattern of dental visits are also related to edentulousness and play a significant role in its prevalence [1, 4, 5]. Edentulousness has been found to increase in old age, which may partly be attributable to physical disabilities that could occur in old age [1, 4]. Also, the prevalence of general and dental diseases increases with aging, leading to edentulousness [4].

Several studies have investigated the prevalence of edentulousness in relation to gender [4–8]. A higher percentage of edentulousness has been seen among females than among males [4, 6, 8]. Possible reasons for this are probably the higher prevalence of dental caries and periodontal diseases in women in addition to other social and economic reasons [8]. However, some studies have reported a higher incidence of edentulousness among males [5, 7, 9].

The prevalence of edentulousness has been used as an indicator to evaluate the efficiency of oral health services as well as to show the oral health of a population [10]. It has been monitored in several countries for decades [1, 4, 10]. The rate of edentulousness has declined particularly in the western countries, which is at least partly attributed to improved oral health services [11]. However, its prevalence is still high in some other countries [6, 11, 12]. Since the number of people advancing into old age is increasing worldwide, more edentulous people are expected, accordingly [2].

Although dental implants are increasingly used to support dental prosthesis, the conventional removable dentures are used in many cases due to financial and/or medical considerations. Patients demand to replace missing teeth is affected by several factors including availability of dental services and educational, financial, and social status of the patients [13, 14]. The demand for prosthodontic care is expected to increase among Saudis [14].

Limited data are available on the prevalence of edentulousness in the Arabic countries, as well as on predisposing factors. We investigated the percentage of completely and partially edentulous patients and their prosthetic treatment at the Department of Substitutive Dental Sciences (SDS), College of Dentistry, University of Dammam, in the Eastern Province of Saudi Arabia, and examined the relationship between tooth loss and age, gender, general health, and smoking. The hypothesis of the present study expected high level of edentulousness among the study group.

2. Materials and Methods

The proportion of completely and partially edentulous patients and their prosthetic treatment received at the Department of Substitutive Dental Sciences (SDS), College of Dentistry, University of Dammam, were investigated using panoramic radiographs and medical records. The total number of patients treated at the SDS Department between 2011 and 2014 was 1016, and of these the study group included 479 patients who were selected using the following inclusion criteria: age 25+ years, available panoramic radiograph, and complete patient record.

The number of male and female patients was 312 and 162, respectively. Their mean age was 45.9 years (SD 13.52, range 25–96 years). A majority of the patients who visited the SDS Department were Saudis ($n = 295$). According to the general authority of statistics of the Kingdom of Saudi Arabia, the number of residents in Dammam in 2010 was 914,493; 55,000 were Saudi residents and 365,000 were non-Saudis. The College of Dentistry, University of Dammam, is the only Dental College in the Eastern Province of the Kingdom of Saudi Arabia. It provides free charged treatment to the patients by the undergraduates (under supervision of faculty members), interns, and faculty staff members. The patients visiting the colleges' clinics are Saudi and from other nationalities who live in the Eastern Province, such as Philippines, Syrians, and Egyptians. The Department of

SDS constitutes both subspecialties: removable and fixed prosthodontics.

2.1. Radiographic Evaluation. Panoramic radiographs of all the patients included in the study were examined by the same specialist dentist (S.F). Radiographs of the patients with all teeth missing in both jaws were recorded as edentulous; also the number of patients with a single edentulous jaw (maxillary or mandibular) was registered. Patients with at least one missing tooth other than the third molar were recorded as partially edentulous. Using the Kennedy classification, the number and location of missing teeth in the upper and lower jaw were categorized into four groups classes I, II, III, and IV [15].

The patients' medical records were reviewed and their age, gender, and nationality (Saudi/non-Saudi) were recorded. Data on the patients' medical condition were also recorded, including presence of diabetes and heart diseases. Patients' smoking habit was determined as smoker (currently smoking) or nonsmoker. The final prosthetic treatment that the partially edentulous patients received was determined to be a removable partial denture (RPD), a fixed partial denture (FPD), or both.

The proportion of completely edentulous patients, patients with a single edentulous jaw, and partially edentulous patients among the study group was determined. Also, a possible correlation between the number of missing teeth and the patient's age, gender, general health, and smoking habits was analyzed.

2.2. Statistics. Statistical Package of Social Sciences (SPSS version 19) was used for data entry and analysis. Cross tabulations and bar graphs were used to present descriptive statistics. For inferential statistics, Students' t-test, chi-square test, and binomial test were employed. Post hoc testing was employed to analyze the statistical significance between the prosthetic treatments provided to the patients with different Kennedy classes of partial edentulousness; significance was tested for each jaw separately.

3. Results

Most of the patients in the study group ($n = 479$) had missing teeth; 6% ($n = 28$) were completely edentulous, 8% ($n = 37$) had a single edentulous arch, 74% ($n = 354$) were partially edentulous, and 12% ($n = 60$) had no missing teeth (Figure 1).

Edentulousness correlated statistically significantly with age, being more common in older age (p value 0.000). All the completely edentulous patients and most of patients with a single edentulous jaw (34/37 patients) were 45 to 74 years old (Table 1). The mean age of completely edentulous patients was 63.7 ($\pm$11.3), while the remaining patients ($n = 451$) were 45.1 ($\pm$12.9) years old. No significant correlation was found between complete edentulousness and the patients' gender and nationality. Complete edentulousness in a single jaw was found to be significantly higher (p value 0.000) in the upper jaw (6%) than in the lower jaw (1%) and higher among males (70.3%) than among females (29.75%) (Figure 2). Edentulous maxilla and mandible were more common in males than in females (Figure 2).

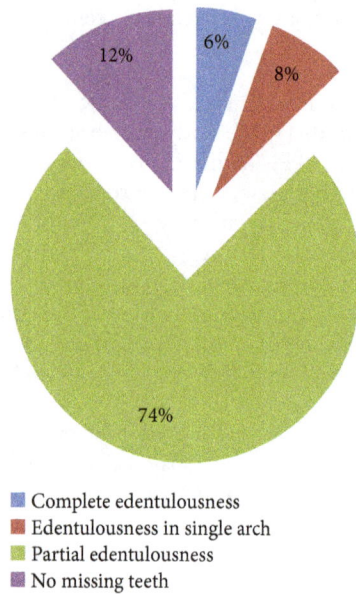

FIGURE 1: Percentage distribution of complete and partial edentulousness in patients ($n = 479$).

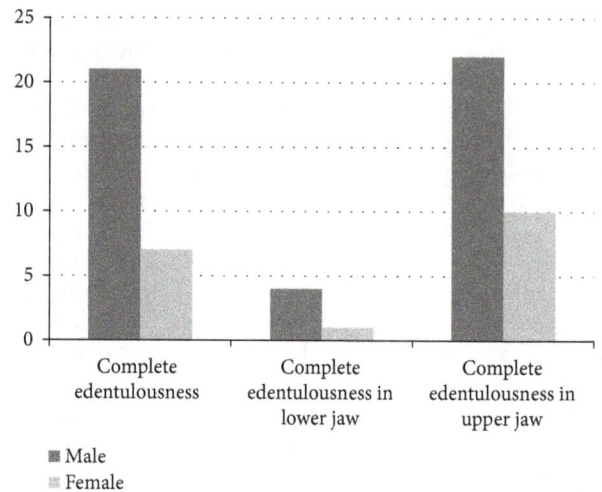

FIGURE 2: Frequency of complete edentulousness in relation to patients' gender.

TABLE 1: Number of missing teeth by age groups in partially edentulous patients ($n = 354$) treated in Dammam.

Missing teeth	Age (years)						Total
	25–34	35–44	45–54	55–64	65–74	75–84	
1–5	70	53	47	20	2	5	197
6–10	16	17	26	19	4	0	82
11–15	2	13	15	11	4	2	47
16–20	3	4	5	6	4	1	23
21–25	0	0	1	3	0	0	4
26–30	0	0	1	0	0	0	1
Total	91	87	95	59	14	8	354

The total number of completely edentulous patients and patients with edentulousness in a single jaw who had a general disease was 65, and almost one-third ($n = 22$) of them had diabetes, 4.6% had a heart disease, and 27.7% were smokers (Table 2). Only diabetes was found to be significantly related to complete edentulousness and edentulousness in a single jaw (p value 0.015).

In the partially edentulous group ($n = 354$), the average number of missing teeth was 6.5 (±5.3). Most of these patients ($n = 197$) missing 1–5 teeth were 25–34 years old (Table 1). The number of missing teeth was significantly higher among males ($p < 0.026$) than among females (Table 2). Partial edentulousness, Kennedy class III, was most usual in single and/or both jaws (p value 0.000) (Table 3).

Of the partially edentulous patients, 15% ($n = 53$) were diabetic, 4% ($n = 14$) had a heart disease, and less than one-quarter ($n = 75$) were smokers. On average, a diabetic patient had 8.1 (±6.7) missing teeth, compared with nondiabetic patients, who had 6.28 (±4.98); the difference in the mean was statistically significant (p value 0.023). Patients with a

heart disease had an average of 6.79 (±5.89) missing teeth compared with patients with no heart disease 6.54 (±5.3); the difference in the mean was not statistically significant. Similarly, the mean number of missing teeth among smokers and nonsmokers was 7.07 (±5.26) and 6.39 (±5.34), respectively, with no significance in the mean difference (Table 2).

The number of patients who had received prosthetic treatment was 237. They had received fixed partial dentures (FPD), removable partial dentures (RPD), or both. One hundred and ten patients (31.1%) had received a RPD, one hundred and eleven (31.4%) a FPD, and sixteen patients (4.2%) both FPD and RPD. The patients with class I and/or class II in the upper and lower jaw were treated most often with a RPD (p value 0.000), while the number of FPD was significantly higher among patients with class III (Table 4).

4. Discussion

The prevalence of edentulousness has significantly decreased in North America and Europe [1, 4, 16]. However, a limited number of studies investigating the prevalence of edentulousness and related factors have been conducted in the Arabic region [9, 13, 17]. The prevalence of edentulousness among the studied group was 6%, which is much lower than in previous studies [4–7, 12]. A higher percentage of edentulousness of 13% and 17% has been reported among patients treated at a faculty hospital or dental clinics [7, 9].

The decreased percentage of edentulous patients among the study group might be because of the age distribution (25–96 years) among the studied sample, which included patients at younger age, compared with previous studies that have included only middle-aged and old patients. Also, it may result from the relatively small size of the sample in comparison with studies of national surveys. The results here are in line with some population based studies, although the sample size and selection are different [16, 18, 19]. A study from Mexico that included adults aged 18 years or more found that 6.3% were edentulous [18]. It was also found that 5% of UK adults

Table 2: Number of missing teeth in partially edentulous patients ($n = 354$) treated in Dammam by gender, smoking, and general health.

	Number of missing teeth						Total
	1–5	6–10	11–15	16–20	21–25	26–30	
Gender							
Male	139 (61.5)	42 (18.6)	26 (11.5)	16 (7.1)	3 (1.3)	0	226
Female	58 (45.3)	40 (31.2)	21 (16.4)	7 (5.5)	1 (0.8)	1 (0.8)	128
Smoking							
Yes	38 (50.7)	20 (26.7)	11 (14.7)	6 (8)	0	0	75
No	159 (57.2)	61 (21.7)	37 (13)	17 (6.2)	4 (1.5)	1 (0.4)	279
Diabetes							
Yes	26 (49)	12 (22.6)	6 (11.3)	6 (11.3)	3 (5.7)	0	53
No	171 (56.7)	70 (23.3)	41 (13.7)	17 (5.7)	1 (0.3)	1 (0.3)	301
Heart disease							
Yes	7 (50)	4 (28.6)	1 (7.1)	2 (14.3)	0	0	14
No	189 (55.8)	79 (23)	46 (13.6)	21 (6.2)	4 (1.2)	1 (0.3)	340

Statistically significant with *p* value (<0.026).

Table 3: Distribution of Kennedy classes in maxillary and mandibular jaws in patients ($n = 354$) treated in Dammam.

Kennedy classes	Maxillary arch	Mandibular arch	Both arches
I	31 (15.2)	26 (12.5)	11 (7.7)
II	48 (23.5)	37 (17.8)	24 (16.8)
III	72 (35.3)	93 (44.7)	107 (74.8)
IV	7 (3.4)	3 (1.4)	1 (0.7)
NO missing teeth	46 (22.5)	49 (23.6)	0
Total	*204*	*208*	*143*

Post hoc test; statistically significant with *p* value = 0.000.

Table 4: Prosthetic treatment according to Kennedy classification in maxilla and mandible in patients ($n = 237$) treated in Dammam.

	RPD	FPD	RPD + FPD
Kennedy classes Maxilla			
I	24 (21.8)	5 (4.5)	0
II	27 (24.5)	12 (10.8)	3 (18.8)
III	51 (46.4)	71 (64)	11 (68.8)
IV	1 (0.9)	2 (1.8)	0
Total	*103*	*90*	*14*
Mandible			
I	22 (20)	4 (3.7)	3 (18.8)
II	32 (29.1)	18 (16.8)	5 (31.3)
III	44 (40)	63 (58.9)	8 (50)
IV	5 (4.5)	1 (0.9)	0
Total	*103*	*86*	*16*

between 55 and 64 years of age and 15% between 65 and 74 years are edentulous; these figures are in line with our findings [19]. Moreover, the prevalence of edentulousness among US adults aged 15 years or more reached 4.9% in 2009–2012 [16]. Conversely, a much lower prevalence of edentulousness has been reported in several African countries [17, 20, 21]. The prevalence of edentulousness in Ghana was reported to be

2.8% among people aged 50 years or more and 1.3% among adults aged 65 years or more in Ibadan Nigeria [20, 21].

Edentulousness was also found to be more frequent among older patients in our study. The highest percentage was observed in the age group above 70 (35.7%). It has been well established in the literature that edentulousness increases with age [4, 9]. The incidence of tooth loss has also been proven to be correlated with old age [22]. This is caused by many factors including difficulty to perform oral hygiene procedures due to systemic diseases or functional disability [23].

In the present study, a higher percentage of edentulousness was seen among males than among females. This finding is in line with the results of previous studies [5, 7, 13], one of them conducted in Saudi Arabia [9]. Regarding the partially edentulous patients, the number of missing teeth was significantly higher among males. A study conducted in Brazil found that men were more prone to lose teeth, which supports our result [22]. However, it disagrees with many studies that have found a higher rate of edentulousness among women [4, 8, 20]. In the present study, diabetes was found to be significantly correlated with partial and complete loss of teeth. Kennedy's class III was found to be the most prevalent class in the maxilla and mandible and also in both jaws together. This result agrees with several previous studies [24, 25].

To our knowledge, this study is the first in Dammam to investigate the percentage of partial and complete edentulousness and the prosthetic treatment of partially edentulous patients in a College of Dentistry, as well as the correlation between tooth loss and age, gender, general health, and smoking. However, the sample in the present study does not represent the population of the Eastern Province in Saudi Arabia, as it included patients seeking treatment at clinics of the College of Dentistry, University of Dammam only. Nevertheless, it provides baseline data for further studies. It also gives information about the most common prosthetic treatment for partially edentulous patients, which is beneficial for an educational institution. In addition, several previous studies have investigated the rate of edentulousness and associated factors among patients treated at faculty and outpatient clinics [7, 9, 13, 17]. The sample in the present study included 479 patients, which is close to the sample size of previous studies [7, 9]. The age of the patients ranged from 25 to 96 years, which is much lower than in most previous studies, which have investigated the prevalence of edentulousness among patients in middle and old age only [4–6]. However, several studies have investigated the rate of edentulousness among patients similar to the age group of the present study [9, 17, 18].

The strengths of this study include the fact that edentulousness was determined after screening the panoramic X-rays of all the participants. The X-rays were examined by the same dentist and did not depend on questionnaires filled in by the patients. However, a limitation is that the sample is not representative of the whole population but only includes patients treated at the College of Dentistry. In addition, the fact that panoramic radiographs were not available for all patients might have influenced the findings. A further study with a larger sample representing the whole population of the Eastern Province of Saudi Arabia will be needed.

5. Conclusions

Edentulousness was significantly more common in older age and the number of missing teeth was found to be higher among males than among females. Partial edentulousness, Kennedy class III, was most usual in single and/or both jaws. The patients with class I and/or class II in the upper and lower jaw were treated most often with RPD, while the number of FPD was significantly higher among patients with class III.

Ethical Approval

The study was approved by the Institutional Review Board (IRB-2014-02-025) of the University of Dammam.

Acknowledgments

The authors wish to acknowledge the Deanship of Scientific Research, University of Dammam, Kingdom of Saudi Arabia, for funding this research.

References

[1] I. Polzer, M. Schimmel, F. Müller, and R. Biffar, "Edentulism as part of the general health problems of elderly adults," *International Dental Journal*, vol. 60, no. 3, pp. 143–155, 2010.

[2] E. B. Øzhayat, S. Åkerman, N. Lundegren, and B. Öwall, "Patients' experience of partial tooth loss and expectations to treatment: a qualitative study in Danish and Swedish patients," *Journal of Oral Rehabilitation*, vol. 43, no. 3, pp. 180–189, 2016.

[3] J. Bouma, D. Uitenbroek, G. Westert, R. M. H. Schaub, and F. van de Poel, "Pathways to full mouth extraction," *Community Dentistry and Oral Epidemiology*, vol. 15, no. 6, pp. 301–305, 1987.

[4] B. Haikola, K. Oikarinen, A. L. Söderholm, T. Remes-Lyly, and K. Sipilä, "Prevalence of edentulousness and related factors among elderly Finns," *Journal of Oral Rehabilitation*, vol. 35, no. 11, pp. 827–835, 2008.

[5] M. V. Eustaquio-Raga, J. M. Montiel-Company, and J. M. Almerich-Silla, "Factors associated with edentulousness in an elderly population in Valencia (Spain)," *Gaceta Sanitaria*, vol. 27, no. 2, pp. 123–127, 2013.

[6] K. Peltzer, S. Hewlett, A. E. Yawson et al., "Prevalence of loss of all teeth (Edentulism) and associated factors in older adults in China, Ghana, India, Mexico, Russia and South Africa," *International Journal of Environmental Research and Public Health*, vol. 11, no. 11, pp. 11308–11324, 2014.

[7] J. N. Hoover and R. E. McDermott, "Edentulousness in patients attending a university dental clinic," *Journal of Canadian Dental Association*, vol. 55, no. 2, pp. 139-140, 1989.

[8] S. L. Russell, S. Gordon, J. R. Lukacs, and L. M. Kaste, "Sex/ gender differences in tooth loss and edentulism. historical perspectives, biological factors, and sociologic reasons," *Dental Clinics of North America*, vol. 57, no. 2, pp. 317–337, 2013.

[9] N. A. Al-Ghannam, N. B. Khan, A. R. Al-Shammery, and A. H. Wyne, "Trends in dental caries and missing teeth in adult patients in Al-Ahsa, Saudi Arabia," *Saudi Dental Journal*, vol. 17, pp. 57–62, 2005.

[10] W. M. Thomson, "Monitoring edentulism in older New Zealand adults over two decades: a review and commentary," *International Journal of Dentistry*, vol. 2012, Article ID 375407, 4 pages, 2012.

[11] P. E. Petersen, "The World Oral Health Report 2003: continuous improvement of oral health in the 21st century—the approach of the WHO Global Oral Health Programme," *Community Dentistry and Oral Epidemiology*, vol. 31, supplement s1, pp. 3–24, 2003.

[12] H. E. Nazliel, N. Hersek, M. Ozbek, and E. Karaagaoglu, "Oral health status in a group of the elderly population residing at home," *Gerodontology*, vol. 29, no. 2, pp. e761–e767, 2012.

[13] Z. N. Al-Dwairi, "Complete edentulism and socioeconomic factors in a jordanian population," *International Journal of Prosthodontics*, vol. 23, no. 6, pp. 541–543, 2010.

[14] E. Al Hamdan and M. Fahmy, "Socioeconomic factors and complete edentulism for female patients at King Saud University, Riyadh, Saudi Arabia," *Tanta Dental Journal*, vol. 11, no. 3, pp. 169–173, 2014.

[15] A. B. Carr and D. T. Brown, *Mccracken's Removable Partial Prosthodontics*, Elsevier Health Sciences, 2015.

[16] G. D. Slade, A. A. Akinkugbe, and A. E. Sanders, "Projections of U.S. edentulism prevalence following 5 decades of decline," *Journal of Dental Research*, vol. 93, no. 10, pp. 959–965, 2014.

[17] N. Khalifa, P. F. Allen, N. H. Abu-bakr, and M. E. Abdel-Rahman, "Factors associated with tooth loss and prosthodontic status among Sudanese adults," *Journal of oral science*, vol. 54, no. 4, pp. 303–312, 2012.

[18] C. E. Medina-Solís, R. Pérez-Núñez, G. Maupomé et al., "National survey on edentulism and its geographic distribution, among Mexicans 18 years of age and older (with emphasis in WHO age groups)," *Journal of Oral Rehabilitation*, vol. 35, no. 4, pp. 237–244, 2008.

[19] J. G. Steele, E. T. Treasure, I. O'Sullivan, J. Morris, and J. J. Murray, "Adult dental health survey 2009: transformations in British oral health 1968-2009," *British Dental Journal*, vol. 213, no. 10, pp. 523–527, 2012.

[20] S. A. Hewlett, B. N. L. Calys-Tagoe, A. E. Yawson et al., "Prevalence and geographic distribution of edentulism among older Ghanaians," *Journal of Public Health Dentistry*, vol. 75, no. 1, pp. 74–83, 2015.

[21] J. O. Taiwo and F. Omokhodion, "Pattern of tooth loss in an elderly population from Ibadan, Nigeria.," *Gerodontology*, vol. 23, no. 2, pp. 117–122, 2006.

[22] R. J. De Marchi, J. B. Hilgert, F. N. Hugo, C. M. D. Santos, A. B. Martins, and D. M. Padilha, "Four year incidence and predictors of tooth loss among older adults in a southern Brazilian city," *Community Dentistry and Oral Epidemiology*, vol. 40, no. 5, pp. 396–405, 2012.

[23] K. Avlund, P. Holm-Pedersen, and M. Schroll, "Functional ability and oral health among older people: a longitudinal study from age 75 to 80," *Journal of the American Geriatrics Society*, vol. 49, no. 7, pp. 954–962, 2001.

[24] O. O. Charyeva, K. D. Altynbekov, and B. Z. Nysanova, "Kennedy classification and treatment options: a study of partially edentulous patients being treated in a specialized prosthetic clinic," *Journal of Prosthodontics*, vol. 21, no. 3, pp. 177–180, 2012.

[25] L. A. Shinawi, "Partial edentulism: a five year survey on the prevalence and pattern of tooth loss in a sample of patients attending King AbdulAziz University—Faculty of Dentistry," *Life Science Journal*, vol. 9, no. 4, pp. 2665–2671, 2012.

21

Efficacy of Dental Bleaching with Whitening Dentifrices

Bruno G. S. Casado ⓘ,[1] **Sandra L. D. Moraes,**[1] **Gleicy F. M. Souza,**[1] **Catia M. F. Guerra,**[2] **Juliana R. Souto-Maior,**[1] **Cleidiel A. A. Lemos ⓘ,**[3] **Belmiro C. E. Vasconcelos,**[1] **and Eduardo P. Pellizzer ⓘ**[3]

[1]*School of Dentistry, University of Pernambuco (UPE), Camaragibe, PE, Brazil*
[2]*School of Dentistry, Pernambuco Federal University (UFPE), Recife, PE, Brazil*
[3]*School of Dentistry, Dental Materials and Prosthodontics, São Paulo State University (UNESP), São Paulo, Araçatuba, Brazil*

Correspondence should be addressed to Bruno G. S. Casado; brunocasado@hotmail.com

Academic Editor: Izzet Yavuz

A systematic review was performed to evaluate whether whitening toothpastes promote tooth whitening when compared to the use of conventional (nonbleaching) dentifrices. This review was registered at PROSPERO (CRD42017065132) and is based on the Preferred Reporting Items for Systematic Reviews and Meta-Analyses. Electronic systematic searches of PubMed/MEDLINE, Scopus, and the Cochrane Library were conducted for published articles. Only randomized clinical trials in adults that compared the use of so-called whitening dentifrices to the use of nonwhitening dentifrices were selected. The outcome was tooth color change. Twenty-two articles from 703 data sources met the eligibility criteria. After title and abstract screening, 16 studies remained, after which a further five studies were excluded. In total, nine studies were qualitatively analyzed. Significant differences in tooth color change were found between the groups using whitening dentifrices and those using nonwhitening dentifrices. Within the limitations of this study, the evidence from this systematic review suggests that bleaching dentifrices have potential in tooth whitening. However, although many whitening dentifrices have been introduced into the dental market for bleaching treatments, it is important to analyze tooth surface and color changes when performing home bleaching.

1. Introduction

Tooth discoloration is one of the most commonly reported complaints in patients seeking aesthetic treatment. Variation in tooth color can be influenced by intrinsic and extrinsic factors, ranging from chemical ingestion to consumption of foods that cause staining [1, 2].

Currently, there are several products on the market that remove stains and claim to whiten teeth. Options range from simple professional prophylaxis and the application of bleaching gels to vital teeth for home use or supervised in a dental office [3]. Bleaching gels normally consist of different concentrations of hydrogen peroxide or carbamide peroxide and involve various forms of application. Furthermore, these different applications result in different mechanisms of activation, which provide dental bleaching through oxi-reduction reactions, based on partial oxidation of the active principle, through which the whitening agent alters the structure of pigment molecules, thus promoting tooth whitening [4, 5].

Several companies have developed bleaching toothpastes, which are considered an alternative to home and/or dental whitening procedures, and which promise bleaching results within 2 to 4 weeks. These toothpastes thus offer increasingly simpler and less costly bleaching methods for those wishing to have whiter teeth [6, 7]. Many of these bleaching toothpastes contain hydrogen peroxide, whereas others contain abrasive components, which promote the removal of extrinsic stains [7, 8].

These abrasives may remove blemishes from the coronary surfaces, giving rise to the idea that alterations in tooth coloration have occurred, which is often used as a marketing strategy by companies to show that teeth are healthy. However, little is known about the efficacy of these bleaching dentifrices compared with conventional (nonbleaching) dentifrices and their effects/alterations on stained teeth regardless of etiology [7, 9, 10].

Therefore, the objective of this systematic review was to evaluate whether whitening toothpastes promote tooth whitening when compared to the use of nonbleaching dentifrices. The hypothesis of the study is that bleaching dentifrices do not promote tooth whitening.

2. Materials and Methods

2.1. Protocol Registration. The current systematic review was performed following the Preferred Reporting Items for Systematic Reviews and Meta-Analyses. The methods used in this review are registered on PROSPERO (CRD42017065132).

2.2. Research Methods. The selection of articles was performed individually by two authors (Bruno G. S. Casado and Cleidiel A. A. Lemos) using published papers found in the Cochrane Library, PubMed/MEDLINE, and Scopus databases from inception to December 2017. The following terms were used in the search strategy: "tooth bleaching and dentifrice OR dental bleaching and dentifrice OR tooth bleaching and toothpaste OR dental bleaching and toothpaste."

Two researchers also manually searched for papers published up to December 2017 in specific journals such as Dental Materials and Journal of Dentistry and Operative Dentistry. A third author (Gleicy F. M. Souza) determined divergences in paper selection by the researchers and a consensus was obtained through discussion.

2.3. Eligibility Criteria. The selection criteria included randomized clinical trials (RCTs) and articles published in English. The exclusion criteria included prospective and retrospective studies, crossover studies, *in vitro* studies, animal studies, mechanical studies, case reports, and literature reviews.

2.4. Search Strategy. Clinical studies were selected from the title and abstract through electronic searches conducted by two independent researchers. In studies where it was not possible to obtain sufficient information, the complete article was downloaded. After reading the title and abstract, the studies that did not meet the inclusion criteria were excluded.

The following specific question was elaborated based on the population, intervention, control, and outcomes criteria: "Do bleaching dentifrices effectively promote tooth whitening?" According to these criteria, the population was composed of patients who used dentifrices, and the intervention was the use of so-called whitening dentifrices compared with the use of nonwhitening dentifrices. The evaluated outcome was the efficacy of bleaching dentifrices on tooth color change.

2.5. Risk of Bias and Evaluation of Study Quality. Two investigators (Bruno G. S. Casado and Cleidiel A. A. Lemos) evaluated the methodological quality of the included studies using bias analyses based on the Cochrane criteria for assessing the risk of bias. This tool assessed the quality and risk of bias of the included studies based on sequence generation, allocation concealment, blinding of participants, personnel or outcome investigator, incomplete outcome data, selective outcome reporting, and other sources of bias and was rated as low/high or unclear risk of bias according to the studies evaluated.

2.6. Data Collection and Analysis. The data collected from the articles were classified as quantitative and qualitative by one researcher (Bruno G. S. Casado) and then verified by another researcher (Gleicy F. M. Souza). All disagreements were resolved by a third researcher (Cleidiel A. A. Lemos) through discussion until a consensus was reached. Quantitative and qualitative data were tabulated to aid the comparison.

2.7. Additional Analysis. An additional analysis was performed using the kappa coefficient, which was calculated to establish the interexaminer agreement in study selection from the three databases. The kappa value was obtained by evaluating the titles and abstracts selected. The Cochrane Library ($K = 0.94$), PubMed/MEDLINE ($K = 0.71$), and Scopus ($K = 0.92$) showed a high level of agreement.

3. Results

The database search identified a total of 703 articles, 287 of which were from PubMed/MEDLINE, 303 from Scopus, and 113 from the Cochrane Library. After removal of duplicate references and a thorough review of titles and abstracts, 16 studies were read in full. After reading, nine studies were excluded (Table 1). Details regarding the search strategy are presented in the flow diagram (Figure 1).

In total, seven studies were selected for qualitative analyses and are summarized in Table 2. All selected studies were RCTs published between 2001 and 2016. A total of 1,399 patients with a mean age of 36.89 years were included in the studies, of which 879 used some type of dentifrice considered to be a bleaching agent by the manufacturer. The groups of patients evaluated varied according to the dentifrice, and the effectiveness of nine products was tested: Arm & Hammer® Advance White® Extreme Whitening Baking Soda and Peroxide Toothpaste ($n = 86$), Arm & Hammer® Truly Radiant Toothpaste ($n = 59$), Crest® 3-D white radiant mint toothpaste ($n = 56$), Crest® Extra whitening ($n = 363$), Colgate® Simple White® Advanced Whitening Toothpaste Sparkling Mint ($n = 21$), Colgate® Baking Soda Peroxide ($n = 216$), Colgate Luminous White® ($n = 32$), Close-Up White Now® ($n = 31$), and Oral B 3D white ($n = 15$).

The bleaching effectiveness of the studied dentifrices was evaluated. Four studies showed that the products evaluated were effective in bleaching teeth using the VITA color scale (subjective method), and three studies showed that the

TABLE 1: Reasons for exclusion of "9" articles.

Author, year	Reason for exclusion
Llena et al. 2016 [11]	Use of gel substance associated with dentifrice for enzymatic activation.
Motta et al. 2013 [12]	Abstract only
Forner et al. 2012 [13]	Use of gel substance associated with dentifrice for enzymatic activation.
Raoufi and Birkhed, 2010 [14]	Another method of analysis
Collins et al. 2008 [15]	Crossover study
Yhudira et al. 2007 [16]	Association of different bleaching methods.
Sharma et al. 2004 [17]	Without control group
Soparkar et al. 2004 [18]	Without control group
Gerlach et al. 2004 [19]	Without conventional toothpaste as a control group

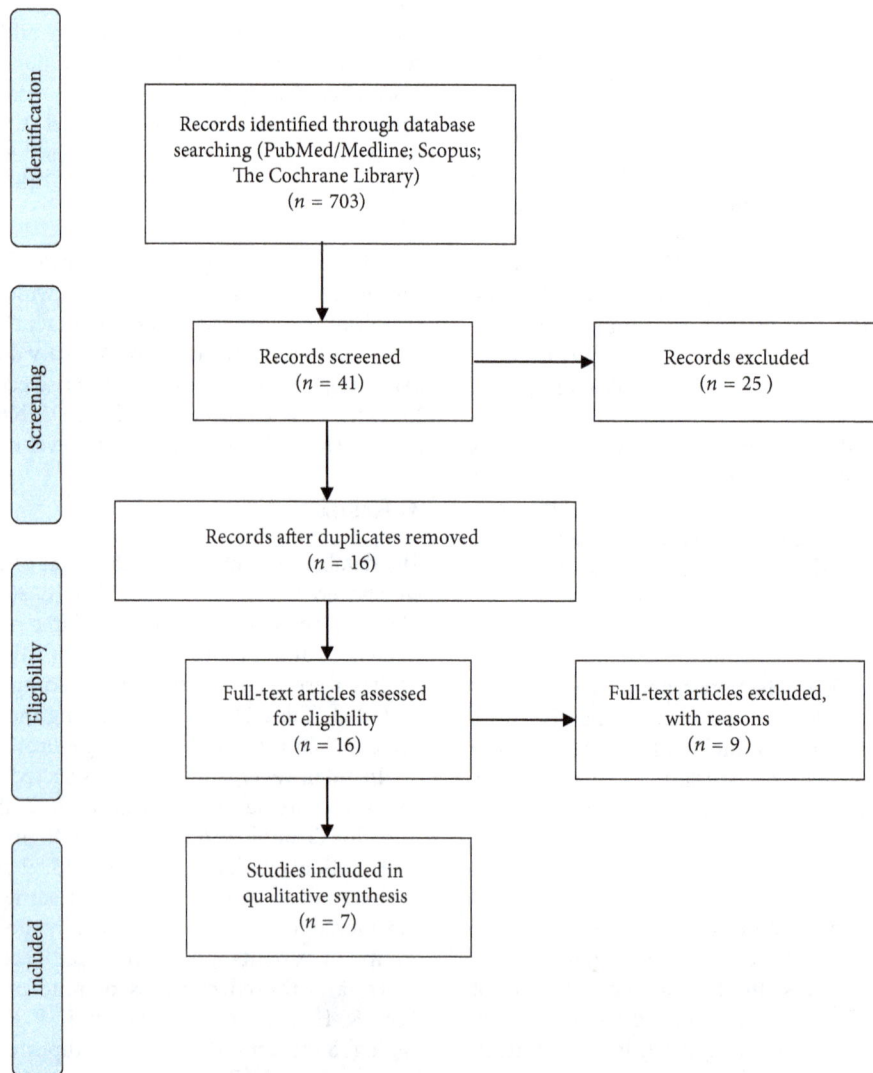

FIGURE 1: Flow chart showing the steps in the literature search.

products were effective in bleaching teeth using spectrophotometry (objective method).

In relation to daily brushing frequency, most studies [20–24] reported that using toothpaste twice a day increased tooth whitening, but two studies indicated that patients who brushed three times a day were more likely to have whiter teeth. In addition, the follow-up period ranged from 5 days to 8 weeks, with the most common period being 4 weeks (six studies). All studies included in this review examined subjects who used conventional toothpaste (not considered to have a bleaching effect by the manufacturers) as the control group.

The relevance of the articles included in this systematic review was considered satisfactory as all studies were RCTs with a low risk of bias (Figure 2). We included Cochrane randomized clinical trial studies to determine the bias scale

TABLE 2: Summary of characteristics of included studies.

Author/year	Design of study	Patients, n	Mean age (range)	Frequency of use (time)	Evaluation time	Evaluation methods	Groups, n	Follow-up period	Color mean (SD): Reduction in score — Whitening dentifrice	Color mean (SD): Reduction in score — Control group	Difference between groups	Effect of whitening dentifrice
Ghassemi et al. 2012 [23]	Randomized controlled trial	135	38,9 (19–70)	Twice daily (1 minute)	4 and 6 weeks	Shade guide	G1: Arm & Hammer advanced white (n = 86); G2: Crest cavity protection toothpaste (n = 49)	Week 4	(G1) 1.82 (0.80)	(G2) 0.07 (0.42)	G1* × G2 $p < 0.0001$	Positive
								week 6	(G1) 2.57 (0.99)	(G2) −0.04 (0.69)	G1* × G2 $p < 0.0001$	Positive
Ghassemi et al. 2015 [24]	Randomized controlled trial	178	38.5 (18–75)	Twice daily (2 minutes)	5 days and 2, 4, and 6 weeks	Shade guide	G1: Truly radiant toothpaste (n = 59); G2: Crest 3D white radiant mint toothpaste (n = 56); G3: Colgate cavity protection toothpaste (n = 63)	Day 5	(G1) 0.597; (G2) 0.324	(G3) −0.08	G1* × G2 $p = 0.0105$; G1/G2* × G3 $p < 0.0001$	Positive
								week 2	(G1) 1.172; (G2) 0.837	(G3) 0.046	G1 × G2 $p = 0.1595$; G1/G2* × G3 $p < 0.0001$	Positive
								week 4	(G1) 1.170; (G2) 1.326	(G3) 0.107	G1 × G2 $p = 0.2409$; G1/G2* × G3 $p < 0.0001$	Positive
								week 6	(G1) 2.081; (G2) 1.467	(G3) 0.038	G1* × G2 $p = 0.0383$; G1/G2* × G3 $p < 0.0001$	Positive
Gerlach et al. 2001 [20]	Randomized controlled trial	278	43,9 (19–79)	Twice daily (NI)	4 and 8 weeks	Shade guide	G1: crest extra whitening (n = 144); G2: Arm & Hammer dental care dentifrice (n = 134)	Week 4	(G1) 1.04	(G2) 0.53	No difference	None
								week 8	(G1) 1.42	(G2) 0.96	G1* × G2 $p < 0.05$	Positive
Isaacs et al. 2001 [21]	Randomized controlled trial	654	43 (NI)	Twice daily (NI)	4 and 8 weeks	Spectroscopy	G1: Crest extra whitening (silica) (n = 219); G2: Colgate baking soda and peroxide (n = 216); G3: Crest cavity protection (n = 219)	Week 4	(G1) 0.05; (G2) 0.08	(G3) −0.14	G1* × G3 $p = 0.007$; G2* × G3 $p = 0.002$	Positive; Positive
								week 8	(G1) 0.03; (G2) 0.10	(G3) −0.25	G1* × G3 $p < 0.001$; G2* × G3 $p < 0.001$; G1 × G2 No difference	Positive; Positive

TABLE 2: Continued.

Author/year	Design of study	Patients, n	Mean age (range)	Frequency of use (time)	Evaluation time	Evaluation methods	Groups, n	Follow-up period	Color mean (SD): Reduction in score: Whitening dentifrice	Control group	Difference between groups	Effect of whitening dentifrice
Kakar et al. 2004 [22]	Randomized controlled trial	44	34,15 (NI)	Twice daily (2 minutes)	2 weeks and 4 weeks	Shade guide	G1: Colgate simply white (n = 21) G2: control dentifrice (n = 23)	Week 2 week 4	(G1) 4.04 (1.40) (G1) 5.17 (1.09)	(G2) 0.41 (0.55) (G2) 0.53 (0.63)	p < 0.05 G1 p < 0.05 G1	Positive Positive
Horn et al. 2014 [25]	Randomized controlled trial	60	NI (19–36)	Three times a day (2-3 minutes)	2 weeks	Spectroscopy	G1: Colgate total 12 (n = 15) G2: Close-Up white now (n = 15) G3: Oral B 3D white (n = 15) G4: Colgate luminous white (n = 15)	Week 2	(G2) −0.7 (G3) −0.3 (G4) −1.7	(G1) −1.1	G1 × G2 or G3 No difference G4* × G1 p = 0.01	None Positive
Pintado-Palomino et al. 2016 [7]	Randomized controlled trial	50	22,9 (19–36)	Three times a day (2-3 minutes)	4 weeks	Spectroscopy	G1: Colgate luminous white (n = 17) G2: Close-Up white now (n = 16) G3: Sorriso (n = 17)	Week 4	(G1) 5.1 (2.8) (G2) 6.8 (3.5)	(G3) 4.4 (3.0)	No difference	None

*Groups with significant statistical difference. NI, not informed.

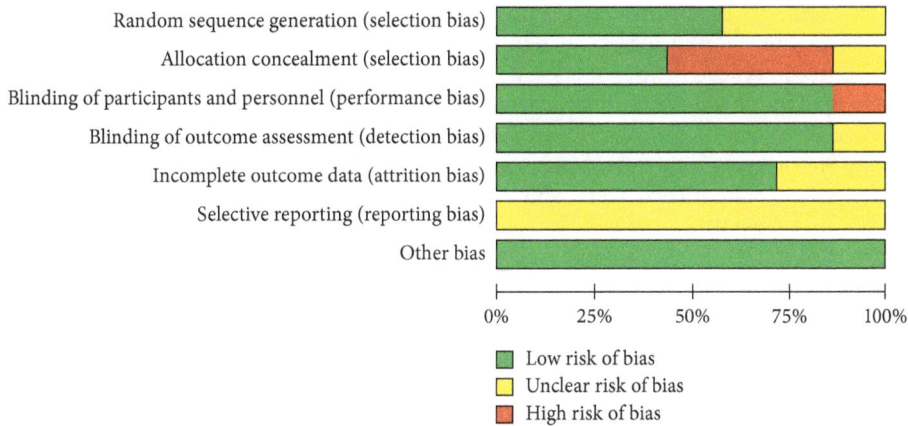

FIGURE 2: Cochrane scale for bias risk.

in each study. All included studies were characterized as double-blind (randomized studies were performed with the patient and the evaluator blinded to the product), which is considered important in understanding responses in experimental clinical research.

3.1. Bleaching Effectiveness. In the four studies that evaluated tooth color change using the VITA shade guide, all studies [20, 22–24] reported that bleaching dentifrices were effective for tooth whitening when compared with regular dentifrices ($p < 0.05$). However, Gerlach et al. [20] found differences between the groups only in the evaluation period following 4 weeks of dentifrice use.

In the studies that used a spectrophotometer to analyze tooth whitening, two studies [21, 25] demonstrated that bleaching dentifrices differed in relation to conventional dentifrices. However, Horn et al. [25] tested three different dentifrices, and found that only the use of Colgate Luminous White® had a tooth-whitening effect after 2 weeks. In agreement, a study by Pintado-Palomino et al. [7] showed that most bleaching and control dentifrices showed similar clinical performances, without a significant chromatic reduction, during a 4-week follow-up period.

4. Discussion

The results of this systematic review indicate that most of the included studies showed a significant change in dental coloration following the use of commercially available bleaching dentifrice agents when used for a period of between 5 days and 8 weeks.

Although peroxide bleaching materials are well-established for aesthetic tooth whitening, the use of these substances in dentifrices is quite limited [25]. In addition to causing alterations in products, high concentrations of hydrogen peroxide need to be counterbalanced by the use of soft tissue protective barriers in order to maintain contact with dental surfaces, which is not the case with bleaching toothpastes [8].

However, Isaacs et al. [21], Kakar et al. [22], and Ghassemi et al. [23] observed that the presence of 1.0% hydrogen peroxide in the chemical formulation of dentifrices caused tooth coloration changes when compared with nonwhitening toothpastes. These findings agreed with those obtained by Sharma et al. [17] who demonstrated the bleaching potential of these dentifrices and concluded that the presence of hydrogen peroxide was able to significantly interfere with dental chromatic alterations over a brushing period of 2 to 6 weeks. Therefore, it is important to consider the concentration of hydrogen peroxide and its contact time as important contributors to effective tooth whitening [19].

On the other hand, studies by Gerlach et al. [20], Horn et al. [25], and Ghassemi et al. [24] tested bleaching dentifrices that were free from any type of peroxide and obtained satisfactory results regarding changes in tooth coloration during the use of these toothpastes. These results may have been due to the presence of high performance abrasive agents contained in the bleaching dentifrices such as silica, which was present in almost all products included in this review [7, 21–25]. These abrasive agents promote the gradual physical removal of extrinsic pigments without effectively whitening teeth. Therefore, these bleaching dentifrices are sometimes considered only as surface spot removers [7, 8, 25].

Interestingly, the studies by Hilgenberg et al. [26] and Özkan et al. [27] showed that bleaching dentifrices promoted morphological changes on the surfaces of tooth enamel. Therefore, it is important to consider that brushing with toothpastes containing abrasive substances should be done with caution, as the indiscriminate use of dentifrices with large quantities of these agents can lead to irreversible damage of hard dental tissues and restorative materials; they can also lead to recession of the gingiva, abrasion in the cervical region, and in some cases, dentin hypersensitivity [8, 26].

Another limiting factor is that these studies did not use similar evaluation methods, making it difficult to compare the parameters studied in the coloration change analyses in this review. Dozic et al. [28] proposed that the spectrophotometer was the most reliable instrument on the market for tooth coloration analysis; the accuracy of the results is related to the positioning of the equipment at the same point of the dental surface at all times of analysis [14].

However, among the studies selected in this review which used spectrophotometry as the evaluation method, only the study by Isaacs et al. [21] demonstrated a significant color change following use of the bleaching dentifrices. This probably occurred because the products tested by Isaacs et al. [21] contained hydrogen peroxide associated with a high performance silica. These results are in agreement with those by Sharma et al. [17], who confirmed that these two substances in a dentifrice were able to remove extrinsic stains, reducing the yellow color pigmentation (b^* parameter) of the teeth, when compared to conventional dentifrices.

The findings of Horn et al. [25] and Pintado-Palomino et al. [7], who also used spectrophotometry as a method of evaluation, did not show a significant difference between bleaching and conventional dentifrices, a factor justified by the absence of hydrogen peroxide in the dentifrices tested. Although in the study by Horn et al. [25], a statistical difference was shown in one of the test groups (Colgate Luminous White dentifrice) by altering the values of L^* (brightness), it was also seen that according to the NBS criterion, the value of ΔE was 1.15, which meant a change in color was not perceived by the human eye. This change in luminosity probably occurred due to the presence of abrasive contents in this dentifrice, such as hydrated silica.

The four studies that used the VITA shade guide observed a statistically significant difference between the test and control groups. These favorable findings may have been attributed to the method used to analyze the color on the total surface of the tooth, without taking into account specific points [14].

The limitations of the present systematic review include the following: the lack of clinical studies using the same method to evaluate the color of dental substrates, in order to allow a comparison of the parameters included in the data analysis; the lack of studies that took into account the durability of color change following discontinuation of the bleaching dentifrices; and the studies did not take into account the frequency of brushing with bleaching dentifrices, as brushing time can influence color change [7]. Thus, future studies are necessary in order to investigate characteristics such as morphological alterations of the dental surface caused by dentifrice materials, in order to establish an effective time-of-use protocol, the influence of dentifrice components on whitening properties, and the durability of tooth whitening after whitening toothpaste is discontinued.

5. Conclusions

Within the limitations of this study, the evidence from this systematic review suggested that bleaching dentifrices have potential in tooth whitening. However, these results should be interpreted with caution before any decision is made, and more randomized clinical trials are required to better determine the efficacy of bleaching dentifrices due to their possible morphological alterations of dental tissues.

References

[1] V. B. Haywood, "Nightguard vital bleaching: current concepts and research," *Journal of the American Dental Association*, vol. 128, pp. 19S–25S, 1997.

[2] C. D. Lynch and R. J. McConnell, "The use of microabrasion to remove discolored enamel: a clinical report," *Journal of Prosthetic Dentistry*, vol. 90, no. 5, pp. 417–419, 2003.

[3] A. Joiner, "The bleaching of teeth: a review of the literature," *Journal of Dentistry*, vol. 34, no. 7, pp. 412–419, 2006.

[4] M. Goldberg, M. Grootveld, and E. Lynch, "Undesirable and adverse effects of tooth-whitening products: a review," *Clinical Oral Investigations*, vol. 14, no. 1, pp. 1–10, 2010.

[5] H. Eimar, R. Siciliano, M. Abdallah et al., "Hydrogen peroxide whitens teeth by oxidizing the organic structure," *Journal of Dentistry*, vol. 40, no. 2, pp. 25–33, 2012.

[6] N. C. A. Claydon, J. Moran, M. L. Bosma, S. Shirodaria, M. Addy, and R. Newcombe, "Clinical study to compare the effectiveness of a test whitening toothpaste with a commercial whitening toothpaste at inhibiting dental stain," *Journal of Clinical Periodontology*, vol. 31, no. 12, pp. 1088–1091, 2004.

[7] K. Pintado-Palomino, C. V. M. Vasconcelos, R. J. Silva et al., "Effect of whitening dentifrices: a double-blind randomized controlled trial," *Brazilian Oral Research*, vol. 30, no. 1, p. 82, 2016.

[8] A. Joiner, "Whitening toothpastes: a review of the literature," *Journal of Dentistry*, vol. 38, no. 2, pp. e17–e24, 2010.

[9] E. Macdonald, A. North, B. Maggio et al., "Clinical Study investigating abrasive effects of three toothpastes and water in a in situ model," *Journal of Dentistry*, vol. 38, no. 6, pp. 509–516, 2010.

[10] C. N. Soraes, F. L. Amaral, M. F. Mesquita, F. M. Franca, R. T. Basting, and C.P. Turssi, "Toothpastes containing abrasive and chemical whitening agents: efficacy in reducing extrinsic dental staining," *General Dentistry*, vol. 63, no. 6, pp. e24–e28, 2015.

[11] C. Llena, C. Oteo, J. Oteo, J. Amengual, and L. Forner, "Clinical efficacy of a bleaching enzume-based toothpaste. A double-blind controlled clinical trial," *Journal of Dentistry*, vol. 44, pp. 8–12, 2016.

[12] R. J. G. Motta, R. Juns Da Silva, L. E. Adami, R. P. Souza, F. C. P. Pires-De-Souza, and C. Tirapelli, "Effectiveness of bleaching dentifrices: a randomized, double-blind, placebo-controlled clinical study," in *Proceedings of the General Session of the International Association for Dental Research*, Seattle, WA, USA, March 2013.

[13] L. Forner, J. Amengual, C. Llena, and P. Riutord, "Therapeutic effectiveness of a new enzymatic bleaching dentifrice," *European Journal of Esthetic Dentistry*, vol. 7, no. 1, pp. 62–70, 2012.

[14] S. Raoufi and D. Birkhed, "Effect of whitening toothpastes on tooth staining using two different colour measuring devices—a 12-week clinical trial," *International Dental Journal*, vol. 60, no. 6, pp. 419–423, 2010.

[15] L. Z. Collins, M. Naeeni, and S. M. Platten, "Instant tooth whitening from a silica toothpaste containing blue covarine," *Journal of Dentistry*, vol. 36, pp. S21–S25, 2008.

[16] R. Yhudira, M. Peumans, M. L. Barker, and R. W. Gerlach, "Clinical trial tooth whitening with 6% hydrogen peroxide whitening strips and two whitening dentifrices," *American Journal of Dentistry*, vol. 20, pp. 32A–36A, 2007.

[17] N. Sharma, H. J. Galustians, J. Qaqish et al., "Comparative tooth whitening and extrinsic tooth stain prevention efficacy

of a new dentifrice and a commercially available tooth whitening dentifrice: six-week clinical trial," *Journal of Clinical Dentistry*, vol. 15, no. 2, pp. 52–57, 2004.

[18] P. Soparkar, K. Rustogi, Y. P. Zhang, M. E. Petrone, W. DeVizio, and H. M. Proskin, "Comparative tooth whitening and extrinsic tooth stain removal efficacy of two tooth whitening dentifrices: six-week clinical trial," *Journal of Clinical Dentistry*, vol. 15, no. 2, pp. 46–51, 2004.

[19] R. W. Gerlach, M. L. Barker, and H. L. Tucker, "Clinical response of three whitening products having different peroxide delivery: comparison of tray, paint-on gel, and dentifrice," *Journal of Clinical Dentistry*, vol. 15, no. 4, pp. 112–117, 2004.

[20] R. W. Gerlach, M. L. Barker, J. D. Hyde, M. B. Jones, and R. E. Cordero, "Effects of tartar control whitening dentifrice on tooth shade in a population with long-standing natural stain," *Journal of Clinical Dentistry*, vol. 12, no. 2, pp. 47–50, 2001.

[21] R. L. Isaacs, R. D. Bartizek, T. S. Owens, P. A. Walters, and R. W. Gerlach, "Maintenance of tooth color after prophylaxis: comparison of three dentifrices," *Journal of Clinical Dentistry*, vol. 12, no. 2, pp. 51–55, 2001.

[22] A. Kakar, K. Rustogi, Y. P. Zhang, M. E. Petrone, W. DeVizio, and H. M. Proskin, "A clinical investigation of the tooth whitening efficacy of a new hydrogen peroxide-containing dentifrice," *Journal of Clinical Dentistry*, vol. 15, no. 2, pp. 41–45, 2004.

[23] A. Ghassemi, W. Hooper, L. Vorwerk, T. Domke, P. DeSciscio, and S. Nathoo, "Effectiveness of a new dentifrice with baking soda and peroxide in removing extrinsic stain and whitening teeth," *Journal of Clinical Dentistry*, vol. 23, no. 3, pp. 86–91, 2012.

[24] A. Ghassemi, L. Vorwerk, A. Cirigliano, W. Hooper, P. DeSciscio, and S. Nathoo, "Clinical effectiveness evaluation of a new whitening dentifrice," *Journal of Clinical Dentistry*, vol. 26, no. 3, pp. 66–71, 2015.

[25] B. A. Horn, B. F. Bittencourt, O. M. Gomes, and P. A. Farhat, "Clinical evaluation of the whitening effect of over-the-counter dentifrices on vital teeth," *Brazilian Dental Journal*, vol. 25, no. 3, pp. 203–206, 2014.

[26] S. P. Hilgenberg, S. C. Pinto, P. V. Farago, F. A. Santos, and D. S. Wambier, "Physical-chemical characteristics of whitening toothpaste and evaluation of its effects on enamel roughness," *Brazilian Oral Research*, vol. 25, no. 4, pp. 288–294, 2011.

[27] P. Özkan, G. Kansu, S. T. Özak, S. Kurtulmuş-Yilmaz, and P. Kansu, "Effect of bleaching agents and whitening dentifrices on the surface roughness of human teeth enamel," *Acta Odontologica Scandinavica*, vol. 71, no. 3-4, pp. 488–497, 2013.

[28] A. Dozic, C. J. Kleverlaan, A. El-Zohairy, A. J. Feilzer, and G. Khashayar, "Performance of five commercially available tooth color-measuring device," *Journal of Prosthodontics*, vol. 16, no. 2, pp. 93–100, 2007.

22

Matrix Metalloproteinase-8 as an Inflammatory and Prevention Biomarker in Periodontal and Peri-Implant Diseases

Ahmed Al-Majid (iD),[1] **Saeed Alassiri,**[2] **Nilminie Rathnayake,**[3] **Taina Tervahartiala,**[2] **Dirk-Rolf Gieselmann,**[4] **and Timo Sorsa** (iD)[2,3]

[1]*Clinic of Preventive Dentistry, Periodontology and Cariology, Center of Dental Medicine, University of Zurich, Zurich, Switzerland*
[2]*Department of Oral and Maxillofacial Diseases, University of Helsinki and Helsinki University Hospital, Helsinki, Finland*
[3]*Karolinska Institutet, Department of Dental Medicine, Division of Periodontology, Stockholm, Sweden*
[4]*Institute of Molecular Diagnostics, Dentognostics GmbH, Solingen and Jena, Germany*

Correspondence should be addressed to Ahmed Al-Majid; ahmedalmajid25@gmail.com

Academic Editor: Saso Ivanovski

Levels of and especially the degree of activation of matrix metalloproteinase (MMP-8) in oral fluids (i.e., saliva, mouth rinse, gingival crevicular fluid (GCF) and peri-implantitis sulcular fluid (PISF)) increase to pathologically elevated levels in the periodontal and peri-implant diseases. This study aimed at collecting and collating data from previously published studies and determining whether active MMP-8 (aMMP-8) could serve as a biomarker for the diagnosis and prevention of periodontal and peri-implant diseases. The literature search identified a total of 284 articles. Out of 284 articles, 61 articles were found to be relevant. Data obtained from the selected studies were combined, and it indicated that aMMP-8 in oral fluids exerts the strong potential to serve as a useful adjunctive diagnostic and preventive biotechnological tool in periodontal and peri-implant diseases. aMMP-8 can be used alone or in combination with other proinflammatory and/or microbiological biomarkers.

1. Introduction

Periodontitis and peri-implantitis, globally common infection-induced oral inflammatory disorders of teeth and dental implants supporting soft and hard tissue, i.e., periodontium and peri-implatium, involve destruction of both soft and hard tissues, as active periodontal and peri-implant degradation (APD). Periodontal/peri-implant tissues are mainly made up of type I collagen. The proteolytic enzyme mainly responsible for the active periodontal/peri-implant soft and hard tissue degeneration (APD) is matrix metalloproteinase (MMP-8), also known as collagenase-2 or neutrophil collagenase. MMP-8 is a member of the MMP family. Structurally related but genetically distinct MMPs are Ca^{2+}- and Zn^{2+}-dependent endopeptidases capable of degradation of almost all extracellular matrix and basement membrane protein components both in physiologic repair and pathologic destruction of tissues, such as a breakdown of extracellular matrix in embryonic development, wound healing, and tissue remodeling [1].

The MMP family is divided into six protease groups: collagenases (MMP-1, MMP-8, and MMP-13), gelatinases (MMP-2 and MMP-9), stromelysins (MMP-3, MMP-10, and MMP-11), matrilysins (MMP-7 and MMP-26), member-type MMPs (MMP-14, MMP-15, MMP-16, MMP-17, and MMP-12), and other nonclassified MMPs, given their auxiliary contrasts [2]. Among all of these groups, the collagenase group is of particular relevance in periodontal disease as it can efficiently cleave native collagen fibers I, II, and III. MMP-8 has been categorized under the interstitial collagenase subgroup of the MMP family. Activities of MMPs are inhibited and regulated by the endogenous or natural tissue inhibitors of tissue inhibitors of MMP (TIMPs) and α2-macroglobulin [3]. The imbalance between MMPs and TIMPs often results in irreversible periodontal and peri-implant destructive pathology involving irreversible APD [3–5].

Recently, an increased level of MMP-8, especially in activated/active form (aMMP-8), in oral fluids is associated with and reflects periodontal and peri-implant inflammation/diseases especially in clinical active phases [3, 6–8]. Periodontal and peri-implant degeneration (APD) is caused by interstitial collagenase MMP-8 and not by bacterial enzymes [9]. MMP-8 is released from neutrophils by selective degranulation triggered by potent periodontopathogenic bacteria and their virulence factors together with host-derived proinflammatory mediators [3, 7]. Gingival fibroblasts, when stimulated by proinflammatory mediators, such as interleukin (IL)-1β and tumor necrosis factor-α, can produce collagenolytic MMPs including MMP-8 [10]. The level of active, but not latent or total, collagenase-2/MMP-8 reflects, predicts, and is related to progressive periodontal and peri-implant disease activity [11]. Elevated levels of aMMP-8 in oral fluids (saliva, mouth rinse, gingival crevicular fluid (GCF), and peri-implant sulcular fluid (PISF)) were found to be associated with clinical periodontal parameters, i.e., probing pocket depth (PPD), bleeding on probing (BOP), and clinical attachment loss (CAL) [12]. The levels of aMMP-8 decrease after successful periodontal and peri-implant treatments [7, 13, 14].

A number of studies that have been performed utilize point-of-care (PoC)/chair-side analysis of elevated aMMP-8 in saliva/oral fluids [15–17]. A study comparing a PoC immunoflow tool with the standard gold laboratory-based one concluded that concentration of aMMP-8 in oral fluids is useful in distinguishing periodontal diseases from healthy subjects [15]. Lateral flow immunoassay of aMMP-8 has been shown to have high sensitivity for at least two sites with BOP and two sites with deepened periodontal pockets [18]. Sorsa et al. demonstrated that immunofluorometric assay (IFMA) and DentoAnalyzer-PoC-test could detect aMMP-8 from GCF samples, and these methods are comparable with the chair-side/PoC aMMP-8 dip-stick test [6]. The Amersham enzyme-linked immunosorbent assay (ELISA) for total MMP-8 immunoactivities was not in line with the PoC/chair-side immune tests, specific for aMMP-8 [6]. Few studies demonstrated the associations of various periodontal pathogens in oral fluids with the levels of aMMP-8 and suggested to use in combination with aMMP-8 with other proinflammatory and microbiological biomarkers that may potentially improve the diagnostic accuracy [6, 7]. The present review aimed at collecting and collating the data from published literature regarding the potential of aMMP-8 in saliva/oral fluids to be used as a biomarker and predictor for periodontal and peri-implant diseases [6, 7, 19, 20].

2. Materials and Methods

2.1. Study Identification. A literature search was performed in two electronic databases PubMed and Cochrane to identify related studies of the past 15 years. In addition to this, other relevant studies were identified by manual searching. Keyword used for study identification in all databases were "MMP-8 and periodontal inflammation," "MMP-8 and peri-implantitis," and "MMP-8 and low-dose doxycycline." The synonyms such as MMP-8, collagenase-2,

and neutrophil collagenase were also searched in combination with periodontitis. The electronic search was done from November 11, 2016, to July 30, 2018.

2.2. Study Selection. All identified studies were screened, and the selection process was done on the basis of inclusion and exclusion criteria.

2.2.1. Inclusion Criteria. Inclusion criteria are as follows:

(1) Randomized controlled trials
(2) Observational studies
(3) Review articles
(4) Studies included low-dose doxycycline/subantimicrobial dose doxycycline (L/SDD) as an adjunctive drug for treatment of periodontal diseases

2.2.2. Exclusion Criteria. Exclusion criteria are as follows:

(1) Written in language other than English
(2) Case reports
(3) Thesis
(4) Animals studies
(5) Diagnosis of periodontal disease was not written
(6) Experimental gingivitis

3. Results

3.1. Study Selection and Data Abstraction. The literature search identified a total of 284 articles. Out of 284 articles, data of 61 articles were selected. Data obtained from selected studies were combined and summarized in the present study (Table 1).

3.2. Sources of MMP-8 in the Oral Cavity. A major source of MMP-8 (neutrophil-type MMP-8) in humans are degranulating triggered neutrophils, but MMP-8 (mesenchymal cell-type MMP-8) is also *de novo* expressed and secreted in small amounts by non-PMN-lineage cells such as epithelial cells, smooth muscle cells, fibroblasts, macrophages, and endothelial cells [74–77]. Neutrophil collagenase/polymorphonuclear leukocyte- (PMN-) derived collagenase-2/MMP-8 differs from interstitial collagenases secreted by other cells in that it is synthesized only during the myelocyte stage of development of neutrophils in the bone marrow and stored as a latent enzyme, i.e., latent pro-MMP-8 (Mr 85 kDa) within the specific granules of PMN. Pro-MMP-8 is rapidly released from activated PMN undergoing selective subcellular granule degranulation and is then activated through the cysteine switch mechanism often, but not always, associated with selective N-terminal proteolysis to yield the active form of the enzyme (Mr 65 kDa) and activation fragments [3, 74–77].

The main source of oral salivary collagenase is PMNs that enter the oral cavity through gingival sulcus [11, 75]. It is evident from the fact that collagenase was only detected in

TABLE 1: Summary of studies related to periodontitis, peri-implantitis, and L/SDD and level of MMP-8 in oral fluids.

	Study title and reference	Reference (year)	Objective	Sample source	Smoker	Form of detected MMP-8 and other markers	Study population	Diagnosis	Result
1	Collagenases in different categories of peri-implant vertical bone loss [21]	Ma et al. (2000) [21]	To investigate if level of collagenase-2 and collagenase-3 in PISF act as mediators in the process of bone destruction in peri-implantitis	PISF samples	N/A	aMMP-8 by IFMA	13 subjects aged from 23 to 89 years old	Peri-implantitis	Gingival Index is not a clinically important marker for bone loss, but aMMP-8 and MMP-13 in PISF are. They might participate in peri-implant osteolysis
2	Levels and molecular forms of MMP-7 (matrilysin-1) and MMP-8 (collagenase-2) in diseased human peri-implant sulcular fluid [22]	Kivelä-Rajamäki et al. (2003) [22]	To identify various isoforms of MMP-8 in PISF and its relationship with MMP-7	PISF samples	N/A	aMMP-8 levels were determined by the western immunoblot method with polyclonal anti-human-MMP-8	13 subjects aged from 21 to 86 years old	Peri-implantitis	The elevated levels of aMMP-8 and MMP-7 were identified in active forms in diseased PISF, but MMP-7 was less prominent. MMP inhibitors, potential future tissue protective drugs, seemingly do not interfere with the defensive antibacterial action of MMP-7 but can inhibit aMMP-8
3	Laminin-5 gamma2-chain and collagenase-2 (MMP-8) in human peri-implant sulcular fluid [23]	Kivelä-Rajamäki et al. (2003) [23]	To investigate the forms and concentration of MMP-8 and laminin-5 gamma2-chain in PISF and to find correlation of these two with clinical parameters (i.e., the recorded gingival and bone resorption) of peri-implantitis	PISF samples	N/A	aMMP-8 levels were determined by western immunoblot	13 subjects aged from 21 to 86 years old	Peri-implantitis	aMMP-8 is a important biomarker of peri-implantitis, but longitudinal studies are required to assess their use, either alone or in combination as molecular biochemical PISF markers, to predict the risk of progression of peri-implantitis, as well as to monitor the impact of treatment of the disease
4	Gingival crevicular fluid collagenase-2 (MMP-8) test stick for chair-side monitoring of periodontitis [24]	Mäntylä et al. (2003) [24]	To develop a test stick for detection of MMP-8 in GCF, to evaluate its diagnostic potential as point-of-care/chair-side test, and to monitor the response to treatment of periodontitis	GCF samples	N/A	aMMP-8 levels were determined by IFMA, and chair-side dip-stick was performed	29 subjects, age not applicable	Healthy, gingivitis, and chronic periodontitis	aMMP-8 GCF levels and chair-side test differentiated periodontitis from gingivitis, and healthy control sites. Scaling and root planing could be followed successfully by both PoC-/chair-side and IFMA
5	The effect of adjunctive low-dose doxycycline therapy on clinical parameters and GCF MMP-8 levels in chronic periodontitis [25]	Emingil et al. (2004) [25]	To compare effectiveness of LDD combined with nonsurgical periodontal therapy alone in reducing levels of MMP-8 in GCF and improving clinical parameters in patients with chronic periodontitis	GCF	12 nonsmokers. none of the subjects was a heavy smoker (i.e., not more than 10 cigarettes/day)	aMMP-8 levels determined by the immunofluorometric assay	30 subjects, 37 to 61 years of age	Chronic periodontitis	Randomized, double blind, placebo-controlled, parallel arm study. LDD improved the effects of nonsurgical periodontal therapy

TABLE 1: Continued.

	Study title and reference	Reference (year)	Objective	Sample source	Smoker	Form of detected MMP-8 and other markers	Study population	Diagnosis	Result
6	Longitudinal analysis of metalloproteinases, tissue inhibitors of metalloproteinases and clinical parameters in GCF from periodontitis-affected patients [26]	Pozo et al. (2005) [26]	Assessment of periodontal disease performed through measurement of extracellular MMP-8, MMP-9, and their TIMP-1 and TIMP-2 in GCF	GCF samples	N/A	aMMP-8 levels were determined by immune-western blotting (Cat. MAB 3316, Chemicon International, Temecula, CA, USA), MMP-9 by zymography, and dot blot of TIMP-1 and TIMP-2 (Cat. sc-6832 and sc-6835, respectively, Santa Cruz Biotechnology, Santa Cruz, CA, USA)	24 subjects, 30 to 35 years old	Healthy, and chronic periodontitis	A different pattern of aMMP-8 in control and patient site was found. The study has established the significant correlation between the severity of periodontal disease and the actual aMMP-8. aMMP-8 and the low level of both TIMP-1 and TIMP-2 were found
7	Is the excessive inhibition of matrix metalloproteinases (MMPs) by potent synthetic MMP inhibitors (MMPIs) desirable in periodontitis and other inflammatory diseases? That is: "Leaky" MMPIs vs excessively efficient drugs [27]	Sorsa and Golub (2005) [27]	Comparison between SDD and tetracycline (non-antibacterial composition) with more potent MMP inhibitors	N/A	N/A	N/A	N/A	N/A	Letter to editor: beneficial clinical efficiency observed only with LDD
8	Monitoring periodontal disease status in smokers and nonsmokers using a gingival crevicular fluid matrix metalloproteinase-8-specific chair-side test [28]	Mäntylä et al. (2006) [28]	To evaluate the efficacy of the aMMP-8-specific chair-side dip-stick test in longitudinally monitoring the periodontal status of smoking and nonsmoking patients with chronic periodontitis, using aMMP-8 concentration in GCF	GCF samples	11 smokers and 5 nonsmokers were included in the study	aMMP-8 levels were determined by chair-side lateral-flow immunotests and IFMA	16 subjects, age not applicable	chronic periodontitis	Persistently elevated GCF aMMP-8 concentration were identified, and they indicated sites at enhanced risk; patients with inadequate response to conventional treatment were identifed by PoC/chair-side test and IFMA
9	Matrix metalloproteinases: contribution to pathogenesis, diagnosis and treatment of periodontal inflammation [3]	Sorsa et al. (2006) [3]	To understand the role of MMPs and their inhibitors in pathogenesis, diagnosis, and treatment of periodontal inflammation	N/A	N/A	N/A	N/A	N/A	Review: beneficial LDD adjunctive medical can be monitored/followed by aMMP-8 PoC/chair-side test

TABLE 1: Continued.

	Study title and reference	Reference (year)	Objective	Sample source	Smoker	Form of detected MMP-8 and other markers	Study population	Diagnosis	Result
10	Salivary biomarkers of existing periodontal disease: a cross-sectional study [29]	Miller et al. (2006) [29]	To determine the correlation between salivary biomarkers specific for periodontal tissue inflammation, collagen degradation, bone turnover, and clinical features of periodontitis	Unstimulated whole expectorated saliva samples	33.3 case subjects and 27.6 control subject smokers were included in the study	Total MMP-8 levels were determined by the ELISA kit (Quantikine, R&D Systems, minneapolis, MN, USA)	57 subjects, 28 to 61 years of age	Healthy, and chronic periodontitis	A salivary level of MMP-8 appears to serve as biomarker of periodontitis
11	Characteristics of collagenase-2 from gingival crevicular fluid and peri-implant sulcular fluid in periodontitis and peri-implantitis patients: pilot study [30]	Xu et al. (2008) [30]	To identify the difference in collagenolytic activity between healthy subjects and subjects with peri-implantitis and to find the correlation between severity of peri-implantitis and collagenase activity	GCF and PISF samples	Nonsmokers were included in the study	Both aMMP-8 and total MMP-8 levels were determined by western blot and DNP-octapeptide assay	29 subjects, 4 healthy, 5 gingivitis patients, 10 chronic periodontitis patients, 5 peri-implants patients, 5 peri-implantitis patients, the age range 23 to 72 years old	Healthy, gingivitis, chronic periodontitis and peri-implantitis	Peri-implantitis PISF contained higher active aMMP-8 levels and activity than GCF from similar deep chronic periodontitis sites. GCF and PISF from severe chronic periodontitis and peri-implantitis exhibited the highest aMMP-8 from PMNs and fibroblasts
12	Host-response therapeutics for periodontal diseases [31]	Giannobile (2008) [31]	To study factors affecting hard and soft tissue degradation around the teeth and dental implants.	N/A	N/A	N/A	N/A	N/A	Review: SSD is a useful/beneficial adjunctive medication in periodontitis
13	Host response modulation in periodontics [32]	Preshaw (2008) [32]	To study the role of SDD in modulation of host response in periodontal disease management	N/A	N/A	N/A	N/A	N/A	Review: MMP-8 is a potential biomarker at periodontitis and LDD is a useful adjunctive medication
14	Matrix metalloproteinase levels in children with aggressive periodontitis [33]	Alfant et al. (2008) [33]	To figure out the MMP-1, -2, -3, -8, -9, -12, and -13 levels in a cohort of African American children with and without aggressive periodontitis	GCF samples	17 nonsmokers were included in the study	Total MMP-1, -2, -3, -8, -9, -12, and -13 levels were determined by the ELISA kit (SenzoLyte 520, AnaSpec, San Jose, CA, USA)	44 subjects with AgP, 7 to 19 years of age, and 12 healthy controls. 17 adults with chronic periodontitis 35 to 65 years of age	Healthy, chronic periodontitis, and aggressive periodontitis	MMP-8 levels were elevated in AgP sites relative to nondiseased sites in the same subjects, in siblings and controls and subjects with chronic periodontitis. MMPs associated with the AgP sites in children were generally elevated compared to an adult cohort with a history of chronic periodontitis

TABLE 1: Continued.

	Study title and reference	Reference (year)	Objective	Sample source	Smoker	Form of detected MMP-8 and other markers	Study population	Diagnosis	Result
15	Matrix metalloproteinase-8 concentration in shallow crevices associated with the extent of periodontal disease [34]	Passoja et al. (2008) [34]	To study association between MMP-8 levels in shallow, gingival crevices and the extent of periodontal disease	GCF samples	20 nonsmokers and 28 smokers were included in the study	Total MMP-8 levels were determined by the ELISA kit (Quantikine, R&D Systems, Minneapolis, MN, USA)	48 subjects, 22 to 75 years old	Chronic periodontitis	Statistically significant association between MMP-8 concentration from shallow crevices and the extent of attachment level (AL) ≥4 mm ($p = 0.028$) and AL≥6 mm ($p = 0.001$), in subjects with moderate to high plaque scores
16	Identification of pathogen and host-response markers correlated with periodontal disease [35]	Ramseier et al. (2009) [35]	To find out the ability of putative host and microbially derived biomarkers to identify periodontal disease status from whole saliva and plaque biofilm	Unstimulated whole saliva samples	0% healthy, 19% gingivitis, 36% mild chronic periodontitis, and 81% severe chronic periodontitis smokers were included in the study	Total MMP-8 and -9, calprotectin, and OPG levels were determined by the ELISA kit (Quantikine, R&D Systems, Minneapolis, MN, USA). A.actinomycetemcomitans, C. rectus, F. nucleatum, P. intermedia, P. gingivalis, T. forsythia, and T. denticola with a quantitative PCR assay, IL-1β, -2, -4, -5, -6, -10, and -13, TNF-α, (FN-γ by protein microarray (Whatman, Florham Park, NJ), and ICTP by radioimmunoassay (Immunodiagnostic Systems, Fountain Hills, AZ)	100 subjects, aged ≥18 years old	Healthy, gingivitis, and chronic periodontitis	Multiple combinations of biomarkers especially MMP-8, 9, and osteoprotegerin combined with red complex bacteria provided highly accurate predictions of periodontal diseases.
17	Association of GCF biomarkers during periodontal maintenance with subsequent progressive periodontitis [36]	Reinhardt et al. (2009) [36]	To find correlation between GCF biomarkers of inflammation and bone resorption and loss of periodontal attachment and bone	GCF	N/A	Total MMP-8 level was determined by the ELISA kit (Biosource, Camarillo, CA)	128 osteopenic postmenopausal females (not taking estrogen) 45 to 70 years of age	Good general health, from healthy and chronic periodontitis patients'	Placebo-controlled clinical trial: SDD targets elevated aMMP-8 with beneficial clinical outcome
18	Oral salivary MMP-8, TIMP-1, and ICTP as markers of advanced periodontitis [37]	Gursoy et al. (2010) [37]	To detect potential markers of advanced periodontitis in saliva. In addition, we compared two MMP-8 detection methods using IFMA and ELISA to differentiate periodontitis subjects from controls	Stimulated whole saliva samples	17.2% healthy and 52.3% chronic periodontitis smokers were included in the study	aMMP-8 levels were determined by IFMA, total MMP-8, MMP-14, and TIMP-1 levels were determined by the ELISA kit (Amersham, GE Healthcare, Buckinghamshire, UK) and ICTP levels were measured by enzyme immunoassay (Orion Diagnostica Oy, Espoo, Finland)	165 subjects, aged ≥30 years old	Healthy and chronic periodontitis	Salivary aMMP-8, when used in combination with TIMP-1 and ICTP is a potential biomarker in the detection of advanced periodontitis. The detection of total MMP-8 by the traditional ELISA method technique is less accurate than the aMMP-8 IFMA technique

TABLE 1: Continued.

	Study title and reference	Reference (year)	Objective	Sample source	Smoker	Study population	Form of detected MMP-8 and other markers	Diagnosis	Result
19	Associations between matrix metalloproteinase-8 and -14 and myeloperoxidase in gingival crevicular fluid from subjects with progressive chronic periodontitis: a longitudinal study [13]	Hernández et al. (2010) [13]	To associate the levels, molecular forms, isoenzyme distribution, and degree of activation of MMP-8 and MMP-14, MPO, and TIMP-1 in GCF from patients with progressive periodontitis at the baseline and after periodontal therapy	GCF samples	N/A	25 subjects, 35 to 62 years old	aMMP-8 levels were determined by western blot and IFMA. MPO levels were determined by the ELISA kit (Immundiagnostik, Bensheim, Germany). MMP-14 and TIMP-1 levels were determined by the ELISA kit (Biotrak, GE healthcare, amersham, Slough, UK)	Chronic periodontitis	High aMMP-8 and MPO levels and a high MPO/MMP-8 positive correlation were found in active and inactive sites at baseline. After treatment, decreases in MPO and aMMP-8 were seen, except for active sites in which MMP-8 differences were not significant
20	Smoking affects diagnostic oral salivary periodontal disease biomarker levels in adolescents [38]	Heikkinen et al. (2010) [38]	To investigate the association between salivary aMMP-8 and PMN elastase with commonly used periodontal health indices in a birth cohort of adolescents accounting for their smoking habits	Stimulated whole saliva samples	61 boys and 66 girls were smokers. 197 boys and 177 girls were nonsmokers	501 subjects, 15 to 16 years old	Active MMP-8 levels were determined by IFMA	Most subjects were chronic periodontitis	Smoking significantly decreased both biomarkers, including aMMP-8 studied
21	Detection of gingival crevicular fluid MMP-8 levels with different laboratory and chair-side methods [6]	Sorsa et al. (2010) [6]	To compare four methods for detection of MMP-8 in GCF	GCF samples	Smokers were included in the study, but exact number of smokers is not mentioned	10 subjects, age not applicable	aMMP-8 levels were determined by DentoAnalyzer (Dentognostics GmbH, Jena, Germany), IFMA, and chair-side lateral-flow immunotests (Medix Biochemica Ltd, Espoo, Finland).Total MMP-8 levels were determined by the ELISA kit (Amersham, GE healthcare, Buckingamshire, UK)	Healthy, gingivitis and chronic periodontitis	IFMA (aMMP-8) and DentoAnalyzer (aMMP-8) results can detect MMP-8 from GCF samples, and these methods are comparable. The chair-side dip-stick test (aMMP-8) results were well in line with these assays. The Amersham ELISA (total MMP-8) results were not in line with tests.
22	Gingival crevicular fluid levels of MMP-8, MMP-9, TIMP-2, and MPO decrease after periodontal therapy [39]	Marcaccini et al. (2010) [39]	To compare the levels of MMP-8, MMP-9, TIMP-1, TIMP-2, and MPO in GCF of chronic periodontitis patients and controls at the baseline and three months after nonsurgical therapy	GCF samples	N/A	42 subjects, 35 to 55 years old	Total MMP-8, MMP-9, TIMP-1, and TIMP-2 levels were determined by the ELISA kit (DuoSet R&D Systems, Inc, Minneapolis, MN, USA), and MPO levels were determined (Sigma chemical, Co, St. Louis, MO, USA)	Healthy, and chronic periodontitis	Level of all the markers except TIMP-1 was found to be higher in GCF of patients compared with controls. The elevated level decreased three months after periodontal therapy

Table 1: Continued.

	Study title and reference	Reference (year)	Objective	Sample source	Smoker	Form of detected MMP-8 and other markers	Study population	Diagnosis	Result
23	Use of host-and bacteria-derived salivary markers in detection of periodontitis: a cumulative approach [40]	Gursoy et al. (2011) [40]	The salivary concentration of three different salivary markers P. gingivalis, IL-1β, and MMP-8 were calculated together to obtain the cumulative risk score for detection of periodontitis	Stimulated whole saliva samples	N/A	P. gingivalis with a quantitative real-time PCR assay, IL-1β levels were determined by the ELISA kit (Amersham), and aMMP-8 levels were determined by IFMA	165 subjects, aged ≥30 years old	Healthy, and chronic periodontitis	The results point to that a cumulative risk score, calculated from the three salivary biomarkers, detects periodontal status more accurately than any of the markers individually. However, it is still sufficient to distinguish the periodontitis patient from the healthy group. However, aMMP-8 is reliable when used alone
24	Smoking and matrix metalloproteinases, neutrophil elastase and myeloperoxidase in chronic periodontitis [41]	Özçaka et al. (2011) [41]	To investigate the possible relationship between smoking and serum concentration of aMMP-8, MMP-9, TIMP-1, MPO, and neutrophil lactase in chronic periodontitis patients relative to periodontally healthy subjects	Serum samples	Healthy subjects (17 smokers) and chronic periodontitis patients (16 smokers) were included in the study	aMMP-8 levels were determined by IFMA; MMP-9 levels were determined by Biotrak ELISA Systems, Amersham Biosciences Ltd, Buckinghamshire, UK; TIMP-1 levels were measured by Duoste ELISA Development Systems, R&D systems, MN, USA; MPO levels were measured by Immunodiagnostic AG, Bensheim, Germany; and neutrophil elastase by Bender MedSystems GmbH, Vienna, Austria	111 subjects, 33 to 65 years	Healthy, and chronic periodontitis	aMMP-8 concentration and aMMP-8/TIMP-1 molar ratios in chronic periodontitis group were not found to be significantly different from those in the periodontally healthy group
25	Oral rinse MMP-8 point-of-care immuno test identifies patients with strong periodontal inflammatory burden [42]	Leppilahti et al. (2011) [42]	To determine if MMP-8 (measured by three different methods), TIMP-1, and elastase activity differentiate subjects with the different periodontal conditions, and second, to find out if MMP-8 levels were comparable among the methods used	Oral-rinse samples	Smokers were included in study, but the exact number of smokers is not mentioned	aMMP-8 levels were determined by DentoELISA (Dentognostics GmbH, Jena, Germany) and IFMA; total MMP-8 levels were measured by the ELISA kit (Amersham, GE Healthcare, Buckingamshire, UK); TIMP-1 levels were determined by the ELISA kit (Amersham); and elastase activity by Sigma Co., St Louis, MO, USA	214 subjects, 44 to 78 years old	Chronic periodontitis	aMMP-8 testing of oral-rinse samples may be beneficial in periodontal diagnostics. Total MMP-8 levels were not useful in diagnosis

TABLE 1: Continued.

	Study title and reference	Reference (year)	Objective	Sample source	Smoker	Form of detected MMP-8 and other markers	Study population	Diagnosis	Result
26	Salivary biomarkers of periodontal disease in response to treatment [43]	Sexton et al. (2011) [43]	To check utility of salivary biomarkers in the monitoring of periodontal disease over time in subjects who received localized periodontal therapy	Unstimulated whole saliva samples	23% of the SRP group, and 33% of the OHI group smokers were included in the study	Total MMP-8 and OPG levels were determined by the ELISA kit (Quantikine, R&D Systems, Minneapolis, MN, USA) and IL-1β, IL-8, MIP-1α, and TNF-α levels were measured by Luminex human cytokine/chemokine multiplex kits (Millipore, St. Charles, MO, USA)	68 subjects, aged ≥ 18 years old	Chronic periodontitis	Salivary levels of biomarkers, i.e., IL-1β MMP-8, OPG, and MIP-1α reflected disease severity and response to therapy suggesting their potential utility for monitoring periodontal disease status
27	Full-mouth profile of active MMP-8 in periodontitis patients [44]	Kraft-Neumärker et al. (2011) [44]	To investigate whether there was a relationship between clinical diagnostic parameters and the concentration of aMMP-8 in GCF in the site level full-mouth analysis	GCF samples	Nonsmokers were included in the study	aMMP-8 levels were determined by IFMA	9 subjects, 35 to 66 years old	Chronic periodontitis	A statistically significant relationship found between level of aMMP-8 and pocket depth
28	Matrix metalloproteinase-8 is the major potential collagenase in active peri-implantitis [45]	Arakawa et al. (2012) [45]	To compare levels of MMP-1, -8, and -13 in PISF of both healthy and diseased sites and to find correlation between these MMPs with bone loss	PISF samples	N/A	Total MMP-8, MMP-1, and MMP-13 levels were determined by Fuji Chemical Industry, Takaoka, Japan	64 subjects, the aged range 59 to 78 years old	Peri-implantitis	This study also showed MMP-8 as a possible marker for progressive bone loss in peri-implantitis
29	Matrix metalloproteinases and inflammatory cytokines in oral fluid of patients with chronic generalized periodontitis and various construction materials [46]	Kushlinskii et al. (2012) [46]	To compare oral fluid of practically healthy subjects with intact periodontium and patient with chronic generalized periodontitis with various structural materials of dental restorations	Oral fluid samples	N/A	Total MMP-8 levels were determined by the ELISA kit (Quantikine, R&D Systems, Minneapolis, MN, USA)	105 subjects, 18 to 52 years old	Chronic periodontitis	The MMP-8 level in oral fluid was found to be higher than the normal only in patients with chronic generalized periodontitis with metal restorations. No significant difference was found in the level of MMP-8 in patients of chronic generalized periodontitis without metal restoration
30	Effect of scaling and root planing on interleukin-1β, interleukin-8 and MMP-8 levels in gingival crevicular fluid from chronic periodontitis patients [47]	Konopka et al. (2012) [47]	To determine amounts of MMP-8, IL-8, and IL-1β in GCF from patients with chronic periodontitis in relation to clinical parameters	GCF samples	Nonsmokers were included in the study	Total MMP-8 and IL-8 and IL-1β levels were determined by the ELISA kit (Quantikine, R&D Systems, Minneapolis, MN, USA)	51 subjects, 30 patients (mean age 48.7 ± 9.1 years old), and 21 healthy subjects (mean age 33.7 ± 8.2 years)	Healthy, and chronic periodontitis	Short-term nonsurgical therapy resulted in significant improvement in periodontal indices and a marked decrease of MMP-8, IL-8, and IL-1β in GCF. However, the level of humoral factors was still higher than those in control group

TABLE 1: Continued.

	Study title and reference	Reference (year)	Objective	Sample source	Smoker	Form of detected MMP-8 and other markers	Study population	Diagnosis	Result
31	Associations of periodontal microorganisms with oral salivary proteins and MMP-8 in gingival crevicular fluid [19]	Yakob et al. (2012) [19]	To investigate in subjects with and without periodontitis, the levels of salivary proteins and aMMP-8 in GCF in relation to the presence of specific periodontal pathogens	Unstimulated and stimulated whole saliva, and GCF samples	15 healthy, and 30 chronic periodontitis smokers were included in the study	aMMP-8 levels were determined by IFMA, A. actinomycetemcomitans, P. intermedia, P. gingivalis T. forsythia, and T. denticola with a quantitative PCR assay; Albumin was analyzed using an immunoturbidimetric Tina-Quant® kit (Roche, Basel, Switzerland); the salivary immunoglobulin concentrations were then analyzed by ELISA [87]; and salivary total protein was measured using the colorimetric Lowry method [49]	101 subjects, mean age 59.2 ± SD 2.9	Healthy, and chronic periodontitis	Salivary albumin and protein concentration were significantly higher in subjects with T. denticola. Level of aMMP-8 was significantly higher in subjects with T. denticola and T. forsythia
32	Treponema denticola associates with increased levels of MMP-8 and MMP-9 in gingival crevicular fluid [50]	Yakob et al. (2013) [50]	To assess the association between the presence of site-specific subgingival microorganisms and the level of aMMP-8 and MMP-9 in GCF	GCF samples	15 healthy and 30 chronic periodontitis were included in the study	aMMP-8 levels were determined by IFMA, A. actinomycetemcomitans, P. intermedia, P. gingivalis, T. forsythia, and T. denticola with a quantitative PCR assay; MMP-9 levels were determined by the ELISA kit (Amersham, Biosciences UK Ltd, Buckinghamshire, UK)	99 subjects, mean age 59.2 ± 2.9	Healthy, and chronic periodontitis	The presence of T. forsythia and T. denticola was associated with increased levels of aMMP-8 in the test sites
33	Cytokine and matrix metalloproteinase expression in fibroblasts from peri-implantitis lesions in response to viable porphyromonas gingivalis [51]	Irshad et al. (2013) [51]	To analyze inflammatory reactions of fibroblasts after in vitro challenge with P. gingivalis	Fibroblasts	All subjects' nonsmokers were included in the study	Total MMP-8, -1 levels were determined by the ELISA kit (Quantikine Human, Pharmacia Biotech, Buckinghamshire, UK) TIMP-1 immunoassay (R&D Systems, Minneapolis, MN, USA), and P. gingivalis with a quantitative real-time PCR assay	Five patients periodontally healthy 54.4 ± (±18.7) years old, nine patients (II) 57.8 (±12.4) years old, seven peri-implantitis patients 54.4 (±9.2) years old	Peri-implantitis	Fibroblasts from peri-implantitis and periodontitis lesions gave a more pronounced inflammatory response to the P. gingivalis challenge than fibroblasts from healthy donors. They may therefore be involved in the development of inflammation in peri-implantitis and periodontitis. Moreover, the sustained upregulation of inflammatory mediators and MMP-1 in peri-implantitis fibroblasts may play a role in the pathogenesis of peri-implantitis

TABLE 1: Continued.

	Study title and reference	Reference (year)	Objective	Sample source	Smoker	Form of detected MMP-8 and other markers	Study population	Diagnosis	Result
34	Salivary biomarkers of oral health: a cross-sectional study [52]	Rathnayake et al. (2013) [52]	Aimed to investigating if known salivary biomarkers could be used for epidemiological studies for detection of periodontitis	Stimulated whole saliva samples	75 smokers were included in the study	Active MMP-8 levels were determined by IFMA; TIMP-1 levels were measured by the ELISA kit; (Amersham); TNF-α, IL-1β, IL-6, and IL-8 were measured by Luminex Chemokine multiplex); lysozyme levels were measured the ELISA kit (Quantikine, R&D Systems, Minneapolis, MN, USA)	966 subjects, 20 to 89 years old	Chronic periodontitis	aMMP-8 could be used as marker of periodontal disease in more significant patient populations
35	Oral salivary type I collagen degradation end-products and related matrix metalloproteinases in periodontitis [53]	Gursoy et al. (2013) [53]	Type I collagen degradation end products and related MMPs were examined aiming at detecting potential markers of periodontitis in saliva with high sensitivity and specificity	Stimulated whole saliva samples	86 smokers were included in the study	Active MMP-8 levels were determined by IFMA; MMP-9 and MMP-13 levels were measured by the ELISA kit (Amersham, GE Healthcare, Buckinghamshire, UK); TRACP-5b levels were measured by BoneTRAP® assay, Immunodiagnostic Systems Ltd, Boldon, UK); ICTP levels were measured by enzyme immunoassay; (Orion Diagnostica UniQ ICTP, EIA; Orion Diagnostica, Espoo, Finland); CTx levels were measured by Serum CrossLaps® ELISA assay (Immunodiagnostic, Systems Ltd, Boldon, UK); and NTx levels were measured by OSTEOMARK® NTx; serum levels were measured by Wampole Laboratories (Princeton, NJ, USA)	230 subjects of ≥30 years old	Chronic periodontitis	aMMP-8 is a reliable biomarker candidate for detecting alveolar bone destruction

TABLE 1: Continued.

	Study title and reference	Reference (year)	Objective	Sample source	Smoker	Form of detected MMP-8 and other markers	Study population	Diagnosis	Result
36	Periodontal treatment reduces matrix metalloproteinase levels in localized aggressive periodontitis [54]	Gonçalves et al. (2013) [54]	To evaluate MMP-1, -2, -3, -8, -9, -12 and -13 levels in the GCF after treatment of LAgP and to correlate these levels with clinical response	GCF samples	Nonsmokers were included in the study	Total MMPs levels were determined by the ELISA kit (SensoLyte 520, AnaSpec, Fremont, CA)	29 subjects of 5 to 21 years old	Aggressive periodontitis	Treatment of LAgP with Conventional mechanical treatment and systemic antibiotics reduced specific MMPs levels effectively. The significant association was observed between MMP-1, -2, -3, -8, -9, -12 and -13 and percentage of sites with PD > 4 mm
37	Patterns of salivary analytes provide diagnostic capacity for distinguishing chronic adult periodontitis from health [55]	Ebersole et al. (2013) [55]	To determine to analyze expression levels in unstimulated whole saliva samples collected from multiple occasions from 30 healthy adults and 50 chronic adult periodontitis patients	Unstimulated whole saliva samples	Only nonsmokers were included in study	Total MMP-8 levels were determined by the ELISA kit (Quantikine, R&D Systems, minneapolis, MN, USA)	80 subjects of 18 to 45 years old	Healthy and chronic periodontitis	Salivary levels of MMP-8 were significantly elevated in periodontitis patients compared with the daily variation observed in healthy adults
38	Clinical correlates of a lateral-flow immunoassay oral risk indicator [18]	Nwhator et al. (2014) [18]	To investigate the clinical correlates of a lateral-flow immunoassay with BOP, oral hygiene, and periodontal probing depth on the first time	Oral-rinse samples	5 smokers and 71 nonsmokers were included in the study	aMMP-8 levels were determined by chair-side lateral-flow immunotests (Dentognostics GmbH, Jena, Germany)	76 subjects, age not applicable	Healthy, and chronic periodontitis	The chair-side aMMP-8 immunoassay showed a high (82.6%) sensitivity for at least two sites with BOP and periodontal pockets. It showed a lower relationship with single-site periodontal pockets and BOP
39	Crevicular fluid biomarkers and periodontal disease progression [56]	Kinney et al. (2014) [56]	Assess the ability of a panel of GCF biomarkers as predictors of periodontal disease progression	Unstimulated whole saliva samples	0% was healthy, 19% were gingivitis, 36% were mild chronic periodontitis, and 81% were severe chronic periodontitis smokers were included in the study	Total MMP-8 levels were determined by the ELISA kit (Quantibody human cytokine array by RayBiotech, Inc., Norcross, GA, USA)	100 subjects, aged ≥ 18 years old	Healthy, gingivitis, and chronic periodontitis	MMP-8 was significantly higher in periodontal disease progression group compared to stable patients
40	Salivary biomarkers associated with gingivitis and response to therapy [57]	Syndergaard et al. (2014) [57]	The primary aim was to compare the concentrations of IL-1β, IL-6, PGE$_2$, MMP-8, and MIP-1α in the whole saliva from patients with gingivitis with concentrations of these substrates in the saliva of patients with a clinically healthy periodontium	Unstimulated whole saliva samples	N/A	Total MMP-8, IL-1β, IL-6, PGE$_2$ and MIP-1α levels were determined by ELISA kit, assay design, Ann Arbor, MI & EMD, millipore, Billerica, MA	80 subjects of 23 to 38 years old	Healthy and gingivitis	Concentrations of IL-1β, IL-6, and MMP-8 cannot distinguish gingivitis from health

TABLE 1: Continued.

	Study title and reference	Reference (year)	Objective	Sample source	Smoker	Form of detected MMP-8 and other markers	Study population	Diagnosis	Result
41	Oral salivary biomarkers of bacterial burden, inflammatory response, and tissue destruction in periodontitis [58]	Salminen et al. (2014) [58]	To investigate the association of selected salivary biomarkers with periodontal parameters and validate the use of a novel salivary diagnostic approach, the cumulative risk score (CRS), in detection of periodontitis in subjects with angiographically verified coronary artery disease diagnosis	Stimulated whole saliva samples	58 were current smokers and 202 former smokers were included in the study	aMMP-8 levels were determined by IFMA, IL-1β was measured by flow cytometry-based Luminex kits, Milliplex, Map Kit; MPXHCYTO-60k, Millipore, Billerica, MA, USA, and *P. gingivalis* with a quantitative PCR assay was performed	493 subjects, age nonapplicable	Chronic periodontitis	The high salivary concentration of aMMP-8, IL-1β, and *P. gingivalis* was associated with deepened periodontal pockets and alveolar bone loss. aMMP-8 performed better compared to BOP%
42	Matrix metalloproteinases and myeloperoxidase in GCF provide site-specific diagnostic value for chronic periodontitis [59]	Leppilahti et al. (2014) [59]	To identify the diagnostic accuracy of GCF candidate biomarkers to discriminate periodontitis from inflamed and healthy sites and to compare the performance of two independent MMP-8 immunoassays	GCF samples	5 subjects healthy (nonsmokers), 3 nonsmokers with gingivitis, and 3 nonsmokers with chronic periodontitis were included in the study	aMMP-8 levels were determined by IFMA, and total MMP-8 was measured by ELISA kits, GE Healthcare, Amersham	25 subjects, healthy (mean age, 48.2 ± 11.2 years) gingivitis (mean age, 35.7 ± 15.4 years) and periodontitis patients (mean age, 46.0 ± 5.0 years)	Healthy, gingivitis, and chronic periodontitis	MMPs are highly discriminatory biomarkers for site-specific diagnosis of periodontitis. The comparison of two quantitative MMP-8 methods demonstrated IFMA to be more accurate than ELISA
43	Gingival crevicular fluid matrix metalloproteinase-8 levels predict treatment outcome among smokers with chronic periodontitis [60]	Leppilahti et al. (2014) [60]	To explore different GCF aMMP-8 patterns in smokers and nonsmokers with chronic periodontitis and test the utility of baseline GCF aMMP-8 levels in predicting categorically assessed treatment outcomes	GCF samples	10 smokers and 5 nonsmokers were included in the study	aMMP-8 levels were determined by IFMA	15 subjects, aged 28 to 64 years	Chronic periodontitis	Baseline aMMP-8 level in GCF strongly predicts how aMMP-8 levels behave during the maintenance period. In this regard, aMMP-8 analysis can be considered more useful than BOP. In smokers' sites, high baseline aMMP-8 levels indicate and predict weak treatment response
44	Targeted salivary biomarkers for discrimination of periodontal health and disease(s) [61]	Ebersole et al. (2015) [61]	Saliva-based diagnostic approach for periodontal health and disease based upon the abundance of salivary analyses coincidence with the disease	Unstimulated whole saliva samples	28 current smokers were included in the study	Total MMP-8 levels were determined by ELISA kit, the MILLIPLEX MAP Kit, EMD millipore, Billerica, MA, USA	209 subjects, aged ≥18 years	Healthy, gingivitis, and chronic periodontitis	Demonstrated the utility of MMP-8 in differentiating periodontitis from health
45	Activated matrix metalloproteinase-8 in saliva as diagnostic test for periodontal disease? a case-control study [62]	Izadi Borujeni et al. (2015) [62]	To evaluate sensitivity and specificity of a chair-side test for aMMP-8 to detect periodontitis	Oral-rinse samples	25 smokers were included in the study	aMMP-8 levels were determined by chair-side lateral-flow immunotests, Dentognostics GmbH, Jena, Germany	60 subjects, aged ≥18 years	Healthy and chronic periodontitis	Positive results of the aMMP-8 test significantly correlate with generalized chronic periodontitis. The test shows 87% sensitivity and 60% specificity in the diagnosis of chronic periodontitis

TABLE 1: Continued.

	Study title and reference	Reference (year)	Objective	Sample source	Smoker	Form of detected MMP-8 and other markers	Study population	Diagnosis	Result
46	The utility of gingival crevicular fluid matrix metalloproteinase-8 response patterns in prediction of site-level clinical treatment outcome [63]	Leppilahti et al. (2015) [63]	To study different response patterns of MMP-8 among smoker and nonsmoker subjects with CP and GAgP to test its utility in predicting site level treatment outcome	GCF samples	86 smokers were included in the study	aMMP-8 levels were determined by IFMA	158 subjects, aged 27 to 49 years	Chronic periodontitis and aggresive periodontitis	Distinct types of MMP-8 response patterns were obtained for smokers and nonsmokers. Optimal cutoff levels of aMMP-8 defined for smokers and nonsmokers, which indicate risk for compromised treatment outcome at baseline and during maintenance
47	Pilot study on oral health status as assessed by an active matrix metalloproteinase-8 chair-side mouth rinse test in adolescents [64]	Heikkinen et al. (2016) [64]	To investigate whether a PoC mouth rinse test based on aMMP-8 immunoassay could identify patients with oral inflammatory burden among adolescents with early pathologic findings	Mouth rinse samples	5 smokers, and 42 nonsmokers were included in the study	aMMP-8 levels were determined by chair-side lateral-flow immunotests (Dentognostics GmbH, Jena, Germany)	47 subjects, aged 15 to 17 years	Chronic periodontitis	PoC/chairside was found to be useful in the online detection/diagnosis of oral inflammatory burden, i.e., periodontitis in adolescents with early, initial signs of periodontitis. Detection of caries is also possible but with less efficiency. The test shows 76.5% sensitivity and 96.7% specificity in the diagnosis of initial chronic periodontitis
48	Host-derived biomarkers at teeth and implants in partially edentulous patients. A 10-year retrospective study [65]	Ramseier et al. (2016) [65]	To compare host-derived biomarkers in PISF and in GCF from adjacent teeth and implants and to analyze their level in both periodontal disease and healthy condition	PISF and GCF samples	Smokers were included in study but exact number of smokers is not mentioned	IL-1β, MMP-3, MMP-8, MMP-1, and MMP-1/TIMP-1 levels were determined by ELISA kits, R&D systems, Europe Ltd, Abingdon, UK	Total 997 samples were evaluated	chronic periodontitis and peri-implantitis	Increased levels of MMP-8 and IL-1β in PISF or GCF may be associated with inflammation around teeth and implants while lower levels of MMP-8/TIMP-1 may be an indicator of disease progression around implants and eased levels of MMP-8 and IL-1β in PISF or GCF may be associated with inflammation around teeth and implants while lower levels of MMP-1/TIMP-1 may be an indicator of disease progression around implants
49	Non-antibacterial tetracycline formulations: host-modulators in the treatment of periodontitis and relevant systemic diseases [66]	Golub et al. (2016) [66]	To address the evidences supporting adjunctive use of host modulation therapy with scaling and root planning in the long-term management of periodontal disease	N/A	N/A	N/A	N/A	N/A	Review: aMMP-8 PoC test is suitable to monitor the adjunctive beneficial SDD in periodontitis

TABLE 1: Continued.

	Study title and reference	Reference (year)	Objective	Sample source	Smoker	Form of detected MMP-8 and other markers	Study population	Diagnosis	Result
50	Analysis of matrix metalloproteinases, especially MMP-8, in GCF, mouth rinse, and saliva for monitoring periodontal diseases [7]	Sorsa et al. (2016) [7]	To review recent studies related to monitoring of periodontal and peri-implant diseases by analyzing systemic and oral fluid biomarkers [7]	N/A	N/A	N/A	N/A	N/A	Review: SDD targets increased aMMP-8 beneficial clinical outcome and no development bacterial resistance
51	Protein biomarkers and microbial profiles in peri-implantitis [67]	Wang et al. (2016) [67]	To assess diagnostic ability of biomarkers when combined with microbial profiles [67]	PICF samples	4 current smokers and 21 past smokers were included in the study	Total MMP-8, OPG, IL-1β, TIMP-2, and vascular endothelial growth factor levels were determined by ELISA kits, custom human Quantibody, arrays, RayBiotech, Inc, Norcross, GA, USA, and *A. actinomycetemcomitans, P. intermedia, P. gingivalis, T. forsythia,* and *T. denticola* with a quantitative PCR assay	68 subjects, age range: 37 to 83 years	Peri-implantitis	The present data suggest that the increased levels of the selected PICF-derived biomarkers of periodontal tissue inflammation, matrix degradation/regulation, and alveolar bone turnover/resorption combined with site-specific microbial profiles may be associated with peri-implantitis and could have potential as predictors of peri-implant diseases
52	Peri-implant sulcus fluid (PISF) matrix metalloproteinase (MMP) -8 Levels in peri-implantitis [14]	Thierbach et al. (2016) [14]	To assess MMP-8 levels in PISF from diseased sites in both smokers and nonsmokers	PISF samples	17 smokers were included in the study	aMMP-8 levels were determined by DentoELISA immunoassay (Dentognostics, Jena, Germany)	29 subjects, 8 healthy patients, 3 gingivitis, and 18 chronic periodontitis	Peri-implantitis	aMMP-8 levels increase in peri-implantitis affected implants both in nonperiodontitis and periodontitis patients, but levels still after treatment of the condition reflect intensified host response around implants and indicate challenges of controlling peri-implantitis with any treatment modality
53	Correlation between peri-implant sulcular fluid rate and expression of collagenase2 (MMP8) [68]	Janska et al. (2016) [68]	To identify correlation between PISF and collagenase-2 level in superficial and fundus area of PI sulcus	PISF samples	N/A	aMMP-8 levels were determined by DentoELISA immunoassay (Dentognostics, Jena, Germany)	15 subjects, the age range 43 to 75 years	Peri-implantitis	Examination of aMMP-8 is a sensitive method when examining early inflammatory changes but depends from the depth of the sample collection in the gingival pocket
54	Rapid assessment of oral salivary MMP-8 and periodontal disease using lateral flow immunoassay [15]	Johnson et al. (2016) [15]	To determine the efficacy of a novel POCID for detecting MMP-8 concentration in oral fluids in comparison with a gold standard laboratory-based immunoassay	Unstimulated whole saliva samples	10 smokers were included in the study	Total MMP-8 levels were determined by rapidassays, ApS, Copenhagen-S, Denmark, EMD Millipore, Billerica, MA and luminex, Austin, TX, USA	41 subjects, aged 18 years or older	Healthy and chronic periodontitis	MMP-8 can be detected by POCID and concentration correlates with luminex for both saliva and rinse fluids. This study confirmed and further extended the original studies of Nwhator et al. [18] and Heikkinen et al. [64]

Table 1: Continued.

	Study title and reference	Reference (year)	Objective	Sample source	Smoker	Form of detected MMP-8 and other markers	Study population	Diagnosis	Result
55	Diagnostic accuracy for apical and chronic periodontitis biomarkers in gingival crevicular fluid: An exploratory study [69]	Baeza et al. (2016) [69]	Assessment of level and diagnostic accuracy of an asset of potential biomarkers in GCF from patients with chronic periodontitis and AAP	GCF samples	19 smokers were included in the study	aMMP-8 levels were determined by IFMA, MPO levels were determined by ELISA kit, immunodiagnostik, AG, Bensheim, Germany, IL-1β, IL-6, TNF-α, Dkk-1, ON, PTN, TRAP-5, and OPG levels were determined by Multiplex detection panels Millipore, St. Charles, MO, USA, Magpix, Millipore, St. Charles, MO, USA, and MMP-2 and -9 levels were determined by gelatin zymography.	106 subjects, aged 44 to 52 years	Chronic periodontitis	aMMP-8 shows diagnostic potential for both chronic periodontitis and AAP. aMMP-8 was found to be higher in chronic periodontitis, followed by AAP
56	Pilot study on the genetic background of an active matrix metalloproteinase-8 test in finnish adolescents [70]	Heikkinen et al. (2017) [70]	To determine whether aMMP-8 chair-side test can detect initial periodontitis and caries with genetic background in adolescents	Oral fluid and DNA samples	5 smokers and 42 nonsmokers were included in the study	aMMP-8 levels were determined by chair-side lateral-flow immunotests (Dentognostics GmbH, Jena, Germany)	47 subjects aged 15 to 17 years	Chronic periodontitis	The aMMP-8 chair-side test has potential to detect initial periodontitis in adolescents with predisposing genetic background. aMMP-8 PoC/chair-side test acts as a gene test
57	Association of oral fluid MMP-8 with periodontitis in swiss adult subjects [12]	Mauramo et al. (2017) [12]	To find association between periodontitis and levels of aMMP-8 in saliva and GCF	Stimulated whole saliva and GCF	Never smokers were 150 (58.1%). Former smokers were 70 (27.1%). Current smokers were 38 (14.7%)	aMMP-8 levels were determined by IFMA	258 subjects, mean age 43.5 (21–58) years	Healthy and chronic periodontitis	Elevated levels of aMMP-8 in saliva and GCF are significantly associated with periodontitis in a systemically healthy adult
58	Association between serum and oral matrix metalloproteinase-8 levels and periodontal health status association between serum and oral matrix metalloproteinase-8 levels and periodontal health status association between serum and oral matrix metalloproteinase-8 levels and periodontal health status [71]	Noack et al. (2017) [71]	To identify the association between extent of circulating aMMP-8 and status of periodontal disease and aMMP-8 levels in oral fluids	Unstimulated whole saliva, stimulated whole saliva, GCF, and serum samples	Smokers were included in study but exact number of smokers is not mentioned	aMMP-8 levels were determined by IFMA, PerioSafe plus, (Dentognostics GmbH, Jena, Germany), and A. actinomycetemcomitans, P. intermedia, P. gingivalis, T. forsythia, and T. denticola with a semiquantitative PCR assay	59 subjects, aged 23 to 58 years	Healthy, gingivitis, and chronic periodontitis	The serum levels correlated significantly with oral aMMP-8 as well as with clinical periodontal parameters in a dose-dependent manner in systematically healthy subjects

TABLE 1: Continued.

	Study title and reference	Reference (year)	Objective	Sample source	Smoker	Form of detected MMP-8 and other markers	Study population	Diagnosis	Result
59	Influence of different forms and materials (zirconia or titanium) of abutments in peri-implant soft-tissue healing using matrix metalloproteinase-8: a randomized pilot study [72]	Kumar et al. (2017) [72]	To compare peri-implant connective tissue response around titanium and zirconia abutments	PISF samples	Nonsmokers were included in the study	Total MMP-8 levels were determined by ELISA, Boster Biological Technology Co Ltd	12 subjects, the age range 20 to 45 years	Healthy	This study suggests the presence of more remodeling and/or inflammatory phenomena around titanium implant abutments than around zirconia abutments of a different design during the early stages but not at 1 year
60	Microbiological and aMMP-8 findings depending on peri-implant disease in patients undergoing supportive implant therapy [73]	Ziebolz et al. (2017) [73]	To study relation of microbiological findings and aMMP-8 level with peri-implant mucositis and peri-implantitis in subjects receiving periodontal or implant therapy	PISF samples	17 smokers with 43 implant sites	aMMP-8 levels were determined by DentoELISA (Dentognostics GmbH, Jena, Germany)	89 subjects with 171 implants. Mean age: 52 ± years, 116 dental implants were healthy, 39 dental implants had mucositis, and 16 dental implant had peri-implantitis	Peri-implantitis, peri-mucositis around implants, and chronic periodontitis	Within the limitations of this study, microbiological findings and aMMP-8 levels are not suitable for a differentiation between healthy, peri-mucositis, and peri-implantitis in patients all undergoing SIT/SPT. No healthy and disease patients without SIT/SPT were involved. Only smoking and the presence of Pi appear to be potential parameters associated with peri-implant disease in SIT/SPT patients. SIT/SPT intervention downregulated aMMP-8 during maintenance
61	Diagnosing peri-implant disease using the tongue as a 24/7 detector [49]	Ritzer et al. (2017) [49]	Anyone, anywhere, and anytime diagnostics were developed for peri-implant disease. The sensors responded to MMPs and provided proof of concept in statistically differentiating patients with peri-implant disease from healthy volunteers	Oral fluid	No-smokers were included in the study	aMMP-8 levels were determined by DentoELISA (Dentognostics GmbH, Jena, Germany) and MMP-8 analyzed by 24/7 chewing gum	33 subjects saliva or sulcus fluid collected from patients with peri-implant disease (defined as mucositis or peri-implantitis; $n = 19$) and healthy control ($n = 14$)	Peri-implantitis	Elevated MMP-8 could be detected in peri-implantitis, oral fluid vs. healthy oral fluid

whole oral saliva of subjects and not in secretions of major oral salivary glands. Furthermore, whole oral saliva collected from edentulous subjects did not show a significant amount of collagenase [75].

Oral fluid (GCF, PISF, mouth rinse, and saliva) collagenases exert similarity with PMN- or neutrophil-type collagenase-2 (MMP-8). It degrades type I and II collagens significantly faster than the type III collagen. Its molecular weight is 65–70 kDa, same as collagenase of the PMNs/neutrophils/MMP-8 and gingival sulcus [3, 7]. It is activated by gold thioglucose, which only activates PMN/neutrophil collagenase [3, 7, 75, 77].

3.3. Active and Latent Forms. Most of the oral salivary collagenase found in a healthy mouth is in the latent form, whereas in case of periodontal or/and peri-implant disease patient(s), it is in active or activated (aMMP-8) form together with activation fragments [3, 43, 75, 77]. Studies done by Gangbar et al. and Lee et al. [11, 76] demonstrated that oral fluid active collagenase, but not latent, is related and reflects to progressive clinical periodontal disease activity, i.e., loss attachment or APD. aMMP-8 in oral fluids precedes, predicts, is associated with, and reflects on on-going or future/developing progressive, often hidden and subclinical, periodontal and peri-implant disease activity, i.e., CAL, APD, and active peri-implant degeneration [3, 6, 7, 17, 76, 77]. Significant correlations have been found between aMMP-8 and progressing severity of periodontal and peri-implant diseases [3, 4, 6, 7, 26]. Successful periodontal and peri-implant treatment significantly reduces aMMP-8 levels in oral fluids [3, 6, 7, 17, 78, 79].

3.4. MMP-8 and Correlation with Periodontal Diseases. It has been documented in several studies that salivary and oral fluids at aMMP-8 levels are higher in subjects with localized and generalized periodontitis than in healthy controls but the levels reduced after nonsurgical periodontal therapy, i.e., scaling and root planning (SRP) [12, 39, 41, 43, 53]. Furthermore, aMMP-8, but not latent/total MMP-8, levels could differentiate between periodontitis and gingivitis as well [59]. A slight increase in MMP-8 levels could be observed in case of gingivitis, which shows a decrease after dental prophylaxis or secondary preventive interventions [57].

Nwhator et al. demonstrated that aMMP-8, measured by lateral flow chair-side/PoC immunoassay (PerioSafe®), is directly proportional to the oral hygiene status [18]. It shows a positive correlation with chronic periodontitis and BOP but only in the presence of two or more sites having the deepened PPD of not less than 5 mm; these aMMP-8 PoC findings indicate that such deepened sites are APD affected. The sensitivity of immunoassay for a single site affected by chronic periodontitis was found to be less [18]. Levels of aMMP-8 in oral fluids have been demonstrated to correlate with clinical periodontal parameters in particularly PPD, and it also reflects the effect of treatment [12, 18, 44, 47, 54, 62]. Levels of aMMP-8 are not only associated with clinical periodontal parameters status but also showed significant association with radiological parameters. aMMP-8 levels have been shown to differentiate subjects with a severe bone loss with those with a slight bone loss [53, 58]. Izadi Boroujeni et al. demonstrated a sensitivity of 87% and specificity of 60% of aMMP-8 in a PoC detection of generalized chronic periodontitis [62].

In children, sites with aggressive periodontitis show higher levels of MMP than adults with chronic periodontitis [33]. Baeza et al. reported in their study that aMMP-8 levels in chronic periodontitis were elevated [69]. When aMMP-8 levels were measured by ELISA, the cutoff point was identified as 13 ng/ml chronic periodontitis case [69].

In number of previous investigations, aMMP-8 levels have been reported to predict periodontal disease progression [3, 7, 76, 77]. aMMP-8 levels differentiate between subjects with stable and progressing periodontitis; these confirmatory findings have been repeatedly recorded by independent immune and catalytic activity assays specific for aMMP-8 [6, 8, 80, 81]. While predicting periodontal disease progression, highest sensitivity was noted with salivary/oral fluid aMMP-8, whereas GCF aMMP-8 showed high specificity [56, 59, 63, 71].

Leppilahti et al. established cutoff levels for smoking and nonsmoking periodontal patients to predict site-specific levels of treatment outcomes [56, 57, 59, 63]. The most optimal cutoff value among smokers was 0.045, whereas for nonsmokers, the calculated value was 0.085. These values can be helpful in longitudinal monitoring of the disease status during the maintenance period [56, 57, 59, 63].

3.5. Study Specimens. Oral fluids, such as mouth rinse, GCF, PISF, and saliva, have been used as specimens [3, 6, 7]. Mouth-rinse samples can be collected quickly, noninvasively, and the collection process is less time-consuming as compared to a collection of GCF and PISF. Mouth-rinse assay is useful for screening purposes mainly, but it does not provide exact information or identification/localization about the sites of clinically active disease. Whole saliva, variation in the salivary flow rate, use of antimicrobial medication, and smoking habits may have an impact on the results. GCF and PISF provide site-specific information, therefore useful in the personalized treatment plan of an individual [53]. Johnson et al. reported that when measured with lateral flow immunoassay, saliva showed 4.1 times higher concentration of MMP-8 in periodontal patients than periodontal healthy controls [15].

Correlation between aMMP-8 levels in serum and oral fluids have been tested in few studies [34, 41, 56, 71]. Noack et al. reported a significant correlation between aMMP-8 concentration in the serum and severity of periodontal disease. In addition, serum MMP-8 concentration was also found to show a positive correlation with a subgingival bacterial load [71]. Differing from findings of Noack et al. [71], others on serum concentration of MMP-8 failed to find any correlation with periodontal disease [34, 41]. These varying associations can also be affected by differences in the use of clinical indices utilized to assess periodontal health and disease as well as systemic assessments of patients and healthy controls. Additionally, various mediations may affect systemic and serum aMMP-8. [34, 41, 56, 71] Only one study reported that fibroblasts were used as a study specimen to evaluate its role in the pathophysiology of peri-implantitis. [34] When proinflammatory and matrix degrading responses of gingival and granulation tissue fibroblasts to an *in vitro* challenge to *Porphyromonas gingivalis* (*P. gingivalis*) were compared between subjects with healthy periodontium and patients with periodontitis and peri-implantitis lesion, MMP-8 expression was found higher in nonchallenged peri-implantitis fibroblasts than in fibroblasts from healthy periodontium. This indicates that the inflammatory response was more pronounced in fibroblasts from periodontitis and peri-implantitis than in fibroblasts from periodontally healthy individuals. These findings suggest that the exposure of prolonged inflammation, i.e., periodontal/peri-implant disease experience and burden, can affect and promote cells' ability to express MMP-8 [34].

Passoja et al. did not find any correlation between periodontal disease and serum MMP-8 levels [34]. A study performed by Özçaka et al. showed that the levels of MMP-8 in the serum of patients with chronic periodontitis did not significantly differ from periodontal healthy subjects [41]. Kinney et al. showed that serum levels of biomarkers did not play any significant role in the diagnosis of periodontitis [56].

3.6. Immunoassays Used to Detect aMMP-8 (IFMA, DentoAnalyzer, DentoELISA, ELISA as Neutrophil Collagenase-2 Immunoassays).

MMP-8 detected by the IFMA technique correlates more strongly with the periodontal and peri-implant status, and better diagnostic accuracy is found higher than that of ELISA [58, 59]. A possible reason is that ELISA mostly detects all forms of MMP-8 (total/latent MMP-8), whereas IFMA selectively identifies activated neutrophil and fibroblast-type isoforms of MMP-8, then particularly in the active form (aMMP-8) [6]. A study done by Leppilahti et al. shows that results of IFMA were comparable with DentoELISA but not with commercial Amersham ELISA; IFMA and DentoELISA utilize the same aMMP-8 antibody [6–8, 18, 24, 28, 42, 64, 70, 82] Total MMP-8 levels measured by the Amersham ELISA test did not correlate with values of periodontal parameters [6–8, 42, 83].

Baeza et al. reported aMMP-8, measured by IFMA, to be less accurate in differentiating periodontitis from healthy sites. Differing from the other studies, the performance of DentoELISA was comparable to IFMA [69]. In chronic periodontitis patients, a positive correlation was observed between PPD and aMMP-8, measured by IFMA. CAL showed a positive correlation with aMMP-8, measured by IFMA and DentoELISA.[69]. Lateral-flow chair-side/PoC-PerioSafe® and ImplantSafe® immunotests (Figure 1), with and without the quantitative reader ORALyzer®, utilized the same aMMP-8 antibody as IFMA and DentoELISA, and they all correlate well with each other [13, 17, 61, 65, 78, 84, 85].

3.7. aMMP-8 Level in Oral Fluids of Smokers.

According to Mäntylä et al., the mean aMMP-8 levels in smokers were found to be lower compared to non-smokers, but sites with the progressive disease show similar or higher levels of aMMP-8 in both smokers and nonsmokers [28]. Heikkinen

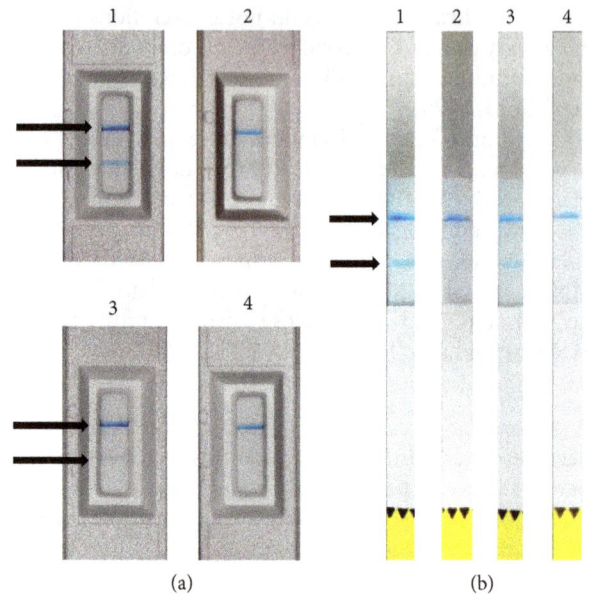

FIGURE 1: Periodontitis (a) results based on PerioSafe®-mouthrinse test: two chronic periodontitis patients (1) and (3) before and (2) and (4) after nonsurgical periodontal treatment, scaling, and root planning (SRP). The appearance of two lines (>20 ng/ml) pointed by arrows in the figure is a considered positive test which indicates elevated risk for periodontitis. The appearance of only one line indicates successful test performance and no risk for periodontitis (aMMP-8 < 20 ng/ml) after SRP treatment. Peri-implantitis (b) results based on ImplantSafe®-PISF-strip-test; two peri-implantitis patients (1) and (3) before and (2) and (4) after peri-implantitis treatment (plastic scaling, oral hygiene instructions, and use of chlorhexidine). Two lines in the result window indicate elevated aMMP-8 in PISF and increased risk for peri-implantitis. The appearance of a single line indicates successful test performance, low aMMP-8 in PISF, and no risk for peri-implantitis after treatment [78, 84].

et al. found similar results when comparing levels of aMMP-8 levels between smokers and nonsmokers, but the difference found was not statistically significant. Levels of aMMP-8 reduced after SRP but sites with exceptionally elevated aMMP-8 concentrations clustered in smokers did not show a significant decrease in aMMP-8 after SRP. These sites with a poor response may indicate sites at elevated risk and were easily identified by the chair-side/PoC aMMP-8 test. [28, 38] Baseline GCF aMMP-8 levels have been shown to predict aMMP-8 levels during maintenance of periodontitis. Particularly in smokers, high levels of aMMP-8 at the baseline indicated a poor response to periodontal treatment [60].

According to Heikkinen et al., smoking affects the biomarker values in a dose-dependent manner. Former smokers were found to have a similar level of aMMP-8 as compared to nonsmokers. Furthermore, obesity was found to be a confounder. Values of aMMP-8 among nonsmokers did not remain statistically significant when body mass index values were taken into account during analysis. However, the values were not affected in case of male smokers [38].

In contrast to these studies, Passoja et al. and Miller et al. did not find any significant correlation of smoking with an elevated aMMP-8 level in their independent studies done on saliva and GCF, respectively [29, 34]. Results of a study by Gursoy et al. showed that aMMP-8 was higher in non-smoking periodontitis patients than controls, and in smokers', only statistically significant parameter was TIMP-1 level that could differentiate between periodontitis patients and control. The ratio of aMMP-8, measured by the IFMA method, and TIMP-1 could successfully differentiate between periodontitis and healthy smoking subjects as well. A possible explanation for this finding, according to the authors, is that MMP-8 is less effective in mediating tissue degradation in the smoker subjects. It also indicates that smoking eventually can affect the detection of the potential biomarkers of periodontal disease [37].

3.8. MMP-8 Levels before and after Nonsurgical Therapy.
Gonçalves et al. demonstrated that SRP and use of systemic antibiotics effectively reduced local levels of specific MMPs in case of localized aggressive periodontitis. [54] Leppilahti et al. showed in their study that in patients who underwent azithromycin antibiotic treatment, the MMP-8 levels in GCF specifically are more stable and remain lower than a pre-defined cutoff level [63].

A study done by Konopka et al. showed that SRP improves all examined clinical periodontal parameters, apart from CAL. However, the GCF levels of MMP-8 after therapy in the periodontitis patient was still found to be higher than a control group [47]. In contrast to this finding, Gonçalves et al., found that level of MMP-8 in GCF was comparable to healthy sites. Most marked reduction in MMP-8 levels was noticed in a short period, i.e., 3–6 months after receiving treatment [54].

Nonsurgical therapy with and without antibiotics can reduce the level of active and total collagenase/MMP-8 [11] At the beginning of the treatment, the total collagenase activity was found similar to that of active collagenase demonstrating that most of the collagenase present at this stage was in an active form [11]. However, Konopka et al. could not find any correlation between clinical parameters and amount of humoral factors after the therapy, while they showed a correlation at the baseline with PPD and a proximal plaque index (PI) [47]. Baseline GCF MMP-8 levels strongly predict the change in level during a maintenance period [59, 63]. Elevated baseline levels of GCF MMP-8 in smokers indicate a weak response to therapy [59, 60, 63].

3.9. Host Response Modulation.
This term is recently introduced in dentistry and means modifying destructive aspects of inflammatory host response that develops in periodontal and peri-implant tissues as a result of inflammatory outcome to chronic subgingival bacterial plaque. The purpose of this therapy was to restore a balance between proinflammatory mediators and anti-inflammatory mediators. Host modulation by low-dose-doxycycline/sub-antimicrobial-dose-doxycycline (L/SDD) medication also efficiently inhibits and reduces gingival tissue and oral fluid aMMP-8 and at the same time ceases the progression of periodontal/peri-implant tissue destruction (APD) [3, 7, 66]. Only L/SDD has been licensed and accepted by FDA as a host response modulator and MMP-

inhibitory drug in humans for the treatment of periodontal disease until now [66]. In L/SDD, doxycycline 20 mg is given orally twice a day or 40 mg once a day to produce serum levels of doxycycline, which is too low to produce any antimicrobial effects but enough effective to inhibit/downregulate aMMP-8 [7]. In contrast to traditional dose (100 mg, once, or twice daily), L/SDD does not cause any bacterial resistance to doxycycline and does not alter normal flora, a composition of bacterial biofilm and their susceptibility to doxycycline and other antibiotics, even after long-term (up to 24 months) daily administration [66]. Furthermore, L/SDD causes a significant reduction in the levels of inflammatory mediators, mediators of collagenolysis (= aMMP-8), collagen degradation products, proinflammatory cytokines, and periodontal connective tissue destruction. [32] It has been shown to inhibit alveolar bone loss during periodontitis due to its ability to reduce gingival oxidative stress and aMMP-8 [32].

Evidence suggests that L/SDD has a strong potential for modulation of host response in beneficially aiding disease management when used as an adjunct medication to conventional mechanical therapy, SRP [27]. L/SDD reduces postsurgical BOP, PPD, and periodontal bone resorption [66]. L/SDD has been shown to support periodontal treatment like SRP as well as reduce the related systemic low-grade inflammation [31].

Emingil et al. concluded in their study that use of L/SDD together with SRP in the chronic periodontitis patient showed better clinical results/treatment outcomes as compared to SRP alone. A significant decrease in gingival inflammation scores at 3 months, and PPD reduction at 9 months was observed in the L/SDD group compared to a placebo group and was maintained until the end of 12 months [25]. In a study, L/SDD caused 36% reduction of bone height loss, when added to periodontal maintenance [36]. Sorsa et al. concluded that L/SDD, when coupled with SRP, could inhibit the activity or decrease expression of host MMPs, especially aMMP-8, by a mechanism that is unrelated to its antimicrobial property [3, 6, 7].

3.10. Effect of Metal Restorations.
According to a study done by Khuslinski et al. on practically healthy subjects with intact periodontium and patients with chronic generalized periodontitis with various structural materials of dental restorations [46], the level of MMP-8 surpassed the normal only in oral fluids of patients with chronic generalized periodontitis with metal restorations. In patients with chronic generalized periodontitis with or without metal dental restorations, obtained correlation coefficients indicate triggered biochemical cascade accompanied by the activation of cytokine production in response to etiological factors. The group of patients with periodontitis and metal restorations demonstrated a reaction that is more marked.

3.11. Association of Periodontal Microorganism with MMP-8.
The presence of subgingival microorganisms, mainly Treponema denticola (T. denticola), seemed to increase the levels of salivary albumin, the total protein contain in saliva, and levels of MMP-8 in GCF. There is a possibility that both T.

denticola and *Tannerella forsythia* (*T. forsythia*) have induced a cascade-type host response with increased release and activation of MMP-8 in GCF [35, 50, 86]. *T. denticola* and *P. gingivalis*-derived proteases (dentosilin and gingipain, respectively) can proteolytically and efficiently activate and convert latent pro-MMP-8 to aMMP-8 [45, 86, 88].

3.12. MMP-8 and Genetic Background. According to Heikkinen et al., genetic polymorphism of MMP-3 and vitamin D receptor found to be linked to initial periodontitis in Finnish adolescents, and aMMP-8 PoC/chair-side immunoassay PerioSafe® mouth-rinse test can be used for on-line PoC detection of initial periodontitis or preperiodontitis in adolescent patients with such type of genetic predisposition. This indicates the preventive potential of the PerioSafe® ORALyzer®-aMMP-8 chair-side/PoC test [70]. Thus, aMMP-8 mouth-rinse chair-side/PoC test positivity and 3 or more >4 mm pockets associated with the vitamin-D receptor and MMP-3 single-nucleotide polymorphisms. No association was found between single nucleotide polymorphism studied with the positivity of aMMP-8 [70].

3.13. MMP-8 in Dental Peri-implantitis. An inflammatory reaction associated with loss of supporting bone beyond initial biological bone remodeling around a dental implant, called peri-implantitis, is commonly reported as one of the significant contributors to dental implant failure [88–91]. The etiopathogenesis in case of peri-implantitis shows considerable similarity to periodontitis and shows comparable bacterial colonization and exudate of immune cells [88]. Similar to the periodontitis, aMMP-8 levels were repeatedly found to be pathologically elevated in diseased PISF as well [21–23, 30, 35, 45, 68, 82]. Both PMN- and non-PMN-type MMP-8 isoforms particularly in active forms have been observed in PISF of peri-implantitis patients [21–23, 30, 82]. However, Wang et al. reported that MMP-8 alone was not able to differentiate peri-implantitis patients from healthy patients [67]. *T. denticola* and *Prevotella intermedia* were reported to show diagnostic ability in case of peri-implantitis [67, 72, 73]. Gingival inflammation showed correlation to aMMP-8 levels in PISF [22, 23]. Ma et al. found that aMMP-8 in PISF, assessed by IFMA, associated with enhanced bone loss indicating that aMMP-8 participated in peri-implant bone loss and osteolysis [21]. Ritzer et al. [49] demonstrated by the 24/7-chewing-gum MMP-8 assay that elevated levels of MMP-8 could be detected in peri-implantitis oral fluids confirming and further extending the findings of Teronon et al., Kivelä-Rajamäki et al., Xu et al., and Kivelä-Rajamäki et al. [21–23, 30, 82].

Ramseier et al. reported a positive correlation between MMP-8, PI, and BOP in both GCF and PISF [65]. Ziebolz et al. have demonstrated that PISF aMMP-8 levels can be kept successfully low during maintenance in patients undergoing successfully supportive implant therapy indicating that successful professional maintenance intervention is associated with low (<20 ng/ml) PISF aMMP-8 levels similar to the healthy peri-implant status [73, 78, 79]. Similar clinical parameters and MMP-8 levels were obtained with both zirconium and titanium abutments at the end of 1 year. However, initially, titanium abutment was reported to show higher PISF MMP-8 levels and probing depth [72].

Thus, elevated levels of aMMP-8 in PISF associate significantly and repeatedly with peri-implant inflammation and bone loss/osteolysis [21–23, 30, 78]. Low (<20 ng/ml) in aMMP-8 levels in PISF reflects and indicates healthy and/or successfully treated status peri-implantium (Figure 1) [73, 78, 79]. Pathologically elevated levels of aMMP-8 (>20 ng/ml) can be conveniently detected by a quantitative lateral flow aMMP-8 dip-stick test, i.e., ImplantSafe® (Figure 1) [17, 78].

3.14. Combining Other Biomarkers to Increase Diagnostic Accuracy. Simultaneous measurement of more than one oral fluid marker may allow more accurate prediction of periodontal inflammatory burden [53]. Combinations of the MMP-8 biomarker and pathogens that correspond with it (such as *T. denticola*) may give a more accurate prediction of periodontitis as compared to a single biomarker alone [35].

Gursoy et al. concluded in their study that proportional or combined use of oral salivary biomarkers increases diagnostic accuracy, particularly in smoker subjects [37]. It was found that the MMP-8/TIMP molar ratio and the combination of two biomarkers, MMP-8 and pyridinoline cross-linked carboxyterminal telopeptide of type I collagen (ICTP), were significantly higher in detecting periodontitis compared to MMP-8 test alone [37]. A study testing accuracy of the cumulative risk score calculated (CRS) from three salivary biomarkers (i.e., *P. gingivalis*, IL-1β, and MMP-8) was more accurate in the diagnosis of advanced periodontitis than any of the markers alone [40]. Leppilahti et al. suggested measurement of MMP-8 and TIMP-1 to obtain higher diagnostic accuracy [42]. A study performed by Rathnayake et al. proposed use of MMP-8/TIMP-1 molar ratio as markers of periodontal disease in a larger patient population [52]. Salminen et al. proposed combination of three biomarkers, i.e., MMP-8, IL-1β, and *P. gingivalis* (CRS) for diagnosis of periodontitis [54] The median concentration of these three was significantly higher in the moderate to severe periodontitis group as compared to controls. In addition, Ebersole et al. reported also that salivary levels of IL-1β, IL-6, and MMP-8 provide high diagnostic accuracy for periodontitis with high sensitivity and specificity [55]. Furthermore, MMP-8 levels were higher in patients diagnosed with chronic periodontitis and diabetic, but *P. gingivalis* did not affect much. Unlike MMP-8, *P. gingivalis* values remain unaffected in edentulous subjects. *P. gingivalis* successfully differentiated current smokers from former smokers and however, did not show correlation with BOP [54].

Therefore, using biomarkers and various pathogens in combination may improve accuracy in diagnosis; however, the complexity and costs to perform such tests routinely will increase considerably. Therefore, simpler, inexpensive, and readily available tests that have been shown to be sufficient alone to detect and quantify aMMP-8, such as PerioSafe® and ImplantSafe®/ORALyzer®, might be more desirable (Figure 1) [78].

3.15. PoC Tests. Chair-side and point-of-care (PoC) lateral flow immunotests for the detection of aMMP-8 in oral fluids are commercially available (i.e., PerioSafe® and ImplantSafe®) with the detection limit of 20 ng/ml (Figure 1). The tests resemble the pregnancy home test (Figure 1). The quantitative reader-equipped ORALyzer® PoC test of oral fluids that measure aMMP-8 is found useful in differentiating active and inactive periodontal and peri-implant sites and patients, predicting disease progression in future, and monitoring the responses to therapy during the maintenance phase [17, 78]. The benefits of using these aMMP-8 tests are that these can be used in clinical settings, are easy to use, are inexpensive, and give prompt quick results with high sensitivity and specificity (i.e., the sensitivity of 90% and specificity of 70–85%) [6, 7, 16, 17, 24, 28, 42, 44, 51, 62, 64, 70, 78].

Alassiri et al. demonstrated that quantitative, PerioSafe® and ImplantSafe® ORALyzer®, PoC/chair-side assays could conveniently diagnose and follow the treatment of periodontitis and peri-implantitis [17, 78]. Thus, these tests can detect subclinical, developing periodontitis and peri-implantitis and related collage degradation even before the appearance of clinical and radiographical signs [14, 16, 17, 73, 82]. These test alarm preperiodontitis and pre-peri-implantitis and identity preventively future periodontal and peri-implantitis breakdown. They thus make invisible destruction or onset of periodontal/peri-implant collagenolysis to be visible and detectable in an enough early and predictive manner allowing the identification and timing of the preventive interactions/treatment such as secondary prevention and/or supportive periodontal/peri-implant treatment [17, 61, 65, 73, 84, 85].

PerioSafe® and ImplantSafe® with digital readers are modern *in vitro* fast immunological diagnostic and prevention professional technologies/tests for examination of the oral/periodontal/peri-implant status of teeth and dental implants at different time intervals (at least once annually) to detect risk of silent or hidden periodontal, peri-implant tissue degeneration and alveolar bone loss even before they can be detected clinically or radiographically [16, 17]. The PoC tests also help in time preventive treatment which is necessary for long-term success of implants, periodontal tissues, and patients. Another aspect of it is that this is also healthy and economical for the patients and society.

Regarding the chair-side/PoC-aMMP-8 lateral flow immune tests (Figure 1), the appearance of only one line indicates the negative result that reveals normal condition/a healthy status (<20 ng aMMP-8 per ml), and appearance of two lines indicates increased risk (>20 ng aMMP-8 per ml) (Figure 1) for periodontitis and/or peri-implantitis, either already existing or developing periodontitis and peri-implantitis, identified by PerioSafe and ImplantSafe, respectively (Figure 1). These PoC tests can be used with the reader for quantitative analysis [17, 78].

For quantitative analysis, dip-stick tests should be placed in the corresponding compartment of the reader. Then, flap is closed, the compartment is pushed into ORALyzer®, and check mark is pressed. The ORALyzer® is designed in such a way that it automatically starts and measures the aMMP-8 levels after 5 min. Thus, the qualitative "eye"-estimated plus/minus test results are quantitatively expressed in ng/ml aMMP-8 PoC/chairside [17, 78].

4. Summary

The current review analyzed the potential of aMMP-8 as a potential diagnostic, predictive, and preventive adjunctive biomarker/biotechnological tool for periodontal and peri-implant diseases. The available evidence suggests that especially aMMP-8 in oral fluids reflect, associate, and predict well with the clinical periodontal parameters and outcomes as well as clinical disease activity of periodontitis and peri-implantitis together with evaluation of treatment outcomes [18, 44, 47, 54]. Only few studies failed to find the correlation between clinical CAL [47], and few others reported that MMP-8 levels are not correlated with BOP [62]. In addition, aMMP-8 levels were reported to be associated with radiological parameters too [53]. Importantly when evaluating these studies, it should be kept in mind that active/activated MMP-8, not MMP-8 or total latent MMP-8, is a biomarker of active and progressive periodontal and peri-implant disease [3, 4, 6–9, 11, 17, 76, 77, 80, 81].

Thus, pathologically and repeatedly elevated of aMMP-8 levels in saliva show the highest sensitivity and in GCF/PISF, the highest specificity [56]. aMMP-8 levels of mouth rinse and oral saliva can be useful for screening, whereas GCF/PISF levels could predict at site-specific level treatment outcomes and may be a useful adjunct in an individual/personalized treatment and monitoring plans. Thus, the aMMP-8 tests represent tools for personalized medicine [56]. aMMP-8 levels reduce after nonsurgical therapy, such as SRP. Most of the studies confirmed the effect of smoking on MMP-8 level, except few [29, 34]. Combination of other biomarkers (TIMP-1, IL-6, and IL-1β) and periodontal pathogens (such as *T. denticola* and *P. gingivalis*) with aMMP-8 in the detection of periodontal inflammation may increase accuracy, but aMMP-8 alone functions quantitatively very well [6, 7, 16, 17, 78]. Both IFMA and DentoELISA were found to be able to differentiate periodontitis from healthy subjects, but in general, IFMA was more accurate [6, 7, 16, 17]. Results obtained from Amersham ELISA were not in line with IFMA and DentoELISA. Lateral flow chair-side/PoC aMMP-8 immunoassay correlated well with clinical parameters of periodontitis but with at least two sites and extended better accuracy than BOP [18, 78]. Notably, invasive aMMP-8 PoC-tests cause always bacteremia, but noninvasive aMMP-8 PoC-tests never [78].

Despite their high sensitivity and specificity, aMMP-8 PoC-assays should be mainly used as adjunct tools to the clinical examination; mouth-rinse/salivary assays are useful for screening and dip-stick for site-specific personlized medical approaches. High levels of oral fluid MMP-8 in subjects with clinically "appearing" healthy periodontium/peri-implantium indicate silent "hidden," developing future preperiodontitis and pre-peri-implantitis indicating early preventive supportive periodontal and peri-implant treatment [16]. In the case, oral fluid aMMP-8 is not treated to be <20 ng/ml, and these preperiodontitis and pre-peri-implantitis phases will often develop to be periodontitis and peri-implantitis with on-going collagenolytic APD.

Elevated oral fluid aMMP-8 thus predicts, reflects, and precedes future APD, i.e., CAL of the teeth and dental implants [3, 7, 17, 76]. Thus, aMMP-8 PoC/chair-side tests make invisible hidden inflammation visible [17, 78].

Our literature review results are in line with previous studies. A review done by Sorsa et al. concluded that MMP-8 is a promising candidate for diagnosis and determination of progressive periodontitis and peri-implantitis and monitoring response to therapy and further extend them also to peri-implantitis and provides diagnostic tests to monitor follow treatment and adjunctive medication such as L/SDD [7].

A systematic review and a recent study were done by de Morais et al. and Alassiri et al. and they concluded the same and recommended use of MMP-8 as a quantitative biomarker of periodontal and peri-implant diseases adjunctive to clinical examination [17, 78, 92].

4.1. Clinical Implications. Repeatedly pathologically elevated levels of aMMP-8, but not total/latent MMP-8, in oral fluids (mouth rinse, saliva, GCF, and PISF) show the positive correlation with the clinical and radiological parameters of periodontitis and peri-implantitis. Oral fluid aMMP-8 levels reduce after periodontal therapy, i.e., SRP combined with host modulation and/or antimicrobial medication [7, 93]. Continuously and sustainably pathologically elevated oral fluid MMP-8 levels indicate and predict sites and patients with compromised disease outcomes regarding course, treatment, and maintenance. Importantly, the oral fluid PoC/chair-side tests can be utilized to predict time preventive interventions before the development of irreversible tissue destruction (APD) in periodontium and peri-implantium by indentifying and alarming the preperiodontitis and pre-peri-implantitis [17, 70].

4.2. Limitations of the Study

(1) Only the articles written in English language were selected.

(2) A literature search was performed in two databases, and additional articles have been chosen by manual searching, but it is possible that some relevant data are left behind.

4.3. Recommendations for Future Research. Further studies, especially longitudinal and perspective ones, should be conducted to explore the relationship between aMMP-8 with other biomarkers. Some factors such as obesity and gender reported as confounding factors should also be addressed more in detail. The relationship between serum concentration of aMMP-8 and periodontitis and peri-implantitis is still not clear and needs further investigations.

Abbreviations

PI:	Plaque index
PPD:	Probing pocket depth
BOP:	Bleeding on probing
CAL:	Clinical attachment loss
SRP:	Scaling and root planning
PISF:	Peri-Implant sulcus fluid
PICF:	Peri-implant crevicular fluid
MMP:	Matrix metalloproteinase
MMP-8, etc.:	Matrix metalloproteinase-8
aMMP-8:	Active form of matrix metalloproteinase-8
AAP:	Asymptomatic apical periodontitis
(IL) IL-6, 8, etc.:	Interleukins
(IL)-1β:	Interleukin-1 beta
OPG:	Osteoprotegerin
Dkk-1:	Dickkopf-related protein 1
PTN:	Periostin
TRAP-5:	Tartrate-resistant acid phosphatase-5
ON:	Osteonectin
TNF-α:	Tumor necrosis factor-alpha
IFN-γ:	Interferon gamma
TRACP-5b:	Tartrate-resistant acid phosphatase serum type-5b
CTx:	C-terminal cross-linked telopeptide of type I collagen
NTx:	N-terminal cross-linked telopeptide of type I collagen
PMN:	Polymorphonuclear leukocyte
P. gingivalis:	*Porphyromonas gingivalis*
A. actinomycetemcomitans:	*Aggregatibacter actinomycetemcomitans* (previously *Actinobacillus actinomycetemcomitans*)
C. rectus:	*Campylobacter rectus*
F. nucleatum:	*Fusobacterium nucleatum*
P. intermedia:	*Prevotella intermedia*
T. forsythia:	*Tannerella forsythia* (previously *Tannerella forsythensis*)
T. denticola:	*Treponema denticola*
PCR:	polymerase chain reaction
GCF:	Gingival crevicular fluid
IFMA:	Immunofluorometric assay
ELISA:	Enzyme-linked immunosorbent assay
TIMP-1:	Tissue inhibitor of matrix metalloproteinase
ICTP:	Pyridinoline cross-linked carboxy-terminal telopeptide of type I collagen
AgP:	Aggressive periodontitis
CRS:	Cumulative risk score
MIP-1α:	Macrophage inflammatory protein
PGE2:	Prostaglandin E2
PI:	Peri-implantitis
CP:	Chronic periodontitis
G:	Gingivitis
GAgP:	

	Generalized aggressive periodontitis
PoC:	Point-of-care
POCID:	Point-of-care immunoflow device
APD periodontal:	Peri-implant degeneration
L/SDD:	Low-dose doxycycline/sub-antimicrobial-dose doxycycline
AUC:	Area under the curve
CRS:	Cumulative risk score.

Disclosure

Periodontal diagnoses and classification of periodontal disease have been performed during the international workshop for classification of periodontal diseases and conditions from October 30 to November 2, 1999 (Periodontol 1999) (type I: gingivitis, type II: chronic periodontitis, and type III: aggressive periodontitis) [85].

Acknowledgments

Prof. Dr. Timo Sorsa has been supported by grants from the Helsinki University Hospital Research Foundation (TYH 2016251, TYH 2017251, TYH2018229, Y101I4SLO17, and Y1014SLOI8), Helsinki, Finland, and Karolinska Institutet, Stockholm, Sweden.

References

[1] D. F. Kinane, "Regulators of tissue destruction and homeostasis as diagnostic aids in periodontology," *Periodontology 2000*, vol. 24, no. 1, pp. 215–225, 2000.

[2] H. Nagase, R. Visse, and G. Murphy, "Structure and function of matrix metalloproteinases and TIMPs," *Cardiovascular Research*, vol. 69, no. 3, pp. 562–573, 2006.

[3] T. Sorsa, L. Tjaderhane, Y. T. Konttinen et al., "Matrix metalloproteinases: contribution to pathogenesis, diagnosis and treatment of periodontal inflammation," *Annals of Medicine*, vol. 38, no. 5, pp. 306–321, 2006.

[4] T. Sorsa, L. Tjaderhane, and T. Salo, "Matrix metalloproteinases (MMPs) in oral diseases," *Oral Diseases*, vol. 10, no. 6, pp. 311–318, 2004.

[5] L. Bernasconi, L. L. Ramenzoni, A. Al-Majid et al., "Elevated matrix metalloproteinase levels in bronchi infected with periodontopathogenic bacteria," *PLoS One*, vol. 10, no. 12, Article ID e0144461, 2015.

[6] T. Sorsa, M. Hernández, J. Leppilahti, S. Munjal, L. Netuschil, and P. Mäntylä, "Detection of gingival crevicular fluid MMP-8 levels with different laboratory and chair-side methods," *Oral Diseases*, vol. 16, no. 1, pp. 39–45, 2010.

[7] T. Sorsa, K. Ulvi, S. Nwhator et al., "Analysis of matrix metalloproteinases, especially MMP-8, in GCF, mouthrinse and saliva for monitoring periodontal diseases," *Periodontology 2000*, vol. 70, no. 1, pp. 142–163, 2016.

[8] T. Sorsa, P. Mäntylä, T. Tervahartiala, P. J. Pussinen, J. Gamonal, and M. Hernandez, "MMP activation in diagnostics of periodontitis and systemic inflammation," *Journal of Clinical Periodontology*, vol. 38, no. 9, pp. 817–819, 2011.

[9] T. Sorsa, V. J. Uitto, K. Suomalainen, M. Vauhkonen, and S. Lindy, "Comparison of interstitial collagenases from human gingiva, sulcular fluid and polymorphonuclear leukocytes," *Journal of Periodontal Research*, vol. 23, no. 6, pp. 386–393, 1988.

[10] S. W. Cox, B. M. Eley, M. Kiili, A. Asikainen, T. Tervahartiala, and T. Sorsa, "Collagen degradation by interleukin-1beta-stimulated gingival fibroblasts is accompanied by release and activation of multiple matrix metalloproteinases and cysteine proteinases," *Oral Diseases*, vol. 12, no. 1, pp. 34–40, 2006.

[11] S. Gangbar, C. M. Overall, C. A. G. McCulloch, and J. Sodek, "Identification of polymorphonuclear leukocyte collagenase and gelatinase activities in mouthrinse samples: correlation with periodontal disease activity in adult and juvenile periodontitis," *Journal of Periodontal Research*, vol. 25, no. 5, pp. 257–267, 1990.

[12] M. Mauramo, A. M. Ramseier, E. Mauramo et al., "Association of oral fluid MMP-8 with periodontitis in swiss adult subjects," *Oral Diseases*, vol. 24, no. 3, pp. 449–455, 2017.

[13] M. Hernàndez, J. Gamonal, T. Tervahartiala et al., "Associations between matrix metalloproteinase-8 and 14 and myeloperoxidase in gingival crevicular fluid from subjects with progressive chronic periodontitis: a longitudinal study," *Journal of Periodontology*, vol. 81, no. 11, pp. 1644–1652, 2010.

[14] R. Thierbach, K. Maier, T. Sorsa, and P. Mäntylä, "Peri-implant sulcus fluid (PISF) matrix metalloproteinase (MMP)-8 levels in peri-implantitis," *Journal of Clinical and Diagnostic Research*, vol. 10, no. 5, pp. ZC34–ZC38, 2016.

[15] N. Johnson, J. L. Ebersole, R. J. Kryscio et al., "Rapid assessment of oral salivary MMP-8 and periodontal disease using lateral flow immunoassay," *Oral Diseases*, vol. 22, no. 7, pp. 681–687, 2016.

[16] D. F. Kinane, P. G. Stathopoulou, and P. N. Papapanou, "Authors' reply: predictive diagnostic tests in periodontal diseases," *Nature Reviews Disease Primers*, vol. 3, article 17070, 2017.

[17] T. Sorsa, D. Gieselmann, N. B. Arweiler, and M. A. Hernández, "A quantitative point of care test for periodontal and dental peri implant diseases," *Nature Reviews Disease Primers*, vol. 3, article 17038, 2017.

[18] S. O. Nwhator, P. O. Ayanbadejo, K. A. Umeizudike et al., "Clinical correlates of a lateral-flow immunoassay oral risk indicator," *Journal of Periodontology*, vol. 85, no. 1, pp. 188–194, 2014.

[19] M. Yakob, K. Kari, T. Tervahartiala et al., "Associations of periodontal microorganisms with oral salivary proteins and MMP-8 in gingival crevicular fluid," *Journal of Clinical Periodontology*, vol. 39, no. 3, pp. 256–263, 2012.

[20] P. Van Lint and C. Libert, "Matrix metalloproteinase-8: cleavage can be decisive," *Cytokine & Growth Factor Reviews*, vol. 17, no. 4, pp. 217–223, 2006.

[21] J. Ma, U. Kitti, O. Teronen et al., "Collagenases in different categories of peri-implant vertical bone loss," *Journal of Dental Research*, vol. 79, no. 11, pp. 1870–1873, 2000.

[22] M. J. Kivelä-Rajamäki, P. Maisi, R. Srinivas et al., "Levels and molecular forms of MMP-7 (matrilysin-1) and MMP-8 (collagenase-2) in diseased human peri-implant sulcular

fluid," *Journal of Periodontal Research*, vol. 38, no. 6, pp. 583–590, 2003.

[23] M. J. Kivelä-Rajamäki, O. P. Teronen, P. Maisi et al., "Laminin-5 gamma2-chain and collagenase-2 (MMP-8) in human peri-implant sulcular fluid," *Clinical Oral Implants Research*, vol. 14, no. 2, pp. 158–165, 2003.

[24] P. Mäntylä, M. Stenman, D. F. Kinane et al., "Gingival crevicular fluid collagenase-2 (MMP8) test stick for chair-side monitoring of periodontitis," *Journal of Periodontal Research*, vol. 38, no. 4, pp. 436–439, 2003.

[25] G. Emingil, G. Atilla, T. Sorsa, H. Luoto, L. Kirilmaz, and H. Baylas, "The effect of adjunctive low dose doxycycline therapy on clinical parameters and GCF MMP-8 levels in chronic periodontitis," *Journal of Periodontology*, vol. 75, no. 1, pp. 106–115, 2004.

[26] P. Pozo, M. A. Valenzuela, C. Melej et al., "Longitudinal analysis of metalloproteinases, tissue inhibitors of metalloproteinases and clinical parameters in GCF from periodontitis affected patients," *Journal of Periodontal Research*, vol. 40, no. 3, pp. 199–207, 2005.

[27] T. Sorsa and L. M. Golub, "Is the excessive inhibition of matrix metalloproteinases (MMPs) by potent synthetic MMP inhibitors (MMPIs) desirable in periodontitis and other inflammatory diseases? that is: 'Leaky' MMPIs vs excessively efficient drugs. Letter to editor," *Oral Diseases*, vol. 11, no. 6, pp. 408–409, 2005.

[28] P. Mäntylä, M. Stenman, D. F. Kinane et al., "Monitoring periodontal disease status in smokers and nonsmokers using a gingival crevicular fluid matrix metalloproteinase-8-specific chair-side test," *Journal of Periodontal Research*, vol. 41, no. 6, pp. 503–512, 2006.

[29] C. S. Miller, C. P. King Jr., M. C. Langub, R. J. Kryscio, and M. V. Thomas, "Oral salivary biomarkers of existing periodontal disease: a cross-sectional study," *Journal of the American Dental Association*, vol. 137, no. 3, pp. 322–329, 2006.

[30] L. Xu, Z. Yu, H. M. Lee et al., "Characteristics of collagenase-2 from gingival crevicular fluid and peri-implant sulcular fluid in periodontitis and peri-implantitis patients: pilot study," *Acta Odontologica Scandinavica*, vol. 66, no. 4, pp. 219–224, 2008.

[31] W. V. Giannobile, "Host-response therapeutics for periodontal diseases," *Journal of Periodontology*, vol. 79, no. 8s, pp. 1592–1600, 2008.

[32] P. M. Preshaw, "Host response modulation in periodontics," *Periodontol 2000*, vol. 48, no. 1, pp. 92–110, 2008.

[33] B. Alfant, L. M. Shaddox, J. Tobler, I. Magnusson, I. Aukhil, and C. Walker, "Matrix metalloproteinase levels in children with aggressive periodontitis," *Journal of Periodontology*, vol. 79, no. 5, pp. 819–826, 2008.

[34] A. Passoja, M. Ylipalosaari, T. Tervonen, T. Raunio, and M. Knuuttila, "Matrix metalloproteinase-8 concentration in shallow crevices associated with the extent of periodontal disease," *Journal of Clinical Periodontology*, vol. 35, no. 12, pp. 1027–1031, 2008.

[35] C. A. Ramseier, J. S. Kinney, A. E. Herr et al., "Identification of pathogen and host-response markers correlated with periodontal disease," *Journal of Periodontology*, vol. 80, no. 3, pp. 436–446, 2009.

[36] R. A. Reinhardt, J. A. Stoner, L. M. Golub et al., "Association of GCF biomarkers during periodontal maintenance with subsequent progressive periodontitis," *Journal of Periodontology*, vol. 81, no. 2, pp. 251–259, 2010.

[37] U. K. Gursoy, E. Könönen, P. Pradhan-Palikhe et al., "Oral salivary MMP-8, TIMP-1, and ICTP as markers of advanced periodontitis," *Journal of Clinical Periodontology*, vol. 37, no. 6, pp. 487–493, 2010.

[38] A. M. Heikkinen, T. Sorsa, J. Pitkaniemi et al., "Smoking affects diagnostic oral salivary periodontal disease biomarker levels in adolescents," *Journal of Periodontology*, vol. 81, no. 9, pp. 1299–1307, 2010.

[39] A. M. Marcaccini, C. A. Meschiari, L. R. Zuardi et al., "Gingival crevicular fluid levels of MMP-8, MMP-9, TIMP-2, and MPO decrease after periodontal therapy," *Journal of Clinical Periodontology*, vol. 37, no. 2, pp. 180–190, 2010.

[40] U. K. Gursoy, E. Kononen, P. J. Pussinen et al., "Use of host- and bacteria-derived salivary markers in detection of periodontitis: a cumulative approach," *Disease Markers*, vol. 30, no. 6, pp. 299–305, 2011.

[41] O. Özçaka, N. Biçakci, P. Pussinen, T. Sorsa, T. Köse, and N. Buduneli, "Smoking and matrix metalloproteinases, neutrophil elastase and myeloperoxidase in chronic periodontitis," *Oral Diseases*, vol. 17, no. 1, pp. 68–76, 2011.

[42] J. M. Leppilahti, M. M. Ahonen, M. Hernández et al., "Oral rinse MMP-8 point-of-care immuno test identifies patients with strong periodontal inflammatory burden," *Oral Diseases*, vol. 17, no. 1, pp. 115–122, 2011.

[43] W. M. Sexton, Y. Lin, R. J. Kryscio, D. R. Dawson, J. L. Ebersole, and C. S. Miller, "Salivary biomarkers of periodontal disease in response to treatment," *Journal of Clinical Periodontology*, vol. 38, no. 5, pp. 434–441, 2011.

[44] M. Kraft-Neumärker, K. Lorenz, R. Koch et al., "Full-mouth profile of active MMP-8 in periodontitis patients," *Journal of Periodontal Research*, vol. 47, no. 1, pp. 121–128, 2012.

[45] H. Arakawa, J. Uehara, E. S. Hara et al., "Matrix metalloproteinase-8 is the major potential collagenase in active peri-implantitis," *Journal of Prosthodontic Research*, vol. 56, no. 4, pp. 249–255, 2012.

[46] N. E. Kushlinskii, E. A. Solovykh, T. B. Karaoglanova et al., "Matrix metalloproteinases and inflammatory cytokines in oral fluid of patients with chronic generalized periodontitis and various construction materials," *Bulletin of Experimental Biology and Medicine*, vol. 153, no. 1, pp. 72–76, 2012.

[47] L. Konopka, A. Pietrzak, and E. Brzezińska-Błaszczyk, "Effect of scaling and root planing on interleukin-1β, interleukin-8 and MMP-8 levels in gingival crevicular fluid from chronic periodontitis patients," *Journal of Periodontal Research*, vol. 47, no. 6, pp. 681–688, 2012.

[48] O. H. Lowry, N. J. Rosebrough, A. L. Farr, and R. J. Randall, "Protein measurement with the Folin phenol reagent," *Journal of Biological Chemistry*, vol. 193, no. 1, pp. 265–275, 1951.

[49] J. Ritzer, T. Lühmann, C. Rode et al., "Diagnosing peri-implant disease using the tongue as a 24/7 detector," *Nature Communications*, vol. 8, no. 1, p. 264, 2017.

[50] M. Yakob, J. H. Meurman, T. Sorsa, and B. Söder, "Treponema denticola associates with increased levels of MMP-8 and MMP-9 in gingival crevicular fluid," *Oral Diseases*, vol. 19, no. 7, pp. 694–701, 2013.

[51] M. Irshad, N. Scheres, D. Anssari Moin et al., "Cytokine and matrix metalloproteinase expression in fibroblasts from peri-implantitis lesions in response to viable porphyromonas gingivalis," *Journal of Periodontal Research*, vol. 48, no. 5, pp. 647–656, 2013.

[52] N. Rathnayake, S. Akerman, B. Klinge et al., "Salivary biomarkers of oral health: a cross sectional study," *Journal of Clinical Periodontology*, vol. 40, no. 2, pp. 140–147, 2013.

[53] U. K. Gursoy, E. Könönen, S. Huumonen, T. Tervahartiala, P. J. Pussinen, and A. L. Suominen, "Salivary type I collagen degradation end-products and related matrix

metalloproteinases in periodontitis," *Journal of Clinical Periodontology*, vol. 40, no. 1, pp. 18–25, 2013.

[54] P. F. Gonçalves, H. Huang, S. McAninley et al., "Periodontal treatment reduces matrix metalloproteinase levels in localized aggressive periodontitis," *Journal of Periodontology*, vol. 84, no. 12, pp. 1801–1808, 2013.

[55] J. L. Ebersole, J. L. Schuster, J. Stevens et al., "Patterns of salivary analytes provide diagnostic capacity for distinguishing chronic adult periodontitis from health," *Journal of Clinical Immunology*, vol. 33, no. 1, pp. 271–279, 2013.

[56] J. S. Kinney, T. Morelli, M. Oh et al., "Crevicular fluid biomarkers and periodontal disease progression," *Journal of Periodontology*, vol. 41, no. 2, pp. 113–120, 2014.

[57] B. Syndergaard, M. Al-Sabbagh, R. J. Kryscio et al., "Oral salivary biomarkers associated with gingivitis and response to therapy," *Journal of Periodontology*, vol. 85, no. 8, pp. e295–e303, 2014.

[58] A. Salminen, U. K. Gursoy, S. Paju et al., "Oral salivary biomarkers of bacterial burden, inflammatory response, and tissue destruction in periodontitis," *Journal of Clinical Periodontology*, vol. 41, no. 5, pp. 442–450, 2014.

[59] J. M. Leppilahti, P. A. Hernández-Ríos, J. A. Gamonal et al., "Matrix metalloproteinases and myeloperoxidase in GCF provide site-specific diagnostic value for chronic periodontitis," *Journal of Clinical Periodontology*, vol. 41, no. 4, pp. 348–356, 2014.

[60] J. M. Leppilahti, A. M. Kallio, T. Tervahartiala, T. Sorsa, and P. Mäntylä, "Gingival crevicular fluid matrix metalloproteinase-8 levels predict treatment outcome among smokers with chronic periodontitis," *Journal of Periodontology*, vol. 85, no. 2, pp. 250–260, 2014.

[61] J. L. Ebersole, R. Nagarajan, D. Akers, and C. S. Miller, "Targeted salivary biomarkers for discrimination of periodontal health and disease(s)," *Frontiers in Cellular and Infection Microbiology*, vol. 5, p. 62, 2015.

[62] S. Izadi Borujeni, M. Mayer, and P. Eickholz, "Activated matrix metalloproteinase-8 in saliva as diagnostic test for periodontal disease? a case-control study," *Medical Microbiology and Immunology*, vol. 204, no. 6, pp. 665–672, 2015.

[63] J. M. Leppilahti, T. Sorsa, M. A. Kallio et al., "The utility of gingival crevicular fluid matrix metalloproteinase-8 response patterns in prediction of site-level clinical treatment outcome," *Journal of Periodontology*, vol. 86, no. 6, pp. 777–787, 2015.

[64] A. M. Heikkinen, S. O. Nwhator, N. Rathnayake, P. Mäntylä, P. Vatanen, and T. Sorsa, "Pilot study on oral health status as assessed by an active matrix metalloproteinase-8 chairside mouthrinse test in adolescents," *Journal of Periodontology*, vol. 87, no. 1, pp. 36–40, 2016.

[65] C. A. Ramseier, S. Eick, C. Brönnimann, D. Buser, U. Brägger, and G. E. Salvi, "Host-derived biomarkers at teeth and implants in partially edentulous patients. A 10-year retrospective study," *Clinical Oral Implants Research*, vol. 27, no. 2, pp. 211–217, 2016.

[66] L. M. Golub, M. S. Elburki, C. Walker et al., "Non-antibacterial tetracycline formulations: host-modulators in the treatment of periodontitis and relevant systemic diseases," *International Dental Journal*, vol. 66, no. 3, pp. 127–135, 2016.

[67] H. L. Wang, C. Garaicoa-Pazmino, A. Collins, H-S. Ong, R. Chudri, and W. V. Giannobile, "Protein biomarkers and microbial profiles in peri-implantitis," *Clinical Oral Implants Research*, vol. 27, no. 9, pp. 1129–1136, 2016.

[68] E. Janska, B. Mohr, and G. Wahl, "Correlation between peri-implant sulcular fluid rate and expression of collagenase2

(MMP8)," *Clinical Oral Investigations*, vol. 20, no. 2, pp. 261–266, 2016.

[69] M. Baeza, M. Garrido, P. Hernández-Ríos et al., "Diagnostic accuracy for apical and chronic periodontitis biomarkers in gingival crevicular fluid: an exploratory study," *Journal of Clinical Periodontology*, vol. 43, no. 1, pp. 34–45, 2016.

[70] A. M. Heikkinen, T. Raivisto, K. Kettunen et al., "Pilot study on the genetic background of an active matrix metalloproteinase-8 test in finnish adolescents," *Journal of Periodontology*, vol. 88, no. 5, pp. 464–472, 2017.

[71] B. Noack, T. Kipping, T. Tervahartiala, T. Sorsa, T. Hoffmann, and K. Lorenz, "Association between serum and oral matrix metalloproteinase-8 levels and periodontal health status," *Journal of Periodontal Research*, vol. 52, no. 5, pp. 1–8, 2017.

[72] Y. Kumar, V. Jain, S. Chauhan, V. Bharati, D. Koli, and M. Kumar, "Influence of different forms and materials (zirconia or titanium) of abutments in peri implant soft-tissue healing using matrix metalloproteinase-8: a randomized pilot study," *Journal of Prosthetic Dentistry*, vol. 118, no. 4, pp. 475–480, 2017.

[73] D. Ziebolz, G. Schmalz, D. Gollasch, P. Eickholz, and S. Rinke, "Microbiological and aMMP-8 findings depending on peri-implant disease in patients undergoing supportive implant therapy," *Diagnostic Microbiology and Infectious Disease*, vol. 88, no. 1, pp. 47–52, 2017.

[74] C. A. Owen, Z. Hu, C. Lopez-Otin, and S. D. Shapiro, "Membrane-bound matrix metalloproteinase-8 on activated polymorphonuclear cells is a potent, tissue inhibitor of metalloproteinase-resistant collagenase and serpinase," *Journal of Immunology*, vol. 172, no. 12, pp. 7791–7803, 2004.

[75] V. J. Uitto, K. Suomalainen, and T. Sorsa, "Oral salivary collagenase: origin, characteristics and relationship to periodontal health," *Journal of Periodontal Research*, vol. 25, no. 3, pp. 135–142, 1990.

[76] W. Lee, S. Aitken, J. Sodek, and C. A. McCulloch, "Evidence of a direct relationship between neutrophil collagenase activity and periodontal tissue destruction in vivo: role of active enzyme in human periodontitis," *Journal of Periodontal Research*, vol. 30, no. 1, pp. 23–33, 1995.

[77] M. Kiili, S. W. Cox, H. Y. Chen et al., "Collagenase-2 (MMP-8) and collagenase-3 (MMP-13) in adult periodontitis: molecular forms and levels in gingival crevicular fluid and immuno-localisation in gingival tissue," *Journal of Clinical Periodontology*, vol. 29, no. 3, pp. 224–232, 2002.

[78] S. Alassiri, P. Parnanen, N. Rathnayake et al., "Ability of quantitative, specific and sensitivity point-of-care/chair-side oral fluid immunotests for aMMP-8 to detect periodontal and per-implant diseases," *Disease Markers*, vol. 2018, Article ID 1306396, 5 pages, 2018.

[79] P. Sahrmann, C. Betschart, D. B. Wiedemeier, A. Al-Majid, T. Attin, and P. R. Schmidlin, "Treatment of peri-implant mucositis with a repeated chlorhexidine chipapplication during SPT-a randomized controlled clinical trial," *Clinical Oral Implants Research*, In press.

[80] S. Mancini, R. Romanelli, C. A. Laschinger, C. M. Overall, J. Sodek, and C. A. McCulloch, "Assessment of a novel screening test for neutrophil collagenase activity in the diagnosis of periodontal diseases," *Journal of Periodontology*, vol. 70, no. 11, pp. 1292–1302, 1999.

[81] R. Romanelli, S. Mancini, C. Laschinger et al., "Activation of neutrophil collagenase in periodontitis," *Infection and Immunity*, vol. 67, no. 5, pp. 2319–2326, 1999.

[82] O. Teronen, Y. T. Konttinen, C. Lindqvist et al., "Human neutrophil collagenase MMP-8 in peri-implant sulcus fluid

and its inhibition by clodronate," *Journal of Dental Research*, vol. 76, no. 9, pp. 1529–1537, 1997.

[83] T. Sorsa, Y. L. Ding, T. Ingman et al., "Cellular source, activation and inhibition of dental plaque collagenase," *Journal of Clinical Periodontology*, vol. 22, no. 9, pp. 709–717, 1995.

[84] N. Rathnayake, D. Gieselmann, A. M. Heikkinen, T. Tervahartiala, and T. Sorsa, "Salivary diagnostics-point-of-care diagnostics of MMP-8 in dentistry and medicine," *Diagnostics*, vol. 7, no. 1, p. 7, 2017.

[85] G. C. Armitage, "Development of a classification system for periodontal diseases and conditions," *Annals of Periodontology*, vol. 4, no. 1, pp. 1–6, 1999.

[86] T. Sorsa, T. Ingman, K. Suomalainen et al., "Identification of proteases from periodontopathogenic bacteria as activators of latent human neutrophil and fibroblast-type interstitial collagenases," *Infection and Immunity*, vol. 60, no. 11, pp. 4491–4495, 1992.

[87] O. P. Lehtonen, E. M. Grahn, T. H. Stahlberg, and L. A. Laitinen, "Amount and avidity of salivary and serum antibodies against streptococcus mutans in 2 groups of human subjects with different dental-caries susceptibility," *Infection and Immunity*, vol. 43, no. 1, pp. 308–313, 1984.

[88] M. T. Nieminen, D. Listyarifah, J. Hagström et al., "Treponema denticola chymotrypsin-like proteinase may contribute to orodigestive carcinogenesis through immunomodulation," *British Journal of Cancer*, vol. 118, no. 3, pp. 1–7, 2017.

[89] A. Mombelli and N. P. Lang, "The diagnosis and treatment of peri-implantitis," *Periodontol 2000*, vol. 17, pp. 63–76, 1998.

[90] N. P. Lang, T. G. Wilson, and E. F. Corbet, "Biological complications with dental implants: their prevention, diagnosis and treatment," *Clinical Oral Implants Research*, vol. 11, no. 1, pp. 146–155, 2000.

[91] T. Berglundh, L. Persson, and B. Klinge, "A systematic review of the incidence of biological and technical complications in implant dentistry reported in prospective longitudinal studies of at least 5 years," *Journal of Clinical Periodontology*, vol. 29, no. s3, pp. 197–212, 2002.

[92] E. F. de Morais, J. C. Pinheiro, R. B. Leite, P. P. A. Santos, C. A. G. Barboza, and R. A. Freitas, "Matrix metalloproteinase-8 levels in periodontal disease patients: a systematic review," *Journal of Periodontal Research*, vol. 53, no. 2, pp. 156–163, 2017.

[93] H. F. Jentsch, A. Buchmann, A. Friedrich, and S. Eick, "Nonsurgical therapy of chronic periodontitis with adjunctive systemic azithromycin or amoxicillin/metronidazole," *Clinical Oral Investigations*, vol. 20, no. 7, pp. 1765–1773, 2016.

23

How Intraday Index Changes Influence Periodontal Assessment

Carlo Bertoldi,[1] Andrea Forabosco,[1] Michele Lalla,[2] Luigi Generali,[1] Davide Zaffe,[3] and Pierpaolo Cortellini[4]

[1]Department of Surgery, Medicine, Dentistry and Morphological Sciences with Transplant Surgery, Oncology and Regenerative Medicine Relevance, University of Modena and Reggio Emilia, Modena, Italy
[2]Department of Economics Marco Biagi, University of Modena and Reggio Emilia, Modena, Italy
[3]Department of Biomedical, Metabolic and Neural Sciences, University of Modena and Reggio Emilia, Modena, Italy
[4]European Research Group on Periodontology (ERGO Perio), Bern, Switzerland

Correspondence should be addressed to Davide Zaffe; davide.zaffe@unimore.it

Academic Editor: Yoshitaka Hara

It is reputed that periodontal indices remain unchanged over a 24-hour period, with great clinical significance. This preliminary study analyzes daily index changes. In 56 selected patients, full-mouth plaque score (FMPS), full-mouth bleeding score (FMBS), periodontal screening and recording (PSR) indices, and periodontal risk assessment (PRA) were recorded at baseline and three times per day (check-I: 08.30, check-II: 11.30, and check-III: 14.30), after appropriate cause-related therapy. Correlation between variables was statistically analyzed by Stata. All periodontal indices improved at the examination phase. Statistical differences were detected for FMPS comparing all thrice daily checks. Statistical differences were detected for FMBS and PRA comparing check-III with check-I and check-II. PSR showed no significant changes. The worst baseline indices produced the widest daily fluctuation at the examination phase. Significant variation of indices is directly related to clinical severity of periodontal conditions at baseline. Patients affected by severe periodontal disease may show significantly greater index changes. As indices are routinely recorded only once per day, the index daily variation has clinical significance. This greatly affects therapeutic strategy as correct periodontal assessment requires multiple evaluations at standardized times, particularly when baseline conditions are severe.

1. Introduction

Maintenance of integrity and of biological rehabilitation, function, and aesthetics are principal objectives in general dentistry and periodontology [1, 2]. Dental health can be jeopardized to varying degrees by different periodontal diseases [3–7]. Periodontal diseases are oral disorders, characterized by gingival and periodontal inflammation, attachment loss, and alveolar bone resorption [4, 6, 7]. Oral microbiota, immune and inflammatory mediation, gene regulation, and hormonal changes play important roles in the onset of periodontal disease [8–10]. However, several additional causes, sometimes linked to systemic diseases, but also linked to psychological aspects or lifestyle, play roles in the progression of periodontal damage. Wide evidence exists in that daily stressors and stress vulnerability factors are associated with inflammatory markers and endocrine and immune functioning [5, 10, 11]. Moreover, it is known, thanks to pioneering work on animals, that response to various pathogens and their by-products including bacterial endotoxins and exotoxins and proinflammatory cytokines is under diurnal control [12–19]. Thaiss et al. [19] report that intestinal microbiota undergoes diurnal oscillation, controlled by host feeding time. Moreover, short-term rhythmic oscillations in intestinal microbiota may be exaggerated or disrupted under various disease conditions, impacting progression of microbiota-mediated diseases with different manifestations or with varying degrees of severity at different times of day [19–21]. The mucosal immune system found inside the mouth is similar to that of the small intestine [22, 23]. Dendritic cells, lymphocytes, and mucosal-associated lymphoid tissue (in the tonsils and lymphoid follicles) help to sample contents entering the mouth and determine "friend or foe." Resident bacteria in the oral cavity are critical to this process. However, outside of dental circles, little attention has been paid to this fact until now [24] or to the 45% overlap of microbes found both in the mouth and in the colon [25]. Sato et al. [26], after studying the oral bacteriome, observed that some bacterial species exhibit significant changes in abundance over time while the majority of species exhibited no periodic changes over the course of a day. However, inter- and intraindividual variability and stability of the human microbiome remain poorly characterized, particularly at the intraday level [26].

Moreover, prevalence of periodontitis in several countries is based upon indices of periodontal treatment screening [27–29]. Consequently, clinical periodontal indices assume particular epidemiological, diagnostic, and prognostic importance in risk assessment and identification of appropriate therapeutic strategy, given the lack of reliable pathogenic criteria based specifically upon interpretation of type of inflammation [4, 5, 30, 31]. Probing depth and clinical attachment levels are used in the diagnosis or prognosis of specific periodontal diseases, but these indicators are liable to misinterpretation, even when correctly measured and even when abundant microbiota deposition or gingivitis is present [32–34]. These situations are frequent mainly during early stages of periodontal therapy. Conservative, orthodontic, and prosthetic issues, individual sensitivity to risk factors, lifestyle, and pathological state requiring treatment, motivate patients and achieve as standardized a periodontal condition as possible. Cause-related periodontal therapy is always performed during the oral hygiene education phase to fulfill this purpose. The cause-related treatment reduces periodontal inflammation and contributes to greater patient status standardization [35].

The community periodontal index of treatment needs (CPITN) and the periodontal screening and recording (PSR) score are indices recommended by both the American Dental Association and the American Academy of Periodontology as screening tools to facilitate early detection and periodontal disease treatment requirements [6, 36]. These indices are not, however, a substitute for periodontal charting during clinical and therapeutic periodontal evaluation but have great importance during the initial stages of patient evaluation. The full-mouth plaque score (FMPS) evidences presence of microbiota [37] while full-mouth bleeding score (FMBS) [38] evidences periodontal inflammation.

Periodontal risk assessment (PRA) consists in a functional diagram that helps the clinician to determine the risk of disease progression in individual patients [39] and is particularly effective in compliant subjects not suffering from aggressive periodontal disease [32, 40].

Treatment needs and management of periodontal disease depend largely upon accurate and reliable index recording, development of an appropriate treatment plan, and subsequent monitoring. However, since pioneering work by Hoover and Lefkowitz [41], gingival inflammation has been considered as a fluctuating disease with a daily cycle of change.

At present, periodontal indices are routinely recorded presupposing that they should not vary significantly, irrespective of the time of day. The aim of this study is to evaluate periodontal FMBS, FMPS, PSR, and PRA indices intraday changes during supportive periodontal therapy.

2. Materials and Methods

2.1. Study Population. The present study population was selected from a list of systemically healthy subjects referred for periodontal treatment, examined, and treated with cause-related therapy.

Checks or improvement studies in health care without external funding, performed by a clinician group working in a single sanitary structure, require no ethical committee approval according to Italian law (standard operating procedure of the provincial ethical committee of Modena, revision November 16, 2010).

All patients signed informed consent in which all procedures of the study were detailed. The research was conducted in full accordance with ethical principles, including the 2013 WMA Helsinki Declaration [42].

Subjects meeting the criteria reported in Table 1 were enrolled.

Enrolled subjects were affected by only mild periodontitis [43, 44] and had not undergone periodontal treatment during the previous year. Additionally, after completion of cause-related therapy, subjects had to be considered good compliers [1, 45, 46].

Each patient in this study had to meet all the above criteria in every phase of the clinical trial.

2.2. Study Design. Before patient examination and treatment, a pretrial calibration session was performed by two examiners on 10 healthy volunteer patients. Number of teeth present in the oral cavity (NoT), FMPS, FMBS, and PSR were recorded three times a day to obtain acceptable intra- and interexaminer clinical periodontal parameter assessment reproducibility.

The first step was the patient screening phase, anamnesis, preliminary dental visit, motivation, and preliminary treatment after patient consent. Gingival tissue sanitization was necessary to achieve a predictive periodontal diagnosis particularly in patients lacking dental supportive therapy or even with no history of regular dental examination for an extended period of time. This step concerned initial dental hygiene treatment and acute and urgent surgical, endodontic, and conservative conditions requiring a short-term solution to stabilize periodontal tissues.

The study opening visit was performed after completion of the first step of causal therapy. The opening visit (baseline, b) was carried out with a flat rhodium-plated dental mirror, dental probe, and periodontal probe with 1-millimeter marks (modified Click-Probe, Kerr Corp., Bioggio, Switzerland). Full-mouth plaque score at baseline (FMPS-b), by plaque disclosing gel detection, and full-mouth bleeding score at baseline (FMBS-b) were assessed at six sites per tooth. Periodontal screening and recording at baseline (PSR-b) was assessed using the World Health Organization (WHO)

TABLE 1: Systemic and specific inclusion criteria.

Systemic criteria	Absence of relevant medical conditions (subjects with a clear medical history and no physical or psychological condition, psychotic disorders, personality disorders, which could affect their conduct in the study).
	Smoking status: nonsmokers or smokers up to 20 cigarettes a day (cigar or pipe smokers or people with a story of alcohol and drug abuse were excluded).
	Education: only patients having almost completed at least compulsory education.
	Pregnant, lactating, and underage patients were excluded.
Local criteria	Subjects having more than 16 teeth, not wearing removable partial dentures, not showing oral parafunctions, and not presenting severe skeletal and occlusal abnormalities or substantial oral dysmorphism were enrolled.
	Oral and periodontal conditions: absence of premalignant lesion of the oral cavity.
	Treatment history: subjects who received scaling root planning, or periodontal surgical treatment in the preceding 6 months, or undergoing recent orthodontic or prosthetic therapy were excluded.
	Level of infection: subjects presenting with severe cariogenicity, stomatitis, acute abscesses, or gingival fistulae were excluded.

periodontal probe. PSR was measured for each tooth and sextant, but only the peak index value for each patient was considered. Finally, PRA-b was calculated.

The following variables were routinely recorded:

(i) age;

(ii) gender;

(iii) body mass index (BMI) as previously described [7];

(iv) number of teeth (NoT) present in the oral cavity;

(v) glycemia (Gly).

Smoking habits (number of cigarettes per day [NoC]; current smoker, nicotinism; former smoker or nonsmoker, and, if smoker, the number of years as smoker) were recorded. Required cause-related therapy, including scaling and root planning, was completed and oral hygiene instructions were given. Indices at baseline were only considered in patients who were subsequently enrolled in the study.

2.3. Study Outcomes and Data Analysis. Five weeks after completion of the previous periodontal therapy, all patients were reevaluated. Patients fulfilling the study inclusion criteria and needing periodontal supportive therapy were enrolled and a new examination (examination phase) was performed the next week.

Each subject would be present at 3 different times (in a single day) at the periodontal examination and maintained usual daily routines. Checks (examination phase) were scheduled (check-I: 08.30, check-II: 11.30, and check-III: 14.30).

FMPS, FMBS, PSR, and PRA were considered during each check. NoT was considered once during examination phase. These data were compared with recorded clinical indices, gender, and smoking habits.

2.4. Statistical Analyses. Inter- and intrarate comparisons were carried out using Spearman coefficients for the number of teeth, PSR, FMBS, FMPS, and PRA.

Comparisons between initial and check-I, check-II, and check-III values for the considered variables were carried out using the Wilcoxon signed-rank statistic (matched data), while, for binary variables gender and smoking habit, comparisons between two independent groups (unmatched data) were carried out using the Mann–Whitney test. Spearman correlation coefficients between variables were calculated and the null hypotheses that no relationship exists between the pairs of variables were tested against the alternative (two-tailed) hypotheses that a relationship exists. FMPS, FMBS, PSR, and PRA were identified as dependent variables. The relationship between dependent and independent (covariates) variables was examined using the seemingly unrelated regression (SUR) model. SUR was used to analyze the effects of covariates on the level of the dependent variables on their maximum observed between the check at the examination phase equal to I, II, and III (that is, Δ-check, the maximum gap between check-I, check-II, and check-III). The level of significance of the applied tests was the standard value $\alpha = 0.05$.

Multivariate analysis of covariance (MANCOVA) for repeated measurement was carried out for examination phases in order to profile index changes over time and to compare SUR results.

Statistical analysis was performed using Stata, version 14.00 (StataCorp LP, Lakeway Drive, College Station, TX, USA) [47].

3. Results

Spearman test analysis of the calibration session, performed by the two examiners on 10 healthy volunteer patients and concerning NoT, FMPS, FMBS, and PSR, produced intrarater agreement ranging between 0.782 and 1.000 ($p < 0.001$) and interrater agreement ranging between 0.771 and 1.000 ($p < 0.001$).

Sixty-seven patients met all requirements of the experimental protocol and study design. However, a total of 11 patients were excluded: 3 patients did not present at maintenance therapy visits conflicting with the study's stringent inclusion criteria; 6 patients (two females and four males) missed the examination phase; 1 patient moved to a distant

TABLE 2: Assessed periodontal indices, grouped by gender and smoker status.

	Baseline	Check-I	Check-II	Check-III
FMPS				
Nonsmokers	48.7 ± 13.4	19.8 ± 8.9	17.0 ± 6.7	16.3 ± 5.2
Female	49.7 ± 14.4	22.5 ± 9.3	17.5 ± 6.5	16.5 ± 4.3
Male	47.7 ± 12.7	17.3 ± 7.9	17.2 ± 7.0	16.1 ± 6.0
Smokers	34.7 ± 15.5	20.6 ± 9.0	18.3 ± 7.9	20.4 ± 7.8
Female	32.8 ± 15.5	18.3 ± 8.7	17.8 ± 9.0	22.3 ± 8.6
Male	36.7 ± 15.9	23.1 ± 9.1	18.9 ± 7.0	18.4 ± 6.7
Overall	42.9 ± 15.8	20.1 ± 8.9	17.7 ± 7.1	18.0 ± 6.6
FMBS				
Nonsmokers	24.2 ± 11.1	9.9 ± 6.4	9.7 ± 6.2	8.9 ± 6.6
Female	25.3 ± 12.2	10.0 ± 5.6	10.2 ± 5.5	9.7 ± 6.7
Male	23.1 ± 10.2	9.9 ± 7.2	9.3 ± 7.0	8.2 ± 6.7
Smokers	18.5 ± 12.1	8.3 ± 5.5	7.0 ± 6.6	6.5 ± 4.9
Female	17.6 ± 12.7	7.7 ± 6.1	8.2 ± 8.4	7.6 ± 5.8
Male	19.4 ± 12.1	9.0 ± 5.1	5.7 ± 3.6	5.3 ± 3.5
Overall	21.8 ± 11.8	9.2 ± 6.0	8.6 ± 6.4	7.9 ± 6.0
PSR				
Nonsmokers	1.63 ± 0.46	0.89 ± 0.26	0.89 ± 0.22	0.86 ± 0.23
Female	1.66 ± 0.49	0.99 ± 0.11	0.97 ± 0.13	0.94 ± 0.12
Male	1.61 ± 0.45	0.79 ± 0.31	0.81 ± 0.26	0.79 ± 0.29
Smokers	1.40 ± 0.46	0.96 ± 0.14	0.86 ± 0.22	0.92 ± 0.15
Female	1.30 ± 0.41	0.96 ± 0.15	0.92 ± 0.18	0.97 ± 0.14
Male	1.51 ± 0.51	0.95 ± 0.13	0.80 ± 0.25	0.86 ± 0.15
Overall	1.54 ± 0.47	0.91 ± 0.22	0.88 ± 0.21	0.89 ± 0.20
PRA				
Nonsmokers	16.8 ± 13.9	10.4 ± 10.3	10.4 ± 10.2	9.7 ± 9.7
Female	19.3 ± 17.5	12.0 ± 13.1	12.2 ± 12.9	11.4 ± 11.8
Male	14.4 ± 9.5	8.9 ± 6.8	8.6 ± 6.5	8.1 ± 7.2
Smokers	31.2 ± 16.2	17.6 ± 6.4	15.9 ± 8.2	14.2 ± 5.2
Female	25.5 ± 12.1	16.4 ± 7.7	16.2 ± 10.0	14.8 ± 5.3
Male	37.4 ± 18.4	18.9 ± 4.8	15.5 ± 6.1	13.5 ± 5.2
Overall	22.7 ± 16.4	13.4 ± 9.5	12.6 ± 9.7	11.5 ± 8.4

Values are expressed as mean ± standard deviation. FMPS: full-mouth plaque score; FMBS: full-mouth bleeding score; PSR: periodontal screening and recording; PRA: periodontal risk assessment.

city; and 1 patient became pregnant. Therefore, 28 females (16 nonsmokers and 12 smokers) and 28 males (17 nonsmokers and 11 smokers), aged 19–91 years (mean ± SD, 43.2 ± 15.7), formed the test population.

3.1. Indices at Baseline. Ranges in nonsmokers were NoT 10–31, FMPS-b 20–67.4%, FMBS-b 2.4–41.3%, PSR-b 1.0–2.5, and PRA-b 2.6–68.4. Ranges in smokers were NoT 10–30, FMPS-b 12.9–68.0%, FMBS-b 2.4–43.1%, PSR-b 0.83–2.0, and PRA-b 8.7–68.4. The greater FMPS-b and the lower PRA-b of nonsmokers were statistically significant in both genders when compared with smokers (Table 2).

3.2. Indices at Examination Phase. At check-I, ranges in nonsmokers were FMPS 6.5–38.5%, FMBS 0.7–25.0%, PSR 0.03–1.2, and PRA 2.6–46.7. At check-I, ranges in smokers

were FMPS 7.0–35.3%, FMBS 1.2–19.2%, PSR 0.7–1.2, and PRA 8.7–29.9 (Table 2).

At check-II, ranges in nonsmokers were FMPS 3.3–35.0%; FMBS 0.5–25.0%; PSR 0.2–1.2; PRA 2.6–46.7. At check-II, ranges in smokers were FMPS 5.0–28.9%; FMBS 1.2–25.6%; PSR 0.8–1.2; PRA 7.8–34.6 (Table 2).

At check-III, ranges in nonsmokers were FMPS 3.3–28.4%, FMBS 0.01–22.8%, PSR 0.01–1.17, and PRA 2.60–43.30. At check-III, ranges in smokers were FMPS 5.6–36.0%, FMBS 2.0–18.5%, PSR 0.67–1.17, and PRA 8.66–25.12 (Table 2).

3.3. Clinical Outcomes. In all patients, FMPS, FMBS, PSR, and PRA (Table 2) highlighted statistically significant clinical improvements from baseline to the examination phase. In all patients, statistically significant differences were recorded between check-I, check-II, and check-III. PSR was almost

TABLE 3: Nonparametric analysis of dental indices.

	Females I	Females II	Males I	Males II	Nonsmokers I	Nonsmokers II	Smokers I	Smokers II	Overall I	Overall II
FMPS										
I	—	—	—	—	—	—	—	—	—	—
II	−2.7	—	n.s.	—	n.s.	—	n.s.	—	−2.7	—
III	n.s.	n.s.	n.s.	n.s.	−2.5	n.s.	n.s.	n.s.	−2.1	n.s.
FMBS										
I	—	—	—	—	—	—	—	—	—	—
II	n.s.	—	−2.7	—	n.s.	—	n.s.	—	n.s.	—
III	n.s.	n.s.	−3.3	n.s.	n.s.	−2.5	−2.5	n.s.	−3.0	−2.3
PSR										
I	—	—	—	—	—	—	—	—	—	—
II	n.s.	—	n.s.	—	n.s.	—	−2.2	—	n.s.	—
III	n.s.	n.s.	n.s.	n.s.	n.s.	n.s.	n.s.	n.s.	n.s.	n.s.
PRA										
I	—	—	—	—	—	—	—	—	—	—
II	n.s.	—	−2.2	—	n.s.	—	−2.0	—	n.s.	—
III	n.s.	n.s.	−3.4	−2.2	−2.0	−2.5	−3.0	n.s.	−3.4	−2.4

Significant coefficients after Mann–Whitney test. FMPS: full-mouth plaque score; FMBS: full-mouth bleeding score; PSR: periodontal screening and recording; PRA: periodontal risk assessment. I: check-I; II: check-II; III: check-III; n.s.: not significant.

TABLE 4: Significance of dental indices at examination phase after Spearman test.

	PRA-III	PSR-III	FMBS-III	FMPS-III	PRA-II	PSR-II	FMBS-II	FMPS-II	PRA-I	PSR-I	FMBS-I
FMPS-I	n.s.	n.s.	0.4	0.4	n.s.	0.4	0.5	0.7	n.s.	0.7	0.6
FMBS-I	0.4	n.s.	0.8	n.s.	0.4	0.3	0.9	0.3	0.4	0.4	
PSR-I	n.s.	0.5	0.4	0.4	n.s.	0.6	0.3	n.s.	n.s.		
PRA-I	0.9	n.s.	0.3	0.3	0.9	n.s.	0.4	n.s.			
FMPS-II	n.s.	0.2	n.s.	0.5	n.s.	0.3	n.s.				
FMBS-II	0.4	n.s.	0.9	n.s.	0.4	0.4					
PSR-II	n.s.	0.7	0.4	n.s.	n.s.						
PRA-II	0.9	n.s.	0.4	n.s.							
FMPS-III	0.3	0.4	n.s.								
FMBS-III	0.4	0.3									
PSR-III	n.s.										

Significant coefficients after Spearman test. Only variables abutting almost one significant correlation are reported. FMPS: full-mouth plaque score; FMBS: full-mouth bleeding score; PSR: periodontal screening and recording; PRA: periodontal risk assessment. I: check-I; II: check-II; III: check-III; n.s.: not significant.

not significant, whereas FMBS, FMPS, and PRA were often significant (Table 3).

Check-I and check-II FMPS values were significantly different in females, whereas check-I FMBS value was significantly different from check-II and check-III FMBS values in males (Table 3). Check-I, check-II and check-III PSR values were not statistically different in either females or males. Check-II and check-III PSR values were significantly greater in females than in males (Table 2). Check-I, check-II and check-III PRA values were statistically different in males, but not in females (Table 3).

Check-I FMPS value was significantly different from check-III FMPS value in nonsmokers (Table 3). Check-III FMBS values were significantly different from check-II FMBS value in nonsmokers and check-I FMBS value in smokers. Check-I PSR value was significantly different from check-II PSR value in smokers. Check-III PRA value was significantly different from check-I and check-II PRA values in nonsmokers, whereas check-I PRA value was significantly different from check-II and check-III PRA values in smokers (Table 3).

Several significant positive correlations between dental indices at examination phases (check-I, check-II, and check-III) were found after the Spearman test was performed (Table 4).

3.4. SUR Analysis. SUR multivariate analysis highlighted several statistically significant relationships between dental, individual, and lifestyle indices versus periodontal indices (Table 5).

Older patients showed a significant decrease of 1.3 units of FMPS-Δ and 0.5 units of FMBS-Δ relative to the expected

TABLE 5: Baseline and maximum gap between check-I, check-II, and check-III of indices after seemingly unrelated regression (SUR) analysis.

	FMPS		FMBS		PSR		PRA	
	b	Δ	b	Δ	b	Δ	b	Δ
Age		−0.13 (0.021)		−0.05 (0.011)				
Female						−0.19 (0.001)		
NoC						−0.02 (0.001)		
FMPS-b	—		−0.07 (0.001)		0.02 (0.001)			
FMBS-b			—	0.16 (0.001)	0.03 (0.001)	−0.01 (0.001)	0.7 (0.001)	0.08 (0.005)
PSR-b	28.2 (0.001)	5.45 (0.002)	14.3 (0.001)		—		−9.1 (0.005)	
PRA-b			0.5 (0.001)		−0.01 (0.001)	0.01 (0.039)	—	
Δ-NoT	−7.0 (0.007)		−10.8 (0.001)		0.45 (0.001)		14.9 (0.001)	

Estimated coefficients and p values (in brackets) for the 4 seemingly unrelated regressions. Only variables abutting almost one significant correlation are reported. FMPS: full-mouth plaque score; FMBS: full-mouth bleeding score; PSR: periodontal screening and recording; PRA: periodontal risk assessment; NoC: number of cigarettes (per day); Δ-NoT: number of hopeless teeth extracted during cause-related therapy. b: baseline; Δ: Δ-check (maximum gap between check-I, check-II, and check-III).

indices of patients 10 years younger. Women showed a significantly decreased PSR-Δ. An increase of 20 cigarettes per day caused a significant PSR-Δ reduction of 0.4 units (Table 5), whereas smokers (nicotinism) showed an increased PRA-Δ of approximately 4 units.

The 20% increase in FMBS at baseline (FMBS-b) produced a significant increase of FMBS-Δ (Δ-check, the maximum gap between check-I, check-II, and check-III) of 3.2%, PRA-Δ of 1.6 units, and a minimal decrease of PSR-Δ. The 2-unit increase of PSR-b produced a significant increase of approximately 11% FMPS-Δ. The 20-unit increase of PRA-b produced a significant increase of PSR-Δ of 0.2 units (Table 5).

SUR analysis of baseline values is reported in Table 5.

4. Discussion

Periodontal screening tests require probing to assess periodontal attachment loss circumferential to each dental element or dental implant. To assess the risk of disease progression, a useful tool can be found in PRA (periodontal risk assessment), consisting of a functional diagram [39]. PSR is a useful test for periodontal screening as it is sensitive, specific, inexpensive, quick, and simple to perform, limiting the number of possible errors associated only with probing procedures [28, 29, 31, 33]. This present study was performed relating to the initial stages of periodontal examination and supportive treatment. PSR is particularly useful during the initial phase and is particularly important in order to determine periodontal treatment requirements [6, 36, 46]. FMBS and FMPS are, respectively, indices of inflammation and of microbiota presence and should be obtained early. Regarding systemic predisposition to inflammatory disorders, several

risks and prognostic factors are probably challenges that trigger or worsen periodontal disorders. Therefore, patients affected by systemic and oral health conditions that could potentially introduce disturbing variables were excluded [5, 48, 49]. Stringent enrollment criteria were applied and the decision to perform the examination phase was made only after and temporally close to a positive response to causal therapy in order to achieve a reliable clinical outcome and an excellent standard of oral clinical settings, thus avoiding potentially perturbing variables.

Enrolled patients were affected by only mild periodontitis, but not by moderate or severe periodontitis [43, 44]. The nosology of periodontitis is complex and currently being developed and studied. In this present study, patients affected by advanced periodontitis were excluded. This decision was made to reduce the impact of major confounding variables resulting from the complexity of severe periodontitis which exacerbates other risk conditions and frequently entails elaborate and significantly different therapeutic strategies [2, 4, 43, 44, 50, 51].

Different forms of periodontal disease require different therapeutic strategies. Furthermore, a specific periodontal lesion may not always be treatable in the same manner, but rather on a case-specific basis [52, 53]. Further research, therefore, may suddenly present new therapeutic strategies [54, 55]. Consequently, it may be more difficult to obtain examiner agreement regarding patients with moderate or severe periodontitis due to haste and/or inaccurate, immoderate assessment [56–59].

The use of specific dental indices, specific periodontal probes, and a preventive calibration session make examiner agreement more obtainable and reliable [56, 59, 60].

Furthermore, patients progressing to the examination phase of this present study were required not to change their daily habits and were examined delicately three times in one day. A large number of exogenous variables potentially able to produce misleading results during the examination phase were eliminated thus creating the necessary conditions to obtain significantly similar measurements. Nevertheless, baseline data recorded using the same accurate method used during the three check phases were included in order to detect possible influences on index fluctuation. The baseline situation is a key factor in both therapeutic decisions and clinical outcomes [51, 61].

Most studies report reproducibility of the same periodontal indices while using different measuring instruments [60, 62, 63], in different clinical situations [31, 33, 59, 60], and evaluating clinical correlation or reproducibility of the same indices [64]. However, only few studies report the daily periodontal indices trend [65].

The results of this present study highlight the clinical effectiveness of cause-related therapy in genders, smokers and nonsmokers, and also additional correlations such as the direct relationship of periodontal indices during the examination phase.

The main aim of this present study is to analyze periodontal indices to ascertain whether or not these indices remain unchanged during the day during the examination phase. In the examination phase, significant changes of FMPS, FMBS, and PRA, but not of PSR, were recorded. Similar significant variations were also observed in nonsmokers. The substantial changes detected in some of the aforementioned periodontal indices have no easy explanation. Periodontal risk assessment variation during the examination phase is significant. However, statistical analysis of PRA changes over time (during the examination phase) showed a statistically similar trend to not only FMBS but also to both FMPS and PSR.

Multivariate analysis can help us to understand these variations by showing that a rise in either PRA-b or PSR-b increases PSR Δ-check (with cumulative effect) and that a rise in either FMBS-b or NoC increases FMBS Δ-checks. Separately, a rise in either PSR-b or female gender increases FMPS Δ-checks, and a rise in either FMBS-b or nicotinism increases PRA Δ-checks (with cumulative effect). Among the considered variables, any one related to either lifestyle or biologic condition of the subject appears to influence Δ-check widths in a different manner. However, many of the measured variables significantly associated with Δ-checks are periodontal indices recorded at baseline and produce an increase of Δ-check widths. Therefore, the worst periodontal indices at baseline produce the widest daily fluctuation at the examination phase, considering the cumulative effect of overall influencing factors. It is probable that, at baseline, subjects suffering from serious periodontal conditions show greater periodontal state instability which is further increased by presence of risk factors such as nicotinism. Nevertheless, patients enrolled in this present study suffered from only mild periodontitis in the worst case. Patients were compliant with study prescriptions and observed the stringent supportive protocol and, on the whole, showed clinically favorable indices during the examination phase.

Biological processes displaying endogenous fluctuation had been widely observed in animals and human beings. It is probable that this fluctuation stimulates physiological mechanisms that promote adjustment to environmental circumstances, favoring systemic requirements [66, 67]. It is hard to separate behavioral and physiological influences on the daily index fluctuation, also considering the mutual correlation between those factors. Different check times during the day may characterize dissimilar situations due to systemic physiology, habits, lifestyle, activities, hygiene, and nutrition. It is known that the alimentary canal macrobiome also shows short-term oscillations related to diet and lifestyle [19–21] and that these oscillations also seem to occur in the oral cavity. However, there are fewer studies and less evidence regarding this [26]. Gingival flow rate and human crevicular fluid flow vary during the day in relation to eating, chewing, and other stimuli [68, 69], particularly in presence of gingival inflammation and the tonicity of saliva increases with saliva flow rate. Additionally, daily oscillations in the expression of inflammatory, immunological, and promigratory molecules have also been described in humans. Several chronic disease symptoms or presentations are known to be exacerbated by daily stressors and worrying which create a stress vulnerability factor [11, 18]. Gene transcription also seems to be time of day dependent in some cases [8]. Even human fibroblasts could have substantial daily variations [70]. Periodontal disease is substantially a set of inflammatory disorders largely supported by microbiota but also supported by other risk and prognostic factors.

The examination phase was performed during three different time slots: early morning, late morning, and early afternoon. These times of day seem to have a neurophysiologic and hormonal meaning in both mammals [71] and humans and are linked to circumstances and different habits related to working rhythms, dietary habits, and lifestyle.

Very few studies comparing the same periodontal indices during the day are found in the literature. In this present study, repeated measurements at different times on the same day were performed in compliant patients affected by mild periodontitis. Repeated measurements performed at different times along several days would introduce greater behavioral and/or physiological effects. This present study observed fluctuations within the same indices on the same day. These fluctuations were significant and significantly proportional with respect to the clinical severity of periodontal damage at baseline but not at examination phase. It is therefore conceivable that these fluctuations are more important in patients affected by severe or serious periodontal disease due to the fact that the pathological substrate may still be active also after stabilization of the clinical condition. It is also possible that daily fluctuations of the oral microbiota, inflammatory and immunological regulation, and even cellular constituents of periodontal tissue amplify indices variation. However, this present study demonstrates that the discrepancy between index measurements seems to be directly related to clinical severity of the periodontal condition at baseline. Therefore, it is conceivable that in patients affected by severe periodontal disease the recognizable variations could become dramatic even if the single index measurement is performed at a second phase after baseline when signs of periodontal damage are much less evident. This could even misdirect the therapeutic strategy due to the fact that the predictive measurement referable to the patients' therapeutic feasibility of recovery could be unknown.

5. Conclusion

Our results showed significant variation within indices directly related to clinical severity of the periodontal condition at baseline. Patients affected by severe periodontal disease may show much larger index changes. Since the indices are routinely recorded only once, the index daily variation may have actual clinical significance. This could greatly affect therapeutic strategy because correct periodontal assessment requires multiple evaluations with standardized timing, particularly when the baseline condition is severe.

Acknowledgments

The authors thank RDHs Valeria Ponzini, Greta Caprara, and Anastasia Nechytaylo (Private Practice, Registered Dental Hygienists, Modena and Reggio Emilia, Italy) and Mrs. Domenica Bussi for technical and organizational assistance during the study. This study was funded by the authors' own institution.

References

[1] S. Renvert and G. Rutger Persson, "Supportive periodontal therapy," *Periodontology 2000*, vol. 36, pp. 179–195, 2004.

[2] C. Bertoldi, C. Pellacani, M. Lalla et al., "Herpes Simplex i virus impairs regenerative outcomes of periodontal regenerative therapy in intrabony defects. A pilot study," *Journal of Clinical Periodontology*, vol. 39, no. 4, pp. 385–392, 2012.

[3] J. J. Hyman and B. C. Reid, "Epidemiologic risk factors for periodontal attachment loss among adults in the United States," *Journal of Clinical Periodontology*, vol. 30, no. 3, pp. 230–237, 2003.

[4] C. Bertoldi, E. Bellei, C. Pellacani et al., "Non-bacterial protein expression in periodontal pockets by proteome analysis," *Journal of Clinical Periodontology*, vol. 40, no. 6, pp. 573–582, 2013.

[5] C. Bertoldi, M. Lalla, J. M. Pradelli, P. Cortellini, A. Lucchi, and D. Zaffe, "Risk factors and socioeconomic condition effects on periodontal and dental health: A pilot study among adults over fifty years of age," *European Journal of Dentistry*, vol. 7, no. 3, pp. 336–346, 2013.

[6] H. F. Wolf, T. M. Hassell, E. M. Rateitschak-Pl?ss, and K. H. Rateitschak, *Color Atlas of Dental Medicine*, Georg Thieme Verlag, Stuttgart, 2005.

[7] C. Bertoldi, D. Bencivenni, A. Lucchi, and U. Consolo, "Augmentation of keratinized gingiva through bilaminar connective tissue grafts: a comparison between two techniques," *Minerva stomatologica*, vol. 56, no. 1-2, pp. 3–20, 2007.

[8] H. R. Ueda, W. Chen, A. Adachi et al., "A transcription factor response element for gene expression during circadian night," *Nature*, vol. 418, no. 6897, pp. 534–539, 2002.

[9] U. Baser, A. Cekici, S. Tanrikulu-Kucuk, A. Kantarci, E. Ademoglu, and F. Yalcin, "Gingival inflammation and interleukin 1-β and tumor necrosis factor-alpha levels in gingival crevicular fluid during the menstrual cycle," *Journal of Periodontology*, vol. 80, no. 12, pp. 1983–1990, 2009.

[10] R. J. Genco and W. S. Borgnakke, "Risk factors for periodontal disease," *Periodontology 2000*, vol. 62, no. 1, pp. 59–94, 2013.

[11] A. W. M. Evers, E. W. M. Verhoeven, H. Van Middendorp et al., "Does stress affect the joints? Daily stressors, stress vulnerability, immune and HPA axis activity, and short-term disease and symptom fluctuations in rheumatoid arthritis," *Annals of the Rheumatic Diseases*, vol. 73, no. 9, pp. 1683–1688, 2014.

[12] M. A. Reynolds, "Modifiable risk factors in periodontitis: At the intersection of aging and disease," *Periodontology 2000*, vol. 64, no. 1, pp. 7–19, 2014.

[13] R. D. Feigin, V. H. San Joaquin, M. W. Haymond, and R. G. Wyatt, "Daily periodicity of susceptibility of mice to pneumococcal infection," *Nature*, vol. 224, no. 5217, pp. 379-380, 1969.

[14] R. D. Feigin, J. N. Middelkamp, and C. Reed, "Circadian rhythmicity in susceptibility of mice to sublethal coxsackie B3 infection," *Nature New Biology*, vol. 240, no. 97, pp. 57-58, 1972.

[15] P. G. Shackelford and R. D. Feigin, "Periodicity of susceptibility to pneumococcal infection: influence of light and adrenocortical secretions," *Science*, vol. 182, no. 4109, pp. 285–287, 1973.

[16] S. D. House, S. Ruch, W. F. Koscienski III, C. W. Rocholl, and R. L. Moldow, "Effects of the circadian rhythm of corticosteroids on leukocyte- endothelium interactions in the AM and PM," *Life Sciences*, vol. 60, no. 22, pp. 2023–2034, 1997.

[17] A. C. Silver, A. Arjona, W. E. Walker, and E. Fikrig, "he circadian clock controls toll-like recept or 9-mediated innate and adaptive immunity," *Immunity*, vol. 36, no. 2, pp. 251–261, 2012.

[18] C. Scheiermann, Y. Kunisaki, and P. S. Frenette, "Circadian control of the immune system," *Nature Reviews Immunology*, vol. 13, no. 3, pp. 190–198, 2013.

[19] C. A. Thaiss, D. Zeevi, M. Levy et al., "Transkingdom control of microbiota diurnal oscillations promotes metabolic homeostasis," *Cell*, vol. 159, no. 3, pp. 514–529, 2014.

[20] X. Liang, F. D. Bushman, and G. A. Fitzgerald, "Time in motion: The molecular clock meets the microbiome," *Cell*, vol. 159, no. 3, pp. 469-470, 2014.

[21] A. Zarrinpar, A. Chaix, S. Yooseph, and S. Panda, "Diet and feeding pattern affect the diurnal dynamics of the gut microbiome," *Cell Metabolism*, vol. 20, no. 6, pp. 1006–1017, 2014.

[22] F. Brito, C. Zaltman, A. T. P. Carvalho et al., "Subgingival microflora in inflammatory bowel disease patients with untreated periodontitis," *European Journal of Gastroenterology and Hepatology*, vol. 25, no. 2, pp. 239–245, 2013.

[23] S. Reichert, A. Schlitt, V. Beschow et al., "Use of floss/interdental brushes is associated with lower risk for new cardiovascular events among patients with coronary heart disease," *Journal of Periodontal Research*, vol. 50, no. 2, pp. 180–188, 2015.

[24] R.-Q. Wu, D.-F. Zhang, E. Tu, Q.-M. Chen, and W. Chen, "The mucosal immune system in the oral cavity-an orchestra of T cell diversity," *International Journal of Oral Science*, vol. 6, no. 3, pp. 125–132, 2014.

[25] N. Segata, S. Kinder Haake, P. Mannon et al., "Composition of the adult digestive tract bacterial microbiome based on seven mouth surfaces, tonsils, throat and stool samples," *Genome Biology*, p. R42, 2012.

[26] Y. Sato, J. Yamagishi, R. Yamashita et al., "Inter-individual differences in the oral bacteriome are greater than intra-day

fluctuations in individuals," *PLoS ONE*, vol. 10, no. 6, Article ID e0131607, 2015.

[27] A. J. Morris, J. Steele, and D. A. White, "The oral cleanliness and periodontal health of UK adults in 1998," *British Dental Journal*, vol. 191, no. 4, pp. 186–192, 2001.

[28] G. E. Rapp, A. D. A. Barbosa Júnior, A. J. D. Mendes, A. C. F. Motta, M. A. D. A. Bião, and R. V. Garcia, "Technical assessment of WHO-621 periodontal probe made in Brazil," *Brazilian Dental Journal*, vol. 13, no. 1, pp. 61–65, 2002.

[29] D. E. Wallace, "PSR and CPITN charting. The need for documentation in patients," *Journal of the New Zealand Society of Periodontology*, vol. 89, pp. 17–21, 2006.

[30] Research Science and Therapy Committee of the American Academy of Periodontology, "Diagnosis of periodontal diseases," *Journal of Periodontology*, vol. 74, no. 8, pp. 1237–1247, 2003.

[31] G. C. Armitage, G. K. Svanberc, and H. Löe, "Microscopic evaluation of clinical measurements of connective tissue attachment levels," *Journal of Clinical Periodontology*, vol. 4, no. 3, pp. 173–190, 1977.

[32] M. Leininger, H. Tenenbaum, and J.-L. Davideau, "Modified periodontal risk assessment score: Long-term predictive value of treatment outcomes. A retrospective study," *Journal of Clinical Periodontology*, vol. 37, no. 5, pp. 427–435, 2010.

[33] C. Fowler, S. Garrett, M. Crigger, and J. Egelberg, "Histologic probe position in treated and untreated human periodontal tissues," *Journal of Clinical Periodontology*, vol. 9, no. 5, pp. 373–385, 1982.

[34] A. Karayiannis, N. P. Lang, A. Joss, and S. Nyman, "Bleeding on probing as it relates to probing pressure and gingival health in patients with a reduced but healthy periodontium: A clinical study," *Journal of Clinical Periodontology*, vol. 19, no. 7, pp. 471–475, 1992.

[35] P. Axelsson, B. Nyström, and J. Lindhe, "The long-term effect of a plaque control program on tooth mortality, caries and periodontal disease in adults: results after 30 years of maintenance," *Journal of Clinical Periodontology*, vol. 31, no. 9, pp. 749–757, 2004.

[36] A. Khocht, H. Zohn, M. Deasy, and K. M. Chang, "Assessment of periodontal status with PSR and traditional clinical periodontal examination," *Journal of the American Dental Association*, vol. 126, no. 12, pp. 1658–1665, 1995.

[37] T. J. O'Leary, "The Impact of Research on Scaling and Root Planing," *Journal of Periodontology*, vol. 57, no. 2, pp. 69–75, 1986.

[38] M. S. Tonetti, G. Pini-Prato, and P. Cortellini, "Periodontal regeneration of human intrabony defects. IV. Determinants of healing response.," *Journal of Periodontology*, vol. 64, no. 10, pp. 934–940, 1993.

[39] N. P. Lang and M. S. Tonetti, "Periodontal risk assessment (PRA) for patients in supportive therapy (SPT)," *Oral Health and Preventive Dentistry*, vol. 1, pp. 7–16, 2003.

[40] A. Meyer-Bäumer, M. Pritsch, R. Cosgarea et al., "Prognostic value of the periodontal risk assessment in patients with aggressive periodontitis," *Journal of Clinical Periodontology*, vol. 39, no. 7, pp. 651–658, 2012.

[41] D. R. Hoover and W. Lefkowitz, "Fluctuation in marginal gingivitis," *Journal of Periodontology*, vol. 36, no. 4, pp. 310–314, 1965.

[42] "WMA Declaration of Helsinki. Ethical principles for medical research involving human subjects," http://www.wma.net/en/30publications/10policies/b3/index.html.

[43] M. S. Tonetti and N. Claffey, "Advances in the progression of periodontitis and proposal of definitions of a periodontitis case and disease progression for use in risk factor research: Group C Consensus report of the 5th European workshop in periodontology," *Journal of Clinical Periodontology*, vol. 32, no. 6, pp. 210–213, 2005.

[44] R. C. Page and P. I. Eke, "Case definitions for use in population-based surveillance of periodontitis," *Journal of Periodontology*, vol. 78, no. 7, pp. 1387–1399, 2007.

[45] L. Checchi, G. A. Pelliccioni, M. R. Gatto, and L. Kelescian, "Patient compliance with maintenance therapy in an Italian periodontal practice," *Journal of Clinical Periodontology*, vol. 21, no. 5, pp. 309–312, 1994.

[46] "SIdP guidelines," http://www.sidp.it/la-societa/linee-guida-sidp/.

[47] "Stata statistical software. Release 9, vol. 1-4, StataCorp LP, College Station TX, 2005".

[48] B. L. Mealey and T. W. Oates, "Diabetes mellitus and periodontal diseases," *Journal of Periodontology*, vol. 77, no. 8, pp. 1289–1303, 2006.

[49] T. Saito and Y. Shimazaki, "Metabolic disorders related to obesity and periodontal disease," *Periodontology 2000*, vol. 43, no. 1, pp. 254–266, 2007.

[50] P. Cortellini and M. S. Tonetti, "Clinical and radiographic outcomes of the modified minimally invasive surgical technique with and without regenerative materials: a randomized-controlled trial in intra-bony defects," *Journal of Clinical Periodontology*, vol. 38, no. 4, pp. 365–373, 2011.

[51] D. E. Deas, A. J. Moritz, R. S. Sagun, S. F. Gruwell, and C. A. Powell, "Scaling and root planing vs. conservative surgery in the treatment of chronic periodontitis," *Periodontology 2000*, vol. 71, no. 1, pp. 128–139, 2016.

[52] U. Pagliaro, M. Nieri, R. Rotundo et al., "Clinical guidelines of the Italian Society of Periodontology for the reconstructive surgical treatment of angular bony defects in periodontal patients," *Journal of Periodontology*, vol. 79, no. 12, pp. 2219–2232, 2008.

[53] R. M. Palmer and P. Cortellini, "Periodontal tissue engineering and regeneration: Consensus Report of the Sixth European Workshop on Periodontology," *Journal of Clinical Periodontology*, vol. 35, no. 8, pp. 83–86, 2008.

[54] P. Cortellini, G. Stalpers, A. Mollo, and M. S. Tonetti, "Periodontal regeneration versus extraction and prosthetic replacement of teeth severely compromised by attachment loss to the apex: 5-year results of an ongoing randomized clinical trial," *Journal of Clinical Periodontology*, vol. 38, no. 10, pp. 915–924, 2011.

[55] T. T. Hägi, O. Laugisch, A. Ivanovic, and A. Sculean, "Regenerative periodontal therapy," *Quintessence international (Berlin, Germany : 1985)*, vol. 45, no. 3, pp. 185–192, 2014.

[56] A. Kingman, H. Löe, A. Anerud, and H. Boysen, "Errors in measuring parameters associated with periodontal health and disease.," *Journal of Periodontology*, vol. 62, no. 8, pp. 477–486, 1991.

[57] S. G. Grossi, R. G. Dunford, A. Ho, G. Koch, E. E. Machtei, and R. J. Genco, "Sources of error for periodontal probing measurements," *Journal of Periodontal Research*, vol. 31, no. 5, pp. 330–336, 1996.

[58] M. A. Espeland, U. E. Zappa, P. E. Hogan, C. Simona, and H. Graf, "Cross-sectional and longitudinal reliability for clinical measurement of attachment loss," *Journal of Clinical Periodontology*, vol. 18, no. 2, pp. 126–133, 1991.

[59] P. Eickholz, F. L. Grotkamp, H. Steveling, J. Mühling, and H. J. Staehle, "Reproducibility of peri-implant probing using a force-controlled probe," *Clinical Oral Implants Research*, vol. 12, no. 2, pp. 153–158, 2001.

[60] P. Guglielmoni, A. Promsudthi, D. M. Tatakis, and L. Trombelli, "Intra- and inter-examiner reproducibility in keratinized tissue width assessment with 3 methods for mucogingival junction determination," *Journal of Periodontology*, vol. 72, no. 2, pp. 134–139, 2001.

[61] L. J. Heitz-Mayfield, L. Trombelli, F. Heitz, I. Needleman, and D. Moles, "A systematic review of the effect of surgical debridement vs non-surgical debridement for the treatment of chronic periodontitis," *Journal of Clinical Periodontology*, vol. 29, supplement 3, pp. 92–102, 2002.

[62] M. Quirynen, A. Callens, D. van Steenberghe, and M. Nys, "Clinical evaluation of a constant force electronic probe.," *Journal of Periodontology*, vol. 64, no. 1, pp. 35–39, 1993.

[63] L. Tupta-Veselicky, P. Famili, F. J. Ceravolo, and T. Zullo, "A clinical study of an electronic constant force periodontal probe," *Journal of periodontology*, vol. 65, no. 6, pp. 616–622, 1994.

[64] J. Miranda, L. Brunet, P. Roset, M. Farré, and C. Mendieta, "Reliability of two measurement indices for gingival enlargement," *Journal of Periodontal Research*, vol. 47, no. 6, pp. 776–782, 2012.

[65] C. Bertoldi, C. Pellacani, L. Generali et al., "Variation of the periodontal indexes during the day. A pilot study carried out during the maintenance phase," *Dental Cadmos*, vol. 80, no. 3, pp. 119–136, 2012.

[66] N. Nader, G. P. Chrousos, and T. Kino, "Circadian rhythm transcription factor CLOCK regulates the transcriptional activity of the glucocorticoid receptor by acetylating its hinge region lysine cluster: potential physiological implications," *The FASEB Journal*, vol. 23, no. 5, pp. 1572–1583, 2009.

[67] P. Kovacic and R. Somanathan, "Cell signaling, receptors, electrical effects and therapy in circadian rhythm," *Journal of Receptors and Signal Transduction*, vol. 33, no. 5, pp. 267–275, 2013.

[68] N. F. Bissada, E. M. Schaffer, and E. Haus, "Circadian periodicity of human crevicular fluid flow.," *Journal of Periodontology*, vol. 38, no. 1, pp. 36–40, 1967.

[69] G. Iorgulescu, "Saliva between normal and pathological. Important factors in determining systemic and oral health," *Journal of Medicine and Life*, vol. 2, pp. 303–307, 2009.

[70] S. A. Brown, D. Kunz, A. Dumas et al., "Molecular insights into human daily behavior," *Proceedings of the National Academy of Sciences of the United States of America*, vol. 105, no. 5, pp. 1602–1607, 2008.

[71] M. Cuesta, D. Clesse, P. Pévet, and E. Challet, "From daily behavior to hormonal and neurotransmitters rhythms: Comparison between diurnal and nocturnal rat species," *Hormones and Behavior*, vol. 55, no. 2, pp. 338–347, 2009.

24

Knowledge of Periodontal Diseases, Oral Hygiene Practices, and Self-Reported Periodontal Problems among Pregnant Women and Postnatal Mothers Attending Reproductive and Child Health Clinics in Rural Zambia

T. M. Kabali [ID][1] **and E. G. Mumghamba** [ID][2]

[1]*Department of Orthodontics, Paedodontics and Community Dentistry, Muhimbili University of Health and Allied Sciences (MUHAS), P.O. Box 65014, Dar-es-Salaam, Tanzania*

[2]*Department of Restorative Dentistry, School of Dentistry, Muhimbili University of Health and Allied Sciences (MUHAS), P.O. Box 65014, Dar-es-Salaam, Tanzania*

Correspondence should be addressed to T. M. Kabali; theodorakmiti@yahoo.com

Academic Editor: Gilberto Sammartino

Aim. To determine the level of knowledge of periodontal diseases, practices regarding oral hygiene, and self-perceived periodontal problems among pregnant and postnatal women attending reproductive and child health clinics in rural districts of Zambia. *Methodology.* This was a quantitative, questionnaire-based, descriptive, and cross-sectional study that recruited 410 women aged 15 to 43 years. Data were analyzed using SPSS v19.0 computer program. *Results.* Participants knowledgeable of periodontal diseases were 62%; gingivitis signs included gum swelling (87.4%) and bleeding (93.3%). Of all participants, 95.6% practiced tooth brushing: twice/day (38.5%), using plastic toothbrush (95.6%), chewing stick (12.2%), toothpick (10.7%), dental floss (2.0%), and tongue cleaning (55.4%). Self-reported periodontal problems were bleeding gums (23.2%), gums that were reddish (10.5%), swollen (11.0%), painful (15.9%), and mobile teeth (3.4%). In logistic regression analysis, painful gums, reddish gums, and toothpick use were 21.9, 4.7, and 4.3 respectively, significantly more likely to cause gum bleeding on tooth brushing. *Conclusions.* Most studied women had general knowledge of periodontal diseases but only few knew the cause. All participants performed tooth cleaning; however, majority did not know appropriate practices, and only few had periodontal problems. Integration of oral health to general health promotion and periodontal therapy to pregnant women at high risk is recommended.

1. Introduction

"Periodontal problems" encompass several conditions that include gingival and periodontal diseases [1]. Periodontal diseases always start as gingivitis which denotes an inflammation of gingival tissue due to microbial challenge [2]. Epidemiological studies show that gingivitis may or may not progress to periodontal disease [3]. However, the most significant factors for gingivitis to progress to periodontal diseases include presence of periodontal pathogens in particular the red complex that includes the *Porphyromonas gingivalis*, *Tannerella forsythensis*, *Treponema denticola*, genetics, and poor oral hygiene in the form of accumulation of oral biofilm that is full of millions of microbes (1 gm contains more than 10^{11} microorganisms) and of different types as gram positive and gram negative [4].

During pregnancy, periodontal tissues' response to biofilm challenge is reinforced as female sex hormones are necessary but not sufficient to produce gingival changes by themselves and usually plaque plays a role [5]. Pregnancy period is accompanied by an increase in the levels of both progesterone and estrogen which by the third trimester, reaches levels 10–30 times more than the one seen during typical menstrual cycle, and changes in the gingiva include an increase in gingivitis that usually starts during the second to third month of pregnancy and increases in severity through the eighth month, where it decreases along with the abrupt decrease in hormone secretion [6, 7]. Pregnancy affects the severity of previously inflamed gingival tissues but does not alter healthy gingiva [8]. Pregnant women with previous chronic gingivitis which attracted no attention before pregnancy become aware of their gingival status as the previously inflamed areas become enlarged and edematous and more noticeably discolored with an increased tendency to bleeding [9].

An intensive approach to plaque removal may be effective to treat pregnancy gingivitis and all forms of gingival enlargements [10]. Improving maternal oral hygiene is important for oral health and may reduce systemic proinflammatory cytokines and improve maternal outcomes [11]. In a study involving 409 postpartum women, only half of the women brushed their teeth more than once a day for about 1–3 minutes; in addition, a substantial proportion of patients (35%) reported seeking oral care from a dentist only when they experience pain, thus making preventive strategies less possible [12].

The impact of periodontal disease on pregnancy outcome is now under scrutiny. Findings from observational studies yielded inconsistent conclusions on the relationship between periodontal disease and various pregnancy outcomes (including early pregnancy loss, preterm birth, low birth weight, and preeclampsia) [13]. A close relationship was shown to exist between lack of oral hygiene and periodontal disease in pregnant women [14]. Most of these ill-effects could be avoided by good oral hygiene practices [15]. Traditionally, tooth brushing using manual or powered toothbrush and flossing have been considered the standard for routine plaque removal and gingivitis reduction [16]. In Zambia, retrievable information on oral hygiene practices and gum/periodontal problems among females at reproductive age in particular pregnant women and mothers for young children is lacking. The aim of this study is to assess knowledge on periodontal diseases, practices regarding oral hygiene, and self-reported periodontal problems among pregnant women and postnatal mothers attending reproductive and child health clinics in rural Zambia.

2. Materials and Methods

2.1. Study Design, Place of Study, and Participants. This was a quantitative, descriptive, cross-sectional health facility-based study. It was conducted in Chibombo and Chisamba rural districts located in the Central Province in Zambia. Five different health facilities participated including four rural health centres (RHC) and one district hospital. These health facilities were readily accessible and thus conveniently selected. Specific health facilities that participated were Chibombo RHC, Twalumba RHC, and Mwachisompola RHC from Chibombo district together with Malombe RHC and Liteta District Hospital from Chisamba district. Recruitment of study participants involved all pregnant women (PW) who were routinely attending 2nd visit antenatal clinic and all postnatal mothers (PM) who were routinely attending postnatal services provided that they were willing and thus gave their consent.

2.2. Sampling. The single stage cluster sampling was utilized to select the five RHC clinics for the study, and the recruitment of study participants was done by registering consecutively every consenting pregnant woman and postnatal mother in the selected health facilities until achieving the required sample size. No random sampling was undertaken rather a convenience sampling approach was used within the clinic setting.

2.3. Data Sources and Collection Procedure. A pretested and validated questionnaire which was prepared in English and translated in Bemba and Lenje, the local languages of the study participants, was used to interview 90% of the participants who could not read and write, and the rest undertook a self-administered questionnaire.

The data collection tool consisted of questions on sociodemographic factors (age, level of education, and marital status), knowledge of periodontal diseases (17 items), oral hygiene practices (9 items), and self-reported periodontal problems (5 items). Correct responses/answers in each section were summed up and divided over the total items for calculation of percentages out of 100% as regards to knowledge of periodontal diseases, oral hygiene practices, and self-reported periodontal problems. The respondents who scored above 50% were graded as "good" and those who scored below 50% were graded as "poor."

2.4. Data Analysis. Data were entered into a computer and analyzed using Statistical Package for Social Sciences (SPSS) version 19.0. Frequency tables were generated. Data transformation was undertaken in particular dichotomization of some variables that had more than two options for example, age (15–24 years versus 25 years and above) and level of education (primary education and lower versus secondary, college, and university education). Furthermore, the type of occupation of the study participants was dichotomized and recoded as informal (none and self-employed) versus formal (employed and business persons), and health facility was dichotomized as hospital versus health centres. The responses to specific oral hygiene practices and self-reported periodontal problems were dichotomized into presence (Yes) or absence (No) of the specific condition. Cross tabulations were processed between dichotomized categorical variables that generated two-by-two contingency tables. The chi-square test or Fisher's exact test (in cross tabulation cases where one or more of the cells had a value of "5" or less) was used to detect statistically significant differences between two groups of any categorical variables under consideration. In all analyses, the statistical significance level was set at "<0.05."

For binary logistic regression analyses, the dichotomized variables were recoded into zero (0) for a code that was assigned to an advantageous or nonproblematic aspect, and a code number of one (1) was given to any previous code number that meant to be in a disadvantageous or problematic aspect. For example, someone who is brushing the teeth twice a day in line with the international recommendation (thus being on an advantageous aspect) were given a code number of zero (0), and anyone who was not brushing according to this recommendation did put him/herself into disadvantageous aspect and thus was given a new code number of one (1). Also, anyone having a sign of a disease or condition under study was given a code number of one (1), whereas a study participant without any sign of that disease or condition was given a code number of zero (0). All those variables that were recoded for the binary logistic regression analyses were subjected to descriptive statistics in particular cross tabulation. Variables with a significant probability (P) value ($P < 0.05$) during cross tabulation were selected and entered into the logistic regression analysis. In addition, all variables that were thought to be important as predisposing factors for the dependent variable (gum bleeding) provided that P value was less than 0.3 (arbitrarily chosen) and were included in the logistic regression analyses. The characteristic of maternal status, meaning that the study participant was either "pregnant" or a "postnatal" woman, was deliberately included in the model although the probability value was far above the selected cutoff point because it was strongly felt that this factor is associated with bleeding gums. The backward stepwise (Wald) logistic regression method was chosen for analysis. The dependent variable was the self-reported condition as experienced "gum bleeding'" and the rest of the variables on oral hygiene practices, knowledge, and other predisposing conditions were considered as categorical "covariates" whereby the contrast was the "indicator" and reference category was set as the "first" category. The options were set at the 95% confidence interval (95% CI) for the exponential (B) whereby the probability for the backward stepwise (Wald) model was set at entry value of 0.05 and removal at value 0.10. The final iteration of the backward stepwise (Wald) model was included as final results.

3. Results

3.1. Distribution of Study Participants. A total of 410 study participants comprising 270 pregnant women and 140 postnatal mothers were recruited (Table 1) with age ranging from 15 to 43 years (Mean age ± standard deviation: 25.72 ± 6.88 years). The median age was 24 years. Majority of the study participants were at 15–24 years of age (65.7%). The ever married women were the majority (83%). Most of the study participants had primary education or less, and generally the employed group was 56%. Health centres had higher number of study participants (75%) as compared to the hospital.

3.2. Oral Hygiene Practices. The prevalence of oral hygiene practices and self-reported periodontal problems among pregnant women and postnatal mothers is shown in Table 2. All participants claimed to practice regular tooth brushing, but frequency of tooth brushing varied among individuals. Tooth brushing once per day was 24.9% and brushing twice per day was 38.5%. Those who brushed three times per day were 36.3%. Duration of tooth brushing was estimated to take about 1–3 minutes (57.1%). Chewing stick users were at 12.2%. Use of a plastic toothbrush to clean teeth (Table 2) was significantly higher among postnatal mothers (100%) than in pregnant women (93.3%, $P = 0.001$, $\chi^2 = 9.672$).

Replacement of tooth brushes once/month was done by 25.4% while 39.3% replaced their toothbrushes after every three months. Slightly more than half of the study participants (55.4%) had the habit of cleaning the tongue regularly. Regular use of toothpaste during tooth brushing was reported by 91.7%, and there were no significant differences between pregnant women and postnatal mothers (Table 2).

Among all the study participants ($n = 410$) who responded to the question whether they had ever heard of the gum or periodontal diseases, 254 (62%) participants answered correctly (Yes), and there were more pregnant women (179/270 (66.3%)) than postnatal mothers (75/140 (53.6%)) ($\chi^2 = 6.333$, $P = 0.012$). Among all respondents ($n = 256$), 222 (86.7%) gave the correct response to the question that gum or periodontal diseases can present itself in a form of gingival swelling, and there were more postnatal mothers (72/75 (96.0%)) than pregnant women (150/181 (82.9%)) (Fisher's exact test, $P = 0.004$). Correct response to the question that gum or periodontal diseases can be prevented by visiting a dentist was given by 207/256 (80.9%) respondents, and there were more postnatal mothers (67/75 (89.3%)) than pregnant women (140/181 (77.3%)) ($\chi^2 = 4.922$, $P = 0.027$). Eating balanced diet was considered to be one of the preventive measures for gum or periodontal diseases by 138/257 (53.7%) study participants where the proportion of postnatal mothers was higher (49/76 (64.5%)) than pregnant women (89/181 (49.2%)) ($\chi^2 = 5.041$, $P = 0.025$). Use of plastic toothbrush was significantly higher among postnatal mothers (100%) than pregnant women (93.3%) ($\chi^2 = 9.762$, $P = 0.001$). Chewing stick users were almost equally distributed among the pregnant women (11.1%) and postnatal mothers (10.0%) ($\chi^2 = 0.119$, $P = 0.865$). Those who opted to use a finger for teeth cleaning were only found among pregnant women (3/270 (1.1%)); there were none from the group of postnatal mothers, and the differences were not statistically significant (Table 2). Two out of three (66.7%) participants who used a finger for teeth cleaning also reported to use toothpaste.

3.3. Self-Reported Periodontal Problems. The prevalence of self-reported periodontal problems included bleeding gums (23.2%), painful gums (15.9%), swollen gums (11.0%), reddish gums (10.5%), and tooth mobility (3.4%), and there was no statistically significant difference between pregnant women and postnatal mothers (Table 2). The differences in the proportion of study participants who have heard about dental plaque among pregnant women (184/270 (68.1%)) versus postnatal mothers (96/140 (68.6%)) as well as about calculus (171/270 (63.3%)) versus (81/140 (57.9%)), respectively, were not statistically significant (table not shown).

The level of knowledge of oral hygiene practices when categorized as "good" or "poor" in relation to different demographic factors among women attending the RHC clinics in rural Zambia is shown in Table 3.

Of all the participants in the category of good knowledge, there were more married women than singles, more of the low level of education, and more from the health centres than their respective counterparts. However, the level of knowledge of oral hygiene practices (good versus poor) did

TABLE 1: Distribution of the study participants by demographic characteristics.

Sociodemographic characteristics	Pregnant women, n (%)	Postnatal mothers, n (%)	All (n = 410), n (%)	χ^2 value	P value
Age group					
15–24 years	136 (50.4)	71 (50.7)	207 (50.5)		
25–45 years	134 (49.6)	69 (49.3)	203 (49.5)	0.004	0.947
Education level					
No/primary education	163 (60.4)	75 (53.6)	238 (58.0)		
Secondary and above	107 (39.6)	65 (46.4)	172 (42.0)	1.750	0.186
Marital status					
Single	47 (17.4)	22 (15.7)	69 (16.8)		
Ever married	223 (82.6)	118 (84.3)	341 (83.2)	0.189	0.664
Employment					
Unemployed	113 (41.9)	69 (49.3)	182 (44.4)		
Employed	157 (58.1)	71 (50.7)	228 (55.6)	2.064	0.151
Health facility					
Hospital	60 (22.2)	40 (28.6)	100 (24.4)		
Health centres	210 (77.8)	100 (71.4)	310 (75.6)	2.015	0.156

TABLE 2: Oral hygiene practices and self-reported periodontal problems among pregnant women and postnatal mothers in rural Zambia.

Oral hygiene practices	Distribution in percentages (%)			χ^2 value	P value
	All (n = 410)	Pregnant women (n = 270)	Postnatal mothers (n = 140)		
Cleaning of teeth and gums	98.3	98.9	97.1	1.675	0.196
Brushing once a day	24.9	23.0	28.6	3.798	0.284
Brushing twice a day	38.5	37.4	40.7	3.798	0.284
Brushing three times a day	36.3	39.3	30.7	3.798	0.284
Brushing once a week	0.2	0.4	0.0	3.798	0.284
Brush less than 1 minute	25.9	26.3	25.0	3.231	0.199
Brush 1–3 minutes	57.1	54.4	62.1	3.231	0.199
Brush more than 3 minutes	17.1	19.3	12.9	3.231	0.199
Use of toothbrush to clean teeth	95.6	93.3	100	9.762	0.001
Use of chewing stick to clean teeth	12.2	11.1	10.0	0.119	0.865
Use of toothpick to clean teeth	10.7	13.0	10.7	0.435	0.509
Use of finger to clean teeth	0.7	1.1	0.0	1.567	0.554
Regular use of toothpaste	91.7	92.2	90.7	0.276	0.600
Tongue brushing	55.4	53.3	59.3	1.322	0.250
Flossing	2.0	2.2	1.4	#	0.721
Use of mouth wash	13.9	16.3	9.3	3.786	0.070
Changes toothbrush (TBR) once/month	25.4	27.4	21.4	6.002	0.199
Changes TBR after 3 months	39.3	37.4	42.9	6.002	0.199
Changes TBR after 1 year	6.8	6.7	7.1	6.002	0.199
Changes TBR when bristles bend	25.6	24.4	27.9	6.002	0.199
Changes not the TBR	2.9	4.1	0.7	6.002	0.199
Bleeding gums	23.2	23.3	22.9	0.012	0.914
Painful gums	15.9	14.8	17.9	0.640	0.424
Swollen gums	11.0	10.7	11.4	0.45	0.833
Reddish gums	10.5	10.4	10.7	0.012	0.914
Tooth mobility	3.4	3.7	2.9	0.212	0.645

#Fisher's exact test (no chi-square value as the chi-square test was not used for this item) as one cell had 2 study participants only that is less than the minimum of 5 subjects.

not statistically differ significantly between age groups, marital status, level of education, employment, and type of health facility attended. There was a significantly higher proportion of pregnant women (Table 3) in the category of poor knowledge (69.8%) as compared to that of good knowledge of oral hygiene practices (59.2%) ($\chi^2 = 4.741$, $P = 0.029$) (Table 3).

The level of knowledge of gum and periodontal diseases in relation to different demographic factors among women attending the RHC clinics in rural Zambia is shown in Table 4. The level of knowledge of gum and periodontal diseases as categorized as "good" or "poor" in various demographic factors including pregnant women and postnatal mothers, low and high education, singles and married women, and employment status was homogeneous in that the difference was not statistically significant (Table 4).

Results of the bivariate analysis regarding self-reported gum bleeding in relation to maternal status (pregnant woman or postnatal mother), sociodemographic factors, lack

TABLE 3: The level of knowledge of oral hygiene practices in different demographic factors among women attending the RHC clinics in rural Zambia.

Demographic factors	Level of knowledge of oral hygiene practices		χ^2 value	P value
	Good n (%)	Poor n (%)		
Age group				
15–24 years	75 (49.3)	132 (51.2)	0.127	0.722
25–45 years	77 (50.7)	126 (48.8)		
Marital status				
Single	23 (15.1)	46 (17.8)	0.497	0.481
Ever married	129 (84.9)	212 (82.2)		
Education level				
No/primary education	86 (56.6)	152 (58.9)	0.214	0.643
Secondary and above	66 (43.4)	106 (41.1)		
Employment				
Unemployed	71 (46.7)	111 (43.0)	0.527	0.468
Employed	81 (53.3)	147 (57.0)		
Health facility				
Hospital	44 (28.9)	56 (21.7)	2.720	0.099
Health centres	108 (71.1)	202 (78.3)		
Study participants				
Pregnant women	90 (59.2)	180 (69.8)	4.741	0.029
Postnatal mothers	62 (40.8)	78 (30.2)		

TABLE 4: The level of knowledge of gum and periodontal diseases in relation to different demographic factors among women attending the RHC clinics in rural Zambia.

Demographic factors	Level of knowledge of gum/periodontal disease		χ^2 value	P value
	Good n (%)	Poor n (%)		
Women attending RHC				
Pregnant women	116 (69.5)	90 (61.6)	2.116	0.146
Postnatal mothers	51 (30.5)	56 (38.4)		
Age group				
15–24 years	87 (52.1)	65 (44.5)	1.790	0.181
25–45 years	80 (47.9)	81 (55.5)		
Education level				
No/primary education	92 (55.1)	85 (58.2)	0.310	0.577
Secondary and above	75 (44.9)	61 (41.8)		
Marital status				
Single	30 (18.0)	23 (15.8)	0.271	0.603
Ever married	137 (82.0)	123 (84.2)		
Employment				
Unemployed	73 (43.7)	67 (45.9)	0.149	0.699
Employed	94 (56.3)	79 (54.1)		
Health facility				
Hospital	45 (26.9)	36 (24.7)	0.213	0.645
Health centres	122 (73.1)	110 (75.3)		

of knowledge on periodontal diseases, oral hygiene practices, and self-reported periodontal problems are shown in Table 5. Prevalence of self-reported gum bleeding was significantly associated with being of older age 25–45 years ($\chi^2 = 4.04$, $P = 0.036$) and lack of knowledge that eating balanced diet can prevent gum and periodontal diseases ($\chi^2 = 5.527$, $P = 0.019$). Other significant factors were as follows: not changing the toothbrush after a period of 1–3 months ($\chi^2 = 10.766$, $P = 0.001$), self-reported presence of swollen gums ($\chi^2 = 97.703$, $P < 0.001$), reddish gums ($\chi^2 = 70.871$, $P < 0.001$), painful gums ($\chi^2 = 98.310$, $P < 0.001$), and shaky (mobile) teeth ($\chi^2 = 18.812$, $P < 0.001$).

The final model of the binary logistic regression analyses (backward stepwise, Wald) for occurrence of self-reported gum bleeding in relation to selected demographic factors and periodontal problems among pregnant women and postnatal mothers is shown in Table 6.

Factors that more likely and significantly associated with self-reported gum bleeding were being a pregnant woman (odds ratio (OR): 6.198, 95% confidence interval (CI): 1.620–23.715, $P = 0.008$), presence of reddish gums (OR: 4.724, 95% CI: 1.375–16.225, $P = 0.014$), painful gums (OR: 21.901, 95% CI: 6.731–71.264, $P < 0.001$), and toothpick use (OR: 4.288, 95% CI: 1.110–16.571, $P = 0.035$).

4. Discussion

The study was a quantitative, descriptive, cross-sectional investigation that took place among pregnant women and postnatal mothers in Chibombo and Chisamba rural districts in Zambia. The sample size and age ranges were almost similar to a study done in Nigeria [9]. This could be due to the fact that this is the reproductive age (15–49 years) in sub-Saharan Africa [17].

In the current study, it showed that majority of the women did not go to school or went up to primary level. This could be due to poverty and early marriages which stands at 31.4% in Zambia [18], especially in rural areas where this study was conducted as well as long distances to a few available schools [19] which led many to drop out of school and end up getting married.

The proportion of study participants that had primary education was similar to a study done in Pakistan [20], where more than half of the participants ended at primary school level (Asia levels at 64% versus sub-Saharan Africa with 65% [21]). The current study found that more than three quarters were married (83%) than the singles. This is different from the study done in south-west Sydney [22], where more than half of the participants were single, and it is speculated that the possible reason might be the difference in culture and lifestyles. Health centres had more RHC clinic attendances than the hospital. This can be attributed to the number of rural health centres included in the study (four) versus one rural hospital as is typical of levels and referral health system in Zambia. Another study done in Nigeria [9] reported that women do not seek professional help if they perceive that their gingival status is normal and that women were more likely to use dental services in pregnancy if married, educated, and had dental insurance. However, for comparability, retrievable reports on oral health among pregnant women in Zambia were scarce.

In the current study, almost all the respondents were brushing their teeth at least once per day and the finding is consistent with what was reported elsewhere in Tanzania [23]. The use of chewing sticks (twigs or roots of certain plants that are chewed until one end is frayed and used to clean teeth) in the current study was slightly more than one

TABLE 5: Bivariate analysis: self-reported gum bleeding in relation to sociodemographic factors, knowledge, oral hygiene practices, and self-assessed periodontal status.

Characteristics of the study participants	Whole sample (n = 410)		Self-reported gum bleeding				χ^2 value	P value
			Yes		No			
	n	%	n	%	N	%		
Maternal status								
Had pregnancy	270	65.9	63	66.3	207	65.7	0.012	0.914
Sociodemographic factors								
Age 25–45 years (not 15–24 years)	203	49.5	56	58.9	147	46.7	4.404	0.036
Had primary education or less	238	58.0	62	65.3	176	55.9	2.643	0.104
Not employed or have petty business	302	73.7	64	67.4	238	75.6	2.521	0.112
Knowledge: lack of knowledge								
Have not heard about plaque	130	31.7	35	36.8	95	30.2	1.506	0.220
Have not heard about calculus	158	38.1	41	43.2	117	37.1	1.115	0.291
On causes of periodontal diseases	146	46.6	37	52.1	109	45.0	1.103	0.294
That PD presents with gum bleeding	19	7.4	2	3.4	17	8.6	1.723	0.189
That PD presents with gum swelling	34	13.3	5	8.6	29	14.6	1.414	0.234
That PD presents with reddish gums	39	15.2	5	8.6	34	17.2	2.540	0.111
That calculus can be removed	107	42.5	27	50.0	80	40.4	1.599	0.206
That good oral hygiene can prevent PD	37	14.6	5	8.8	32	16.2	1.983	0.159
That eating balanced diet can prevent PD	119	46.3	19	32.8	100	50.3	5.527	0.019
That visiting a dentist can prevent PD	49	19.1	8	13.8	41	20.7	1.386	0.239
Oral hygiene practices								
Not using plastic toothbrush	18	4.4	7	7.4	11	3.5	2.613	0.106
Not changing toothbrush 1–3 months	145	35.4	47	49.5	98	31.1	10.766	0.001
Uses toothpick	50	12.2	17	17.9	33	10.5	3.751	0.053
Self-reported periodontal problems								
Had swollen gums	45	11.0	36	37.9	9	2.9	91.703	<0.001
Had reddish gums	43	10.5	32	33.7	11	3.5	70.871	<0.001
Had painful gums	65	15.9	46	48.4	19	6.0	98.310	<0.001
Had shaky teeth	14	3.4	10	10.5	4	1.3	18.812	<0.001

#Each condition presented in this table has basically ""Yes and No" alternatives with numerical values corresponding to each individual situation. Only the numerical values corresponding to "Yes" have been presented in this table and the counterpart alternative ("No") numerical values have been left out. For example, if have swollen gums ("Yes versus No"), only the numerical values for "Yes" have been presented in this table while the ones corresponding to "No" have been left out; PD = periodontal diseases.

TABLE 6: Final model of logistic regression backward stepwise (Wald) analyses: binary logistic regression analyses in relation to self-reported gum bleeding versus demographic factors and periodontal problems among the study participants.

Characteristics of the study participant	B	SE	Odds ratio	95% confidence interval	P value
Had pregnancy	1.824	0.685	6.198	1.620–23.715	0.008
Had reddish gums	1.553	0.630	4.724	1.375–16.225	0.014
Had gum pains	3.087	0.602	21.901	6.731–71.264	<0.001
Uses toothpicks	1.456	0.690	4.288	1.110–16.571	0.035

Key: B = beta weights (regression coefficient), SE = standard error.

to ten (1 : 10), and the possible explanation might be due to difficult affordability within the rural constraint economy and these results are consistent with the studies done in Nigeria and Tanzania, respectively [2, 23]. In the present study, a minority of the subjects use dental floss, unlike the study done in Australia [6] where the majority were using dental floss with an understanding that it would help prevent gum disease. This shows that the participants in the current study in rural Zambia had insufficient knowledge on interdental space cleaning and were limited to toothbrushes as cleaning aids [24]. Most of the study participants pointed out that plaque can be controlled by maintaining good oral hygiene, and this is achieved by brushing the teeth at least twice daily and this is in line with what is recommended

worldwide [21]. Serious attention to this important preliminary understanding emphasis on oral hygiene instruction, for example, systematic tooth brushing for two minutes [25] and interdental cleaning might be a good area to begin with when launching customized oral health program in Zambia. The most used tooth cleaning aids were plastic toothbrush, followed by chewing stick, whereby the latter is believed to be an effective oral hygiene aid by which different cultures have attached functional value since ancient times [26]. It happened that about one percent of the pregnant women used a finger for cleaning teeth whereas their level of education was above primary school. This could be due to extreme poverty as most of them were unemployed. Also, the issue of beliefs cannot be underestimated because these participants, for example, could have used chewing sticks that were readily available in rural areas.

The proportion of knowledge of periodontal diseases displayed by women in the age group less than 30 years was moderately higher compared to those above 30 years, and further, it was higher among the singles as compared to the married; however, the differences did not reach a statistically significant level. The study participants who had attained secondary education were more knowledgeable than the ones who were primary school leavers or below. This simply shows that education plays a part in terms of knowledge and exposure [27]; however, the difference was statistically insignificant. The proportion of pregnant women that had knowledge of periodontal disease was moderately higher than the postnatal mothers. The reason could be that pregnant women were able to identify themselves with the features of periodontal diseases that are modified by the presence of high levels of circulating hormones during pregnancy; however, the differences did not reach a statistically significant level. Even though the pregnant women and the postnatal mothers were knowledgeable about periodontal diseases, only a minority were aware of the causative factor and dental plaque. This may point to a serious need for proper oral health education to the pregnant women and postnatal mothers in the studied rural population. Slightly less than three quarters of the participants knew what plaque was and how it could be removed, and this is consistent with the Saudi Arabia study [28], but inconsistent with the findings from elsewhere [6] where the majority knew about dental plaque and did not know about periodontal disease. The possible explanation for this might be the differences in the availability of oral health education and health promotion programs in these populations [29]. The majority of the pregnant women and postnatal mothers knew the presentation of periodontal disease as well as the prevention. Proper nutrition and healthy lifestyle also play a key role in the general well-being of the mother to be, and this includes periodontal health [30].

Regarding self-reported gum and periodontal problems, a minority of the study participants reported having bleeding gums, and the findings are similar to those reported by women attending a tertiary health institution in Nigeria [31]. On the other hand, our findings differ from the ones reported in Nigerian women [32] and Ghanaian women [33] where bleeding of gums was much higher than what was found in our study, and the most probable explanation is the difference in methodology. The current study has a low proportion of women reporting painful gums, swollen gums, and bleeding gums as compared to other studies which revealed that hormonal changes in pregnancy combined with neglected oral hygiene tend to increase the gingivitis which is characterized by increased redness, edema, and higher tendency toward bleeding [34, 35].

Use of plastic toothbrush in our study was significantly higher among pregnant mothers than postnatal women, and this difference might be accounted by possible exposure to oral health education session during antenatal visits. The results in the current study are similar to the study done in Nigeria [36] where most of the participants used plastic toothbrushes and paste.

Likewise, there were no statistically significant differences on the level of knowledge of gum and periodontal diseases in relation to different demographic factors between pregnant women and postnatal mothers in our study, thus showing a similar experience between the groups. These results are in agreement with Bangalore report where awareness of gum disease among pregnant women was not associated with age and educational qualifications [37].

Lack of knowledge that eating balanced diet can prevent gum and periodontal diseases was in the bivariate analysis found to be a significant factor as regards to the self-reported gum bleeding on tooth brushing. Lack of knowledge on the importance of balanced diet was higher in our study than in Bilaspur, India [38], and the possible reason among others was that our study was done in rural area alone while the latter was in both urban and rural. In comparison with postnatal mothers, pregnant women were significantly more likely to experience gum bleeding on tooth brushing, and this might be explained by the inflammatory reaction of the gingival due to hormonal changes coupled with presence of poor oral hygiene [34, 35]. Findings from a similar study in India revealed that less than one third of the studied pregnant women had experienced bleeding from gums during pregnancy, and that, slightly less than a quarter did not brush their teeth when they experienced bleeding, instead, they cleaned using fingers [39].

The results of this study must be viewed in the light of certain limitations. Due to constraint in resources especially time and funds to collect data for this elective study, the rural area was selected for convenience. This approach limits the inference of the findings to be much more applicable to the rural districts studied population and not to the whole RHC clinic attendees in the country. This study relied on self-reported information and therefore the data are subject to some form of bias. Furthermore, the face-to-face interview with most of the study participants might have provoked "socially desirable responses" instead of what was the real practice in daily life [40, 41].

5. Conclusions

In this study, most pregnant women and postnatal mothers had general knowledge of periodontal diseases but only few knew the cause and their prevention. All participants were engaged in tooth cleaning procedures; however, the majority did not know the appropriate practices. Self-reported signs of gingival and periodontal diseases were experienced by the minority.

6. Recommendations

In view of the ever growing evidence that periodontal diseases are associated with various systemic conditions including adverse pregnancy outcomes, it is recommended that oral health be integrated into general health care of pregnant women in all reproductive and child health clinics in the country.

Ethical Approval

Ethical clearance was granted by the Research and Publication Committee of the School of Dentistry empowered by MUHAS Ethical Committee.

Disclosure

This work was an elective research study which was part of the requirement for the Doctor of Dental Surgery (DDS) undergraduate training at Muhimbili University of Health and Allied Sciences (MUHAS).

Authors' Contributions

T. M. Kabali participated in developing the proposal and data collection tool, performed all the data collection, data entry into the computer, and some data analysis under guidance, and was responsible for interpretation, write-up, and submission of the manuscript. E. G. Mumghamba conceived the study, supervised the development of proposal and data collection tool, performed data entry into the computer, data cleaning, guided data analysis, and logistic regression analyses, was responsible for interpretation and write-up, and gave final approval to submission of the manuscript.

Acknowledgments

This study was sponsored by the Ministry of Health (Zambia) as an undergraduate (T. M. Kabali) "elective study" research work at the Muhimbili University of Health and Allied Sciences.

References

[1] G.C. Armitage, "Development of a classification system for periodontal diseases and conditions," *Annals of Periodontology*, vol. 4, no. 1, pp. 1–6, 1999.

[2] L. Shaw, U. Harjunmaa, R. Doyle et al., "Distinguishing the signals of gingivitis and periodontitis in supragingival plaque, a cross-sectional study in Malawi," *Applied and Environmental Microbiology*, vol. 82, no. 19, pp. 6057–6067, 2016.

[3] M.S. De Franceschi, L. Fortunato, C. Carallo et al., "Periodontal disease and carotid atherosclerosis: mechanisms of the association," in *Oral Health Care-Prosthodontics, Periodontology, Biology, Research and Systemic Conditions*, InTech, London, UK, 2012.

[4] N. Silva, L. Abusleme, D. Bravo et al., "Host response mechanisms in periodontal diseases," *Journal of Applied Oral Science*, vol. 23, no. 3, pp. 329–355, 2015.

[5] A. F. E. Carillo-de-Albornoz, D. C. P. Herrera, and A. Bascones-Martinez, "Gingival changes during pregnancy: III. Impact of clinical, microbiological, immunological and socio-demographic factors on gingival inflammation," *Journal of Clinical Periodontology*, vol. 39, no. 3, pp. 272–283, 2011.

[6] N. J. Thomas, P. F. Middleton, and C. A. Crowther, "Oral and dental health care practices in pregnant women in Australia: a postnatal survey," *BMC Pregnancy and Childbirth*, vol. 8, no. 1, p. 13, 2008.

[7] R. Ovadia, R. Zirdok, and R. M. Diaz-Romero, "Pregnancy outcomes influenced by periodontitis," *Medicine and Biology*, vol. 14, no. 1, pp. 10–14, 2007.

[8] J. Otomo-Corgel, "Periodontal therapy in the female patient," in *Carranza's Clinical Periodontology*, F. A. Carranza, P. R. Klokkevold, H. H. Takei, and M. J. Newman, pp. 412–421, Elsevier Saunders, 11th edition, 2012.

[9] J. U. Ifesanya and G. A. Oke, "Self-report of adverse gingival conditions among pregnant south-western Nigerian women," *Journal of Dentistry and Oral Hygiene*, vol. 5, no. 2, pp. 13–20, 2013.

[10] M. L. Geisinger, M. Robinson, M. Kaur et al., "Individualized oral health education improves oral hygiene compliance and clinical outcomes in pregnant women with Gingivitis," *Journal of Oral Hygiene and Health*, vol. 1, no. 2, pp. 1–9, 2013.

[11] A. Srivastava, K. K. Gupta, S. Srivastava, and J. Garg, "Effects of sex hormones on the gingiva in pregnancy: a review and report of two cases," *Journal of Periodontology and Implant Dentistry*, vol. 3, no. 2, pp. 83–87, 2011.

[12] A. Villa, S. Abati, L. Strohmenger, M. Cargnel, and I. Cetin, "Self-reported oral hygiene habits and periodontal symptoms among postpartum women," *Archives of Gynecology and Obstetrics*, vol. 284, no. 1, pp. 245–249, 2011.

[13] X. Xiong, P. Buekens, W. D. Fraser, J. Beck, and S. Offenbacher, "Periodontal disease and adverse pregnancy outcomes: a systematic review," *An International Journal of Obstetrics and Gynaecology*, vol. 113, no. 2, pp. 135–143, 2006.

[14] J. Silness and H. Loe, "Periodontal disease in pregnancy II. Correlation between oral hygiene and periodontal condition," *Journal Acta Odontologica Scandinavica*, vol. 22, no. 1, pp. 121–135, 1964.

[15] M. A. Laine, "Effects of pregnancy on periodontal and dental health," *Journal Acta Odontologica Scandinavica*, vol. 60, no. 5, pp. 257–264, 2002.

[16] C. M. Barness, C. M. Russel, R. A. Reinhardt, J. B. Payne, and D. M. Lyle, "Comparison of irrigation to floss as an adjunct to tooth brushing: effects on bleeding, gingivitis and supragingival plaque," *Journal of Clinical Dentistry*, vol. 16, no. 3, pp. 71–77, 2005.

[17] C. Ronsmans and W. J. Graham, "Maternal mortality, who, when, where and why," *The Lancet*, vol. 368, no. 9542, pp. 1189–1200, 2006.

[18] UNFPA and Government of the Republic of Zambia, *Policy Brief, Child Marriage in Zambia, Lusaka, Zambia*, Population Council, New York, NY, USA, 2017.

[19] UNICEF ESARO and UIS, "Global initiative on out-of-school children," ESAR Regional Report, pp. 1–106, UNICEF, Nairobi, Kenya, 2014.

[20] S. Shabbir, M. Zahi, and A. Qazi, "Oral hygiene among pregnant women, practices and knowledge," *Professional Medical Journal*, vol. 22, no. 1, pp. 106–111, 2015.

[21] L. Zhu, P.E. Peterson, H. Wang, J. Bian, and B. Zhang, "Oral health knowledge attitude and behavior of adults in China," *International Dental Journal*, vol. 55, no. 4, pp. 231–241, 2005.

[22] A. George, M. Johnson, A. Blinkhorn et al., "The oral health status, practices and knowledge of pregnant women in south-west Sydney," *Australian Dental Journal*, vol. 58, no. 1, pp. 26–33, 2013.

[23] E. G. Mumghamba, K. P. Manji, and J. Michael, "Oral health practices, periodontal conditions status and self-reported bad mouth breath among mothers, Tanzania," *International Journal of Dental Hygiene*, vol. 4, no. 4, pp. 166–173, 2006.

[24] J. Ramamurthy and F. Irfana, "Assessment of knowledge and awareness about periodontal oral health among pregnant women-a questionnaire study," *International Journal of Current Pharmaceutical Review and Research*, vol. 9, no. 1, pp. 9–12, 2017.

[25] J. Asadoorian, "CDHA position paper on tooth brushing," *Canadian Journal of Dental Hygiene*, vol. 40, no. 5, pp. 232–248, 2006.

[26] F. N. M. Nordin, S. R. A. S. Mohsain, and S. M. Tamizi, "A review on the Sunnah of Miswak (Salvadora Persica) and its potentiality to improve oral health," *Revelation and Science*, vol. 2, no. 1, pp. 33–41, 2012.

[27] A. Duha, C. Colin, and M. Naci, "The impact of education on health knowledge," *Economics of Education Review*, vol. 30, no. 5, pp. 792–812, 2011.

[28] F. A. Asaad, G. A. I. Rahman, N. A. I. Mahmoud, E. Shamasi, and A. Alkhuwailerdj, "Periodontal disease awareness among pregnant women in the central eastern region of Saudi Arabia," *Journal of Investigative and Clinical Dentistry*, vol. 6, no. 1, pp. 8–15, 2015.

[29] P. D. Nakre and A. G. Harikiran, "Effectiveness of oral hygiene education progress: a systematic review," *Journal of International Society of Preventive and Community Dentistry*, vol. 3, no. 2, pp. 103–115, 2013.

[30] S. Najeeb, M. S. Zafar, Z. Khurshid, S. Zohaib, and K. Almas, "The role of nutrition in periodontal health: an update," *NCBI Resources*, vol. 8, no. 9, p. 530, 2016.

[31] B. O. Bishiru and I. N. Anthony, "Oral health awareness and experience among pregnant women in Nigerian Tertiary Health Institution," *Journal of Dental Research and Review*, vol. 1, no. 2, pp. 66–69, 2014.

[32] O. O. Onigbinde, M. E. Sorunke, M. O. Braimoh, and A. O. Adeniyi, "Periodontal status and some variables among pregnant women in a Nigeria Tertiary Institution," *Annals of Medical and Health Sciences Research*, vol. 4, no. 6, pp. 852–857, 2014.

[33] I. Nuamah and B. D. Annan, "Periodontal status and oral hygiene practices of pregnant and non-pregnant women," *East African Medical Journal*, vol. 75, no. 12, pp. 712–714, 1998.

[34] M. R. Hasan, A. B. Dithi, N. A. Nomann, J. Nessa, and T. Saito, "Self-reported oral and dental health status among pregnant women of a selected hospital in Dhaka city," *Bangladesh Journal of Dental Research and Education*, vol. 4, no. 2, pp. 61–64, 2015.

[35] J. Chandropooja, R. Gayathri, and V. vishnupri, "Oral health during pregnancy-a systematic review," *Journal of Pharmaceutical Sciences and Research*, vol. 8, no. 8, pp. 841–843, 2016.

[36] J. U. Ifesanya, A. O. Ifesanya, M. C. Asuzu, and G. A. Oke, "Determinants of good oral hygiene among pregnant women in Ibadan, south-western Nigeria," *Annals of Ibadan Postgraduate Medicine*, vol. 8, no. 2, pp. 95–100, 2010.

[37] S. Singh, K. Dagrus, P. B. Kariya, S. Singh, J. Darmina, and P. Hase, "Oral periodontal health knowledge and awareness among pregnant females in Bangalore, India," *International Journal of Dental and Medical Research*, vol. 1, no. 6, pp. 7–10, 2015.

[38] R. Nagi, S. Sahu, and R. Nagaraju, "Oral health, nutritional knowledge, and practices among pregnant women and their awareness relating to adverse pregnancy outcomes," *Journal of Indian Academy of Oral Medicine and Radiology*, vol. 28, no. 4, pp. 396–402, 2016.

[39] P. Sajjan, J. I. Pattanshetti, C. Padmini, V. M. Nagathan, M. Sajjanar, and T. Siddiqui, "Oral health related awareness and practices among pregnant women in Bagalkot district, Karnataka, India," *Journal of International Oral Health*, vol. 7, no. 2, pp. 1–5, 2015.

[40] J. H. Abramson and Z. H. Abramson, *Survey Methods in Community Medicine, Epidemiological Research, Program Evaluation and Clinical Trials*, Churchill Livingstone, Edinburgh, 5th edition, 1999.

[41] L. A. Sanzone, J. Y. Lee, K. Divaris, D. A. DeWalt, A. D. Baker, and W. F. Vann Jr., "A cross sectional study examining social desirability bias in caregiver reporting of children's oral health behaviors," *BMC Oral Health*, vol. 13, no. 1, p. 24, 2013.

25

The Role and Impact of Salivary Zn Levels on Dental Caries

Milaim Sejdini,[1] **Agim Begzati** ⓘ**,**[2] **Sami Salihu,**[3] **Sokol Krasniqi,**[1] **Nora Berisha** ⓘ**,**[1] **and Nora Aliu**[1]

[1]*Faculty of Medicine, Orthodontic Clinic, University of Pristina, Pristina, Kosovo*
[2]*Faculty of Medicine, Paediatric Dentistry Clinic, University of Pristina, Pristina, Kosovo*
[3]*Faculty of Medicine, Maxillofacial Surgery Clinic, University of Pristina, Pristina, Kosovo*

Correspondence should be addressed to Agim Begzati; agim.begzati@uni-pr.edu

Academic Editor: Ali I. Abdalla

Introduction. Minimal attention has been given to the role of salivary microelements, the importance they have in reducing the intensity of caries, and the effect of caries prophylaxes. *Aim.* This research aimed to determine the concentration and quantity of Zn and its impact on the prevention and the reduction of the intensity of caries in schoolchildren aged 12-13 years with permanent dentition. *Methods.* For this research, we analyzed the stimulated and nonstimulated full saliva of 106 schoolchildren divided into three groups by mean decayed, missing, and filled teeth (DMFT) index. The control group consisted of 25 caries-free children, the second group had 47 children with mean DMFT index of 1 to 6, and the third group had 34 children with DMFT index of ≥ 6. Complete saliva was collected from all children in a sterile test tube. *Results.* The concentration of Zn in saliva before stimulation in caries-free children has variations of the order of 0.001+ to 0.01 mmol/l. The maximum concentration after stimulation is 6.72 mmol/l, while the maximum value is 64.38 mmol/l. *Conclusion.* The Zn concentration in the stimulated saliva showed a significant increase in the group of caries-free children and could be described as a positive value for the reduction of caries.

1. Introduction

A number of theories attempt to explain the mechanism of initiation of the appearance of caries. Recent research shows that caries have multicausal aetiology, mostly under the influence of general factors but especially under the influence of local factors.

Dental caries is perhaps the most ubiquitous disease that has afflicted mankind. While it is not normally a fatal condition, it can cause a great deal of pain and distress, and the loss of teeth has profound consequences in terms of eating, speaking, and social behavior in general [1]. In recent years, particular importance in the appearance of caries has been devoted to saliva because of the impact of its chemical components and immunology [2, 3].

Although it is known that the basic prerequisites for the appearance of cavities are defined by the presence of microorganisms, the substrate, and the tooth itself for a certain period of time, all of this occurs under the influence of the liquid media of the mouth saliva. In their researches, Gamershtein and Maksimovski [4] and Tvinnereim et al. [5] showed that the appearance of caries is directly affected by the presence of salivary components, specifically the amount of microelements that are present. Saliva, with the presence and composition of its immunochemistry, enables a large number of functions within oral homeostasis such as maintenance of oral cavity humidity and its self-cleaning ability, buffer of oral media, stabilization and preservation of bacterial flora, maintenance and preservation of the surrounding tooth minerals, digestive activity, control of pH, and many other functions.

According to Dawes [6], Mason and Chisholm [7], and Schmidt [8], during high salivary flow, osmolarity can reach plasma osmolarity, while the flow of nonstimulated saliva can be so low that it can reach 1/20 of the plasma osmolarity. Research regarding salivary electrolytes shows that the saliva is saturated with some of the ions. Between the components of salivary electrolytes and those deposited in the enamel of the tooth, it has been found that there are certain equilibrium and controlled report [6–8].

The most important microelements that are present include calcium, sodium, magnesium, zinc, and fluoride; these are of great importance for the mineralization and maturation of hard tooth tissue [9].

The relationship that trace elements in saliva might have with dental caries activity has interested scientists for many years [10].

Qualitative and quantitative analysis (EDS X-rays) shows evidence that the lowest content of the macroelements Ca, P, C, and O and the microelements Al, Cl, In, Mg, Si, Na, S, and W was found in carious enamel layers compared with normal enamel layers [11].

There is an evident difference in salivary electrolyte concentrations from different sources of saliva. Parotid saliva contains fewer Zn electrolytes of Zn and is the opposite of the concentration of Zn^{2+} in the mixed saliva; the concentration of Zn^{2+} varies significantly. The research regarding mineral components in saliva is scarce and has contradictory results with respect to their role in the process of demineralization, remineralization, and dental maturity [12]. In saliva, Zn plays multiple roles and affects many metabolic processes. Its role in the metabolism of protein is so important that it is compared with essential amino acids. It is found in the composition of many enzymes where their activation depends on the presence of Zn. The impact and the amount of Zn in the tooth enamel are more in the outer layer (200–900 ppm) compared to the inner layer (up to 200 ppm) [13–15]. Curzon has noted that zinc and calcium showed promise as antiplaque agents, whereas Sr and Zn may enhance remineralization in enamel [16].

Research has shown that Zn is easily incorporated as a substitute for Ca^{++} ions. Its incorporation in the enamel helps decrease its solubility. In many publications, the role of Zn in dental plaque and oral tissue has been described as an important factor in reducing the ability of bacteria, especially anaerobic bacteria [2, 9].

Zinc salts have antibacterial actions due to their ability to inhibit bacterial adhesion, metabolic activity, and growth [17].

Relatively large amounts of zinc are incorporated into enamel prior to eruption, but after eruption, zinc concentration at the surface of the teeth apparently increases further, suggesting that some incorporation does occur during posteruptive exposure to the oral fluids [18].

Zinc competes with calcium for bacterial-binding sites in model biofilms, and it has been proposed that half of the bound zinc would be released under cariogenic conditions through, for example, protonation of carboxylate and phosphate groups in bacterial lipoteichoic acid [19].

The aim of this research was to find the Zn values in a group of caries-free children and two other groups with vulnerability to caries to determine the concentration and volume of Zn in the full stimulated and nonstimulated saliva through chemical and immunochemical analysis.

Also, this research aimed to define the influence of this microelement in preventing or reducing the rate of the incidence of caries in schoolchildren aged 12-13 years with permanent dentition.

2. Materials and Methods

This research was conducted on 106 schoolchildren aged 12 to 13 years with permanent dentition. This was a cross-sectional study where all children were divided into three groups (control group and two groups with vulnerability). The control group was composed of children with all caries-free teeth (DMFT index = 0), healthy oral tissues, and good oral hygiene (25 children). The second group were children with a mean DMFT index of 1 to 6 (47 children), and the third group were children with a mean DMFT index of > 6 (34 children). Nonstimulated saliva was taken from all of the children in the morning because of the circadian rhythm for five-minute duration. For obtaining the stimulated saliva, a clean paraffin wax bone was used for chewing for the duration of five minutes. All samples were taken in sterile test tubes that were graded; until the analysis, the samples were stored in chambers at a temperature of −20°C. Chemical and immunochemical tests were conducted at the Faculty of Science, Ss. Cyril and Methodius University in Skopje. Analyses were performed by flame atomic absorption spectrometer model Solar S4 from Thermo Elemental (UK), at a wavelength of 213.9 nm, spectral slit of 0.5 nm, and lamp current of 10 mA, representing a method with relatively high sensitivity. For the determination of zinc, 1 ml of saliva was diluted with redistilled water in a 10 ml volumetric flask. Statistical analyses were processed with Statistics for Windows/Release 7.0, at the Institute of Statistics of the Faculty of Medicine in Skopje. We obtained permission for this research from the corresponding institutions of our country.

3. Results and Discussion

Publications describing the mineral composition of native nonstimulated saliva are few; in the research that has been published, the results are often contradictory. Fluctuations of the volumetric physiological sphere of studied electrolytes are caused by the speed of saliva flow and the composition changes of the various secretions of salivary glands.

Table 1 shows the concentration values of the examined samples and the amount of Zn in saliva before and after stimulation with paraffin. The first group (control) had a concentration of Zn in stimulated saliva that varied in the interval of 0.01 ± 0.01 mmol/l, with a confidence interval of −0.01 + 0.01, a minimum value of 0.0002, and a maximum value of 0.03 mmol/l. The Zn concentration in the stimulated saliva showed variations in the interval of 0.28 ± 1.35, with a confidence interval of −0.27 + 0.83 mmol/l. The minimum value was 0.002, while the maximum value was 6.78 mmol/l. The Zn amount before stimulation was 0.02 ± 0.02 μmol/l. The minimum value is 0.0001 μmol/l, while the maximum value is 0.07 μmol/l. The amount of Zn after stimulation showed a more pronounced change with values of 2.65 μmol/l, with a standard deviation of ± 12.86,

TABLE 1: Concentration and quantity of Zn before and after stimulation in caries-free children.

Parameters	N	Mean	Confidence −95.00%	Confidence 95.00%	Minimum	Maximum	SD
Zn concentration, mmol/l (before the stimulation)	25	0.01	−0.01	0.01	0.0002	0.03	0.01
Zn concentration, mmol/l (after the stimulation)	25	0.28	−0.27	0.83	0.002	6.78	1.35
Zn quantity (μmol/l): before the stimulation	25	0.02	−0.01	0.03	0.0001	0.07	0.02
Zn quantity (μmol/l): after the stimulation	25	2.65	−2.66	7.96	0.02	64.38	12.86

TABLE 2: Zn concentration before and after the stimulation.

Parameters	N	T	Z	Found p	p	Sig./N. sig.
Zn concentration (before/after stimulation)	25	142	0.55	0.58	>0.05	N. sig.
Zn quantity (before/after stimulation)	25	30	3.56	0.0003	<0.001	Sig.

Sig = significant, N. sig = not significant.

TABLE 3: Concentration and quantity of Zn before and after stimulation in children with DMFT index of 1–6.

Parameters	N	Mean	Confidence −95.00%	Confidence 95.00%	Minimum	Maximum	SD
Zn concentration, mmol/l (before the stimulation)	47	0.01	0.009	0.01	0.0002	0.08	0.01
Zn concentration, mmol/l (after the stimulation)	47	0.01	0.005	0.01	0.0005	0.07	0.01
Zn quantity (μmol/l): before the stimulation	47	0.02	0.01	0.03	0.0005	0.16	0.03
Zn quantity (μmol/l): after the stimulation	47	0.07	0.03	0.11	0.002	0.71	0.12

a confidence interval of −2.66 + 7.96, and a maximum value of 64.38 μmol/l.

Table 2 shows the differences in the concentration and quantity of Zn before and after stimulation. The concentration of Zn after stimulation was $Z = 0.55$ and showed no increase compared with that prior to stimulation ($p < 0.05$), while the amount of Zn was $Z = 3.56$ and showed a significant increase after salivary stimulation ($p < 0.001$).

A reported decrease in the molarities of Ca and Zn that are found in caries can be very important in acknowledging the risk of caries, namely, to have an important role in the demineralization process of tooth decay. A relative surplus of Zn over Ca can be more closely associated with the occurrence of caries because it is validated with statistical tests.

Table 3 shows the values of Zn concentration and the quantity before and after stimulation in children with DMFT index of 1–6. The Zn concentration varies before stimulation at intervals of 0.01 ± 0.01 mmol/l, with a confidence interval of −0009 + 0.01, a minimum value of 0.0002, and a maximum value of 0.08 mmol/l. The Zn concentration after stimulation has variations with intervals of 0.01 ± 0.01 mmol/l, with a confidence interval of −0005 + 0.01, a minimum value of 0.0005, and a maximum value of 0.07 mmol/l. The Zn amount before the stimulation varied at intervals of 0.02 ± 0.03 μmol/l, with a confidence interval of −0.01 + 0.03, a minimum value of 0.0005, and a maximum value of 0.16 μmol/l. The amount of Zn after stimulation varies, ranging between 0.07 ± 0.12 μmol/l, with a confidence interval of −0.03 + 0.11, a minimum value of 0.002, and a maximum value of 0.71 μmol/l.

The highest incidence of enamel lesions was observed in the mandibular molars in rats fed with Zn-deficit diets compared with mice doubly fed with supplementary Zn diets. Furthermore, the effects of Zn deficiencies in caries in young mice were observed in a greater mass in the smooth surface of molar zinc. Dietary Zn may be a trace mineral that is important during the posteruptive process of enamel mineralization; it could reduce a tooth's sensitivity to caries.

Table 4 shows the differences in Zn concentration and quantity before and after saliva stimulation. For $Z = 1.84$, no significant changes were observed in the Zn concentration after stimulation ($p < 0.05$). The amount of Zn for $Z = 3.36$ is significantly higher after stimulation with high valuation ($p < 0.001$).

Table 5 shows the values of Zn concentration and quantity before and after stimulation of the third group of researched children with a mean DMFT index of > 6.

The Zn concentration before and after stimulation in the saliva did not show significant differences; the amount of Zn before and after stimulation showed significance in the saliva after stimulation for the interval of 0.04 ± 12.08 μmol/l, with a confidence interval of −0.01 + 0.07, a minimum value of 0.0006, and a maximum value of 12.48 μmol/l.

Differences between Zn concentration and quantity before and after stimulation are presented in Table 6. The concentration of Zn after stimulation for $Z = 0.84$ did not show important differences ($p < 0.05$); the amount of Zn for $Z = 3.65$ significantly increased, showing statistical significance ($p < 0.001$).

Differences were observed among the three groups in this research (Table 7) for $H = 2.54$ ($p < 0.05$); for $H = 3.56$, no significant difference was found in the Zn concentration before and after saliva stimulation nor in the nonstimulated saliva (for $H = 5.66$ and $p < 0.05$). A difference was observed among the three groups in the Zn amount after stimulation for $H = 7.99$ ($p < 0.05$).

The amount of Zn for $U = 568.00$ (Table 8) among the groups before stimulation is obviously higher in the second

TABLE 4: Zn concentration before and after the stimulation in children with DMFT index of 1–6.

Parameters	N	T	Z	Found p	p	Sig./N. sig.
Zn concentration (before/after stimulation)	47	390	1.84	0.065	> 0.05	N. sig.
Zn quantity (before/after stimulation)	47	246	3.36	0.0007	< 0.001	Sig.

TABLE 5: Concentration and quantity of Zn before and after stimulation with mean DMFT index of >6.

Parameters	N	Mean	Confidence −95.00%	Confidence 95.00%	Minimum	Maximum	SD
Zn concentration, mmol/l (before the stimulation)	34	0.008	0.005	0.01	0.0002	0.03	0.008
Zn concentration, mmol/l (after the stimulation)	34	0.007	0.003	0.01	0.0002	0.05	0.009
Zn quantity, μmol/l (before the stimulation)	34	0.01	0.007	0.02	0.0005	0.07	0.01
Zn quantity, μmol/l (after the stimulation)	34	0.04	0.01	0.07	0.0006	0.49	0.08

TABLE 6: Zn concentration before and after stimulation in children with mean DMFT index of >6.

Parameters	N	T	Z	Found p	p	Sig./N. sig.
Zn concentration (before/after stimulation)	34	248	0.84	0.39	> 0.05	N. sig.
Zn quantity (before/after stimulation)	34	84	3.65	0.0002	< 0.001	Sig.

TABLE 7: Statistical significance for the analyzed parameters between 3 groups.

Parameters	DMFT index	H	Found p	p	Sig./N. sig.
Zn concentration, mmol/l (before stimulation)	<1 / 1–6 / >6	2.54	0.28	> 0.05	N. sig.
Zn concentration, mmol/l (after stimulation)	<1 / 1–6 / >6	3.56	0.16	> 0.05	N. sig.
Zn quantity, μmol/l (before stimulation)	<1 / 1–6 / >6	5.66	0.05	> 0.05	N. sig.
Zn quantity, μmol/l (after stimulation)	<1	7.99	0.01	< 0.05	Sig.

TABLE 8: Significant differences among analyzed groups.

Parameters	Compartments between groups	U	Found p	p	Sig/N. sig
Zn quantity, μmol/l (before the stimulation)	Gr_2/Gr_3	568.0	0.02	< 0.05	Sig.
Zn quantity, μmol/l (after the stimulation)	Gr_1/Gr_3	240.0	0.004	< 0.01	Sig.

group compared to the third group ($p < 0.05$), while for $U = 240$, the amount of Zn after stimulation has had an ascendance of great importance in the first group compared to the third group ($p < 0.01$).

Although we expected that there will be differences in the three groups for $H = 5.66$, we did not find a statistical significance during the comparison. Differences for $U = 568$ and $U = 240$ in the three groups showed a statistical significance at $p < 0.01$ and $p < 0.05$, respectively.

During the research, we saw that Zn was easily incorporated in the hydroxyapatite, exchanging with the Ca^{+2} ions. With the incorporation of Zn, the dissolution of enamel decreases, but this does not affect the appearance of caries [20]. Insufficient data to describe the role of Zn in the process of caries have been presented in the literature. Quantitative analysis of ions released into solution following the demineralization of samples confirmed that Zn reduces the rate of demineralization as a function of concentration. To influence enamel demineralization under cariogenic conditions, Zn must be available in the plaque fluid at a concentration sufficient to reduce or inhibit tooth mineral loss [21]. Contrary to the research done by Mohammed et al. [21], a study by Duggal et al. found that the concentration of Zn had no relationship with dental caries [22].

The results of Bales and Freeland-Graves [23], Fang et al. [14], and Gregory et al. [24] showed that, in the mice fed with a diet deficient in Zn, the incidence of caries has been high in the molars compared to the mice fed with normal food. This shows a close connection of Zn with proteins. Although there is little research on the role of Zn in the process of decay, in our research, the concentration of Zn is significantly higher in the saliva of children with caries where quantitative growth of Zn is evident in the two groups of children; this could, together with the "empty spaces," have the potential to show the demineralization role of saliva. It is assumed that Zn is easily released from the crystalline structure by leaving "empty space." Our results are similar to those of Tvinnerein et al. [25]. Regarding the clinical effects of zinc on de- and remineralization, it seems unlikely that potentially beneficial effects, such as reductions in solubility and enhanced/prolonged lesion porosity to mineral ingress, will counter any possible negative effects [26]. In light of the current findings, it would appear that there is scope for exploring and optimizing the therapeutic potential of zinc, not only as an antibacterial agent but also as a possible preventive treatment for caries [21]. Distinguished from the results of other authors [27, 28], our data do not match since they have worked in selective saliva (from the saliva of the selected gland, with incomplete saliva) and because of the indirect influence of saliva on dental plaque. Differences were also prescribed to children's age and the presence of mixed dentition. According to Hussein et al., salivary Cu and Zn levels were significantly higher in children with dental caries compared to those who were caries-free [29]. Also, it is found that the use of toothpaste containing nanocrystals of carbonate hydroxyapatite replaced with Zn can produce mimicking effect of morphology, structure, and composition of biological hydroxyapatite of enamel [30].

4. Conclusion

Based on the results obtained with the chemical and immunochemical analysis of whole saliva, we can obtain the following conclusions:

(i) After the stimulation, we found that the Zn concentration in the first group was higher.

(ii) The quantity of Zn before and after the stimulation in the second and third groups with caries showed statistically significant differences.

(iii) The quantity of Zn after the stimulation showed significant differences among the three groups. These differences are higher in the first group in comparison to the second and third groups.

(iv) The increase in Zn concentration and quantity in the first group (caries-free) in comparison with the second and third groups indicates the positive effect on reducing caries.

From these findings, we can conclude that Zn has an impact in reducing the appearance of caries that is proved with the Zn quantity differences found in the three groups that were investigated.

Ethical Approval

The protocols and human data that the authors used in this study were approved by the Ethical Board of the Faculty of Chemistry at the University of "St. Cyrus and Methodius" in Skopje, which gave permission for this research.

References

[1] C. R. Robinson, S. J. Shore, S. Brookes, S. R. Strafford, and J. Wood Kirkham, "The chemistry of enamel caries," *Critical Reviews in Oral Biology and Medicine*, vol. 11, no. 4, pp. 481–495, 2000.

[2] C. Dawes, "Saliva and dental caries," *Understanding Dental Caries. 1. Etiology and Mechanism, Basic Clinical Aspects*, G. Nikiforuk, Ed., vol. 1, pp. 236–260, Basel, Switzerland, Karger, 1985.

[3] S. Alaluusua, "Longitudinal study of salivary IgA in children from 1 to 4 years old with reference to dental caries," *European Journal of Oral Sciences*, vol. 91, pp. 163–168, 1983.

[4] K. A. Gamershtein and J. M. Maksimovski, "Zinc and caries," *Stomatologia*, vol. 68, pp. 54–64, 1989.

[5] H. M. Tvinnereim, R. Eide, T. Riise, G. Fosse, and G. R. Wesenberg, "Zinc in primary teeth from children in Norway," *Science of The Total Environment*, vol. 226, no. 2-3, pp. 201–212, 1999.

[6] C. Dawes, "Physiological factors affecting salivary flow rate, oral sugar clearance, and the sensation of dry mouth in man," *Journal of Dental Research*, vol. 66, no. 1, pp. 648–653, 1987.

[7] D. K. Mason and D. M. Chisholm, *Salivary Glands in Health and Disease*, W. B. Saunders Company, Philadelphia, PA, USA, 1975.

[8] H. Schmidt, *Biochemie fur Stomatologen*, Johann Ambrosius Barth, Leipzig, Germany, 1982.

[9] W. M. Edgar and D. M. O. Mullane, *Saliva and Oral Health*, British Dental Association, London, UK, 2nd edition, 1996.

[10] I. Green, "Copper and manganese in saliva of children," *Journal of Dental Research*, vol. 49, no. 4, pp. 776–782, 1970.

[11] A. Adabache-Ortiz, M. Silva-Briano, M. R. Campos-Esparza, and J. Ventura-Juárez, "Comparison of chemical elements on carious & normal premolar's enamel layers using energy dispersive X ray spectrometer (X Ray-EDS)," *Microscopy Research*, vol. 2, no. 4, pp. 81–91, 2014.

[12] J. Buczowska-Radlindka, "Factors that modify de and remineralization in dental enamel from the aspect of caries susceptibility," *Annales Academiae Medicae Stetinensis*, no. 47, pp. 1–89, 1999.

[13] A. D. Abdazimov, "Changes in the trace elements composition of the hard dental tissues, dental calculus, saliva and gingival biopsies in walkers under the influence of unfavorable factors in the manufacture of Cu, Zn and Pb," *Stomatologija*, vol. 70, no. 3, pp. 22–25, 1991.

[14] M. M. Fang, K. Y. Lei, and L. T. Kilgore, "Effects of zinc deficiency on dental caries in rats," *Journal of Nutrition*, vol. 110, no. 5, pp. 1032–1036, 1980.

[15] J. Tenovuo, "Antimicrobial function of human saliva—how important is it for oral health?," *Acta Odontologica Scandinavica*, vol. 56, no. 5, pp. 250–256, 1998.

[16] M. E. J. Curzon, P. C. Specter, F. L. Losee, and W. D. McHugh, *Trace Elements and Dental Caries. Variation of Strontium Content of Surface Enamel with Geography, Age and Caries*, p. 22, Eastman Dental Center, Rochester, NY, USA, 1976.

[17] C. A. Saxton, G. J. Harrap, and A. M. Lloyd, "The effect of dentifrices containing zinc citrate on plaque growth and oral zinc levels," *Journal of Clinical Periodontology*, vol. 13, no. 4, pp. 301–306, 1986.

[18] F. Brudevold, L. T. Steadman, M. A. Spinelli et al., "A study of zinc in human teeth," *Archives of Oral Biology*, vol. 8, no. 2, pp. 135–144, 1963.

[19] R. K. Rose, "Competitive binding of calcium, magnesium and zinc to *Streptococcus sanguis* and purified *S. sanguis* cell walls," *Caries Research*, vol. 30, no. 1, pp. 71–75, 1996.

[20] G. N. Jenkins, "Current concepts concerning the development of dental caries," *International Dental Journal*, vol. 22, no. 3, pp. 350–362, 1972.

[21] N. R. Mohammed, M. Mneimne, R. G. Hill, M. Al-Jawad, R. J. M. Lynch, and P. Anderson, "Physical chemical effects of zinc on *in vitro* enamel demineralization," *Journal of Dentistry*, vol. 42, no. 9, pp. 1096–1104, 2014.

[22] M. S. Duggal, H. S. Ciuwla, and M. E. J. Curzon, "A study of relationship between trace elements in saliva and dental caries in children," *Archives of Oral Biology*, vol. 36, no. 12, pp. 881–884, 1991.

[23] C. W. Bales and J. H. Freeland-Graves, "Zinc, magnesium, copper and protein concentration in human saliva: age- and sex- related differences," *American Journal of Clinical Nutrition*, vol. 51, no. 3, pp. 462–469, 1990.

[24] R. L. Gregory, L. C. Hobbs, J. C. Kindlc, T. Vonto, and H. S. Molmsstrom, "Immunodominant antigens of *Streptococcus mutans* in dental caries-resistant subjects," *Human Antibodies and Hybridomas*, vol. 1, no. 3, pp. 132–136, 1990.

[25] H. M. Tvinnerein, R. Eide, and T. Ruse, "Heavy metals in human primary teeth: some factors influencing the metals concentrations," *Science of the Total Environment*, vol. 255, no. 1-3, pp. 21–27, 2000.

[26] J. M. Richard Lynch, "Zinc in the mouth, its interactions with dental enamel and possible effects on caries a review of the literature," *International Dental Journal*, vol. 61, no. 3, pp. 46–54, 2011.

[27] G. Sortino and U. Palazzo, "Zinc and experimental caries in the rat," *Rivista Italiana Di Stomatologia*, vol. 26, no. 7, pp. 509–513, 1971.

[28] G. He, E. l. F. Pearce, and C. H. Sissons, "Inhibitory effect of $ZnCl_2$ on glycolysis in human oral microbes," *Archives of Oral Biology*, vol. 47, no. 2, pp. 117–129, 2002.

[29] A. S. Hussein, H. F. Ghasheer, N. M. Ramli, R. J. Schroth, and M. I. Abu-Hassan, "Salivary trace elements in relation to dental caries in a group of multi-ethnic schoolchildren in Shah Alam, Malaysia," *European Journal of Paediatric Dentistry*, vol. 14, no. 2, pp. 113–118, 2013.

[30] M. Lelli, A. Putignano, M. Marchetti et al., "Remineralization and repair of enamel surface by biomimetic Zn-carbonate hydroxyapatite containing toothpaste: a comparative *in vivo* study," *Frontiers in Physiology*, vol. 5, p. 333, 2014.

26

Validity of Digital Imaging of Fiber-Optic Transillumination in Caries Detection on Proximal Tooth Surfaces

Marja-Liisa Laitala,[1] **Liina Piipari,**[1] **Noora Sämpi,**[1] **Maria Korhonen,**[1] **Paula Pesonen,**[2] **Tiina Joensuu,**[3] **and Vuokko Anttonen**[1,4]

[1]*Research Unit of Oral Health Sciences, Department of Cariology, Endodontology and Paediatric Dentistry,*
 University of Oulu, Oulu, Finland
[2]*Research Unit of Oral Health Sciences, University of Oulu, Oulu, Finland*
[3]*Kuopio University Hospital, Kuopio, Finland*
[4]*Medical Research Center, University of Oulu, Oulu University Hospital, Oulu, Finland*

Correspondence should be addressed to Marja-Liisa Laitala; marja-liisa.laitala@oulu.fi

Academic Editor: Ali I. Abdalla

Objective. The aim of our study was to evaluate the validity of the digital imaging fiber-optic transillumination (DIFOTI) method in comparison with clinical visual examination (CV) and bitewing (BW) radiography on detecting caries lesions on proximal surfaces of teeth. *Materials and Methods.* Proximal tooth surfaces of premolars and molars ($n = 2,103$) of 91 voluntary university students aged from 18 to 30 years were examined with CV, BW radiography, and the DIFOTI method. *Results.* DIFOTI detected more initial and manifested caries lesions compared with CV and BW. Of the analyzed tooth surfaces, 69.8% were classified as sound by DIFOTI, 80.3% by BW, and 91.6% by CV. Initial caries lesions were found in 21.2% of the surfaces by DIFOTI, in 14.1% by BW, and in 6.2% by CV, whereas the proportions for manifested dental caries lesions were 9.0%, 5.6%, and 2.2%, respectively. The interexaminer agreement regarding the DIFOTI findings between an experienced clinician and a fifth-year dental student was high: $\kappa = 0.67$ for initial and $\kappa = 0.91$ for manifested caries lesions. *Conclusions.* The noninvasive DIFOTI method seems to offer a potential tool for everyday clinical practice. In clinical use, DIFOTI finds well even initial caries lesions on proximal surfaces, thus providing an instrument for detecting lesions potential for arresting as well as for monitoring the outcome after preventive measures.

1. Introduction

Diagnosing caries lesions, especially initial lesions, is challenging [1, 2]. However, detection of caries lesions as early as possible is a cornerstone in a recent schema of caries controlling [3]. Diagnosing the disease in its early stages enables arresting the progress of initial lesions [3]. Visual-tactile has a long history as the most common diagnostic tool in caries detection. Currently, clinical visual examination (CV) including classifications of the progression and the depth of lesions [4, 5] as well as estimation of the lesion activity [6] is recommended. As a result of this improvement in caries detection protocol, the sensitivity of visual examination has improved [7, 8]. Conventional additional diagnostic methods for CV include bitewing (BW) radiography and fiber-optic transillumination (FOTI). Combined with BW, CV leads to more favorable diagnostic results than CV alone, especially with respect to proximal caries lesions [9–12]. BW images cannot be replaced by the FOTI method [13].

A need for additional tools for early caries detection is clear. During recent decades, research on caries detection has mainly focused on validating methods aiming to detect visually caries lesions of different degrees and evaluating early diagnostics tools [2, 14]. Digital imaging fiber-optic transillumination (DIFOTI) is among the most recent caries detection methods. In DIFOTI, the course of the near-infrared light beam is different in sound tissue compared to damaged tissue. With DIFOTI, the findings can be stored as digital images and displayed on a monitor. Fibers lead the light on the tooth surface and the tooth is transilluminated from both sides through a tip or a sensor in a plastic handgrip of the device. The tip has a tiny camera, and a digital image of the tooth is transmitted to the monitor online. Captured images can be saved in the database. The commercial application has been in use since the early 2000s [14], but scientific evidence on the clinical validity and clinical relevance of the DIFOTI method in caries detection is so far vague [15–19].

The aim of our study was to evaluate the validity of the DIFOTI method in caries detection on the proximal tooth surfaces in comparison with clinical visual examination and bitewing radiography, as well as its feasibility in association with work experience.

2. Materials and Methods

2.1. Participants. All 18–30-year-old university students who had reserved an appointment for a dental examination between October 2013 and February 2014 at the dental clinic of the Finnish Students' Health Service (FSHS) in Oulu, Finland, were invited to participate. Participation was voluntary, and altogether 137 participants were recruited. Of those, 91 participants had caries data on CV, BW radiographs, and DIFOTI images.

2.2. Methodology. Findings of CV, BW radiography, and DIFOTI were analyzed separately.

2.2.1. Clinical Visual Examination. The clinical visual inspection was carried out in a fully equipped dental unit with light using a WHO probe and an oral mirror. Caries clinical staging was recorded by using ICDAS-classification (1–6) as follows: Score 0 = sound tooth surface, Score 1 = first visual change in enamel, Score 2 = distinct visual change in enamel, Score 3 = localised enamel breakdown, without visible dentine exposure, Score 4 = underlying dentine shadow, Score 5 = distinct cavity with visible dentine, and Score 6 = extensive cavity with visible dentine. In case of doubt dentists were advised to choose the higher option.

2.2.2. Bitewing Radiographs and DIFOTI Images. Bitewing radiographs were taken according to the Finnish Current Care Guidelines for Controlling Dental Caries criteria only when clinically indicated (at least one caries lesion with dentin exposure or if the last BW radiographs had been taken more than three years earlier) [20]. All the radiographs were analyzed together by three of the authors, that is, experienced clinicians VA, M-LL, and TJ. Consensus was achieved on all the findings by the team.

A representative of the manufacturer provided education on the use of the DIFOTI device in hands-on sessions. The clinicians were advised to scan all the 1st and 2nd premolars and molars of the participants. A dental nurse at FSHS recorded the findings to the database according to the instructions of the device used. The images were saved for later analyses by using a specific programme offered by the manufacturer.

In the analyses, the distal and mesial surfaces of molars and premolars in BW and DIFOTI images were classified as follows: Score 0 = no caries; Score 1 = caries lesion in outer surface of the enamel; Score 2 = caries lesion extending into the inner enamel or dentoenamel-junction; Score 3 = dentinal caries lesion in the external half of dentin; Score 4 = deep dentinal caries lesion extending into the dentin half near the pulp. In the analyses, missing and failed images were analyzed separately and reported elsewhere.

To calculate the interexaminer agreement for DIFOTI, images of the 91 participants (altogether 2083 tooth surfaces) were analyzed by VA and a fifth-year dental student (NS) separately but at the same time to avoid bias caused by not being able to recognize the tooth or tooth surface correctly.

2.2.3. Examiners. Before the present study, all the dentists ($n = 7$) working at the FSHS in Oulu were trained and calibrated by two of the authors (VA and M-LL) who had previous experience of introducing the protocol and training and calibrating examiners from several similar clinical studies. The training comprised PowerPoint presentations and hands-on in vitro training on caries detection with ICDAS criteria [5] to estimate caries lesion depth and activity. All the dentists participating in the clinical examinations were experienced. One dentist carried out all clinical examinations for one patient: the clinical visual inspection, BW radiographs, and DIFOTI scanning. A dental nurse recorded the findings on structured forms.

The calibration of the examiners was carried out using ICDAS criteria with caries activity assessment on extracted teeth. For the purposes of quality assurance of the clinical examination, the gold standard (M-LL) performed repeated clinical examinations to the patients of each examiner.

2.3. Statistical Analyses. The data were described as frequencies and proportions. To evaluate the findings regarding different tooth groups (upper and lower premolars and molars), cross tabulation was used. Detection rate (sensitivity) and specificity for DIFOTI were calculated by using BW radiographs as the gold standard method; the cut-off points used were initial caries lesions (lesions clinically restricted to enamel/without dentin exposure) and manifested caries lesions (lesions with clinical dentin exposure). Additionally, DIFOTI findings were evaluated by using CV as the gold standard, and CV was compared with BW.

To investigate the interexaminer agreement of the findings between the two examiners analyzing DIFOTI images, kappa values were calculated. For the analyses, SPSS (version 22.0, SPSS, Inc., Chicago, IL, USA) was used.

2.4. Ethical Considerations. The Regional Ethics Committee of the Northern Ostrobothnia Hospital District (EETTMK: 102/2013) and the board of FSHS gave their approval for the study. Participation was voluntary, and all the participants gave their written consent. Data were collected and analyzed without personal IDs.

3. Results

Altogether 1162 teeth were analyzed. Of those, 591 were molars (292 upper, 299 lower) and 571 premolars (293 upper and 278 lower, resp.). DIFOTI detected more initial and

TABLE 1: Distribution of surfaces with different stages of dental caries. Findings of the clinical visual method (CV), bitewing (BW) radiographs, and fiber-optic transillumination (DIFOTI) are presented separately for upper and lower premolars and molars. The total number of analyzed tooth surfaces was $n = 2,103$.

	Proportions (%) of tooth surfaces with different stages of caries lesions								
	Sound			Initial			Manifested		
	CV	BW	DIFOTI	CV	BW	DIFOTI	CV	BW	DIFOTI
Upper premolars $n = 566$	89.2	78.3	69.4	6.4	13.3	20.5	4.4	8.5	10.1
Lower premolars $n = 521$	95.6	87.3	82.1	3.6	10.7	13.6	0.8	1.9	3.6
Upper molars $n = 507$	90.7	76.1	60.4	7.5	16.8	28.0	1.8	7.1	11.6
Lower molars $n = 509$	91.2	79.4	66.4	7.3	16.1	23.0	1.6	4.5	10.6
Total $n = 2,103$	91.6	80.3	69.8	6.2	14.1	21.2	2.2	5.6	9.0

manifested caries lesions compared with the CV and BW methods (Table 1). Of the analyzed proximal tooth surfaces of premolars and molars ($n = 2,103$), about 90% ($n = 1,927$) were classified as sound by CV, 80% ($n = 1,688$) by BW, and 70% ($n = 1,468$) by DIFOTI. Initial caries lesions were found in one-fifth of the surfaces by DIFOTI; the proportion was more than three times higher when compared with findings by CV and almost double when compared with BW. DIFOTI found manifested caries lesions in 9% of the tooth surfaces; respective figures for CV and BW were 2% and 6%.

With respect to the tooth group, the majority of the manifested caries lesions detected by using the CV and BW methods were found in the upper premolars (CV: $n = 25$, BW: $n = 48$, DIFOTI: $n = 57$), whereas by DIFOTI, the majority of the manifested lesions were in the upper molars (CV: $n = 9$, BW: $n = 36$, and DIFOTI: $n = 59$). The number of initial caries lesions in the upper molars ($n = 142$) detected by using DIFOTI was the double of the number detected in the lower premolars ($n = 71$). The corresponding figures using DIFOTI for upper premolars were $n = 116$ and for lower premolars $n = 117$. For CV and BW, the distributions of the initial caries findings were more even: CV upper premolars $n = 36$, lower premolars $n = 19$, upper molars $n = 38$, and lower molars $n = 37$ and BW upper premolars $n = 75$, lower premolars $n = 56$, upper molars $n = 85$, and lower premolars $n = 82$, respectively. However, with all three methods lower premolar teeth showed higher number of sound surfaces (Table 1).

Comparing DIFOTI findings with BW findings, the detection rate was 54.2% when using initial caries lesions as the cut-off point and 46.2% when using manifested caries lesions as the cut-off point. Specificity was 75.7% for initial caries lesions and 93.2% for manifested caries lesions (Table 2(a)). When comparing DIFOTI findings with CV findings, the detection rate was 55.1% and specificity 72.1% with initial caries lesions as the cut-off point, while the respective figures for manifested caries lesions were 47.8% and 93.0%, respectively (Table 2(b)).

Of the methods used, CV found the least initial and manifested caries lesions (Table 2(c)), the difference being more distinct between CV and DIFOTI compared with CV

and BW. The interexaminer agreement concerning DIFOTI findings between the experienced clinician and the fifth-year dental student was high (0.67). When using manifested caries as the cut-off point, the agreement was excellent (0.91) (Table 3).

4. Discussion

In our clinical study, the digital fiber-optic transillumination method, DIFOTI, detected significantly more initial and manifested caries lesions on proximal surfaces compared with CV and BW radiography. Furthermore, the agreement in caries detection was not dependent on the work experience.

Research on the validity of DIFOTI in caries detection is limited. Our results support the outcomes of two recent clinical studies, which concluded that DIFOTI may reduce the need for BW radiography when detecting caries on proximal tooth surfaces [18, 19]. In their in vitro study with histological validation, Astvaldsdóttir et al. [16] reported outcomes similar to ours: DIFOTI was superior in detecting initial caries lesions compared with both CV and BW radiography.

Value of BW radiography has been widely studied clinically. Hietala-Lenkkeri et al. [10] compared CV and BW and reported BW to be beneficial for 14-year-olds in a population with low caries prevalence. In the study of Poorterman et al. [9], the number of surfaces in need of restorative treatment (due to caries or an inadequate restoration) was doubled based on an additional BW examination compared with visual examination alone, BW being most beneficial among 17-year-olds. However, in their study, the same was not true for the 14-year-olds. Our results are somewhat similar, but the DIFOTI method is clearly superior to BW radiography.

Gold standard is always a problem in in vivo studies investigating the validity of caries detection methods. The low values concerning sensitivity and specificity of DIFOTI are explained by the fact that BW radiography and CV were used as the gold standard, a "true finding," for DIFOTI. Here, the "false positive" findings are most likely true additional positive findings. DIFOTI detected significantly more initial

TABLE 2: Comparison of the findings of the fiber-optic transillumination (DIFOTI) method with bitewing (BW) radiographs and the clinical visual method (CV). Numbers and proportions (%) of tooth surfaces with different stages of caries lesions.

(a) DIFOTI versus BW

| | | DIFOTI | | | |
		Sound	Initial	Manifested	Total (%)
BW	Sound	1,278 (75.5)	329 (19.5)	81 (4.8)	1,688 (80.3)
	Initial	157 (52.7)	87 (29.2)	54 (18.1)	298 (14.2)
	Manifested	33 (28.2)	30 (25.6)	54 (46.2)	117 (5.6)
	Total (%)	1,468 (69.8)	446 (21.2)	189 (9.9)	2,103

(b) DIFOTI versus CV

| | | DIFOTI | | | |
		Sound	Initial	Manifested	Total (%)
CV	Sound	1,389 (72.1)	391 (20.3)	147 (7.6)	1,927 (91.6)
	Initial	68 (52.3)	42 (32.3)	20 (15.4)	130 (6.2)
	Manifested	11 (23.9)	13 (28.3)	22 (47.8)	46 (2.2)
	Total (%)	1,468 (69.8)	446 (21.2)	189 (9.9)	2,103

(c) CV versus BW

| | | CV | | | |
		Sound	Initial	Manifested	Total (%)
BW	Sound	1,595 (94.5)	75 (4.4)	18 (1.1)	1,688 (80.3)
	Initial	251 (84.2)	39 (13.1)	8 (2.7)	298 (14.2)
	Manifested	81 (69.2)	16 (13.7)	20 (17.1)	117 (5.6)
	Total (%)	1,927 (91.6)	130 (6.2)	46 (2.2)	2,103

TABLE 3: Findings of fiber-optic transillumination (DIFOTI) images by a fifth-year dental student and an experienced clinician; numbers and proportions of tooth surfaces.

| | | Numbers and proportions (%) of tooth surfaces with different stages of caries lesions | | | |
| | | DIFOTI (fifth-year dental student) | | | |
		Sound	Initial	Manifested	Total (%)
DIFOTI (experienced clinician)	Sound	1,308	106	12	1,426 (68.5)
	Initial	132	278	32	442 (21.2)
	Manifested	15	56	144	215 (10.3)
	Total (%)	1,455 (69.8)	440 (21.2)	188 (9.0)	2,083 (100.0)

caries lesions and more manifested lesions than BW. When using CV as the gold standard, the respective figures were even higher.

In an *in vivo* study, a 2-day temporary separation of the teeth increases the accuracy of the clinical visual examination. This was not possible in our study design and can be considered as a limitation. It must be kept in mind that the quality of DIFOTI images and also of BW radiographs can influence the outcome of caries detection. Under- and overestimation in either case may have caused bias. However, the influence of the limitations on the methods can only be speculated. Despite these uncertainties, the good interexaminer agreement of DIFOTI also supports the validity of the method. Nevertheless, longitudinal studies would be valuable in this respect.

Our study population comprised young adults with fairly low caries prevalence and in most cases only a few restorations. The DIFOTI method easily detects even tooth-colored restorations, which is a benefit. On the other hand, large composite and amalgam restorations may hinder secondary caries detection. In the present study, the study population was appropriate for this type of a study focusing on comparing methods. The study group could have been larger, but it is in line with a recent clinical study on the topic with similar outcomes [19].

While analyzing the images, we found that DIFOTI reveals not only carious lesions but also macro- and microfractures. This provides an additional benefit to use DIFOTI. In their recent systematic review, Innes and Schwendicke [21] found noteworthy heterogeneity in the treatment decisions and restorative thresholds among clinicians; a significant proportion of the caries lesions which should be noninvasively treated are intervened restoratively. Good-quality DIFOTI images show clearly the depth of the caries lesions in the tissue, which helps the clinician to decide whether to choose a noninvasive or invasive treatment. This may reduce unnecessary restorations and give a possibility of implementing successful preventive measures. Because DIFOTI images show only one tooth at a time, the images provide more detailed information than BW radiography, provided that the DIFOTI images are of high quality. The quality of the DIFOTI images and challenges in the technique should be recognized and research of this topic would be valuable.

Compared to FOTI, the advantage of the DIFOTI method is that the image can be stored and that it is easy to use for monitoring lesion progression and effects of preventive measures. The real-time view is also useful to illustrate the condition of the dentition tooth by tooth, not only to the dentist but also to the patient. It could be an easy and efficient tool to motivate patients towards better home care. So far, we have not found any clinical studies comparing these two methods.

The most significant advantage of the method is that it does not cause any extra radiation exposure to the patient. Therefore, it is a safe option even when radiographs are susceptive or contraindicated. In addition, it can be speculated that DIFOTI may cause less discomfort for the patient than BW radiography, when the patients sometimes find the BW film plate uncomfortable. The present DIFOTI device (DIAGNOCam, KaVO, Biberach, Germany) has two sizes of sensors, and selecting the right size makes imaging more comfortable to the patient. Being portable, the device can be shared by several dentists. When comparing the advantages of DIFOTI with BW radiography, also costs and other economic aspects have to be considered. This would be an interesting topic for the future research.

There are some crucial aspects to consider when using DIFOTI. The labelling of the tooth in the saved DIFOTI image must be exact and clear to ensure the right diagnosis and to enable consultation between clinicians. It is impossible for other users compared to the examiner to analyze DIFOTI images later, if the tooth is not properly labelled. Even if the tooth can be recognized, determining the right surface is challenging. This aspect must be kept in mind when evaluating the reliability of the DIFOTI method. Not being able to identify the tooth/tooth surface may cause bias when comparing the outcome. In our study, only the images which were properly labelled and standardized as for tooth surfaces were included in the analyses. Scanning with the DIFOTI device can also be challenging. Proper and thorough training on the use of the DIFOTI device is necessary to assure good image quality.

5. Conclusions

The noninvasive DIFOTI method seems to offer a potential tool in everyday clinical practice for the detection and assessment of caries lesions in proximal surfaces. Specifically, young populations with fairly low caries prevalence seem to benefit from the use of DIFOTI, because the method is at its best when there are none or just a few fillings in the dentition.

In clinical use, DIFOTI finds well initial caries lesions, thus providing an instrument for detecting lesions potential for arresting as well as for monitoring the outcome after preventive measures. It can also be useful in motivating the patient towards good oral self-care.

Acknowledgments

The authors wish to thank all the dentists and other staff at the FSHS in Oulu, Finland, for their valuable input and participation. For providing the device KaVo DIAGNOCam for this study, the manufacturer and KaVo Scandinavia AB are acknowledged.

References

[1] V. Baelum, "What is an appropriate caries diagnosis?" *Acta odontologica Scandinavica*, vol. 68, no. 2, pp. 65–79, 2010.

[2] S. Twetman, S. Axelsson, G. Dahlén et al., "Adjunct methods for caries detection: A systematic review of literature," *Acta Odontologica Scandinavica*, vol. 71, no. 3-4, pp. 388–397, 2013.

[3] A. G. Schulte, N. B. Pitts, M. C. D. N. J. M. Huysmans, C. Splieth, and W. Buchalla, "European core curriculum in cariology for undergraduate dental students," *Caries Research*, vol. 45, no. 4, pp. 336–345, 2011.

[4] K. R. Ekstrand, G. Bruun, and M. Bruun, "Plaque and gingival status as indicators for caries progression on approximal surfaces," *Caries Research*, vol. 32, no. 1, pp. 41–45, 1998.

[5] N. Pitts, "'ICDAS'—An international system for caries detection and assessment being developed to facilitate caries epidemiology, research and appropriate clinical management," *Community Dental Health*, vol. 21, no. 3, pp. 193–198, 2004.

[6] B. Nyvad, V. Machiulskiene, and V. Baelum, "Construct and predictive validity of clinical caries diagnostic criteria assessing lesion activity," *Journal of Dental Research*, vol. 82, no. 2, pp. 117–122, 2003.

[7] A. I. Ismail, W. Sohn, M. Tellez et al., "The International Caries Detection and Assessment System (ICDAS): an integrated system for measuring dental caries," *Community Dentistry and Oral Epidemiology*, vol. 35, no. 3, pp. 170–178, 2007.

[8] A. Jablonski-Momeni, V. Stachniss, D. N. Ricketts, M. Heinzel-Gutenbrunner, and K. Pieper, "Reproducibility and accuracy of the ICDAS-II for detection of occlusal caries in vitro," *Caries Research*, vol. 42, no. 2, pp. 79–87, 2008.

[9] J. H. G. Poorterman, I. H. A. Aartman, J. A. Kieft, and H. Kalsbeek, "Value of bite-wing radiographs in a clinical epidemiological study and their effect on the dmfs index," *Caries Research*, vol. 34, no. 2, pp. 159–163, 2000.

[10] A.-M. Hietala-Lenkkeri, M. Tolvanen, P. Alanen, and K. Pienihäkkinen, "The additional information of bitewing radiographs in the detection of established or severe dentinal decay in 14-year olds: A cross-sectional study in low-caries population," *The Scientific World Journal*, vol. 2014, Article ID 175358, 2014.

[11] A. Wenzel, "Radiographic display of carious lesions and cavitation in approximal surfaces: Advantages and drawbacks of conventional and advanced modalities," *Acta Odontologica Scandinavica*, vol. 72, no. 4, pp. 251–264, 2014.

[12] T. Gimenez, C. Piovesan, M. M. Braga et al., "Clinical relevance of studies on the accuracy of visual inspection for detecting caries lesions: A systematic review," *Caries Research*, vol. 49, no. 2, pp. 91–98, 2015.

[13] J. Vaarkamp, J. J. Ten Bosch, E. H. Verdonschot, and E. M. Bronkhorst, "The real performance of bitewing radiography and fiber-optic transillumination in approximal caries diagnosis," *Journal of Dental Research*, vol. 79, no. 10, pp. 1747–1751, 2000.

[14] G. K. Stookey and C. González-Cabezas, "Emerging methods of caries diagnosis," *Journal of Dental Education*, vol. 65, no. 10, pp. 1001–1006, 2001.

[15] M. Bin-Shuwaish, P. Yaman, J. Dennison, and G. Neiva, "The correlation of DIFOTI to clinical and radiographic images in class II carious lesions," *Journal of the American Dental Association*, vol. 139, no. 10, pp. 1373–1381, 2008.

[16] Á. Astvaldsdóttir, K. Åhlund, W. P. Holbrook, B. De Verdier, and S. Tranæus, "Approximal caries detection by DIFOTI: In vitro comparison of diagnostic accuracy/efficacy with film and digital radiography," *International Journal of Dentistry*, Article ID 326401, 2012.

[17] M. Abdelaziz and I. Krejci, "DIAGNOcam–a Near Infrared Digital Imaging Transillumination (NIDIT) technology," *The international journal of esthetic dentistry*, vol. 10, no. 1, pp. 158–165, 2015.

[18] J. Kühnisch, F. Söchtig, V. Pitchika et al., "In vivo validation of near-infrared light transillumination for interproximal dentin caries detection," *Clinical Oral Investigations*, vol. 20, no. 4, pp. 821–829, 2016.

[19] C. Lara-Capi, M. G. Cagetti, P. Lingström et al., " Digital transillumination in caries detection ," *Dentomaxillofacial Radiology*, vol. 46, no. 4, p. 20160417, 2017.

[20] Finnish Current Care Guidelines for Controlling Dental Caries, "Current Care Guidelines," http://www.kaypahoito.fi/web/english/guidelineabstracts/guideline?id=ccs00105/.

[21] N. Innes and F. Schwendicke, "Restorative thresholds for carious lesions: systematic review and meta-analysis," *Journal of Dental Research*, vol. 96, no. 5, pp. 501–508, 2017.

27

Knowledge, Attitude, and Barriers to Fluoride Application as a Preventive Measure among Oral Health Care Providers

Aqdar A. Akbar [ID],[1] Noura Al-Sumait,[2] Hanan Al-Yahya,[2] Mohammad Y. Sabti [ID],[1] and Muawia A. Qudeimat [ID][3]

[1]Department of General Dental Practice, Kuwait University, Kuwait City, Kuwait
[2]Ministry of Health, Kuwait City, Kuwait
[3]Department of Developmental and Preventive Sciences, Kuwait University, Kuwait City, Kuwait

Correspondence should be addressed to Aqdar A. Akbar; aqdar@hsc.edu.kw

Academic Editor: Izzet Yavuz

Objective. To investigate the knowledge, attitude, and possible barriers to fluoride application among oral health-care providers in Kuwait. *Methods*. A validated self-administered questionnaire was distributed to a random sample of 291 dentists. The questionnaire included four categories: dentists' characteristics, knowledge of and attitude towards fluoride application, factors influencing decision-making on prescription of fluoride, and the clinician's perception of own knowledge. Means, group differences, and logistic regression were calculated. *Results*. 262 completed the questionnaire (response rate of 90%). Half of the participants (49%) reported that water fluoridation is the best method for caries prevention in children. Majority of the participants (80%) acknowledged that topical fluoride prevents dental caries, but only 40% frequently use it in their practices. Fear of overdose was a concern in 57% of the participants. About 31% believed that caries is a multifactorial disease and cannot be prevented. In addition, 32% of the dentists who thought caries is multifactorial and cannot be prevented stated that restorations take precedence over preventive therapy. *Conclusion*. Despite the participants being in favor of topical fluoride application and believing in its effectiveness, certain barriers were apparent such as knowledge deficiencies, products labelling flaw, and lack of participation in effective continuing educational activities.

1. Introduction

A major decline in the prevalence of dental caries has been observed over recent decades. This decline has been attributed to the widespread use of daily fluoride toothpaste [1]. Kuwait is considered a nonfluoridated community since water fluoridation was discontinued in 1980 [2]. In addition, salt, milk, and juice are not fluoridated, and individuals have access to both fluoridated and nonfluoridated toothpaste. Despite the preventative effort from the Ministry of Health and the School Oral Health programs, caries is still considered a major problem [2, 3]. Al-Mutawa et al. [3] found that only 24–32% of 4- and 5-year-old children were caries-free, and the decayed score of the dft/dfs was the major component of the mean scores. Similar scores were reported for DFT/DFS in 12- and 14-year-olds [4].

The sizable amount of available dental literatures in addition to frequent controversies among clinicians and researchers has made decision-making for dental care and treatment planning very complex [5, 6]. Decision-making on caries diagnosis and management is primarily based on factors related to the dentist's characteristics, knowledge and experience, and to patient and practice factors [5, 7]. Dentists' knowledge and attitudes toward evidence-based clinical practices are very important to the profession to be able to offer the best possible care to the patient and to effectively influence their oral health behavior [8–10].

The American Dental Association (ADA) and the National Institute of Health and Care Excellence (NICE) place emphasis on the prevention and early detection of dental caries as the most important elements in any health-care program [11, 12]. With the current level of evidence, fluoride is well documented as an effective preventative method against dental caries for people at risk of developing dental caries via enhancing remineralization and inhibiting demineralization [13–19]. The application of this knowledge in clinical practice seems deficient and not well adopted [9, 10, 20, 21]. Bansal et al., reported that dentists showed a lack of understanding of fluorides' main mechanism of action which could lead to inappropriate judgement on the effectiveness of its use in different age groups [20]. Another study demonstrated a positive attitude towards preventative dental care but a deficiency in the knowledge regarding the role of fluoride in caries prevention as well as underestimation of fluoridated toothpaste role in caries control and reduction [9]. Investigators concluded that many dentists are not prepared well neither to prescribe the right fluoride regimen nor to council patients/parents about the appropriate fluoride use [22]. The aim of this study was to assess the knowledge, attitude, and possible barriers to fluoride application among dentists in Kuwait.

2. Material and Methods

Ethical approval was granted from the Health Science Center Ethical Clearance Committee, Kuwait University, and the Ethics and Research Committee, Kuwait Ministry of Health. All participants provided a signed informed consent. The study was conducted in full accordance with ethical principles, including the Declaration of Helsinki. A questionnaire was designed to investigate knowledge and attitudes as well as barriers to fluoride use as a preventative measure among dentists in Kuwait. The questionnaire was developed according to previous surveys, ADA guidelines, and the most recent available evidence [9, 14, 16, 17, 21]. A pilot study was performed on ten dentists (later excluded from the final sample) working at the Faculty of Dentistry, Kuwait University. This was done to assure that the survey questions were well formulated relating to the objectives of the study and that questions are well understood by the targeted dentists. Face validity was measured against a construct definition. Twenty-four items received 10 out of 10, and five items received 6 out of 10 and were removed mainly because the dentists thought they were unrelated to the objectives of the study. The validated survey was then readministered to the same 10 dentists, and all 24 questions were correctly answered by all participants.

The questionnaire was divided into 4 sections and consisted of 24 questions. In the first section, the dentists reported on their demographics, dental training, and practice after graduation. The second and third sections investigated the dentists' knowledge and attitude towards fluoride and its application. The last section examined the dentists' perception of their own knowledge regarding fluoride applications and the best methods for obtaining new evidence-based information.

The final sample size was calculated based on a confidence level of 90% and marginal error of 5%. At the time of carrying out this study, there were 1160 registered general dentists and specialists working in Kuwait (as per the latest manpower statistics of the Kuwait Ministry of Health) [23]. Therefore, the required sample size was estimated at 219 participants. To account for a possible 25% drop out/refusal, 291 dentists were met in person and invited to participate in

TABLE 1: Participants' characteristics.

Characteristics	n (%)
Sex	
Male	179 (67)
Female	86 (33)
Age	
≤30 years	107 (43)
31–45	114 (46)
≥46	27 (11)
Nationality	
Kuwaiti	147 (57)
Non-Kuwaiti	111 (43)
Region of undergraduate dental education	
North America	38 (16)
Europe	40 (16)
Asia	59 (24)
Middle East	109 (44)
Year of practice	
≥10	155 (61)
<10	101 (39)
Specialty	
General dental practitioners	147 (57)
Specialist (PD, ORTHO, and DPH)	39 (15)
Other specialists	71 (28)
Work place	
Primary care clinics	97 (38)
Specialty care clinics	120 (46)
Private clinics	42 (16)
Area of practice	
Rural	113 (44)
Urban	142 (56)

this study. The study population was randomly selected by a multistage random-sampling method.

A total of 291 dentists working in the six health districts of the country from primary care clinics, specialty care clinics, and the private sector were invited to participate and complete the self-administered questionnaire.

Data were coded, verified, and analyzed using SPSS (version 18; SPSS Inc., Chicago, IL, USA). The logistic regression and chi-square tests were used for the analysis. A probability level of less than 0.05 was considered as statistically significant.

3. Results

A total of 291 dentists were invited to participate, and 262 (176 males and 86 females) completed the questionnaire, giving a response rate of 90%. Table 1 summarizes the participants' characteristics, in which specialty was further divided into three groups: general dental practitioner, specialist caring for children (including pediatric dentists, orthodontists, and dental public health), and a third group of other specialties.

The participants' perception of the most effective methods for caries prevention in children and adults is shown in Table 2. Almost half of the participants (49%) stated that the most effective methods for caries prevention were water fluoridation for children and fluoridated toothpaste for adults. In addition, a few of the dentists believed that caries

TABLE 2: Participants' beliefs regarding the most effective fluoride regimen to prevent dental caries in children and adults.

	Children n (%)	Adult n (%)
Water fluoridation	98 (49)	30 (15)
Fluoride toothpaste	23 (11)	101 (49)
Fluoride rinses	1 (1)	10 (5)
Professionally applied topical fluoride	61 (30)	44 (21)
Fluoride supplements (tablets and drops)	10 (5)	4 (2)
Caries cannot be prevented	8 (4)	17 (8)

cannot be prevented in both children and adults (4% and 8%, resp.).

Table 3 shows results of the logistic regression model for dentists who chose water fluoridation as the most effective fluoride regimen to prevent dental caries in children. Undergraduates from dental schools of Northern America region were found to be more in favor of water fluoridation than undergradutes from other regions.

Table 4 illustrates the participants' belief of topical fluoride benefits and risks. The majority believed that topical fluorides can prevent caries (80%), make enamel more resistant to caries attacks (95%), and that it is safe in recommended concentrations (91%).

When asked about the application of professional topical fluoride, 40% reported frequent use, 47% claimed using it occasionally, whereas 13% never used it. Fluoride gel was reported by 65% of participants to be the most frequently used form of professional topical fluoride application, followed by rinses (5%) and varnish (3%). In addition, 35% of the participants reported the correct application time of 4 minutes for the gel form. Reasons for not supporting topical fluoride application in clinical practice are listed in Table 5.

Table 6 shows results of logistic regression models for the odds of favoring restorative treatment over prevention, which was significantly higher for dentists who believed that caries is a multifactorial disease and cannot be prevented.

Table 7 shows results of logistic regression models for dentists who believed that caries is a multifactorial disease and cannot be prevented. Few dentists who graduated from Asian undergraduate programs agree that caries cannot be prevented.

When participants were asked about their perception of their own knowledge, 60% claimed that they have adequate knowledge regarding topical fluorides. The majority (69%) stated that they needed further information regarding topical fluorides. In addition, 63% of the total participants reported attending topical fluoride continuing education (CE) sessions in the past 5 years or less, and 45% of the participants reported that the best method to obtain new information is through special courses.

4. Discussion

Topical fluoride application in the form of toothpastes, mouth rinses, varnishes, and gels has been shown to prevent dental caries [13, 14, 16, 17]. In this questionnaire, when dentists were asked about the most effective methods of fluoride regimens to prevent dental caries for both children and adults, the responses varied. Surprisingly, 49% stated that for children, water fluoridation is the most effective method; whereas for adults, 49% reported fluoridated toothpaste as being the most effective. Only 11% thought that fluoridated toothpaste is more effective for children compared to other application forms. This suggests that for children, dentists believe that the main effect of fluoride is primarily during the preeruptive stage. Similar findings were also reported in a previous study, where only 5% of participants identified that the posteruptive effect of fluoride surpasses any preeruptive effects [20]. Yoder et al. [21] also found that the majority of dental professionals were unaware of the fluoride's predominant posteruptive mode of action. Understanding the mechanism of action of any therapeutic agent—in this case fluoride—is critical since it will help in providing the best preventive programs for the patient, which will eventually maximize disease control [13, 20, 21]. In addition, believing that water fluoridation is the most effective method of caries prevention in children may affect parents counseling and education of tooth brushing methods and frequency by causing them to underestimate the importance of these methods [20, 21, 24].

In the logistic regression model, dentists who graduated from a Northern American undergraduate dental program were in favor of water fluoridation as the most effective fluoride regimen to prevent dental caries in children. One explanation could be that undergraduate curricula from different universities were suggested to have an influence on dentists' knowledge as reported by different studies [25, 26]. Some authors found that most dentists depend on knowledge gained from their undergraduate studies as the main source of information for their daily practice [26]. Different clinical guidelines and protocols as well as clinical training can also contribute to such beliefs [25, 26]. It is also possible that some participants confused the terms "cost-effectiveness" and "most effective", which might have affected their choice.

Most of the dentists in this study (80%) reported that topically applied fluoride has a beneficial effect in caries prevention for both children and adults. Almost 95% stated that professionally applied topical fluoride in the form of varnishes, gels, and foams makes enamel more caries resistant. Still, only 36% believed that it is more beneficial than systemic fluoridation, which clearly shows the confusion in fluoride's predominant mode of action. Even though 91% of participants believed that it is safe in recommended concentrations and application protocols, 57% still have fear of overdose. This developed fear may be due to that studies and trials rarely provide information on toxicity and adverse effects [14, 20].

When it comes to clinical application, 65% of the participants reported that topical fluoride in gel form was their preferable method of choice. However, 65% of those were unfortunately unaware of the optimal application time of the gel form and will use it for less than 4 minutes, which may minimize the overall effectiveness and benefits. Even though some of the manufacturers recommend an application time of only 1 minute, this duration of application was not supported by the literature [20]. Some studies suggested that flaws in product-labelling and manufacturer instructions

TABLE 3: Logistic regression model for dentists who believed (dependent variable) that water fluoridation is the most effective fluoride regimen to prevent dental caries in children.

Variables	Systemic (%)	Topical (%)	Caries cannot be prevented (%)	Odds ratio	CI (95%)	P
Gender						
Males	55.1	39.0	5.9	0.26	0.46–0.98	0.48
Females (reference)	50.8	49.2	0.0	—	—	—
Age group (years)						
≤30	51.8	43.5	4.7	0.66	1.11–2.43	0.46
31–45	53.8	41.8	4.4	0.90	0.51–2.32	0.21
≥46 (reference)	55.6	44.4	0.0	—	—	—
Region of undergraduate dental education						
North America	71.0	29.0	0.0	1.55	2.58–0.52	0.003
Europe	63.3	33.3	3.3	0.90	1.88–0.07	0.07
Asia	54.5	43.2	2.3	0.66	1.67–0.35	0.20
Middle East (reference)	44.7	48.2	7.1	—	—	—
Specialty						
General dental practitioner	50.4	44.3	5.2	0.05	1.22–1.12	0.93
Specialists caring for children	62.1	37.9	0.0	0.53	1.54–0.49	0.31
Other specialists (reference)	55.6	40.7	3.7	—	—	—
Years of practice						
≥10	51.6	43.4	4.9	0.25	−0.81–1.31	0.65
<10 (reference)	58.1	39.2	2.7	—	—	—
Area of practice						
Rural	50.0	43.9	6.1	0.18	0.50–0.85	0.61
Urban (reference)	55.4	41.5	3.1	—	—	—
Work place						
Primary care clinics	51.2	47.5	1.2	0.25	0.91–1.42	0.67
Specialty care clinics	52.7	40.7	6.6	0.54	0.48–1.55	0.30
Private (reference)	65.5	34.5	0.0	—	—	—
Topically applied fluoride has no risk of overdosing						
Agree	54.8	38.7	6.5	0.50	1.81–0.81	0.45
Disagree	54.7	43.6	1.7	0.32	1.56–0.93	0.62
Not sure	47.4	42.1	10.5	—	—	—

TABLE 4: Participants' beliefs regarding benefits and risks of professional topical fluoride application.

	Agree n (%)	Disagree n (%)	Not sure n (%)
Can prevent caries	205 (80)	27 (10)	25 (10)
Has a beneficial effect on children's oral health	239 (93)	6 (2)	13 (5)
Has a beneficial effect on adults' oral health	183 (72)	37 (14)	36 (14)
Makes enamel more caries resistant	241 (95)	6 (2)	8 (3)
Is preferable to systemic fluoridation (water, tablets, or drops)	91 (36)	109 (43)	53 (21)
Is preferable to brushing twice a day with fluoride toothpaste	64 (25)	173 (68)	17 (7)
Decreases the interest in tooth brushing	31 (12)	199 (78)	25 (10)
Is safe in recommended concentration and application	230 (91)	9 (4)	14 (5)
Has no adverse effects	82 (32)	145 (57)	29 (11)

TABLE 5: Reasons for not applying professional topical fluoride application in clinical practice.

Factors	Agree n (%)	Disagree n (%)	Not sure n (%)
Restorative treatment should take precedence over prevention	40 (16)	186 (78)	13 (6)
Busy in practice, no time for topical fluoride application	44 (18)	186 (77)	13 (5)
Caries cannot be prevented since it is a multifactorial disease	75 (31)	145 (59)	24 (10)

may play a role in the dentist's ability to correctly use many of the available fluoride products which will affect their effective use and counseling with patients [21]. In other studies, the matter of labelling confusion was also raised for varnish products. Varnish products are FDA-approved to be used as cavity liners and not as a preventive agent [22]. The recommendation of using varnish to prevent caries is described as "off the label" [22]. This imprecise labelling of

TABLE 6: Logistic regression model for dentists who believed (dependent variable) that restorative therapy should take precedence over preventative therapy.

Variables	Agree (%)	Disagree (%)	Not sure (%)	Odds ratio	CI (95%)	P
Gender						
Males	16.5	78.7	4.9	−0.30	−1.13–0.53	0.48
Females (reference)	16.0	76.5	7.4	—	—	—
Age group (years)						
≤30	21.2	72.7	6.1	0.58	−1.19–2.35	0.52
31–45	12.0	85.2	2.8	0.05	−1.36–1.46	0.95
≥46 (reference)	16.7	75.0	8.3	—	—	—
Region of undergraduate dental education						
North America	11.1	88.9	0.0	0.67	−0.52–1.86	0.27
Europe	13.9	80.6	5.6	0.85	−0.32–2.02	0.16
Asia	1.8	94.6	3.6	1.28	−0.51–2.61	0.06
Middle East (reference)	26.0	68.3	5.8	—	—	—
Specialty						
General dental practitioners	21.2	72.3	6.6	−0.03	−1.31–1.26	0.97
Specialists caring for children	7.7	89.7	2.6	0.21	−1.01–1.43	0.74
Other specialists (reference)	12.3	84.6	3.1	—	—	—
Years of practice						
≥10	20.1	74.3	5.6	−0.66	−1.89–0.57	0.29
<10 (reference)	10.4	84.4	5.2	—	—	—
Area of practice						
Rural	14.3	78.6	7.1	0.06	−0.73–0.84	0.88
Urban (reference)	17.2	77.7	5.1	—	—	—
Work place						
Primary care clinics	19.8	74.7	5.5	−0.14	−1.48–1.22	0.85
Specialty care clinics	15.8	78.9	5.3	−0.30	−1.51–0.90	0.62
Private (reference)	10.5	84.2	5.3	—	—	—
Dental caries cannot be prevented because caries is a multifactorial disease						
Agree	32.4	58.1	9.5	−2.34	−3.94–0.73	0.004
Disagree	9.7	88.3	2.1	−1.16	−2.68–0.36	0.14
Not sure (reference)	8.3	75.0	16.7	—	—	—

different topical fluoride agents may cause confusions and eventually barriers to its application. In addition, the handling properties of topical fluoride agents can play a role in its application. Participants reported using topical fluoride irregularly in their clinic, in which only 40% frequently apply it to their patients. Since the majority of our participants are using fluoride gel, it could be the handling properties of the gel that hinder their frequent use. As documented in the literature, fluoride gel is very effective as an anticaries agent; however, it has some drawbacks such as the bitter taste, as well as the 4-minute waiting experience with an ill-fitting tray, which can be an unpleasant experience [22].

In this era, with all the advancements in research, knowledge, and dental technologies, it was surprising to see that 31% of our participants did not support topical fluoride application for caries prevention because they believed that caries is a multifactorial disease and cannot be prevented. The acceptance of the classical term "multifactorial disease" could influence dentists' choice and affect their decision of adopting preventative measures in their routine dental practice.

A logistic regression model showed a significant association between dentists who believed that restorative treatment should take precedence over prevention and those who believed that caries is a multifactorial disease and cannot be prevented. Dental caries is frequently described as a multifactorial disease process [27, 28]. Recent reviews suggested that with broader understanding of the disease's process, we can consider the dietary sugars to be the main cause of the disease and the other factors as causal factors that speed the disease process [29, 30]. By understanding the disease's process in its broader definition, we can conclude that treatment of dental caries can be achieved through nonoperative procedures that include dietary and plaque control along with remineralization therapy [31, 32]. In addition, the philosophy of "drill and fill" to treat the disease in early stages could dictate the dentist's treatment decision-making, and the concept of minimally invasive dentistry is still facing some obstacles to its application by some dentists [8]. Moreover, undergraduate dental education from different universities was found to significantly play a role in the dentists' belief that caries is a multifactorial disease and

Table 7: Logistic regression model for dentists who believed (dependent variable) that caries cannot be prevented because it is a multifactorial disease.

Variables	Agree (%)	Disagree (%)	Not sure (%)	Odds ratio	CI (95%)	P
Gender						
Males	30.7	58.3	11.0	0.23	0.89–0.43	0.49
Females (reference)	30.9	61.7	7.4	—	—	—
Age group (years)						
≤30	31.3	56.6	12.1	1.01	0.38–2.39	0.16
31–45	29.2	63.2	7.5	0.33	1.40–0.74	0.55
≥46 (reference)	32.0	56.0	12.0	—	—	—
Country of undergraduate dental education						
North America	19.4	75.0	5.6	0.67	0.24–1.57	0.15
Europe	22.9	68.6	8.6	0.88	0.02–1.77	0.06
Asia	14.3	73.2	12.5	1.05	0.10–2.01	0.03
Middle East (reference)	45.7	43.8	10.5	—	—	—
Specialty						
General dental practitioners	35.0	56.9	8.0	0.18	1.20–0.84	0.73
Specialists caring for children	17.9	71.8	10.3	0.54	0.34–1.43	0.23
Other specialists (reference)	31.2	57.8	10.9	—	—	—
Years of practice						
≥10	32.6	57.6	9.7	0.48	1.45–0.50	0.34
<10 (reference)	28.4	61.1	10.5	—	—	—
Area of practice						
Rural	39.3	52.4	8.3	0.42	1.04–0.20	0.18
Urban (reference)	26.3	62.8	10.9	—	—	—
Work place						
Primary care clinics	36.3	56.0	7.7	0.50	1.54–0.53	0.34
Specialty care clinics	30.1	57.5	12.4	0.59	1.50–0.32	0.20
Private (reference)	18.4	73.7	7.9	—	—	—
Restorative treatment should take precedence over prevention						
Agree	60.0	35.0	5.0	1.61	3.49–0.27	0.09
Disagree	22.8	67.7	9.5	0.05	1.82–1.72	0.96
Not sure	50.0	21.4	28.6	—	—	—

cannot be prevented, to which few Asian undergraduates agreed. It could be that the Asian curriculum is more affiliated with the European system that has been described for many years to adopt a preventative treatment philosophy [33]. Also, differences in education had an effect on both preventative knowledge and preventative dental behaviors amongst Asians as reported by Soh [34].

Contradiction amongst our participants was evident when the majority (60%) claimed that they had adequate knowledge regarding topical fluorides but still 67% reported that they needed further information. In addition, 63% reported attending topical fluoride continuous education (CE) sessions in the past 5 years or less. Hence, there seems to be some doubts and uncertainties when it comes to the knowledge and use of fluoride.

In our study, 45% of the participants stated that the best method to obtain new information is through special courses, lectures and seminars; 23% through scientific journals; 17% through newsletter; and 15% through the World Wide Web. The literature shows that interactive educational meetings through attending workshops and participation in active discussions with the lecturers is the most effective intervention to diffuse certain knowledge and

thus changing clinical practice [35]. However, distribution of passive educational material like guidelines and publications, didactic educational meetings, and lectures have little or no effect on changing practitioners' knowledge or attitude and eventually cause a change in their routine dental practice [35]. To overcome the deficient knowledge among dentists working in Kuwait, an annual interactive workshop that highlights the importance of dental caries prevention, effective strategies, and available materials is highly needed to influence the change and improve the current dental knowledge, attitude, and practice.

In conclusion, despite the belief in topical fluoride effectiveness, certain barriers were apparent to its application. Knowledge deficiencies and attitude of practitioners play a major role. Clinical uncertainty as a result of labelling flaws, outdated undergraduate education, inappropriate continuous education, and lack of participation in effective educational activities are barriers too, and they can hinder clinicians from practicing evidence-based dentistry in their routine dental practice.

References

[1] N. B. Pitts, D. T. Zero, P. D. Marsh et al., "Dental caries," *Nature Reviews Disease Primers*, vol. 3, p. 17030, 2017.

[2] E. S. Akpata, J. Behbehani, J. Akbar, L. Thalib, and O. Mojiminiyi, "Fluoride intake from fluids and urinary fluoride excretion by young children in Kuwait: a non-fluoridated community," *Community Dental Oral Epidemiology*, vol. 42, no. 3, pp. 224–233, 2014.

[3] S. A. Al-Mutawa, M. Shyama, Y. Al-Duwairi, and P. Soparkar, "Dental caries experience of Kuwaiti kindergarten school-children," *Community Dental Health*, vol. 27, no. 4, pp. 213–217, 2010.

[4] S. A. Al-Mutawa, M. Shyama, Y. Al-Duwairi, and P. Soparkar, "Dental caries experience of Kuwaiti schoolchildren," *Community Dental Health*, vol. 23, no. 1, pp. 31–36, 2006.

[5] C. A. Evans and D. V. Kleinman, "The surgeon general's report on America's oral health: opportunities for the dental profession," *Journal of the American Dental Association*, vol. 131, no. 12, pp. 1721–1728, 2000.

[6] I. M. Haron, M. Y. Sabti, and R. Omar, "Awareness, knowledge and practice of evidence-based dentistry amongst dentists in Kuwait," *European Journal of Dental Education*, vol. 16, no. 1, pp. e47–e52, 2012.

[7] D. S. Brennan and A. J. Spencer, "The role of dentist, practice and patient factors in the provision of dental services," *Community Dentistry and Oral Epidemiology*, vol. 33, no. 3, pp. 181–195, 2005.

[8] E. L. Gaskin, S. Levy, S. Guzman-Armstrong, D. Dawson, and J. Chalmers, "Knowledge, attitudes, and behaviors of federal service and civilian dentists concerning minimal intervention dentistry," *Military Medicine*, vol. 175, no. 2, pp. 115–121, 2010.

[9] H. Ghasemi, H. Murtomaa, H. Torabzadeh, and M. M. Vehkalahti, "Knowledge of and attitudes towards preventive dental care among Iranian dentists," *European Journal of Dentistry*, vol. 1, no. 4, pp. 222–229, 2007.

[10] A. F. Al-Mobeeriek, S. M. Al-Shamrani, A. J. Al-Hussyeen, H. Z. Bushnag, and R. A. Al-Waheib, "Knowledge and attitude of dental health workers towards fluoride in Riyadh area," *Saudi Medical Journal*, vol. 22, no. 11, pp. 1004–1007, 2001.

[11] American Dental Association, *Action for Dental Health: Bringing Disease Prevention into Communities. 2013*, February 2018, http://www.ada.org/ADA/PublicPrograms/Files/bringing-disease-prevention-to-communities_adh.ashx.

[12] *NICE Public Health Guideline PH55-Oral health: Local Authorities and Partners*, February 2018, https://www.nice.org.uk/guidance/ph55.

[13] P. Jacobsen and D. Young, "The use of topical fluoride to prevent or reverse dental caries," *Special Care in Dentistry*, vol. 23, no. 5, pp. 177–179, 2003.

[14] V. C. Marinho, "Evidence-based effectiveness of topical fluorides," *Advances in Dental Research*, vol. 20, no. 1, pp. 3–7, 2008.

[15] M. Aspiras, P. Stoodley, L. Nistico, M. Longwell, and M. de Jager, "Clinical implications of power toothbrushing on fluoride delivery: effects on biofilm plaque metabolism and physiology," *International Journal of Dentistry*, vol. 2010, Article ID 651869, 7 pages, 2010.

[16] R. J. Weyant, S. L. Tracy, T. T. Anselmo et al., "Topical fluoride for caries prevention: executive summary of the updated clinical recommendations and supporting systematic review," *The Journal of the American Dental Association*, vol. 144, no. 11, pp. 1279–1291, 2013.

[17] V. C. Marinho, H. V. Worthington, T. Walsh, and J. E. Clarkson, "Fluoride varnishes for preventing dental caries in children and adolescents," *Cochrane Database Systematic Review*, vol. 11, no. 7, 2013.

[18] A. Satyanegara, R. R. Darwita, F. Setiawati, M. Adiatman, and R. Muhammad, "An in vitro study of caries arresting effect of propolis fluoride and silver diamine fluoride on dentine carious lesions," *Journal of International Dental and Medical Research*, vol. 10, pp. 751–756, 2017.

[19] R. Anggraini, R. R. Darwita, and M. Adiatman, "The effectiveness of silver diamine fluoride and propolis fluoride in arresting caries on primary teeth: a study on kindergarten students in west Jakarta Indonesia," *Journal of International Dental and Medical Research*, vol. 10, pp. 668–672, 2017.

[20] R. Bansal, K. A. Bolin, H. M. Abdellatif, and J. D. Shulman, "Knowledge, attitude and use of fluorides among dentists in Texas," *Journal of Contemporary Dental Practice*, vol. 13, no. 3, pp. 371–375, 2012.

[21] K. M. Yoder, G. Maupome, S. Ofner, and N. L. Swigonski, "Knowledge and use of fluoride among Indiana dental professionals," *Journal of Public Health Dentistry*, vol. 67, no. 3, pp. 140–147, 2007.

[22] J. W. Bawden, "Fluoride varnish: a useful new tool for public health dentistry," *Journal of Public Health Dentistry*, vol. 58, no. 4, pp. 266–269, 1998.

[23] Ministry of Health, *Annual Report of the Ministry of Health-Dental Administration*, MOH, Kuwait City, Kuwait, 28th edition, 2010.

[24] J. T. Wright, N. Hanson, H. Ristic, C. W. Whall, C. G. Estrich, and R. R. Zentz, "Fluoride toothpaste efficacy and safety in children younger than 6 years: a systematic review," *Journal of the American Dental Association*, vol. 145, no. 2, pp. 182–189, 2014.

[25] M. A. Qudeimat, F. A. Al-Saiegh, Q. Al-Omari, and R. Omar, "Restorative treatment decisions for deep proximal carious lesions in primary molars," *European Archives of Paediatric Dentistry*, vol. 8, no. 1, pp. 37–42, 2007.

[26] J. T. Autio-Gold and S. L. Tomar, "Dental students' opinions and knowledge about caries management and prevention," *Journal of Dental Education*, vol. 72, no. 1, pp. 26–32, 2008.

[27] H. Achmad and Y. F. Ramadhany, "Effectiveness of chitosan tooth paste from white shrimp (Litopenaeusvannamei) to reduce number of Streptococcus mutans in the case of early childhood caries," *Journal of International Dental and Medical Research*, vol. 10, no. 2, pp. 358–363, 2017.

[28] K. I. Olga, J. Mira, M. E. Zabokova-Bilbilova, M. Pavlevska, and G. Todorovska, "The ultrastructural changes of the initial lesion at early childhood caries," *Journal of International Dental and Medical Research*, vol. 10, no. 1, pp. 36–41, 2017.

[29] J. E. Frencken, M. C. Peters, D. J. Manton, S. C. Leal, V. V. Gordan, and E. Eden, "Minimal intervention dentistry for managing dental caries-a review," *International Dental Journal*, vol. 62, no. 5, pp. 223–243, 2012.

[30] A. Sheiham and W. P. T. James, "Diet and dental caries: the pivotal role of free sugars reemphasized," *Journal of Dental Research*, vol. 94, no. 10, pp. 1341–1347, 2015.

[31] I. Uzel, O. Ulukent, and D. Cogulu, "The effect of silver di-amine fluoride on microleakage of resin composite," *Journal of International Dental and Medical Research*, vol. 6, no. 3, pp. 105–108, 2013.

[32] S. S. Karabekiroğlu and N. Ünlü, "Effectiveness of different preventive programs in cariogram parameters of young adults at high caries risk," *International Journal of Dentistry*, vol. 2017, Article ID 7189270, 10 pages, 2017.

Knowledge, Attitude, and Barriers to Fluoride Application as a Preventive Measure...

201

[33] N. B. Pitts, "Are we ready to move from operative to non-operative/preventive treatment of dental caries in clinical practice?," *Caries Research*, vol. 38, no. 3, pp. 294–304, 2004.

[34] G. Soh, "Racial differences in perception of oral health and oral health behaviours in Singapore," *International Dental Journal*, vol. 42, no. 4, pp. 234–240, 1992.

[35] P. McGlone, R. Watt, and A. Sheiham, "Evidence-based dentistry: an overview of the challenges in changing professional practice," *British Dental Journal*, vol. 190, no. 12, pp. 636–639, 2001.

28

Assessing the Correlation between Skeletal and Corresponding Soft-Tissue Equivalents to Determine the Relationship between CBCT Skeletal/Dental Dimensions and 3D Radiographic Soft-Tissue Equivalents

Da In Kim[1] and Manuel O. Lagravère [ID][2]

[1]School of Dentistry, Faculty of Medicine and Dentistry, University of Alberta, ECHA, 11405-87 Avenue, Edmonton, AB, Canada T6G 1C9
[2]School of Dentistry, Faculty of Medicine and Dentistry, University of Alberta, Edmonton, AB, Canada T6G 1C9

Correspondence should be addressed to Manuel O. Lagravère; mlagravere@ualberta.ca

Academic Editor: Vahid Rakhshan

Objective. Compare measurements of skeletal and dental areas on the CBCT to the corresponding soft-tissue measures taken from a 3D Facial Scanner. *Methods.* 30 patients with CBCT and 3D Facial scanner photos were selected from the orthodontic program database. 30 different distance measurements were obtained from CBCT and facial scan. OrthoInsight software was used to obtain the measurements from the facial scan images, and AVIZO software was used for corresponding CBCT landmarks. The Euclidean distance formula was used to determine the distances for the corresponding *x*, *y*, and *z* coordinates of the CBCT. Reliability for CBCT and Facial Scanner was completed by calculating 30 distances for 10 patients, 3 times. Once reliability was determined, all 30 distances were calculated once for CBCT and facial scanner on each patient and descriptive statistics and paired *t*-test were applied. *Results.* All distances measured presented excellent reliability, the lowest one being the left eye width for the facial scanner (ICC 0.847). The landmark with the highest mean error on the CBCT was 2.0 ± 1.6 mm on the *z*-axis for the spinal level landmark. The Facial Scanner's largest mean measurement error was 1.5 ± 0.9 mm for the distance of the left corner of the mouth to gonion. All data except width between outer eye corners were statistically significant ($p < 0.05$). The average differences between facial scan and CBCT measurements ranged between 0.77 mm (left canine to cheekbone) to 26.94 mm (left subnasale to gonion) and are thus comparable. All measurements show a reasonable standard deviation between 2.57 mm (left eye width) to 9.91 mm (left gnathion to EAM). *Conclusion.* Distances obtained from CBCT and facial scan present mild differences giving the perspective of a relationship between them. Understanding this difference and relationship can make it plausible to expect certain underlying skeletal distances under soft-tissue structures.

1. Introduction

Since the development of dental photographic tools, much emphasis is put on skeletal landmarks as a tool for measurement in orthodontic analysis. In addition to skeletal evaluation, facial soft tissue evaluation plays a relevant role in treatment planning [1], since facial changes must be estimated while a patient undergoes long-term treatment. Both soft- and hard-tissue analyses as well as a more exact prediction of hard and soft tissue changes are important

tools to help the clinician assess treatment outcomes and give added diagnostic information about the patient [2].

2D lateral cephalometric imaging has been the routine method of obtaining hard-tissue information of the patient [3]. In recent years, high precision of three-dimensional (3D) cone-beam computed tomography (CBCT) scanners and their clinically insignificant errors has gauged interest in many clinicians to use this as a routine tool for hard-tissue investigation during treatment planning and diagnosis [4]. However, 3D hard-tissue analysis alone is inadequate for proper treatment planning. Since soft-tissue profile reflects underlying skeletal tissue, visual inspection and examination of the patient can give insightful information of the underlying dental tissue [5]. Conventional methods for facial soft-tissue analysis include 2D measurement methods, such as taking photos of the patient at different angles [6]. These photos are then used to measure certain distances via computational analysis. Over the years, 3D facial soft-tissue analysis has been introduced to provide a more accurate description of the patient's soft-tissue profile [6]. These 3D facial scanners use a strip of laser light to record the contour of the patient's face and cranium and project their recordings onto a computer. With this 3D information, clinicians are able to obtain information such as cranial growth changes and treatment outcomes in a more realistic fashion. This ultimately allows the clinician to undergo prediction planning for the patient [7].

As such, both 3D soft- and hard-tissue analyses are essential in obtaining precise measurements for treatment planning. However, precise facial measurements can only be made when the clinician truly understands the relationship between these two imaging modalities and by obtaining a truthful 3D model of the soft tissues and underlying skeletal structures [7]. By determining relationships and assessing imaging tendencies between CBCT and facial scanner, clinicians will be able to deliver diagnoses with increased exactness: if the soft-tissue distance is highly correlated with that of the hard tissue, the clinician can conclude that this particular distance on the skin can highly reflect its underlying hard-tissue distance. Also, these would be the initial steps towards verifying the effects of treatments (orthodontic or surgical) on soft tissues when viewing in three-dimensions. The objective of this study is therefore, to analyze different landmark relations obtained from 3D facial scanner and CBCT for comparison and prediction planning, for use as a diagnostic tool.

2. Materials and Methods

CBCTs and 3D facial scans from 30 patients that were seen in the University of Alberta Graduate Orthodontic Clinic were selected for analysis. The basis for this sample size was based on availability of the images needed for the purpose of this study, since the CBCT and facial scan images were all taken retrospectively and were chosen amongst a main database. The reasoning of the full field of view CBCTs for these patients was for diagnostic and treatment planning purposes of the orthodontists in charge of the individual patient cases and was not taken for the purpose of this study. The University of Alberta's Human Research Ethics Board approved of this study (Pro00057947). CBCT scans of 0.3 mm voxel size were taken with the I-CAT Next generation device (9 sec exposure time, 13 cm x 16 cm FOV, 0.3 mm voxel size, Imaging Sciences International, Hatsfield, PA) at 120 kV, 5 mA with 8 mm aluminum filtration according to manufacturer's settings. 3D facial scans were obtained on the same day as the CBCTs, using Ortho Insight 3D Scanner (Motion View LLC., United States of America). All images chosen with patients in their natural upright head position, with the Frankfort plane parallel to the floor. As all data were collected retrospectively, strict positioning of the head was not available

to be controlled. CBCTs were analyzed using a third party software called AVIZO (Thermo Fisher Scientific, Hillsboro, United States of America), which helped to obtain the 3D reconstruction of the image for landmark positioning.

In relation to a reference point, each CBCT landmark (Tables 1 and 2) was given coordinates in x, y, and z format. This reference point was an arbitrary position placed amongst the coordinates of the software program. Since the distance between two specific points were to be measured, the initial reference point for each distance was different for each patient and distance, as it was all relative to where the second point was to be placed. The Euclidean distance formula was used to determine the linear distances for the corresponding x, y, and z coordinates.

$$d = \sqrt{(x_1 - x_2)^2 + (y_1 - y_2)^2 + (z_1 - z_2)^2}. \quad (1)$$

The facial scanning machine along with its corresponding third party software, OrthoInsight, was used to obtain the 3D soft-tissue profile of the patient. Soft-tissue distances between landmarks (Table 3) were calculated by the software to obtain landmark measurements in millimetres.

CBCTs and 3D facial scans from 10 patients out of the main sample were selected for reliability analysis (Figures 1 and 2). For the CBCT, reliability analysis was performed by initially obtaining 30 preselected distances (Table 1) based off of well-defined landmarks on soft and hard tissues (Table 2), for each of these 10 sets of patient images for both imaging modalities. All 30 distances were measured repeatedly, 3 times in total, for all 10 selected patient images for the CBCT and facial scan. A time span of one week took place after each of those three trials, in order to minimize any errors regarding the researcher's subjectivity of the placement of landmarks, especially those that were not too precise to locate on the images. Coordinates of the CBCT were analyzed for reliability calculations. For the facial scan, the same 30 distances (Table 1) were measured on 10 different facial scans, 3 times. Landmark distances were measured 3 times, leaving a week in between trials. Reliability calculations were performed from this data. Following landmark reliability calculations, the true data set of CBCT and facial scan images of the 30 selected patients were analyzed. Each of the 30 chosen distances was measured once on these patients for both imaging modalities. Descriptive statistics and paired t-test calculations were applied in order to obtain information regarding the relationships between distances on the skeletal and those on the facial tissue. The gold standard imaging modality is the CBCT, as it claims to have high precision (1:1 image to reality ratio), minimum deviation, and is highly reliable when evaluating linear distances for craniofacial analysis [4, 8–13].

3. Results

All measured distances presented excellent reliability, the lowest one being the left eye width of the facial scanner, with an intraclass correlation coefficient (ICC) of 0.847 (Tables 4 and 5). For CBCTs, the landmark with the highest mean error was 2.0 ± 1.6 mm on the z-axis for the spinal level

TABLE 1: Measured and defined distances depending on the image used.

	Landmarks	Description of distances on CBCT	Description of distances on facial scanner
1	Width of nose	Left bottom-most skeletal corner under the nasal aperture to the right bottom-most skeletal corner	Left alar curvature point (the most lateral part of the curved base of the ala) to the right alar curvature point
2	Left canine to left outer eye	Most tip of left canine crown to left frontozygomatic suture	Most tip of left canine (patient smiling) to left lateral canthus
3	Right canine to right outer eye	Most tip of right canine crown to right frontozygomatic suture	Most tip of right canine (patient smiling) to right lateral canthus
4	Gnathion to throat	Lowest point of the midline of the mandible to C3-C4 cervical vertebrae	Lowest point of the midline of the mandible to the most indented location of the throat between the chin and neck
5	Gnathion to left gonion	Lowest point of the mandibular midline to the lowest, most posterior, and lateral point of the left mandibular angle	Lowest point of the mandibular midline to the lowest, most posterior, and lateral point of the left mandibular angle
6	Gnathion to right gonion	Lowest point of the mandibular midline to the lowest, most posterior, and lateral point of the right mandibular angle	Lowest point of the mandibular midline to the lowest, most posterior, and lateral point of the right mandibular angle
7	Left canine to left cheekbone	Most tip of left canine crown to most prominent frontal portion of the left zygomatic bone	Most tip of left canine crown (patient smiling) to most prominently raised point of left cheek area, most likely an area under the left lateral canthus
8	Right canine to right cheekbone	Most tip of right canine crown to most prominent frontal portion of the right zygomatic bone	Most tip of right canine crown (patient smiling) to most prominently raised point of right cheek area, most likely an area under the right lateral canthus
9	Nasion to gnathion	Distinctly depressed area between the intersection of the frontal bone and two nasal bones to the lowest point of the mandibular midline.	Distinctly depressed area directly between the eyes and superior to the bridge of the nose to the lowest point of the mandibular midline
10	Gnathion to left external auditory meatus (EAM)	Lowest portion of the mandibular midline to lowest bony portion of the left hollow canal of the tympanic portion of the temporal bone, posterior to the condylar process of the mandible	Lowest portion of the mandibular midline to the left lowest portion of the hollow ear canal
11	Gnathion to right EAM	Lowest portion of the mandibular midline to lowest bony portion of the right hollow canal of the tympanic portion of the temporal bone, posterior to the condylar process of the mandible	Lowest portion of the mandibular midline to the right lowest portion of the hollow ear canal
12	Corners of mouth	Tip of left canine crown to tip of right canine crown	Left cheilion (left labial commissure) to right cheilion (right labial commissure)
13	Left EAM to left outer eye corner	Lowest bony portion of the left hollow canal of the tympanic portion of the temporal bone, posterior to the condylar process of the mandible, to the left lateral canthus of eye	Left lowest portion of the hollow ear canal to the left lateral canthus of eye
14	Right EAM to right outer eye corner	Lowest bony portion of the right hollow canal of the tympanic portion of the temporal bone, posterior to the condylar process of the mandible, to the right lateral canthus of eye	Right lowest portion of the hollow ear canal to the right lateral canthus of eye
15	Bottom of nose to nasion	Anterior nasal spine to the distinctly depressed area between the intersection of the frontal bone and two nasal bones	Subnasale (the midpoint of the angle at the nasal base where the lower border of the nasal septum and the upper lip surface meets) to the distinctly depressed area directly between the eyes and superior to the bridge of the nose
16	Width of left eye	Left frontozygomatic suture to left frontomaxillary suture	Left lateral canthus to left medial canthus
17	Width of right eye	Right frontozygomatic suture to right frontomaxillary suture	Right lateral canthus to right medial canthus
18	Left inner eye to left canine	Left frontomaxillary suture to tip of left canine crown	Left medial canthus to tip of left canine crown (patient smiling)
19	Right inner eye to right canine	Right frontomaxillary suture to tip of right canine crown	Right medial canthus to tip of right canine crown (patient smiling)

TABLE 1: Continued.

	Landmarks	Description of distances on CBCT	Description of distances on facial scanner
20	Left gonion to left EAM	Lowest, most posterior, and lateral point of the left mandibular angle to the lowest bony portion of the left hollow canal of the tympanic portion of the temporal bone, posterior to the condylar process of the mandible	Most posterior and lateral point of the left mandibular angle to the left most lowest portion of the hollow ear canal opening
21	Right gonion to right EAM	Lowest, most posterior, and lateral point of the right mandibular angle to the lowest bony portion of the right hollow canal of the tympanic portion of the temporal bone, posterior to the condylar process of the mandible	Most posterior and lateral point of the right mandibular angle to the right most lowest portion of the hollow ear canal opening
22	Bottom of nose to left EAM	Anterior nasal spine to the lowest bony portion of the left hollow canal of the tympanic portion of the temporal bone, posterior to the condylar process of the mandible	Subnasale (the midpoint of the angle at the nasal base where the lower border of the nasal septum and the upper lip surface meets) to the left most lowest portion of the hollow ear canal opening
23	Bottom of nose to right EAM	Anterior nasal spine to the lowest bony portion of the right hollow canal of the tympanic portion of the temporal bone, posterior to the condylar process of the mandible	Subnasale (the midpoint of the angle at the nasal base where the lower border of the nasal septum and the upper lip surface meets) to the right most lowest portion of the hollow ear canal opening
24	Left corner of mouth to left EAM	Tip of left canine crown to the lowest bony portion of the left hollow canal of the tympanic portion of the temporal bone, posterior to the condylar process of the mandible	Left cheilion (left labial commissure) to the left most lowest portion of the hollow ear canal opening
25	Right corner of mouth to right EAM	Tip of right canine crown to the lowest bony portion of the right hollow canal of the tympanic portion of the temporal bone, posterior to the condylar process of the mandible	Right cheilion (right labial commissure) to the right most lowest portion of the hollow ear canal opening
26	Width between outer eye corners	Left frontozygomatic suture to right frontozygomatic suture	Left lateral canthus to right lateral canthus
27	Left corner of mouth to left gonion	Tip of left canine crown to the lowest, most posterior, and lateral point of the left mandibular angle	Left cheilion (left labial commissure) to the most posterior and lateral point of the left mandibular angle
28	Right corner of mouth to right gonion	Tip of right canine crown to the lowest, most posterior, and lateral point of the right mandibular angle	Right cheilion (right labial commissure) to the most posterior and lateral point of the right mandibular angle
29	Bottom of nose to left gonion	Anterior nasal spine to lowest, most posterior, and lateral point of the left mandibular angle	Subnasale (the midpoint of the angle at the nasal base where the lower border of the nasal septum and the upper lip surface meets) to most posterior and lateral point of the left mandibular angle
30	Bottom of nose to right gonion	Anterior nasal spine to lowest, most posterior, and lateral point of the right mandibular angle	Subnasale (the midpoint of the angle at the nasal base where the lower border of the nasal septum and the upper lip surface meets), to most posterior and lateral point of the right mandibular angle

landmark. The facial scanner's largest mean measurement error was 1.5 ± 0.9 mm for the distance of the left corner of the mouth to the left gonion.

When comparing the difference between facial scanner and CBCT measurements via the paired t-test, all data except that of the width between outer eye corners were statistically significant ($p < 0.05$). Although the p value of the width between outer eye corners is $p = 0.44$, a very small facial scan to CBCT mean difference of 0.71 mm makes this measurement comparable.

Most measurements had a mean facial scan to CBCT difference of less than 9 mm. Such means indicate that distances measured on the CBCT and facial scan are very similar and thus comparable. However, measurements containing the left and right gonion, throat, corners of mouth, and subnasale had large facial scan to CBCT mean differences ranging from 16.66 mm (right corner of mouth to gonion) to 23.32 mm (left subnasale to gonion). Even though these means were relatively large, paired measurements with left and right sides had similar means. For example, the left gnathion to gonion measurement had a mean of 21.76 mm, while the right gnathion to gonion measurement had a mean of 20.79 mm, giving a difference in measurement of only 0.97 mm; although the mean is relatively large, both left and right sides are similar, indicating that they are comparable.

TABLE 2: Definition of landmarks used for measuring specific distances, depending on the imaging modality used.

	Landmark	Description of landmark on CBCT	Description of landmark on soft tissue
1	Sides of nose	Left/right bottom most skeletal corner under the nasal aperture	Left/right alar curvature (most lateral part of the curved base of the ala)
2	Canine	Most tip of the left/right canine crown	Most tip of the left/right canine crown
3	Outer eye	Left/right frontozygomatic suture	Left/right lateral canthus
4	Gnathion	Lowest point of the midline of the mandible	Lowest point of the midline of the mandible
5	Throat	C3-C4 cervical vertebrae location	Most indented location of the throat between the chin and neck
6	Gonion	Most posterior and lateral point of the left/right mandibular angle	Most posterior and lateral point of the left/right mandibular angle on the skin
7	Cheekbone	Most prominent frontal portion of the left/right zygomatic bone	Most prominently raised point of the left/right cheek area, most likely an area under the left/right lateral canthus
8	Nasion	Distinctly depressed area between the intersection of the frontal bone and two nasal bones	Distinctly depressed area directly between the eyes and superior to the bridge of the nose
9	External auditory meatus (EAM)	Lowest bony portion of the left/right hollow canal of the tympanic portion of the temporal bone, posterior to the condylar processes of the mandible	Left/right lowest portion of the hollow ear canal
10	Corners of mouth	Tip of left/right canine crowns	Left/right cheilion (left/right labial commissures)
11	Bottom of nose	Anterior nasal spine	Subnasale (midpoint of the angle at the nasal base where the lower border of the nasal septum and upper lip surface meets)
12	Inner eye	Left/right frontomaxillary suture	Left/right medial canthus

4. Discussion

Hard- and soft-tissue analyses are both critical tools for patient treatment planning and diagnosis and analysis of the patient over a long period of time. In contrary to conventional soft tissue and skeletal imaging tools such as patient photos and 2D analog films, 3D images of the patient are considered the ideal method of representing the face, and thus gives added information to the clinician, which in turn will give more realistic analyses [7]. Unlike using traditional 2D imaging to analyze 3D structures, which can have limited significance [7, 14, 15], comparing 3D hard to 3D soft tissue structures can be an improved alternate for the clinician to assess and evaluate cranial changes over time. Recently, several studies have adopted similar approaches in comparing 3D photography to CBCT concepts and have concluded that there is a close relationship between patient images taken by these two modalities.

In the present study, all measurements show a reasonable standard deviation between 2.57 mm (left eye width) to 9.91 mm (left gnathion to EAM). This shows that over a large sample size, these measurements are very similar, and less variable. However, the standard deviation for the gnathion to throat measurement is comparably large at 23.34 mm. This shows that there is lot of variation between the gnathion to throat measurement within a large sample.

The ratio between the soft tissue and CBCT measurements indicate their close correlation and any amount of variation or difference between them. The ratio percentages presented on Table 3 indicate the percentage of the CBCT distance measurements compared to that of the soft tissue measurements. Most ratio measurements are ±20%, but those that include the left and right gonion have a tendency to have smaller ratios, except for that of the left gonion to left

EAM (+49.76%) and that of the right gonion to right EAM (+52.92%). These small ratios indicate that the CBCT, when measuring distances including the left and right gonion, tend to measure shorter than the soft tissue distances. A similar finding is seen in a study conducted by Naudi et al. [7], who evaluated the registration exactness of the simultaneous capture between a CBCT scan and a 3D surface of the face. Unlike the present study, the CBCT scans of this study captured soft-tissue measures to compare their superimposition with the 3D image capture. Naudi et al. concluded that in most of the facial surfaces, the level of superimposition in designated facial patches was 0.4 mm for simultaneous captures, denoting that superimpositions of the CBCT were smaller than those of the 3D image capture. The study also concluded that the most significant difference of superimposition between the CBCT and 3D image capture was in the chin area, with the mobile nature of the mandible being a large contributing factor of this result. It was mentioned that the relaxing atmosphere of the 3D image capture rooms may have led to patients slightly opening their jaws and bringing their teeth apart, leading to a slight increase in the degree of mouth opening and spatial changes of the related soft tissue. It can therefore be extrapolated that a larger degree of mouth opening of the soft tissue scans leads to a large superimposition, and thus, a larger difference compared to the CBCT image. These findings of Naudi et al. agree with the present study, as it was found that the tendency of losing measurement similarity, and thus having less of an intimate relationship between CBCT and facial scans was most prominent along the lateral portions of the face.

The tendency of having a lower correlation along the lateral portions of the face can be due to the variability of amounts of subcutaneous tissue present on each patient, but it may also be attributed to the increased amounts of larger,

TABLE 3: Statistics of soft tissue distances and their CBCT equivalents, including average mean measurements, standard deviation, the difference between the average mean measurements, and the ratio of the CBCT distances to the soft-tissue distances in percentage format, p values, and 95% confidence intervals of the differences between the facial scan and CBCT.

Landmarks		Soft tissue measurements		CBCT hard tissue measurements		p value	95% confidence interval of the differences (facial scan-CBCT)		Facial scanner and CBCT mean difference (mm)	Ratio of soft tissue and CBCT distances (%)
		Average mean (mm)	Standard deviation	Average mean (mm)	Standard deviation		Lower	Upper		
1	Width of nose	25.26	2.53	21.65	3.33	0.001	−15.04	9.43	3.61	−14.29
2	Left canine to left outer eye	70.05	3.97	78.60	5.62	0.001	−17.70	−5.79	−8.55	+12.21
3	Right canine to right outer eye	70.47	4.49	77.90	5.33	0.001	−9.17	−5.68	−7.43	+10.54
4	Gnathion to throat	68.68	24.07	79.67	10.09	0.019	−20.88	−0.42	−10.99	+16.00
5	Gnathion to left gonion	101.68	8.37	79.92	7.72	0.001	21.59	31.86	21.76	−21.40
6	Gnathion to right gonion	100.56	8.33	79.77	6.03	0.001	21.11	31.55	20.79	−20.67
7	Left canine to left cheekbone	48.18	3.28	43.51	3.62	0.001	−7.04	8.58	4.67	−9.69
8	Right canine to right cheekbone	49.09	4.07	42.07	6.32	0.001	−20.36	16.31	7.02	−14.30
9	Nasion to gnathion	116.51	8.51	111.41	8.58	0.003	0.18	14.99	5.10	−4.38
10	Gnathion to left external auditory meatus (EAM)	128.58	12.71	120.86	9.25	0.001	−4.89	15.28	7.72	−6.00
11	Gnathion to right EAM	127.69	12.15	120.30	9.25	0.001	3.47	15.03	7.39	−5.79
12	Corners of mouth	47.43	4.80	35.67	3.74	0.001	−6.24	17.90	11.76	−24.79
13	Left EAM to left corner eye	80.71	5.52	72.88	5.10	0.001	0.29	10.71	7.83	−9.70
14	Right EAM to right corner eye	80.80	5.59	72.87	5.00	0.001	−1.95	10.40	7.93	−9.81
15	Bottom of nose to nasion	47.71	4.32	54.05	6.19	0.001	−8.87	−4.29	−6.34	+13.29
16	Width of left eye	30.94	2.28	38.43	2.79	0.001	−26.87	−1.01	−7.49	+24.21
17	Width of right eye	31.19	2.38	38.48	2.62	0.001	−8.30	−6.27	−7.29	+23.37
18	Left inner eye to left canine	63.27	4.46	70.51	5.48	0.001	−20.34	−2.78	−7.24	+11.44
19	Right inner eye to right canine	63.63	4.63	70.44	5.72	0.001	−43.33	5.63	−6.81	+10.70
20	Left gonion to left EAM	35.25	5.90	52.79	6.53	0.001	−26.02	−14.41	−17.54	+49.76
21	Right gonion to right EAM	34.88	5.17	53.34	7.38	0.001	−27.41	−14.06	−18.46	+52.92
22	Bottom of nose to left EAM	119.07	8.82	101.26	9.21	0.001	14.00	24.11	17.81	−14.96
23	Bottom of nose to right EAM	120.17	8.80	101.29	8.81	0.001	−11.12	30.86	18.88	−15.71
24	Left corner of mouth to left EAM	98.68	7.96	95.78	7.54	0.015	−6.78	6.25	2.90	−2.94
25	Right corner of mouth to right EAM	98.86	8.03	94.92	7.70	0.001	−0.19	7.08	3.94	−3.99
26	Width between outer eye corners	94.88	5.42	94.18	11.69	0.437	−7.03	10.41	0.70	−0.74
27	Left corner of mouth to left gonion	85.72	6.76	68.43	8.44	0.001	7.96	23.08	17.29	−20.17
28	Right corner of mouth to right gonion	84.42	7.15	67.76	6.11	0.001	15.41	20.23	16.66	−19.73
29	Bottom of nose to left gonion	109.42	8.33	86.10	9.35	0.001	21.29	32.56	23.32	−21.31
30	Bottom of nose to right gonion	110.41	8.98	87.26	8.93	0.001	19.84	33.63	23.15	−20.97

curved, bony surface areas on the lateral profile of the face. Toma et al. [16] indicated that due to the difficulty of placing points accurately on a patient's lateral profile, soft-tissue landmarks on both left and right lateral sides of the face are not highly reproducible. Such findings agree with the present study, since it was also found in this investigation that the left and right gonions have a tendency to elicit relatively large differences amongst soft tissue and CBCT landmark sites, whereas some of the smallest CBCT to soft tissue ratios were found along landmarks near the center of the face, including the width between outer eye corners (−0.74%) and the measurement between the nasion to gnathion (−4.38%).

Baumrind and Frantz [17] also found that the gonion was one of the least reliable landmarks to identify, whereas the nasion had a relatively smaller skeletal landmark estimating error. Although this study focused on 2D films, their findings can be extrapolated to 3D skeletal measurements on CBCT films. The study acknowledged that as a boney structure has a gradually curving edge, such as the gonion, the mean error of incorrect landmarking tends to be larger, leading to the large measurement error. Their findings agree with the present study, because in this investigation, landmark distances including either the left or right gonion were interpreted as those with the least amount of correlation between CBCT and 3D facial scanner (Table 3). The difficulty of locating the exact landmark of the left and right gonions may have lead to the large CBCT to soft tissue ratio difference, since landmarks may have been unintentionally placed along different areas of this largely curved boney edge. Additionally, despite the precise definition given to the gonion on the soft tissue (Table 1), the structure itself was found to be very challenging to visualize on facial images of

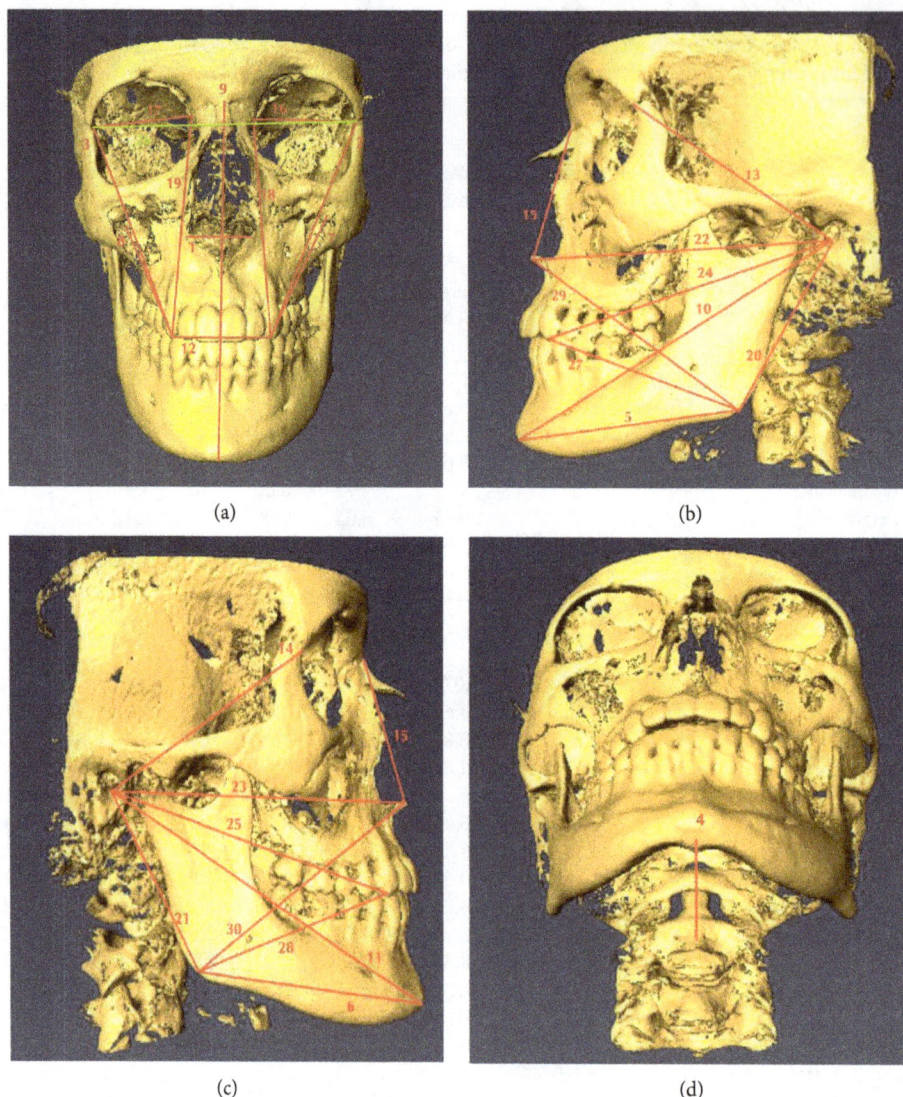

FIGURE 1: Front, left lateral profile, right lateral profile, and inferior views of the CBCT image, with numbered areas corresponding to landmarks. (a) Frontal view. (b) Left lateral profile view. (c) Right lateral profile view. (d) Inferior view.

the patient, as it is a structure that is easily hidden by subcutaneous tissue underneath.

As mentioned previously, measurements containing the left and right gonion, throat, corners of mouth, and subnasale had large facial scanner to CBCT mean differences. These measurements, along with others that had large means between facial scanner and CBCT data were those that had slightly different landmarks on the face between the two imaging modalities. Another study conducted by Maal et al. [18] had similar findings. This group investigated image fusion between soft tissue CBCT images and 3D photographs. It was found in their study that registration errors between CBCT and 3D images were largest at the lateral neck, mouth, and areas around the eyes. One of the causes of such dissimilarities was accredited to the fact of the inability of the CBCT to capture exact soft-tissue surfaces. Although this study focused on soft tissue comparison, the present study agrees with the concept that more registration error is

found when there are different locations and definitions present for the same area on the face between two different imaging modalities. Soft-tissue CBCTs of Maal et al. were not of the same quality of comparison to that of the 3D images, and thus less precise locations would have been compared between these two imaging modalities. Similarly in this project, landmarks with a significant soft tissue to CBCT ratio > 20% are mainly due to the different definitions of the landmarks of the CBCT and soft tissue images, as defined in Table 1. The different definitions were created because it was acknowledged that hard- and soft-tissue landmarks are distinctly different in some definitions. For example, the large ratio percentage of the measurement of the width of the left eye (+24.21%) and the width of the right eye (+23.37%) raises mostly due to the different landmarking positions. The definition given for the "width of eye" is completely different: the CBCT defines this landmark as a distance between the frontozygomatic suture and the frontomaxillary suture,

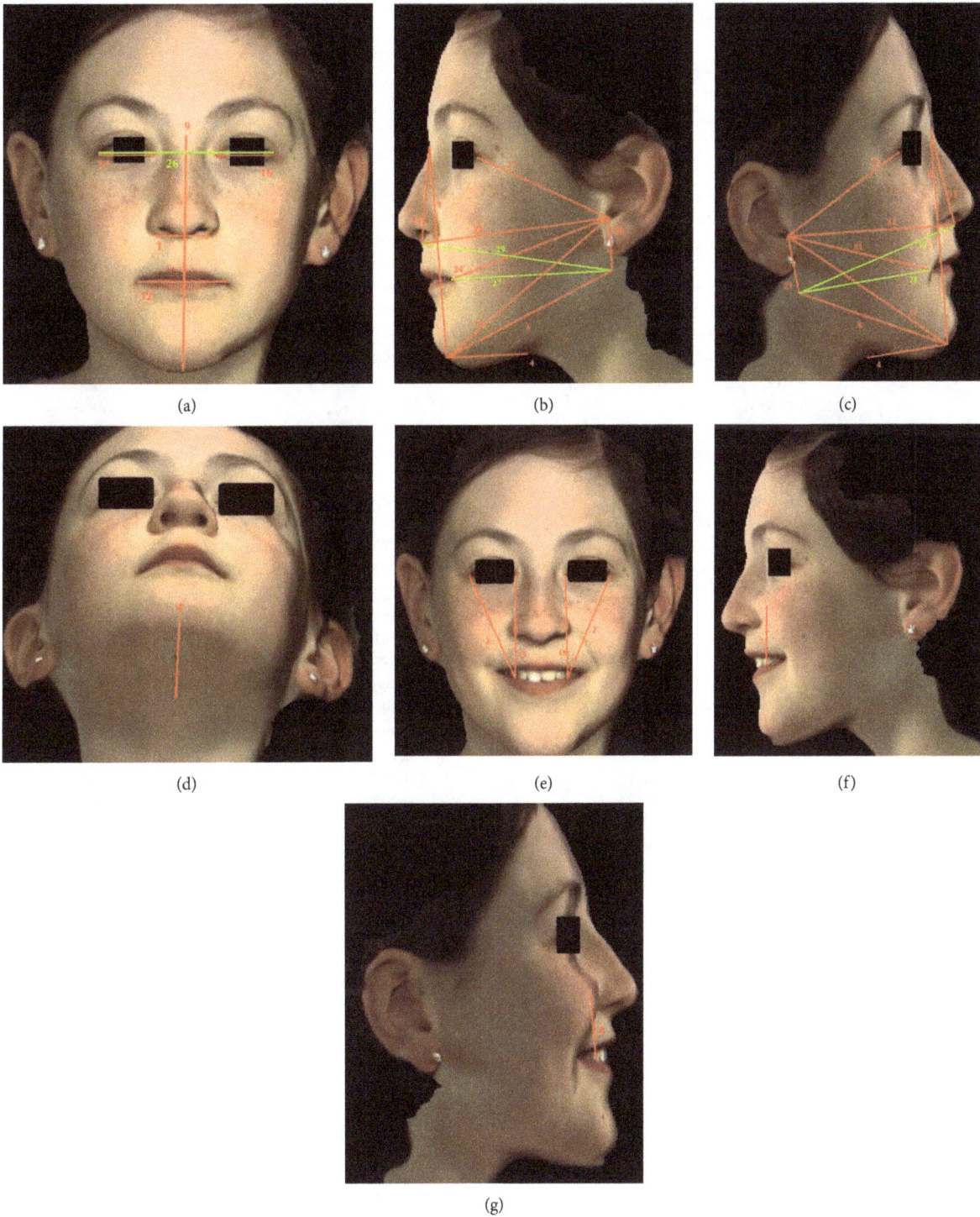

FIGURE 2: Frontal, left lateral profile, right lateral profile, inferior, frontal smiling, left lateral profile smiling, and right lateral profile smiling views of the facial scanner image, with numbered areas corresponding to landmarks. (a) Frontal View. (b) Left lateral profile view. (c) Right lateral profile view. (d) Inferior view. (e) Frontal view, smiling. (f) Left lateral profile view, smiling. (g) Right lateral profile view, smiling.

whereas the same landmark on the facial scanner is defined to be the distance from the lateral canthus to the medial canthus. Since both skeletal sutures extend beyond the lateral and medial canthi, this may be the cause of the CBCT's ratio being much higher. The larger discrepancy of the ratio due to different definitions is also seen in the

"corners of mouth" landmark (−24.79%). The CBCT definition of the distance between the corners of the mouth is from one tip of the canine crown to the other, whereas the soft tissue definition is that of one cheilion to the other. Since individuals may have extended lip commissures, which potentially go further beyond the location of their canines,

TABLE 4: Intraclass correlation coefficients (ICC) of facial scan landmarks, lower and upper limits of their 95% confidence intervals, and their corresponding p values.

	Landmarks	Intraclass correlation coefficient	95% confidence intervals of soft tissue ICC		p value
			Lower	Upper	
1	Width of nose	0.960	0.883	0.989	0.001
2	Left canine to left outer eye	0.965	0.900	0.991	0.001
3	Right canine to right outer eye	0.990	0.970	0.997	0.001
4	Gnathion to throat	0.999	0.997	1.000	0.001
5	Gnathion to left gonion	0.999	0.998	1.000	0.001
6	Gnathion to right gonion	0.999	0.998	1.000	0.001
7	Left canine to left cheekbone	0.947	0.846	0.986	0.001
8	Right canine to right cheekbone	0.971	0.918	0.992	0.001
9	Nasion to gnathion	1.000	0.999	1.000	0.001
10	Gnathion to left external auditory meatus (EAM)	1.000	0.999	1.000	0.001
11	Gnathion to right EAM	1.000	0.999	1.000	0.001
12	Corners of mouth	0.974	0.925	0.993	0.001
13	Left EAM to left corner eye	0.971	0.914	0.992	0.001
14	Right EAM to right corner eye	0.972	0.921	0.992	0.001
15	Bottom of nose to nasion	0.989	0.968	0.997	0.001
16	Width of left eye	0.847	0.539	0.959	0.001
17	Width of right eye	0.875	0.643	0.966	0.001
18	Left inner eye to left canine	0.993	0.979	0.998	0.001
19	Right inner eye to right canine	0.993	0.980	0.998	0.001
20	Left gonion to left EAM	0.994	0.983	0.998	0.001
21	Right gonion to right EAM	0.991	0.974	0.998	0.001
22	Bottom of nose to left EAM	0.998	0.994	0.999	0.001
23	Bottom of nose to right EAM	0.996	0.990	0.999	0.001
24	Left corner of mouth to left EAM	0.996	0.990	0.999	0.001
25	Right corner of mouth to right EAM	0.996	0.989	0.999	0.001
26	Width between outer eye corners	0.989	0.968	0.997	0.001
27	Left corner of mouth to left gonion	0.982	0.950	0.995	0.001
28	Right corner of mouth to right gonion	0.992	0.978	0.998	0.001
29	Bottom of nose to left gonion	0.994	0.982	0.998	0.001
30	Bottom of nose to right gonion	0.991	0.975	0.998	0.001

TABLE 5: Intraclass correlation coefficients (ICC) of CBCT landmarks, lower and upper limits of their 95% confidence intervals, and their corresponding p values.

	Landmark	Intraclass correlation coefficient	95% confidence intervals of CBCT ICC		p value
			Lower	Upper	
1	Left nose radiolucency	0.990	0.971	0.997	0.001
2	Right nose radiolucency	0.967	0.908	0.991	0.001
3	Left canine	0.993	0.980	0.998	0.001
4	Right canine	0.997	0.989	0.999	0.001
5	Gnathion	0.979	0.940	0.994	0.001
6	Throat (spinal level)	0.987	0.964	0.997	0.001
7	Left gonion	0.999	0.997	1.000	0.001
8	Right gonion	0.998	0.995	1.000	0.001
9	Left zygomatic process	0.975	0.927	0.993	0.001
10	Right zygomatic process	0.969	0.910	0.991	0.001
11	Left external auditory meatus	0.998	0.995	1.000	0.001
12	Right external auditory meatus	0.992	0.977	0.998	0.001
13	Left frontozygomatic suture (outer corner of eye)	0.987	0.963	0.997	0.001
14	Right frontozygomatic suture (outer corner of eye)	0.988	0.967	0.997	0.001
15	Subnasale	0.992	0.978	0.998	0.001
16	Nasion	0.991	0.973	0.997	0.001
17	Left frontonasal suture (inner corner of eye)	0.962	0.891	0.990	0.001
18	Right frontonasal suture (inner corner of eye)	0.977	0.934	0.994	0.001

this may cause the CBCT to be seemingly shorter than that of the soft-tissue distances, even though this difference was due to a dissimilar definition.

Considering anterior-posterior (AP) and vertical measurements, left and right gonion landmarks were easily found on the CBCT but were difficult to locate on the facial scanner. Depending on the patient's size, the location of the gonion was easily or not easily found on the facial scanner. If not found, approximate landmarks were taken for the location of the gonion, which may have contributed to a larger difference in location compared to the CBCT. The measurement involving the throat (gnathion to throat, −10.99 mm) also had a relatively large facial scanner to CBCT mean difference, since slightly different landmarks were taken between the facial scanner and CBCT. On the facial scanner, the throat was defined and landmarked as the deepest part of the neck when viewed from the left and right sides. On the CBCT, the "throat" was landmarked as the spinal level that corresponded to the area of the throat, approximately at C2. Such different landmarks may have possibly contributed to a larger difference in the mean, with the CBCT measurement being larger than that of the facial scanner. Large mean differences of the throat may be related to low reproducibility of landmarks, since soft tissue anatomical features of the throat are much less clear than the hard tissue definition of this landmark. This may ultimately lead to low intraobserver reproducibility of this landmark [19].

Considering transverse measurements, the corners of the mouth also lead to a relatively large mean difference of 11.76 mm. On the facial scanner, the corner of each side of the mouth was landmarked to the furthest corner of the lips when the patient was not smiling. On the CBCT, the landmark for each corner of the mouth was taken as the canine for left and right sides. With some patients having a shifted or rotated canine, no canine, or orthodontic brackets, landmarking the canine on the CBCT had to be approximated, and for some cases, maxillary lateral incisors were used as landmarks instead. Distractions such as metal artefacts may reduce the exactness of the superimposition between the two imaging modalities [20]. The landmark for subnasale also had slightly different locations. On the facial scanner, the soft tissue subnasale point was used, which is the point of convergence of the nose and upper lip, directly beneath the nose. However on the CBCT, the central, most dense area directly under and between the two nasal sinuses was used for landmarking. Since the CBCT subnasale landmark was close to the anterior nasal spine, its measurements were more superior on the face compared to that of the facial scanner. A study conducted by Ayoub et al. [15] which investigated the superimposition of 3D data gathered from a CT scanner and a stereophotogrammetry tool found errors within an acceptable range of ±1.5 mm, with relatively large errors around the eyelid area. It was noted that the eyelid and eyebrow area is subject to surface shape differences when taken via these different imaging modalities, leading to this registration error. Additionally, Hwang et al. [19] stated that some anatomical structures such as the midlateral orbit do not clearly represent the actual anatomical structure of the soft tissues. The findings of both

studies agree with the present study, as it was found that measurements containing outer and inner eyes generally had relatively large mean differences. The outer eye landmark on the facial scanner was defined as the most outer sharp part of the eye, and the inner eye landmark was also defined as the most inner sharp part seen on the eye. On the CBCT, the outer eye was defined as the suture between the frontal and zygomatic bones, and the inner eye landmark was located and the suture between the frontal bone and maxilla, near the nasal bone. Since these sutures are more superior on the face than the actual soft tissue outer and inner eye corners, a slightly different mean between the facial scanner and CBCT can be seen; CBCT values are slightly larger, and thus mean difference measurements for left canine to outer eye (−8.55 mm), right canine to outer eye (−7.43 mm), left eye width (−7.49 mm), right eye width (−7.29 mm), left inner eye to canine (−7.25 mm), and right inner eye to canine (−6.81 mm) are negative. As such, these findings indicate that soft- and hard-tissue landmarks of the eye are difficult to reproduce.

Nahm et al. [21] also similarly found the registration relationship between CBCT and facial surfaces to be very close and concluded that merging CBCT and facial scans can produce a much truthful image of the patient to give the orthodontist enhanced diagnostic information and lessen errors in diagnosis. These findings agree with the present study, since it was found that other than some of the few distances mentioned above, many other ratios have excellent soft tissue to CBCT ratio percentages, such as the width between outer eye corners (−0.74%), left (−2.94%) and right (−3.99%) corners of the mouth to EAM, and the nasion to gnathion (−4.38%) measurement. This indicates that the CBCT has a tendency to superimpose very closely to distances of the facial scanner.

Limitations to this study exist which warrant changes to be made for further improvement of this study. Due to the data being collected in a retrospective fashion, there was no method in which head positions for the facial scan and CBCT could have been strictly controlled. Patients were only advised to keep their head in the natural position, with their Frankfort plane parallel to the floor. The result of such minor head position changes of each patient may lead to changes in the position of mobile facial structures, such as the mandible. This will lead to slight changes in landmark positioning of areas such as the gonion, causing a greater difference between the two imaging modalities.

The fact that this study was based off of retrospective data also serves as a limitation in that it limited the sample size. A high-enough sample size is needed based on *a priori* calculations, but such calculations were not performed, since there were only a few patient files within the database that included both facial scans and full field of view CBCTs. Thus, within the small given number of available data to work with, the number 30, was chosen, which was the highest number based on availability of data.

In this study, the gold standard was considered to be the CBCT. This assumption was made based on multiple, high-quality research papers and articles [4, 8–13]. Although it is an educated assumption, this assumption serves as a limitation to this study. In order to improve clinical precision, it is important to complete real distance measurements on the patient's face and compare them very carefully with both digital methods.

Most measurements have a reasonably small facial scanner to CBCT mean difference. Even if the difference is relatively large, this can be explained by knowing that some landmarks were slightly different in terms of location on the CBCT and facial scanner. Additionally, even if the means and standard deviations may be large, all paired measurements with left and right sides have similar values within at most 2.35 mm from each other, indicating that such measurements are still comparable.

5. Conclusion

The mean soft tissue to CBCT facial distances tend to be within ±20%, with a tendency for the facial scan measurements to be slightly larger than CBCT equivalents. In general, correlation between the facial scan and CBCT tends to be smaller at lateral and mobile areas of the face such as the gonion. Right and left gonions were areas of the face with a high level of difference between landmark sites of the two imaging modalities. There is a general tendency of obtaining less correlation on boney structures as they increase in dimensional size and increase their curvature. Other significant measurement dissimilarities were due to differences in landmark definition between CBCT and facial scan, in areas such as the throat, corners of mouth, and outer/inner eyes. Areas of the face that have a tendency to have high differences between surface shapes, such as the eyelid and eyebrow region, had relatively low correlation between their soft tissues and corresponding hard-tissue landmarks. Some of the limitations of this study, which may lead to lower correlation in some facial landmarks, may include data from a retrospective database, nonspecific head positions of the patient, as well as an indefinite gold standard imaging modality.

References

[1] S. Anicy-Milosevicy, M. Lapter-Varga, and M. Slaj, "Analysis of the soft tissue facial profile by means of angular measurements," *European Journal of Orthodontics*, vol. 30, no. 2, pp. 135–140, 2008.

[2] E. G. Kaklamanos and O.-E. Kolokitha, "Relation between soft tissue and skeletal changes after mandibular setback surgery: a systematic review and meta-analysis," *Journal of Cranio-Maxillofacial Surgery*, vol. 44, no. 4, pp. 427–435, 2016.

[3] P. A. Zecca, R. Fastuca, M. Beretta, A. Caprioglio, and A. Macchi, "Correlation assessment between three-dimensional facial soft tissue scan and lateral cephalometric radiography in orthodontic diagnosis," *International Journal of Dentistry*, vol. 2016, Article ID 1473918, 8 pages, 2016.

[4] H. M. Pinsky, S. Dyda, R. W. Pinsky, K. A. Misch, and D. P. Sarment, "Accuracy of three-dimensional measurements using cone-beam CT," *Dentomaxillofacial Radiology*, vol. 35, no. 6, pp. 410–416, 2006.

[5] R. A. Holdaway, "A soft-tissue cephalometric analysis and its use in orthodontic treatment planning. Part I," *American Journal of Orthodontics*, vol. 84, no. 1, pp. 1–28, 1983.

[6] Y.-j. Zhao, Y.-x. Xiong, and Y. Wang, "Three-dimensional accuracy of facial scan for facial deformities in clinics: a new evaluation method for facial scanner accuracy," *PLoS One*, vol. 12, no. 1, Article ID e0169402, 2017.

[7] K. B. Naudi, R. Benramadan, L. Brocklebank, X. Ju, B. Khambay, and A. Ayoub, "The virtual human face: superimposing the simultaneously captured 3D photorealistic skin surface of the face on the untextured skin image of the CBCT scan," *International Journal of Oral and Maxillofacial Surgery*, vol. 42, no. 3, pp. 393–400, 2013.

[8] M. O. Lagravère, J. Carey, R. W. Toogood, and P. W. Major, "Three-dimensional accuracy of measurements made with software on cone-beam computed tomography images," *American Journal of Orthodontics and Dentofacial Orthopedics*, vol. 134, no. 1, pp. 112–116, 2008.

[9] N. Zamora, R. Cibrian, J. Gandia, and V. Paredes, "A new 3D method for measuring cranio-facial relationships with cone beam computed tomography (CBCT)," *Medicina Oral Patología Oral Y Cirugia Bucal*, vol. 18, no. 4, pp. e706–e713, 2013.

[10] C. Lascala, J. Panella, and M. Marques, "Analysis of the accuracy of linear measurements obtained by cone beam computed tomography (CBCT-NewTom)," *Dentomaxillofacial Radiology*, vol. 33, no. 5, pp. 291–294, 2004.

[11] R. Marmulla, R. Wörtche, J. Mühling, and S. Hassfeld, "Geometric accuracy of the NewTom 9000 cone beam CT," *Dentomaxillofacial Radiology*, vol. 34, no. 1, pp. 28–31, 2005.

[12] D. Periago, "Comparative linear accuracy and reliability of cone beam ct derived 2-dimensional and 3-dimensional images constructed using an orthodontic volumetric rendering program," Master's thesis, University of Louisville, Louisville, Kentucky, 2007.

[13] S. Stratemann, J. Huang, K. Maki, A. Miller, and D. Hatcher, "Comparison of cone beam computed tomography imaging with physical measures," *Dentomaxillofacial Radiology*, vol. 37, no. 2, pp. 80–93, 2008.

[14] W. E. Harrell, "3D diagnosis and treatment planning in orthodontics," *Seminars in Orthodontics*, vol. 15, no. 1, pp. 35–41, 2009.

[15] A. F. Ayoub, Y. Xiao, B. Khambay, J. P. Siebert, and D. Hadley, "Towards building a photo-realistic virtual human face for craniomaxillofacial diagnosis and treatment planning," *International Journal of Oral and Maxillofacial Surgery*, vol. 36, no. 5, pp. 423–428, 2007.

[16] A. M. Toma, A. Zhurov, R. Playle, E. Ong, and S. Richmond, "Reproducibility of facial soft tissue landmarks on 3D laser-scanned facial images," *Orthodontics and Craniofacial Research*, vol. 12, no. 1, pp. 33–42, 2009.

[17] S. Baumrind and R. C. Frantz, "The reliability of head film measurements," *American Journal of Orthodontics*, vol. 60, no. 5, pp. 505–517, 1971.

[18] T. J. J. Maal, J. M. Plooij, F. A. Rangel, W. Mollemans, F. A. C. Schutyser, and S. J. Bergé, "The Accuracy of matching three-dimensional photographs with skin surfaces derived from cone-beam computed tomography," *International Journal of Oral and Maxillofacial Surgery*, vol. 37, no. 7, pp. 641–646, 2008.

[19] H.-S. Hwang, S.-Y. Choe, J.-S. Hwang et al., "Reproducibility of facial soft tissue thickness measurements using cone-beam ct images according to the measurement methods," *Journal of Forensic Sciences*, vol. 60, no. 4, pp. 957–965, 2015.

29

Peripheral Exophytic Oral Lesions: A Clinical Decision Tree

Hamed Mortazavi,[1] **Yaser Safi,**[2] **Maryam Baharvand,**[1]
Somayeh Rahmani,[1] **and Soudeh Jafari**[1]

[1]*Department of Oral Medicine, School of Dentistry, Shahid Beheshti University of Medical Sciences, Tehran, Iran*
[2]*Department of Oral and Maxillofacial Radiology, School of Dentistry, Shahid Beheshti University of Medical Sciences, Tehran, Iran*

Correspondence should be addressed to Maryam Baharvand; m.baharvand@gmail.com

Academic Editor: Chia-Tze Kao

Diagnosis of peripheral oral exophytic lesions might be quite challenging. This review article aimed to introduce a decision tree for oral exophytic lesions according to their clinical features. General search engines and specialized databases including PubMed, PubMed Central, Medline Plus, EBSCO, Science Direct, Scopus, Embase, and authenticated textbooks were used to find relevant topics by means of keywords such as "oral soft tissue lesion," "oral tumor like lesion," "oral mucosal enlargement," and "oral exophytic lesion." Related English-language articles published since 1988 to 2016 in both medical and dental journals were appraised. Upon compilation of data, peripheral oral exophytic lesions were categorized into two major groups according to their surface texture: smooth (mesenchymal or nonsquamous epithelium-originated) and rough (squamous epithelium-originated). Lesions with smooth surface were also categorized into three subgroups according to their general frequency: reactive hyperplastic lesions/inflammatory hyperplasia, salivary gland lesions (nonneoplastic and neoplastic), and mesenchymal lesions (benign and malignant neoplasms). In addition, lesions with rough surface were summarized in six more common lesions. In total, 29 entities were organized in the form of a decision tree in order to help clinicians establish a logical diagnosis by a stepwise progression method.

1. Introduction

Lesions in the oral cavity generally present as ulcerations, red-white lesions, pigmentations, and exophytic lesions. Clinical classification of oral lesions is of great importance in the diagnostic process [1, 2]. The term oral exophytic lesions is described as pathologic growths projecting above the normal contours of the oral mucosa [2]. There are several underlying mechanisms responsible for oral exophytic lesions such as hypertrophy, hyperplasia, neoplasia, and pooling of the fluid [1], which makes it difficult to approach such lesions clinically [3, 4]. According to a national epidemiologic study by Zain et al., exophytic lesions account for 26% of all oral lesions [3]. Therefore, attempts should be done to arrive at a timely diagnosis via more logical routes like decision trees rather than test-and-error methods [3, 4]. Exophytic lesions can be classified according to their surface texture (smooth and rough), type of base (pedunculated, sessile, nodular, and dome shape), and consistency (soft, cheesy, rubbery, firm,

and bony hard) [1, 4]. This narrative review paper, however, focuses on the surface shapes of the lesions as the main clinical feature in order to build a diagnostic decision tree. In this regard, oral peripheral exophytic lesions are classified as lesions with rough surface and those with smoothly contoured shape [1, 5, 6].

2. Methodology

General search engines and specialized databases including PubMed, PubMed Central, Medline Plus, EBSCO, Science Direct, Scopus, Embase, and authenticated textbooks were used by the first author and the corresponding author to find relevant topics by means of MeSH keywords such as "oral soft tissue lesion," "oral tumor like lesion," "oral mucosal enlargement," and "oral exophytic lesion." Related English-language articles published since 1988 to 2016 in both medical and dental journals including reviews, meta-analyses, original papers (randomized or nonrandomized

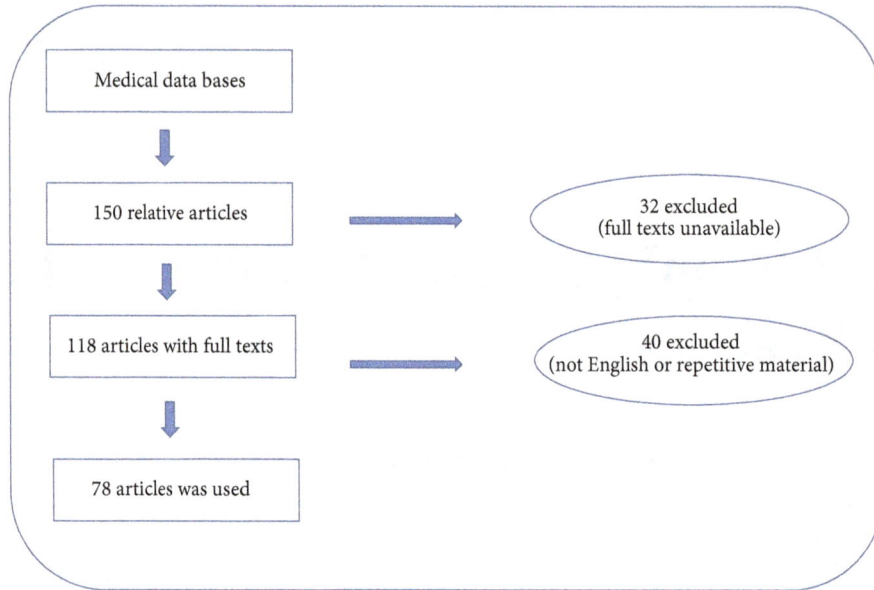

FIGURE 1: Flowchart for choosing eligible articles.

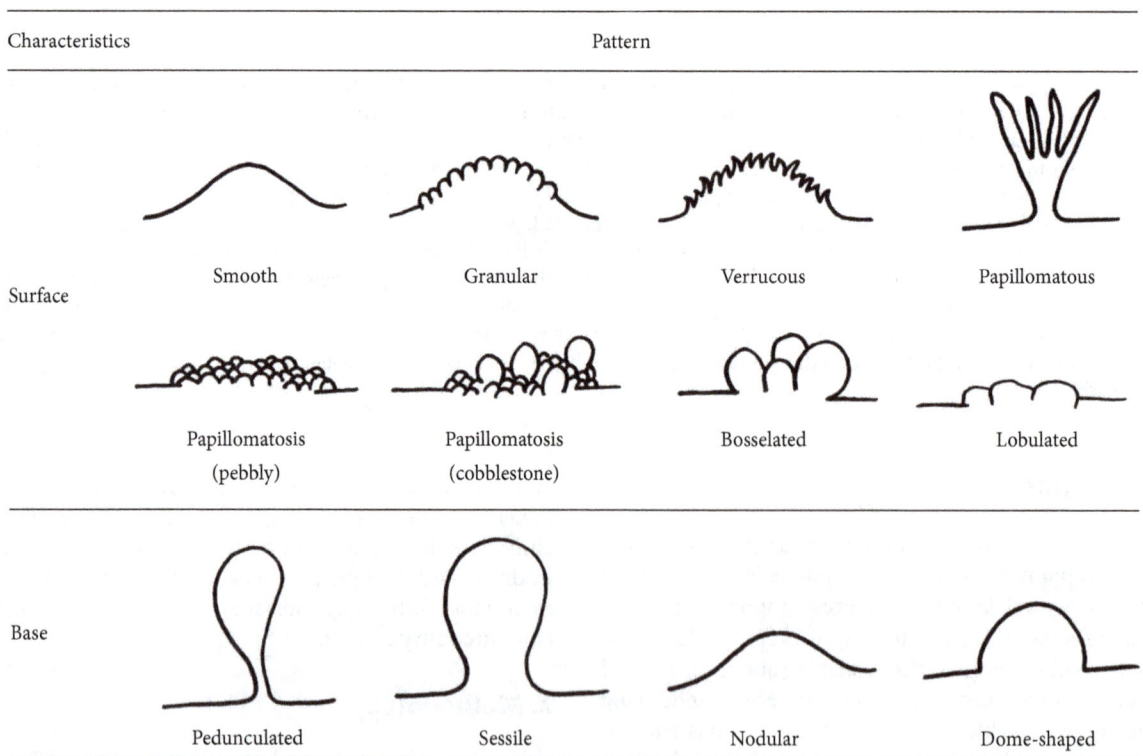

Characteristics	Pattern			
Surface	Smooth	Granular	Verrucous	Papillomatous
	Papillomatosis (pebbly)	Papillomatosis (cobblestone)	Bosselated	Lobulated
Base	Pedunculated	Sessile	Nodular	Dome-shaped

FIGURE 2: Schematic view of surface and base characteristics of oral exophytic lesions.

clinical trials; prospective or retrospective cohort studies), case reports, and case series on oral disease were appraised.

Out of about 150 related articles, 72 were excluded due to lack of full texts, being written in languages other than English or containing repetitive material. Finally, three textbooks and 78 papers were selected including 13 reviews,

55 case reports or case series, and 10 original articles (Figure 1). In this article, peripheral oral exophytic lesions were categorized into two major groups according to their surface texture: smooth (mesenchymal or nonsquamous epithelium-originated) and rough (squamous epithelium-originated) (Figure 2). Lesions with smooth surface were also

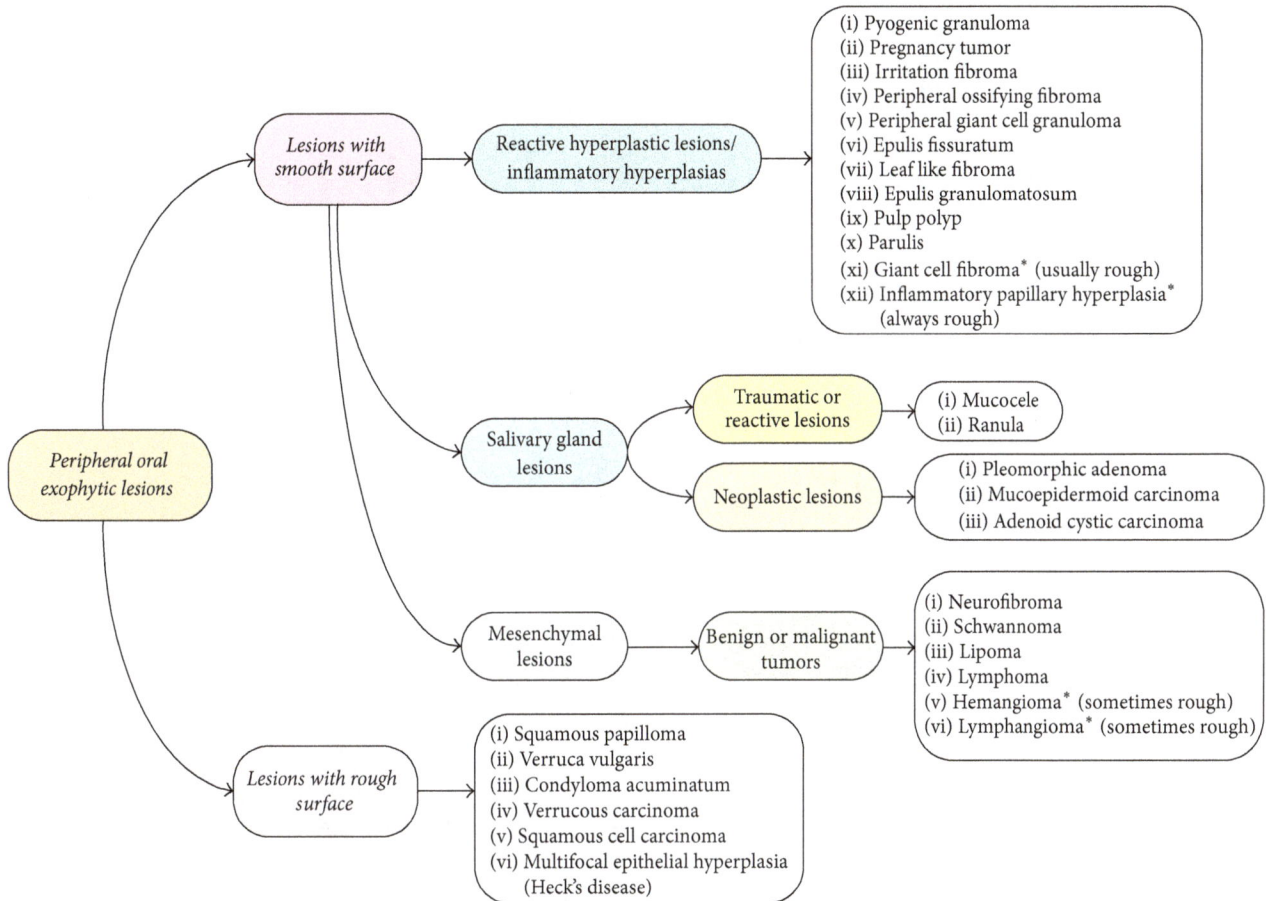

FIGURE 3: Decision tree for peripheral oral exophytic lesions.

categorized into three subgroups according to their general frequency: reactive hyperplastic lesions/inflammatory hyperplasia, salivary gland lesions (nonneoplastic and neoplastic), and mesenchymal lesions (benign and malignant neoplasms). In addition, lesions with rough surface were summarized in six more common lesions. In total, 29 entities were organized in the form of a decision tree (Figure 3) in order to help clinicians establish a logical diagnosis by a stepwise progression method.

3. Lesions with Smooth Surface

3.1. Reactive Hyperplastic Lesions/Inflammatory Hyperplasias. Reactive hyperplasia is the most frequent phenomenon responsible for exophytic lesions in the oral cavity (Table 1). These lesions represent a reaction to some kind of chronic trauma or low grade injuries such as fractured tooth, calculus, chewing, and iatrogenic factors including overextended flange of dentures and overhanging dental restorations [7]. Reactive lesions are usually seen on the gingivae followed by the tongue, buccal mucosa, and floor of the mouth. Clinically, they appear as pedunculated or sessile masses with smooth surface. Lesions are varied from pink to red and soft to firm in terms of color and consistency [7, 8]. However, the clinical features resemble neoplastic lesions in

some instances, which cause a diagnostic dilemma. The most common entities of reactive nature are pyogenic granuloma, pregnancy epulis, irritation fibroma, peripheral ossifying fibroma, peripheral giant cell granuloma, epulis fissuratum, leaf-like fibroma/fibroepithelial polyp, parulis, pulp polyp, epulis granulomatosum, giant cell fibroma, and inflammatory papillary hyperplasia/palatal papillomatosis [1, 4, 7].

3.1.1. Pyogenic Granuloma. Pyogenic granuloma is a common tumor-like lesion in the oral cavity appearing as a smooth or lobulated, asymptomatic mass that is usually pedunculated or sessile. The surface is characteristically ulcerated and friable, which may be covered by a yellow fibrinous membrane (Figure 4) [4, 9]. Depending on the duration of the lesion, its color ranges from shiny red to pink to purple with soft to firm in palpation. It often bleeds easily because of its extreme vascularity. Approximately in one-third of the lesions a history of trauma can be detected [10]. Pyogenic granuloma may exhibit a rapid growth, but it usually reaches its maximum size within weeks or months. The size of the lesion varies from a few millimeters to several centimeters in diameter. In 75% of all cases, the most frequently affected site is the gingivae followed by the lips, tongue, and buccal mucosa. Maxillary gingivae are more affected than mandibular gingivae, and anterior areas more

TABLE 1: General characteristics of smooth-surfaced oral exophytic lesions of reactive origin.

Entity	Age	Gender	Site of involvement	Surface texture	Type of base	Consistency	Color	Size	Symptom & sign	Treatment	Recurrence
Pyogenic granuloma	Children/young adult	Female	Gingivae	Smooth/lobulated	Pedunculated/sessile	Soft to firm	Shiny red/pink/purple	A few mm to several cm	Asymptomatic	Conservative surgical excision	+
Pregnancy tumor	Pregnancy period	Female	Gingivae	Smooth/lobulated	Sessile	Soft to firm	Shiny red/pink/purple	A few mm to several cm	Asymptomatic	Conservative surgical excision	+
Irritation fibroma	4–6 decades	Female	Buccal mucosa	Smooth	Pedunculated/sessile	Firm or soft	Similar to adjacent mucosa	≤1.5 cm	Asymptomatic	Conservative surgical excision	Rare
Peripheral ossifying fibroma	10–19 years old	Female	Exclusively gingivae	Smooth	Pedunculated/sessile	Firm to hard	Red to pink	<2 cm	Tooth mobility Tooth migration Bone loss	Surgical excision down to periosteum	8–20%
Peripheral giant cell granuloma	5–6 decades	Female	Exclusively edentulous ridge & gingivae	Smooth	Pedunculated/sessile/nodular	Firm	Bluish purple	<2 cm or >2 cm	Bone loss Root resorption	Complete surgical excision	+
Epulis granulomatosum	>40 years	Female	Dental socket	Smooth	–	Soft to firm	Similar to adjacent mucosa	<1 cm to massive lesions	Asymptomatic	Conservative treatment/surgery	Not uncommon
Leaf-like fibroma	–	–	Palate	Smooth	Pedunculated/sessile	Firm	Pink	Up to several cm	Asymptomatic	Denture adjustment & surgical removal	Not uncommon
Epulis fissuratum	–	–	Maxillary alveolar ridge	Smooth/ulcerative	Pedunculated/sessile	Firm	Reddish	Up to several cm	Nontender/easily bleeding	Surgical excision & curettage	–
Pulp polyp	Children/young adults	–	Carious lesions of deciduous teeth & first permanent molars	Smooth	Pedunculated/sessile	Soft to firm	Red to pink	<1 cm to large masses	Discomfort	Root canal therapy/extraction	–
Giant cell Fibroma	3rd decade	Female	Gingivae	Rough surface	Pedunculated/sessile	Firm	Pink	<1cm (often)	Asymptomatic	Conservative surgical excision	Rare
Inflammatory papillary hyperplasia	3–5th decades	Male	Palate	Pebbly/cobblestone	–	Soft to firm	Red to pink	Up to several cm	Asymptomatic/symptomatic	Removal of denture at night/antifungals/surgery	–

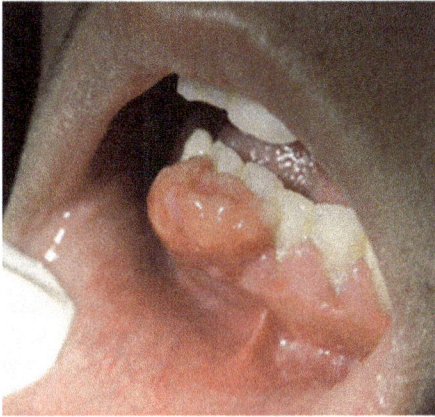

FIGURE 4: Pyogenic granuloma as a sessile lesion on mandibular labial gingivae with an ulcerated smooth surface.

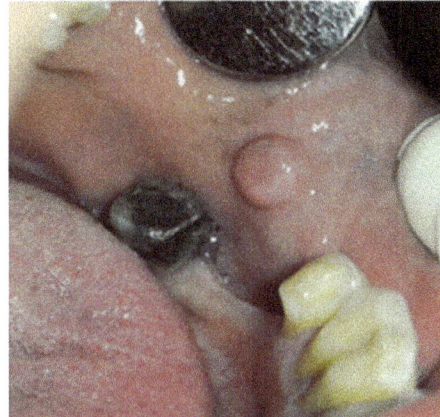

FIGURE 5: Irritation fibroma on the buccal mucosa with a smooth surface and dome-shaped base.

frequently involved than posterior areas [9–11]. There is a female predilection and a tendency to affect children and young adults. Patients with pyogenic granuloma are treated by conservative surgical excision. However, recurrence is not uncommon [9].

3.1.2. Pregnancy Tumor. Pregnancy tumor or granuloma gravidarum is a reactive lesion with the same clinical features to pyogenic granuloma. The lesion may emerge during the first trimester with a gradual increasing incidence to the seventh months of pregnancy, which is presumably related to the rising levels of estrogen and progesterone. Some of these lesions resolve spontaneously after delivery or undergo fibrous maturation mimicking an irritation fibroma [4, 10]. The lesions do not occur in people with optimum oral hygiene suggesting local irritation as an important etiologic factor [4]. Patients with small isolated lesions and otherwise healthy gingivae might be monitored for shrinkage after delivery, but large lesions or generalized pregnancy gingivitis or periodontitis warrants the need for treatment during pregnancy [4].

3.1.3. Irritation Fibroma. Irritation fibroma or focal fibrous hyperplasia is the most common tumor-like lesion of the oral cavity with the prevalence of 1-2% in general population. It appears as an asymptomatic, pedunculated, or sessile exophytic lesion with a smooth surface and being similar to the surrounding mucosa in color (Figure 5). However, the surface may show hyperkeratosis from secondary trauma. It can be firm and resilient or soft with spongy consistency. Although fibromas usually reach to 1.5 cm or less in diameter they might appear as very tiny to quite large lesions. The most commonly affected site is the buccal mucosa along the line of occlusion; however it can occur anywhere in the oral cavity. The labial mucosa, tongue, and gingivae can be involved as well. It is likely that many fibromas represent fibrous maturation of a preexisting pyogenic granuloma. There is a female predilection with female to male ratio of 2 : 1 with the majority of cases being reported in the fourth to sixth

decades of life. Conservative surgical excision is the treatment of choice for irritation fibroma with a low recurrence rate.

3.1.4. Peripheral Ossifying Fibroma. Peripheral ossifying fibroma also called peripheral fibroma with calcification, ossifying fibroid epulis, and calcifying fibroblastic granuloma is a reactive gingival enlargement [10]. It represents 2% to 9% of all gingival lesions and 3% of all oral lesion biopsy samples [12, 13]. The lesion appears as a smooth, pedunculated, or sessile, firm to hard mass that usually emanates from the interdental papilla. It is a red to pink lesion often less than 2 cm in diameter, but lesions up to 8 cm have been reported as well [10, 13]. Tooth mobility, tooth migration, and bone destruction have been noticed in some cases [13]. This lesion occurs exclusively on the gingivae with up to 60% of cases being reported in the anterior areas of the maxilla (incisor-cuspid region) [12, 13]. Two theories have been proposed to explain the pathogenesis of the lesion: it might originate from a calcified pyogenic granuloma, or it may arise from an overgrowth and proliferation of different components of connective tissue in the periodontium, but the main etiology is yet to be elucidated [12, 14]. Peripheral ossifying fibroma is predominantly a lesion of teenagers and young adults with a peak prevalence being between 10 to 19 years [10]. Females are more affected than males, mainly during their second decade of life, due to fluctuations of estrogen and progesterone [12]. Treatment usually involves surgical excision, and the lesion should be excised down to the periosteum. The recurrence rate has been estimated to be between 8% and 20% [10, 12].

3.1.5. Peripheral Giant Cell Granuloma. Peripheral giant cell granuloma is a common tumor-like lesion of the oral cavity that conveys a reactive response in the periodontium, periodontal ligament and gingivae. It occurs exclusively on the edentulous alveolar ridge and gingivae as a smooth, reddish-blue, pedunculated, sessile, or nodular mass, which is firm to palpation. In some cases the clinical appearance of the lesion is similar to pyogenic granuloma; however peripheral giant cell granuloma is more bluish-purple colored

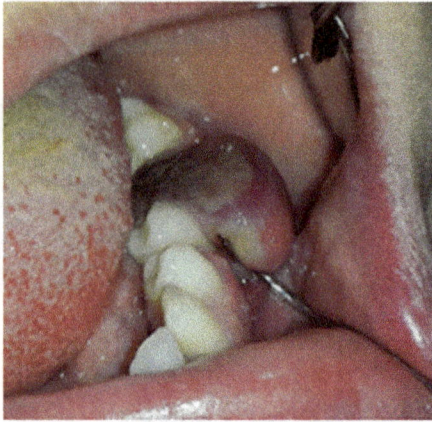

FIGURE 6: PGCG with an ulcerated, smooth surface and purplish color located buccolingually on the left mandibular ridge.

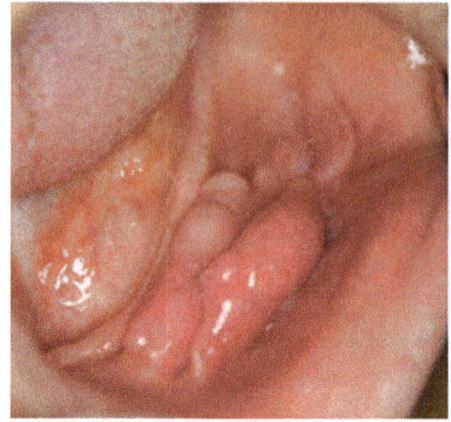

FIGURE 7: Massive epulis fissuratum presenting as an exophytic lesion with smooth surface associated with an ill-fit mandibular denture.

as compared with bright red color of pyogenic granuloma (Figure 6) [10, 15]. It is usually less than 2 cm in diameter, but larger sizes are seen occasionally. Progressive growth in some cases may lead to bone and root resorption [16]. The mandible is more affected than the maxilla, and there is a female predilection with female to male ratio of 2 : 1 [15, 16]. As the giant cells are found to act as a potential target for estrogen, it is not surprising that the lesions are triggered by sex hormones [17]. The lesions can develop at any age; however peak prevalence was found in the fifth and sixth decades of life [10]. Hyperparathyroidism should be considered in differential diagnosis in case of multiple lesions especially with a history of recurrences. In spite of adequate treatment, children with hypophosphatemic rickets are also at a higher risk for developing such lesions [16, 17]. Complete surgical excision with elimination of the entire base of the lesion is the accepted treatment plan for this lesion [15–17].

3.1.6. Epulis Fissuratum. Epulis fissuratum or denture-induced hyperplasia is a reactive lesion of the oral cavity caused by low grade chronic trauma from dentures [18]. About 70% of patients wear ill-fit dentures continuously all day long for more than 10 years [19]. The lesion appears as an asymptomatic single fold or multiple folds of hyperplastic tissues in the alveolar vestibule along denture flanges with a smooth surface, soft to firm consistency, and a normal coloration (Figure 7) [18, 20]. In some cases, severe inflammation or ulceration may be seen in the bottom of the folds [18]. It has been reported in 5% to 10% of the jaws fitted with dentures and is more prevalent in the maxilla than the mandible, especially on the facial aspect of the alveolar ridges [18, 19]. The anterior portions of the jaws are more often affected; however epulis fissuratum of the soft palate has been reported in the literature [20]. Two-thirds to three-fourths of all cases have been found in females [19, 20]. In women, postmenopausal hormonal imbalance makes the oral mucosa susceptible to a hyperplastic growth [18]. It is more frequent in patients over 40 years; however this entity has been reported in patients from childhood to elderly [1].

The size of the lesion varies from less than 1 cm in diameter to massive lesions involving extensive areas on the vestibule [19, 20]. Epulis fissuratum can be treated conservatively or surgically depending on the size of the lesion.

3.1.7. Leaf-Like Fibroma. Ill-fit dentures worn for many years can cause benign hyperplastic fibrous growths or epulides. When a fibrous epulis forms underneath the palatal base of a denture, it is known as a leaf-like denture fibroma or fibroepithelial polyp [21]. It is characterized as a pain less, flattened, pink, firm mass attached to the palate by a narrow stalk or a broad base (pedunculated or sessile) which can reach to several centimeters in diameter. The edge of the lesion is serrated resembling a leaf. In most cases, the flattened mass is closely located to the palate and sits in a slightly cupped-out depression [10, 22]. Treatment is accomplished by means of conservative surgical removal and fabrication of new dentures. While altering the denture may decrease the size of the lesion, adjustment alone will not lead to complete regression due to dense nature of the scar tissue. Recurrence is not uncommon [21].

3.1.8. Epulis Granulomatosum. Epulis granulomatosum or epulis hemangiomatosis—a variant of pyogenic granuloma—presents as an overgrowth arising from a recently extracted tooth socket [23–25]. The precipitating factor in most patients is sharp specula of the alveolar bone left in the walls of the socket [1]. Clinically, it is characterized by reddish, smooth, pedunculated or sessile, nontender, rapidly growing mass with soft to firm in palpation. Surface of the lesion may be ulcerative due to secondary trauma [23, 24]. It often bleeds easily because of its high vascular content [23]. The growth may become apparent in one or two weeks after tooth extraction [1]. Lesions of larger sizes were also incidentally seen as an oral finding in patients with Klippel-Trenaunay syndrome [23]. Evaluation of socket and removal of any bony spicules or tooth fragments at the time of extraction prevent formation of an epulis granulomatosum. Excision of the raised mass and curettage of the alveolus to ensure the

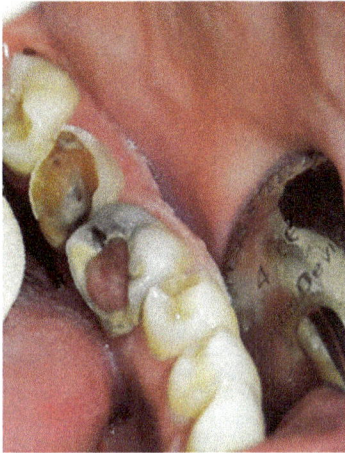

FIGURE 8: Pulp polyp associated with carious first mandibular molar with smooth surface and sessile base.

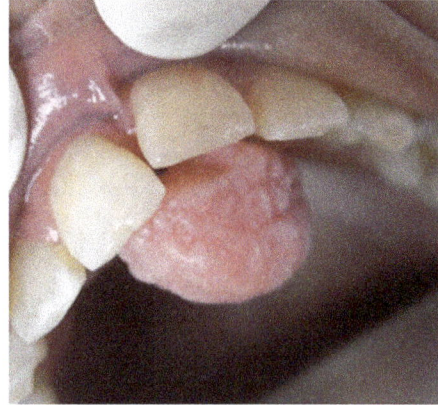

FIGURE 9: Pedunculated lesion of giant cell fibroma with granular surface on the palatal gingivae of maxillary central incisors.

elimination of irritating particles is needed to treat the lesion [23–25].

3.1.9. Pulp Polyp. Pulp polyp or chronic hyperplastic pulpitis or pulpitis aperta is an uncommon reactive lesion, which occurs when caries have destroyed the tooth crown [1]. It appears as a smooth, soft to firm, red to pink, pedunculated, or sessile mass occupying the entire carious cavity in the affected tooth resembling an enlarged gingival tissue (Figure 8) [26, 27]. The size of the lesion varies from less than 1 cm in diameter to large masses (about 4 cm) [26, 27]. It is most frequently found in the deciduous and permanent first molars of children and young adults and is a rare phenomenon in the middle-aged adults [1, 28]. It is usually asymptomatic, but discomfort can occur during mastication. Response to electrical and thermal stimuli may be normal [28]. Periapical radiographs may show an incipient chronic apical periodontitis when pulp involvement is extensive or lingering [28]. The polyp may cover most of the remaining crown of the tooth, giving the lesion an appearance of a flashy mass [29]. A similar hyperplastic mass around a draining sinus tract of a tooth with pulpoperiapical pathology is called parulis [4]. The treatment plan of this lesion includes endodontic treatment or tooth extraction [28].

3.1.10. Giant Cell Fibroma. Giant cell fibroma is a fibrous hyperplastic soft tissue lesion classified as an inflammatory hyperplasia [1]. However, a controversy exists about the origin and etiology of this entity [30]. It represents approximately 2% to 5% of all oral fibrous lesions and 0.4% to 1% of all oral biopsy samples [31]. Clinically, it appears as an asymptomatic, sessile, or pedunculated mass with rough surface (papillary or granular) and firm in palpation (Figure 9) [30, 31]. Despite previously mentioned reactive lesions, giant cell fibroma did not have a completely smooth surface; hence it may clinically be mistaken with lesions of squamous epithelium origin such as papilloma [10]. The color of the lesion is pink or similar to the surrounding normal

mucosa and is usually less than 1 cm in diameter [10, 31]. In about 60% of cases, the lesion is diagnosed in the second to third decade of life with only 4% to 17% of giant cell fibromas being found in children younger than 10 years [31, 32]. There is a slight female predilection and gingivae are the most affected site (about 50% of cases) followed by the tongue, palate, buccal mucosa, lips, and floor of the mouth [10, 31]. Moreover, mandibular gingivae are affected twice as often as the maxillary gingivae [32]. Giant cell fibroma usually is treated by conservative surgical excision. Electrosurgery and laser therapy have been suggested as alternative modalities especially in children. Recurrence is rare [10, 28].

3.1.11. Inflammatory Papillary Hyperplasia. Inflammatory papillary hyperplasia (palatal papillomatosis and denture papillomatosis) is a reactive lesion seen most often in patients with an ill-fit denture wearing all-day-long and poor oral hygiene [10, 33]. This condition is encountered in 10% to 20% of denture wearers [1, 10]. It is featured by exophytic masses with pebbly or cobblestone appearance on the hard palate beneath a denture base with or without symptoms [10]. Although these lesions appear as red, soft masses in the inflammatory stage they convert to pink and firm when they mature to fibrous stage [1]. In some cases, denture papillomatosis develops on the edentulous mandibular alveolar ridge or on the surface of an epulis fissuratum [10]. It can occur at any age. However, it is most frequently encountered in the third to fifth decade of life with a male predilection [33]. In addition to frictional irritation provoked by loose-fit dentures, *Candida albicans* has an etiologic role in this entity [1]. On rare occasions, this condition occurs on the palate of patients without denture especially in people who habitually breathe through their mouth or have a high palatal vault [10]. Less extensive lesions are resolved by removing the denture at night and improving oral hygiene. Patients can also benefit from antifungal agents. Various surgical methods have been suggested for the treatment of this lesion such as partial thickness or full thickness surgical blade excision, curettage, electro surgery, and cryosurgery [10, 34, 35].

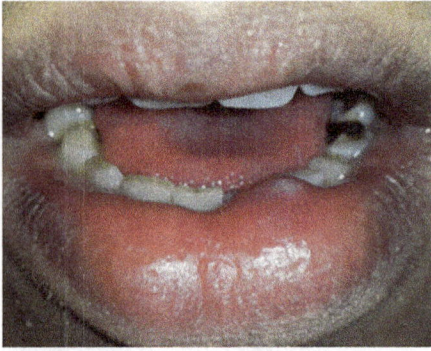

FIGURE 10: Nodular mucocele of the lower lip with smooth surface.

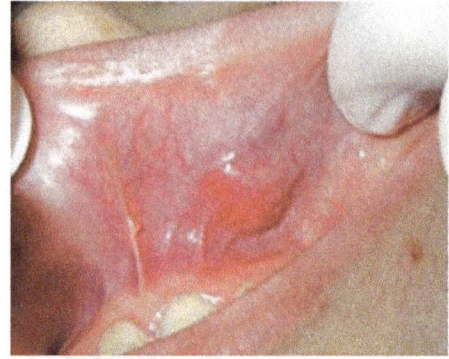

FIGURE 11: Pleomorphic adenoma involving upper lip presented as a dome-shaped exophytic lesion with smooth surface.

3.2. Salivary Gland Lesions. A wide range of lesions arise from intraoral salivary glands, which are categorized as nonneoplastic and neoplastic entities. According to a 15-year-retrospective study by Mohan et al., 55% of lesions were nonneoplastic and 45% were neoplastic [36]. When salivary gland lesions appear as an exophytic lesion they are usually characterized by a dome-shaped or nodular mass with a smooth surface and fluctuant to firm in palpation [1]. The most common lesions of salivary gland origin are as follows (Table 2).

3.2.1. Mucocele and Ranula. Mucocele is a common nonneoplastic lesion of salivary gland origin resulting from breaking or dilation of salivary ducts secondary to obstruction or local trauma [37]. Clinically, it appears as an asymptomatic, fluctuant to firm, bluish to pink, nodular, or dome-shaped mass with a smooth surface (Figure 10) [1, 37]. The size of the lesion varies from 1-2 mm to several centimeters but remains smaller than 1.5 cm in diameter [37]. The incidence is pretty high, 2.5 cases per 1000 persons with no sex predilection [38]. Lesions last from a few days to several months. Many patients mention a history of recurrent swelling with periodic rupture and release of fluid content [10, 38]. The majority of cases have been reported in the first three decades of life, and it is rare among children younger than 1 year of age [37, 38]. The lower lip is the most frequently (60%) affected site followed by buccal mucosa, anterior ventral tongue, floor of the mouth, and upper lip [10]. In some cases, mucoceles rupture and heal spontaneously; however conventional surgical treatment may be suggested in large lesions. Some alternative modalities such as cryosurgery, intralesional injection of steroids, and laser therapy have been implemented as well [37].

When a mucocele occurs in the floor of the mouth it is called ranula featuring as a bluish, dome-shaped or nodular; fluctuant exophytic lesion with a smooth surface usually located lateral to the midline [10]. Fluctuation in size considered as a pertinent feature noticed in the history of ranula. The lesion measures its smallest size early in the morning and reaches to the largest scale at the time of meals [1]. A prevalence of 0.2 cases per 1000 persons has been found, and it accounts for 6% of all oral sialocysts [39]. Most of the patients are young adults with peak frequency being in the second decade of life [39]. This lesion is treated by

marsupialization or removal of the feeding sublingual gland; however marsupialization leads to recurrence in 25% of cases [1, 10].

3.2.2. Pleomorphic Adenoma. Pleomorphic adenoma or mixed tumor is a benign salivary gland tumor which constitutes 3% to 10% of head and neck neoplasms and about 1% of all body tumors [40, 41]. It is the most common (73%) tumor of both minor and major salivary glands [41, 42]. Corresponding to minor salivary glands, the palate is the most affected site followed by lips, buccal mucosa, tongue, floor of the mouth, pharynx, retromolar area, and the nasal cavity [41]. It is suspected when a clinician encounters a unilateral, asymptomatic, slow growing, firm, nodular, or dome-shaped mass covered by a normal-colored mucosa (Figure 11) [40, 41]. The surface of the lesion is usually intact, but ulceration of the overlying mucosa has been reported in some instances [40]. The size of the lesion varies from 1 to 5 cm with the average of 2.6 cm in diameter [41]. In large cases bone resorption has been reported [40]. It can occur at any age, but majority of patients have been reported in their fifth to sixth decades of life [41, 42]. Lip lesions tend to occur at an earlier age than that of other locations [41]. There is a female predilection with female to male ratio of 7 : 3 [41]. Malignant transformation to pleomorphic adenocarcinoma has been noticed in about 6% of cases [42]. Surgical excision usually yields promising results treated with good prognosis. A recurrence rate of 2% to 44% has been reported, and patients younger than 30 years are more likely to have relapsing lesions [41]. Risk for recurrence seems to be lower in the minor salivary gland tumors than that of major salivary glands [41].

3.2.3. Mucoepidermoid Carcinoma. Mucoepidermoid carcinoma or mucoepidermoid tumor is the most common malignant salivary gland neoplasm. It accounts for about 3% of all head and neck tumors [10, 43]. Two-thirds of the lesions arise within the parotid gland and one-third within the minor salivary glands. Intraorally, palate is the most affected site followed by retromolar area, floor of the mouth, buccal mucosa, lips, and tongue. Intraosseous lesions have been also reported in some cases [10, 43, 44]. The tumor can occur at

TABLE 2: General characteristics of smooth-surfaced oral exophytic lesions of salivary origin.

Entity	Age	Gender	Site of involvement	Surface texture	Type of base	Consistency	Color	Size	Symptom & sign	Treatment	Recurrence
Mucocele & ranula	First 3 decades of life	No sex predilection	Lower lip/floor of the mouth	Smooth	Nodular/dome shaped	Fluctuant to firm	Bluish to pink	<1.5 cm	Asymptomatic	Marsupialization	25%
Pleomorphic adenoma	5-6th decades	Female	Palate	Smooth	Nodular/dome shaped	Firm	Normal colored	1-5 cm	Asymptomatic	Surgical excision	2-44%
Mucoepidermoid carcinoma	3-6th decades	Female	Palate	Smooth	Nodular/dome shaped	Firm	Pink/bluish to red or normal colored	Up to several cm	Asymptomatic/Painful in high Grades	Wide surgical excision	Up to 60%
Adenoid cystic carcinoma	5-6th decades	Female	Palate	Smooth/ulcerative	Nodular	Firm	Pink/normal colored	Up to several cm	Pain is common/bone destruction/distant metastasis	Local radical excision + radiotherapy/chemotherapy	—

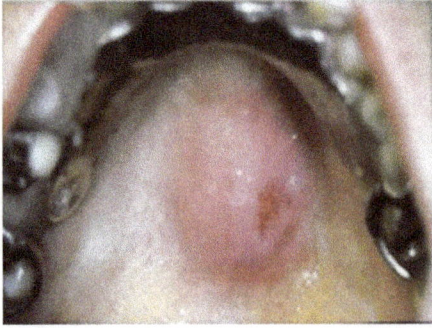

FIGURE 12: Mucoepidermoid carcinoma of the palate, presented as an exophytic lesion with smooth, ulcerated surface, and nodular base.

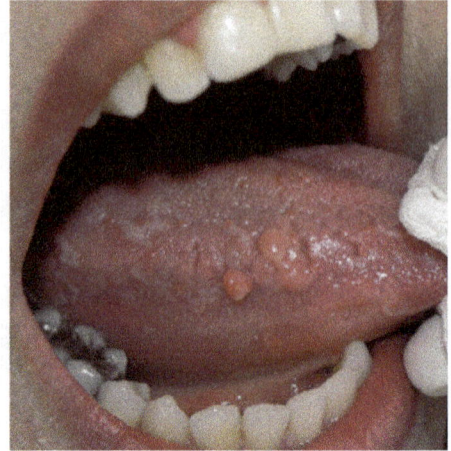

FIGURE 13: Sessile-based and smooth-surfaced exophytic lesions of neurofibroma involving dorsal and lateral border of the tongue.

any age, but the majority of patients have been diagnosed between the third and sixth decade of life with a female predilection. Although it is rare in children, mucoepidermoid carcinoma is the most common malignant salivary gland neoplasm in childhood [10, 43–45]. Clinically, it appears as a smooth-surfaced nodular or dome-shaped, firm mass with a diameter up to several centimeters. The color of the lesion may be pink, bluish to red, or even similar to the surrounding normal mucosa (Figure 12) [1, 10, 43]. Patients are usually asymptomatic, but high grade tumors might be painful [44]. Palatal neoplasms cause bone resorption, and an ulcerative surface might be found in some tumors. [10, 44]. Low grade neoplasms are treated by surgical excision with free surgical margins. High grade ones require wide surgical excision, neck dissection, and postoperative radiotherapy. Recurrence rate is up to 60%, which mostly occurs within 1 year after treatment [45].

3.2.4. Adenoid Cystic Carcinoma.

Adenoid cystic carcinoma is the most common malignant tumor originated from the submandibular and minor salivary glands. It comprises 5% to 10% of all salivary gland neoplasms and 2% to 4% of all head and neck malignancies [4, 46]. It can occur in any salivary gland, but approximately 50% to 60% of cases develop within minor salivary glands. The palate is the most frequently affected site in the oral cavity. Clinically, it is characterized by a slow growing, pink to normal-colored nodular mass with a smooth surface and firm consistency [1, 46, 47]. An intraoral adenoid cystic carcinoma may exhibit mucosal ulceration, a feature that helps distinguish it from a benign pleomorphic adenoma [4]. Pain is a common finding and usually occurs early in the course of the disease before an apparent swelling develops [10]. In cases arising in the palate or maxilla, there is an evidence of bone destruction adjacent to the tumor [4, 47]. Local recurrences, perineural spreading, and distant metastases have been also reported as important features of this entity [4]. The peak prevalence of this tumor is in the fifth and sixth decades, and it is rare in people younger than 20 years [10, 46]. An almost equal sex distribution has been mentioned; however some studies showed a female predilection [10, 46, 47]. Because of the ability of this lesion to spread along the nerve sheets, radical surgical excision

is suggested as the accepted treatment plan. The tumors of the minor salivary glands should be treated by local radical excision and postoperative radiotherapy. Chemotherapy is also recommended in the management of advanced and metastatic salivary gland tumors [47].

3.3. Mesenchymal Lesions.

Peripheral oral mesenchymal tumors are considered among uncommon lesions of the oral cavity (Table 3). According to a 10-year-retrospective study by Mendez, only 4% of oral lesions were of mesenchymal origin [48]. Clinically, these lesions present as asymptomatic, slow growing, nodular, or dome-shaped masses with a smooth surface and firm consistency. These lesions are usually covered with normal mucosa unless chronically traumatized. They can be involved any site of the oral cavity [1]. The most common oral lesions with mesenchymal origin are lipoma, neurofibroma, schwannoma, lymphoma, hemangioma, and lymphangioma [49].

3.3.1. Neurofibroma.

Neurofibroma is the most common peripheral nerve tumor; however it is rarely seen in the oral cavity. Most cases of oral neurofibroma are multiple and as a part of neurofibromatosis syndrome, but it rarely appears as a solitary mass without visceral manifestations [10, 50]. It has been demonstrated that solitary neurofibroma is a hyperplastic hamartomatous malformation rather than a neoplastic lesion [51]. It appears as an asymptomatic, slow growing, soft to firm, nodular, or sessile mass with a smooth surface (sometimes lobulated) and pink in coloration (Figure 13) [50, 51]. It most commonly develops on the tongue followed by palate, mandibular ridge/vestibule, maxillary ridge/vestibule, buccal mucosa, lips, floor of the mouth, and gingivae with up to several centimeters in diameter [50, 51]. Intraosseous lesions have been also reported in the posterior mandible as a well-defined or poorly defined unilocular or multilocular radiolucency [51, 52]. It is most commonly observed in young adults with a peak prevalence in the third decade of life with the sex predilection being still debatable [50, 51]. The tumor is usually treated by complete excision

TABLE 3: General characteristics of smooth-surfaced oral exophytic lesions of mesenchymal origin.

Entity	Age	Gender	Site of involvement	Surface texture	Type of base	Consistency	Color	Size	Symptom & sign	Treatment	Recurrence
Neurofibroma	3rd decade	No sex predilection	Tongue	Smooth	Nodular/sessile	Soft to firm	Pink	Up to several centimeters	Asymptomatic	Complete excision	Rare
Schwannoma	Average: 34 years	Female	Tongue	Smooth	Nodular/sessile	Rubbery	Same to normal mucosa	0.5–4 cm	Asymptomatic	Surgical excision	Rare
Lipoma	>40 years	Male	Buccal mucosa/vestibule	Smooth	Nodular/sessile/pedunculated	Soft/fluctuant	Pink to yellowish	<3 cm (often)	Asymptomatic	Conservative surgical excision	High in intramuscular lesions
Lymphoma	Average: 59 years	Male	Buccal vestibule & postpalate	Smooth/ulcerative	Nodular	Soft to firm	Pink/purplish/normal	Up to several cm	Nontender painful in intraosseous lesions	Chemotherapy/radiotherapy	—
Hemangioma	Early infancy	Female	Lips	Smooth/lobulated	Sessile	Soft	Pink to red purple	Up to several cm	Asymptomatic	Sclerotherapy/surgical excision/laser therapy/cryotherapy	—
Lymphangioma	1st decade	No sex predilection	Tongue	Smooth/pebbly	Sessile	Soft	Pink to yellowish or normal color	Up to several cm	Macroglossy/airway obstruction/sialorrhea/jaw deformity	Surgical excision/cryotherapy/electrocautery/steroid administration/sclerotherapy	—

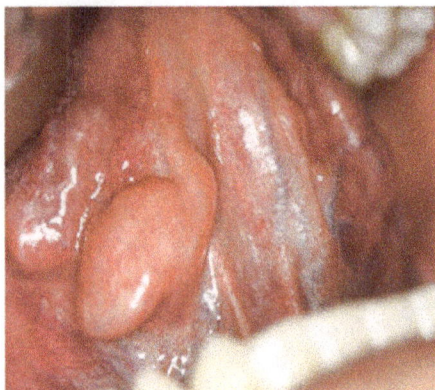

FIGURE 14: A dome-shaped schwannoma on the ventral surface of the tongue with smooth surface.

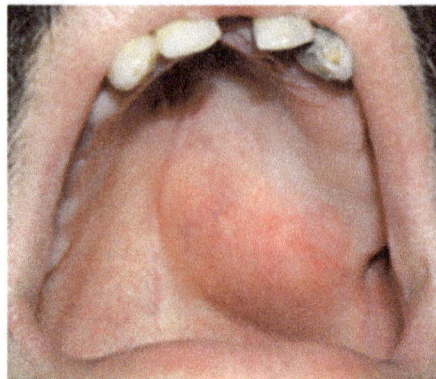

FIGURE 15: Lymphoma presented as a nodular exophytic lesion with smooth surface on the palate.

with a low recurrence rate. However, neurofibroma may convert to neurofibrosarcoma in 5% to 15% of cases especially in multiple lesions [51].

3.3.2. Schwannoma. Schwannoma, also called neurilemmoma, neurinoma, or perineural fibroblastoma, is a benign tumor of neuroectodermal origin [53, 54]. Approximately 25% to 45% of lesions are seen in the head and neck with 1% being reported in the oral cavity as well [53]. Clinically, it is characterized by solitary, asymptomatic, rubbery, nodular, or sessile mass with a smooth surface and is similar to the normal mucosa in coloration (Figure 14). The size of the lesion varies from 0.5 to 4 cm in diameter [53, 54]. Intraoral lesions are frequently located in the tongue followed by palate, floor of the mouth, buccal mucosa, gingivae, lips, and vestibular mucosa [55]. Schwannoma can occur as an intraosseous lesion, which accounts for 1% of all benign primary bony tumors [54, 55]. Intrabony lesions appear as either unilocular or multilocular radiolucencies [53]. Peripheral lesions are usually painless, but tenderness may occur in some instances [10]. Pain and paresthesia are not uncommon for intrabony tumors [10]. Schwannoma has been reported in the age range of 8 to 72 years with an average age of 34 years with a slight female predilection (female to male ratio of 1.6 : 1) [53, 55]. Surgical excision is the treatment of choice and recurrence and malignant transformation are extremely rare [55].

3.3.3. Lipoma. Lipoma is a benign tumor, which seldom occurs in the mouth. It constitutes 4% to 5% of all benign tumors in the body representing about 1% to 5% of all neoplasms of the oral cavity [56]. Generally, the prevalence of the lesion is balanced in both genders; however a slight male predilection has been reported. Lipoma is a rare entity in children, and most of the patients are over 40 years [57]. It presents as a slow growing, nodular, sessile, or even pedunculated mass with a smooth surface and fluctuant to soft in palpation. The superficial lesions usually show yellowish hue, while more deeply seated ones appear as a pink mass [10, 56, 57]. Lipoma varies in size from small to large masses mostly measuring less than 3 cm in diameter [10, 56]. The buccal mucosa and buccal vestibule are the most

commonly affected sites, which accounts for about 50% of all cases [10]. Less affected sites include the tongue, floor of the mouth, and lips [10]. Lipoma is treated by conservative surgical excision and usually does not recur. Intramuscular lipoma has a somewhat higher recurrence rate because of problems to remove completely [4].

3.3.4. Lymphoma. Lymphomas are heterogeneous malignant neoplasms of the lymphocyte cell lines. They can be divided as Hodgkin and non-Hodgkin lymphoma (HL and NHL). Hodgkin lymphoma rarely shows extra-nodal disease (1% of cases) unlike NHL, which arises from extra-nodal sites in 20% to 30% of patients [58, 59]. Extra-nodal lymphoma is the second most commonly encountered neoplasm after squamous cell carcinoma in the head and neck region, which accounts for 5% of all malignancies of head and neck [59–61]. Oral lymphomas usually occur secondary to a more widespread involvement through the body; however it can present as a primary lesion in the oral cavity with the prevalence of 0.1% to 2% [60]. Clinically, it appears as a nontender, smooth surface, soft to firm mass in the mouth (Figure 15) [10, 58–60]. The size of lesion varies from small to large with a pink, purplish, or normal coloration. The surface of lesion may be intact or ulcerative [10, 59, 60]. The mean age of patients with lymphoma is 56 years, and there is a male predilection [60, 61]. The most affected site for oral lesions is buccal vestibule, posterior palate, and gingivae [10, 60]. Intraosseous lesions were also reported in some cases. Bony lesions often present with low grade pain, which can mimic toothache [60]. Radiotherapy plus chemotherapy is recommended for intermediate and high grade tumors. A failure rate of 30% to 50% was demonstrated in intermediate grade lesions; however high grade lesions show a 60% mortality rate [10].

3.3.5. Hemangioma. Hemangioma is a benign common tumor in the head and neck region, but relatively rare in the mouth. In the oral cavity, it can cause esthetic and functional impairment depending on its location and size [62]. The peak prevalence of this entity is described soon after birth or in early infancy; however some cases have been reported

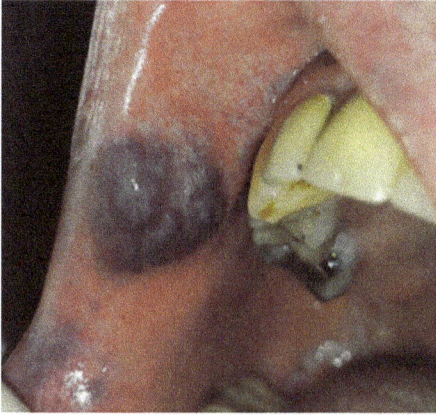

FIGURE 16: Lobulated hemangioma involving the right upper lip.

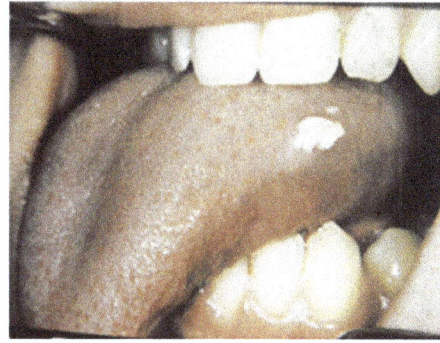

FIGURE 17: Squamous papilloma involving lateral border of the tongue with a sessile base and papillomatous surface.

in adulthood [10, 62]. It is noted that hemangioma is the most common tumor of infancy, occurring in 5% to 10% of one-year-old children [10]. Oral lesions are most common in the lips, gingivae, tongue, and buccal mucosa [62, 63]. Eighty percent of cases occur as a single lesion, but 20% of affected patients present multiple tumors [10]. Clinically, it is characterized by an asymptomatic, soft, smooth, or lobulated, sessile mass with various sizes from a few millimeters to several centimeters (Figure 16). The color of the lesions ranges from pink to red purple, and tumor blanches on the application of pressure [63, 64]. Gingival lesions which arise from the interdental papillae can spread laterally to involve adjacent teeth [63]. There is a female predilection with female to male ratio of 3:1, and they usually occur in whites more often than other racial groups [10]. Treatment of hemangioma depends on its size and location. Small lesions are treated by sclerotherapy, conventional surgical excision, laser therapy, and cryotherapy. In large cases, treatment should include embolization or obliteration of the lesion and the adjacent vessels [62].

3.3.6. Lymphangioma. Lymphangioma is a benign, hamartomatous tumor of lymphatic vessel origin. It has a marked tendency for the head and neck region in a way that 75% of all cases occur in this area. Almost half of the lesions are noted at birth and about 90% developed by two years of age [65]. In the oral cavity, lymphangioma mostly occurs on the dorsal surface and lateral borders of the tongue followed by gingivae, buccal mucosa, and lips [65, 66]. Pathognomonic features of tongue lymphangioma are irregular nodularity of the surface with gray to pink projections and macroglossia [66]. There is no sex predilection, and oral lesions are most common in the first decade of life [66]. The clinical manifestation of the lesion varies based on whether it is superficial or deep. Superficial lesions appear as soft exophytic masses with rough (papillary or pebbly) surface and pink to yellowish coloration. Deeper lesions are described as soft diffuse masses with normal color and smooth surface [65, 67]. Massive lesions might cause macroglossia, obstruction in upper air way, sialorrhea, and jaw deformity as well as difficulties in mastication, speech, and oral hygiene [65]. Lymphangioma is treated by surgical

excision, cryotherapy, electrocautery, sclerotherapy, steroid administration, embolization, laser surgery, and radiation therapy [65].

3.4. Lesions with Rough Surface. This group of lesions most frequently occurs as a result of epithelial proliferation due to reaction to human papilloma virus or a neoplastic process (Table 4).

3.4.1. Squamous Papilloma. Oral squamous papilloma is a benign proliferation of the stratified squamous epithelium. It occurs in one of every 250 adults and constitutes approximately 3% of all oral biopsy lesions [10, 68]. The etiologic factor is the human papillomavirus (HPV), and viral subtypes 2 and 11 have been isolated from up to 50% of oral papillomas [10]. Clinically, it appears as a single, asymptomatic, pedunculated or sessile, soft to firm mass with verrucous, granular, or papillomatous surface (Figure 17). The lesion may be white, slightly red, or normal in color [4, 68–70]. Papilloma usually enlarges rapidly to a maximum size of 5 mm with little or no change in diameter thereafter [10]. The most affected sites in the oral cavity are palatal mucosa and the tongue, but any oral surface may be involved [69]. Although papilloma can involve patients at any age it is diagnosed most often in people between 30 and 50 years [10]. Surgical excision by either scalpel or laser ablation is the treatment of choice. However, other modalities such as electro cautery, cryosurgery, and intralesional injection of interferon have been suggested [70]. Recurrence is uncommon, except for patients infected with human immunodeficiency virus [70].

3.4.2. Verruca Vulgaris. Verruca vulgaris is a benign virus-induced hyperplasia of stratified squamous epithelium. It is usually encountered in children with a peak incidence between 12 and 16 years. However, about 10% of general population affect the disease in their middle age [71, 72]. Most of oral lesions are located on the vermilion border, labial mucosa, or anterior tongue [4, 10]. Clinically, it appears as an exophytic, sessile, or pedunculated lesions with papillary projections (verrucous or papillomatous) or a rough pebbly surface [10, 71]. The lesions are asymptomatic and may be pink, yellowish, or white in coloration [10]. It usually

TABLE 4: General characteristics of rough-surfaced oral exophytic lesions.

Entity	Age	Gender	Site of involvement	Surface texture	Type of base	Consistency	Color	Size	Symptom & sign	Treatment	Recurrence
Squamous papilloma	30–50 years	No sex predilection	Palate & tongue	Verrucous/granular/ papillomatous	Pedunculated/sessile	Soft to firm	White/slightly red/normal	Maximum 5 mm	—	Surgical excision/electrocautery/ cryosurgery/intralesional interferon	Uncommon except for patients with HIV infection
Verruca vulgaris	12–16 years	—	Vermilion border/labial mucosa	Verrucous/ papillomatous/ Pebbly	Sessile/pedunculated	Soft to firm	Pink/yellowish/ white	Few mm	Asymptomatic	Conservative surgical excision	Low
Verrucous carcinoma	>6th decade	Male	Vestibular mucosa	Verrucous	—	Firm	White to normal	Up to several cm	Asymptomatic	Wide surgical excision/ radiotherapy/ chemotherapy	—
Squamous cell carcinoma	62 years	Male	Tongue	Verrucous	—	Firm to hard	White/pink/red	Up to several cm	Painless/moth-eaten radiolucency	Wide surgical excision/radiotherapy	33%
Multifocal epithelial hyperplasia	Childhood	Female	Labial and buccal mucosa	Cobblestone	—	Soft to firm	White to normal	Up to several cm	Nontender	Surgery/laser/ cryosurgery/ electrosurgery	Minimum

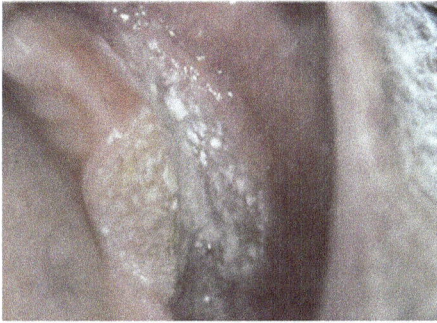

FIGURE 18: Broad-based verrucous carcinoma involving maxillary vestibular mucosa, with verrucous surface.

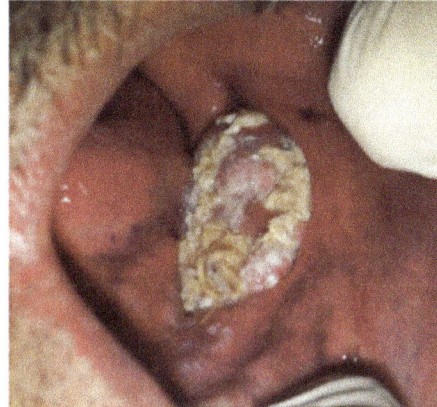

FIGURE 19: Exophytic SCC with a verrucous, necrotic, and ulcerative surface, extended from vestibule of the mandible to floor of the mouth.

enlarges rapidly to its maximum size and remains constant for months or years thereafter [71, 72]. Approximately 23% of lesions show spontaneous regression in two months and the remaining lesions within 2 years [72]. Oral lesions are usually treated by conservative surgical excision. Meanwhile, laser therapy, cryotherapy, or electrosurgery has been also recommended. A small proportion of treated lesions show recurrence [4, 10].

3.4.3. Verrucous Carcinoma.

Verrucous carcinoma which also called Ackerman tumor, Buschke-Lowenstein tumor, florid oral papillomatosis, epithelioma cuniculatum, or snuff dipper's cancer is a nonmetastasizing low grade variant of oral squamous cell carcinoma [68, 73]. The incidence rate has been estimated as one lesion per 1.000.000 of the population each year. The etiology of the lesion is not clear, but oral lesions predominantly occur in patients habituated to areca chewing, alcohol drinking, smoking, and having poor oral hygiene. However, 15% to 51% of the lesions have been found in people without these habits [10, 68]. The most common affected sites in the oral cavity are vestibular mucosa, buccal mucosa, gingivae, and the tongue [10, 68, 73]. There is a male predilection with the majority of lesions being reported in the sixth decade [4, 68, 73]. The lesion is featured by an asymptomatic, broad-based, well-circumscribed, thick, pink to white plaque resembling a cauliflower with verruciform surface (Figure 18) [10]. Similarly simultaneous oral and genital lesions of larger sizes would suggest condyloma acuminatum [10]. Malignant transformation has been detected in 20% of the lesions [73]. Wide surgical excision, radiotherapy, and chemotherapy have been recommended for treatment.

3.4.4. Squamous Cell Carcinoma.

Squamous cell carcinoma (SCC) accounts for 90% of all oral cancers and is considered as the eighth most frequent cancer globally [74]. Males are affected more frequently than females with a male to female ratio of 3 : 1 [10]. The median age of diagnosis is 62 years. However, the incidence of oral SCC in persons younger than 45 is increasing [75–77]. Tongue is the mostly affected site in the oral cavity followed by floor of the mouth, gingivae, palate, retromolar area, buccal, and labial mucosa [10, 75–78]. In young patients and those with congenital oral squamous cell carcinoma the tongue is the mostly affected site of

involvement as well [10]. Warning signs of oral cancer include red-white lesions, ulcer lasting more than three weeks, pain of the tongue due to its mobility and sensitive nature, lump in the oral cavity or in the neck area, discomfort with speech or swallowing, mobile teeth in the absence of periodontitis, anesthesia, and earache without apparent disease. The most frequent complaints among oral cancer patients are swelling, pain, and ulceration [74]. Clinically, it can appear in various forms such as a red or white plaque, a solitary chronic ulcer or an exophytic mass [75]. Approximately 55% of the tongue lesions were exophytic-type. This type of lesions has a rough surface (verrucous) and usually is irregular in shape (Figure 19). The lesion has a broad base and it is white, pink, or red in color. Ulceration may be present in larger fungating lesions with necrotic and multicolored surface. In addition, oral SCCs are painless and firm to hard in palpation and bleeding is not an early characteristic feature [1, 10, 75]. However, in cases with destruction of the underlying bone pain may be reported, and a "moth-eaten radiolucency" with ill-defined or ragged borders is found [10]. Despite early oral cancer whose manifestations are not definitive late-stage oral SCC show quite prominent signs such as a large mass with irregular margins, ulceration, nodularity, and fixation to the surrounding tissues [74]. The treatment of intraoral SCC is guided by the clinical stage of the disease and consists of wide surgical excision, radiation therapy, or a combination of surgery and radiation therapy [10]. The recurrence rate is estimated about 33% within 2 to 96 months [79].

3.4.5. Multifocal Epithelial Hyperplasia.

Multifocal epithelial hyperplasia, also known as focal epithelial hyperplasia, multifocal epithelial papilloma, virus epithelial hyperplasia, and Heck disease, is a virus-induced proliferation of oral squamous epithelium [10]. Although this entity is usually a childhood condition other age groups may also be affected. The frequency of the lesion ranges from 0.002 to 35% in different populations and 70% of patients are in first two decades of their life [79]. In addition, there is a female predilection with female to male ratio of 3 : 1 [79]. It appears

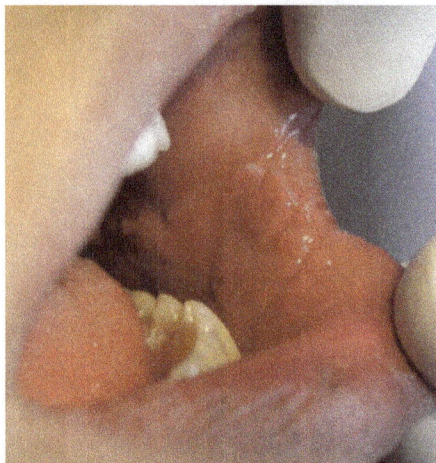

FIGURE 20: Multifocal epithelial hyperplasia presented as numerous exophytic lesions with flat surface distributed in the buccal mucosa and lower lip.

as multiple, soft, circumscribed, nontender, flattened, or rounded papules, with either whitish color or color similar to the normal mucosa and cobblestone appearance (Figure 20) [10, 79, 80]. Most of the lesions are less than 0.5 cm, but lesions with several centimeters in size have been reported as well [10, 79]. The most frequent affected sites are labial, buccal, and lingual mucosa followed by gingivae, palate, and tonsillar mucosa [10]. There is no potential for malignant transformation [79, 80]. However, Niebrügge et al. showed malignant transformation in a female patient with long-standing Heck disease [81]. It is a self-limiting disease; hence it is recommended that only lesions located in areas subjected to trauma be excised. Risk of recurrence after therapy is minimal. There are several treatment modalities like scalpel surgery, cryosurgery, electrosurgery, and carbon dioxide laser vaporization [10, 79].

4. Discussion

In this review article we proposed a practical diagnostic decision tree for oral peripheral exophytic lesions as well as a brief overview about each entity. Although this group of lesions comprises a constellation of heterogeneous origins and pathogeneses, some clinical features help us categorize them to come arrive a more timely and precise differential diagnosis. We used surface texture for clinical classification of the lesions into two major groups: "lesions with smooth surface" and "lesions with rough surface." Furthermore, the former was divided into three subgroups constituting 23 entities, and the latter constituting six lesions. While general characteristics guide to a certain group of lesions, special features point to a unique entity.

In regard to reactive hyperplastic lesions, detecting the insult factor through history taking or physical examination plays the key role for definite diagnosis.

For example, a bright red color in a soft and easily bleeding mass suggests a pyogenic granuloma, which is called a pregnancy tumor in a pregnant woman. However a peripheral

giant cell granuloma presents as a more bluish, buccolingually located mass exclusively on the gingivae or alveolar ridge with a firm consistency. Meanwhile, it has a potential to cause root and bone resorption. Similarly, peripheral ossifying fibroma has a tendency to induce tooth mobility and bone destruction, but it is firm to hard in palpation with a pale pink coloration [4, 9, 10, 12, 13, 15].

Moreover, some lesions can be identified primarily by their region such as those relating to ill-fit dentures. Epulis fissuratum is seen along denture flanges as single or multiple folds, inflammatory papillary hyperplasia is located mostly on the hard palate with a pebbly or cobblestone appearance, and leaf-like fibroma presents with a narrow stalk and serrated borders beneath the base of maxillary dentures [10, 18–21].

Some exophytic lesions are found in close approximation to a tooth such as pulp polyp proliferating inside a large tooth cavity, epulis granulomatosum emanating from an extraction socket, and parulis on the alveolar mucosa or attached gingivae of a necrotic tooth [23, 25, 28].

Oral exophytic lesions of nonneoplastic salivary origin such as mucocele and ranula appear as soft and fluctuant dome-shaped lesions on oral mucosa containing salivary minor glands with a history of periodic rupture and release of fluid content. Therefore, they should not be suspected when a lesion is located on the hard palate or gingivae due to lack of submucosal salivary glands. On the other hand, a dome-shaped or nodular lesion on the posterolateral portion of the hard palate with a soft to firm consistency and slow growth rate would prompt the clinician to consider a benign salivary neoplasm such as pleomorphic adenoma in higher rankings of differential diagnosis. Moreover, accompanying pain raises the possibility of a malignant counterpart like adenoid cystic carcinoma or mucoepidermoid tumor. While a dome-shaped lesion on the lower lip is usually suggestive of a mucocele, such lesion in the upper lip should be suspected as a salivary neoplasm [37, 41, 43, 45, 46].

Peripheral oral exophytic lesions of mesenchymal origin are quite infrequent as compared with reactive or salivary lesions. Although they might show similar clinical features special characteristics such as location help differentiate them.

Neoplasms of neuronal origin mostly appear on the tongue as asymptomatic, soft to firm masses with neurofibroma being mostly multiple contrary to solitary schwannoma. In addition, concomitant eye and skin manifestations indicate neurofibromatosis. A soft fluctuant mass with a yellowish hue especially in the buccal mucosa points out a tumor of adipose tissue (lipoma). Non-Hodgkin lymphoma in the oral cavity produces a nodular pink or purplish mass with an intact or ulcerated surface on the buccal vestibule or palate with a potential for progressive growth and local destruction. Hemangioma and lymphangioma most frequently happen on the tongue sometimes with a rough surface despite their connective tissue origin. Hemangioma is characterized by a pink or purplish color and blanching on pressure, whereas lymphangioma causes macroglossia and gray to pink projections [1, 4, 10].

As a general rule, lesions originating from the epithelium present with a rough surface. An exception in this regard is focal epithelial hyperplasia with numerous small flat-end papules scattered on the oral mucosa most commonly in children and adolescence. Small finger-like projections on lesion surface are invariably seen in viral-induced lesions such as squamous papilloma, verruca vulgaris, and condyloma acuminatum. Papilloma tends to occur as a single lesion rarely exceeding 1 cm in diameter. On the other hand, verruca vulgaris and Heck disease mostly appear in multiple forms with the former being coexisted with cutaneous lesions. Coincidence of large verruca vulgaris-form lesions in the genitalia and oral cavity as well as high-risk sexual behavior refer to a condyloma acuminatum.

Squamous cell carcinoma when appears as a broad-based exophytic lesion involves the lateral border of the tongue with a rough nonhomogenous or sometimes ulcerative or necrotic surface and a progressive potential to unlimited growth. On the other hand, its nonmetastasizing counterpart—verrucous carcinoma—is mostly encountered on the vestibular or buccal mucosa in a snuff-dipper patient with a homogenous cauliflower appearance and an association with smokeless tobacco use.

5. Conclusion

We proposed a diagnostic decision tree regarding oral peripheral exophytic lesions divided into lesions with smooth surface and rough-surfaced lesions. Upon confronting a peripheral exophytic mass in the oral cavity a clinician should consider some features such as surface texture, shape of base, color, and consistency in order to categorize the lesion and progress along the decision tree to reach a logistic differential diagnosis.

References

[1] N. K. Wood and P. W. Goaz, *Differential Diagnosis of Oral And Maxillofacial Lesions*, Mosby, St. Louis, Mo, USA, 5th Edition edition, 1997.

[2] A. B. R. Santosh, D. Boyd, and K. K. Laxminarayana, "Proposed clinico-pathological classification for oral exophytic lesions," *Journal of Clinical and Diagnostic Research*, vol. 9, no. 9, pp. ZE01–ZE08, 2015.

[3] R. B. Zain, N. Ikeda, I. A. Razak et al., "A national epidemiological survey of oral mucosal lesions in Malaysia," *Community Dentistry and Oral Epidemiology*, vol. 25, no. 5, pp. 377–383, 1997.

[4] M. Glick, *Burket's Oral Medicine*, People's medical publishing house, 12th edition edition, 2015, 147-172, 175-188, 236-237.

[5] A. Bermejo-Fenoll and P. López-Jornet, "Differential diagnosis of exophytic lesions of soft oral tissue," *Medicina Oral, Patologia Oral y Cirugia Bucal*, vol. 10, no. 5, pp. 470-471, 2005.

[6] N. G. Nikitakis, "Oral soft tissue lesions: a guide to differential diagnosis part II: surface alterations," *Brazilian Journal of Oral Sciences*, vol. 4, no. 13, pp. 707–715, 2005.

[7] V. Reddy, S. Saxena, S. Saxena, and M. Reddy, "Reactive hyperplastic lesions of the oral cavity: a ten year observational study on North Indian population," *Journal of Clinical and Experimental Dentistry*, vol. 4, no. 3, pp. e136–e140, 2012.

[8] H. Kadeh, S. Saravani, and M. Tajik, "Reactive hyperplastic lesions of the oral cavity," *Iranian Journal of Otorhinolaryngology*, vol. 27, no. 79, pp. 137–144, 2015.

[9] H. Jafarzadeh, M. Sanatkhani, and N. Mohtasham, "Oral pyogenic granuloma: a review," *Journal of Oral Science*, vol. 48, no. 4, pp. 167–175, 2006.

[10] B. W. Neville, D. D. Damm, C. M. Allen, and J. E. Bouquot, *Oral and Maxillofacial Pathology*, Saunders-Elsevier. China, 3rd edition, 2009.

[11] S. R. Gomes, Q. J. Shakir, P. V. Thaker, and J. K. Tavadia, "Pyogenic granuloma of the gingiva: a misnomer?: a case report and review of literature," *Journal of Indian Society of Periodontology*, vol. 17, no. 4, pp. 514–519, 2013.

[12] M. J. Franco-Barrera, M. G. Zavala-Cerna, R. Fernández-Tamayo, I. Vivanco-Pérez, N. M. Fernández-Tamayo, and O. Torres-Bugarín, "An update on peripheral ossifying fibroma: case report and literature review," *Oral and Maxillofacial Surgery*, vol. 20, no. 1, pp. 1–7, 2016.

[13] T. Farquhar, J. Maclellan, H. Dyment, and Anderson R. D., "Peripheral ossifying fibroma: a case report," *Canadian Dental Association*, vol. 47, no. 9, 809 pages, 2016, 812.

[14] M. B. Mishra, K. A. Bhishen, and S. Mishra, "Peripheral ossifying fibroma," *Journal of Oral and Maxillofacial Pathology*, vol. 15, no. 1, pp. 65–68, 2011.

[15] A. Nekouei, A. Eshghi, P. Jafarnejadi, and Z. Enshaei, "A review and report of peripheral giant cell granuloma in a 4-year-old child," *Case Reports in Dentistry*, vol. 2016, Article ID 7536304, 4 pages, 2016.

[16] C. M. Flaitz, "Peripheral giant cell granuloma: a potentially aggressive lesion in children," *Pediatric Dentistry*, vol. 22, no. 3, pp. 232-233, 2000.

[17] G. S. Letterman, "Peripheral giant cell granuloma," *Plastic and Reconstructive Surgery*, vol. 46, no. 3, p. 320, 1970.

[18] K. Veena, H. Jagadishchandra, J. Sequria, S. Hameed, L. Chatra, and P. Shenai, "An extensive denture-induced hyperplasia of maxilla," *Annals of Medical and Health Sciences Research*, vol. 3, no. 5, p. 7, 2013.

[19] E. M. Canger, P. Celenk, and S. Kayipmaz, "Denture-related hyperplasia: A clinical study of a Turkish population group," *Brazilian Dental Journal*, vol. 20, no. 3, pp. 243–248, 2009.

[20] H. Mortazavi, H. R. Khalighi, S. Jafari, and M. Baharvand, "Epulis fissuratum in the soft palate: Report of a case in a very rare location," *Dental Hypotheses*, vol. 7, no. 2, pp. 67–69, 2016.

[21] I. M. Brook and D. J. Lamb, "Surgical/prosthetic problems of a large leaf fibroma," *Dental Update*, vol. 15, no. 3, p. 126, 1988.

[22] N. G. Nikitakis and J. K. Brooks, "Sessile nodule on the palate. Leaflike denture fibroma," *General Dentistry*, vol. 59, no. 1, pp. 76-77, 2011.

[23] B. Manovijay, P. Rajathi, S. M. Fenn, and B. Sekar, "Recurrent epulis granulomatosa: a second look," *Journal of Advanced Clinical & Research Insights*, vol. 2, pp. 140–142, 2015.

[24] S. Ghadimi, N. Chiniforush, M. Najafi, and S. Amiri, "Excision of epulis granulomatosa with diode laser in 8 years old boy," *Journal of Lasers in Medical Sciences*, vol. 6, no. 2, pp. 92–95, 2015.

[25] S. Palanivelu, P. Jayanthi, U. K. Rao, E. Joshua, and K. Ranganathan, "Rapidly enlarging mass following dental extraction," *Journal of Oral and Maxillofacial Pathology*, vol. 15, no. 2, pp. 223–227, 2011.

[26] J. Faryabi and S. Adhami, "Unusual presentation of chronic hyperplastic pulpitis: a case report. Iran Endod J," *Winter*, vol. 2, no. 4, p. 156, 2008.

[27] N. S. A. Jabbar, J. M. Aldrigui, M. M. Braga, and M. T. Wanderley, "Pulp polyp in traumatized primary teeth: a case-control study," *Dental Traumatology*, vol. 29, no. 5, pp. 360–364, 2013.

[28] K. Anilkumar, S. Lingeswaran, G. Ari, R. Thyagarajan, and A. Logaranjani, "Management of chronic hyperplastic pulpitis in mandibular molars of middle aged adults: a multidisciplinary approach," *Journal of Clinical and Diagnostic Research*, vol. 10, no. 1, pp. ZD23–ZD25, 2016.

[29] M. Gorduysus, *Hyperplastic Pulpitis Development in a Bridge Abutment Tooth*, vol. 32, Hacettepe Diş Hekimliği Fakültesi Dergisi, Ankara, Turkey, 1 edition, 2008, 35–37.

[30] H. R. Khalighi, M. Hamian, F. M. Abbas, and S. Farhadi, "Simultaneous existence of giant cell fibroma and squamous papilloma in the oral cavity," *Indian Journal of Medical Specialities*, vol. 2, no. 2, 2011.

[31] N. G. Nikitakis, D. Emmanouil, M. P. Maroulakos, and M. V. Angelopoulou, "Giant cell fibroma in children: report of two cases and literature review," *Journal of Oral and Maxillofacial Research*, vol. 4, no. 1, article e5, pp. 1–7, 2013.

[32] V. K. K. Reddy, N. Kumar, P. Battepati, L. Samyuktha, and S. P. Nanga, "Giant cell fibroma in a paediatric patient: a rare case report," *Case Reports in Dentistry*, vol. 2015, Article ID 240374, 3 pages, 2015.

[33] M. S. Thwaites, T. E. Jeter, and O. Ajagbe, "Inflammatory papillary hyperplasia: review of literature and case report involving a 10-year-old child," *Quintessence International*, vol. 21, no. 2, pp. 133–138, 1990.

[34] J. R. Antonelli, F. V. Panno, and A. Witko, "Inflammatory papillary hyperplasia: supraperiosteal excision by the blade-loop technique." *General dentistry*, vol. 46, no. 4, pp. 390–397, 1998.

[35] P. Infante-Cossio, R. Martinez-de-Fuentes, E. Torres-Carranza, and J. L. Gutierrez-Perez, "Inflammatory papillary hyperplasia of the palate: treatment with carbon dioxide laser, followed by restoration with an implant-supported prosthesis," *British Journal of Oral and Maxillofacial Surgery*, vol. 45, no. 8, pp. 658–660, 2007.

[36] H. Mohan, A. Tahlan, I. Mundi, R. P. S. Punia, and A. Dass, "Non-neoplastic salivary gland lesions: a 15-year study," *European Archives of Oto-Rhino-Laryngology*, vol. 268, no. 8, pp. 1187–1190, 2011.

[37] H. Mortazavi, M. Baharvand, S. Alirezaei, and R. Noor-Mohammadi, "Combination therapy in a large lower lip mucocele: a non-invasive recommended technique," *Dental Hypotheses*, vol. 5, no. 3, pp. 127–129, 2014.

[38] H. Mortazavi, H. R. Khalighi, M. Baharvand, M. Eshghpour, and R. Singh, "Bilateral symmetrical mucocele of the lower lip: report of a rare clinical presentation," *International Journal of Experimental Dental Science*, vol. 3, pp. 92–94, 2014.

[39] R. Prakash, B. B. Kushwaha, and S. Gautam, "Airway management in a child with oral ranula," *International Journal of Biomedical Research*, vol. 5, no. 2, p. 148, 2014.

[40] S. Moghe, A. K. Pillai, S. Prabhu, S. Nahar, and U. K. Kartika, "Pleomorphic adenoma of the palate: report of a case," *International Journal of Scientific Study*, vol. 2, pp. 54–56, 2014.

[41] H. Mortazavi, S. Alirezaei, S. Azari-Marhabi, M. Baharvand, and M. Eshghpour, "Upper lip pleomorphic adenoma: comparison of reported cases between," *Journal of Dental materials and Techniques*, vol. 2, no. 4, pp. 125–129, 1990.

[42] M. Rahnama, U. Orzedala-Koszel, L. Czupkallo, and M. Lobacz, "Pleomorphic adenoma of the palate: a case report and review of the literature," *Wspolczesna Onkologia*, vol. 17, no. 1, pp. 103–106, 2013.

[43] S. J. Jarde, S. Das, S. Narayanswamy, A. Chatterjee, and C. Babu, "Mucoepidermoid carcinoma of the palate: a rare case report," *Journal of Indian Society of Periodontology*, vol. 20, no. 2, pp. 203–206, 2016.

[44] P. Ritwik, K. G. Cordell, and R. B. Brannon, "Minor salivary gland mucoepidermoid carcinoma in children and adolescents: a case series and review of the literature," *Journal of Medical Case Reports*, vol. 6, article no. 182, 2012.

[45] N. Shah, A. Mahjan, H. Patel, R. Shah, and S. Shah, "Mucoepidermoid carcinoma of palate: a case repor," *Scholars journal of dental sciences*, vol. 2, no. 3, pp. 222–224, 2015.

[46] K. Triantafillidou, J. Dimitrakopoulos, F. Iordanidis, and D. Koufogiannis, "Management of adenoid cystic carcinoma of minor salivary glands," *Journal of Oral and Maxillofacial Surgery*, vol. 64, no. 7, pp. 1114–1120, 2006.

[47] P. J. Bradley, "Adenoid cystic carcinoma of the head and neck: a review," *Current Opinion in Otolaryngology & Head and Neck Surgery*, vol. 12, no. 2, pp. 127–132, 2004.

[48] M. Mendez, V. C. Carrard, A. N. Haas et al., "A 10-year study of specimens submitted to oral pathology laboratory analysis: lesion occurrence and demographic features," *Brazilian Oral Research*, vol. 26, no. 3, pp. 235–241, 2012.

[49] M. Ali and D. Sundaram, "Biopsied oral soft tissue lesions in Kuwait: a six-year retrospective analysis," *Medical Principles and Practice*, vol. 21, no. 6, pp. 569–575, 2012.

[50] P. Dalvi, K. Vandana, S. Prakash, and K. Mohan, "Solitary neurofibroma of the gingiva: a rare case report," *Indian Journal of Multidisciplinary Dentistry*, vol. 6, no. 2, p. 111, 2016.

[51] J. P. George and N. Sai Jyothsna, "Solitary neurofibroma: a rare occurrence on gingiva," *General Dentistry*, vol. 64, no. 3, pp. 28–31, 2016.

[52] T. Shimoyama, T. Kato, D. Nasu, T. Kaneko, N. Horie, and F. Ide, "Solitary neurofibroma of the oral mucosa: a previously undescribed variant of neurofibroma." *Journal of oral science*, vol. 44, no. 1, pp. 59–63, 2002.

[53] P. Prasanna Kumar and K. Meghashri, "Schwannoma of the hard palate: a case report and review of literature," *Journal of Oral Research and Review*, vol. 3, no. 1, pp. 23–27, 2012.

[54] J.-M. Sanchis, C.-M. Navarro, J.-V. Bagán et al., "Intraoral schwannomas: presentation of a series of 12 cases," *Journal of Clinical and Experimental Dentistry*, vol. 5, no. 4, pp. 192–196, 2013.

[55] S. Parhar, H. Preet Singh, A. Nayyar, and A. S. Manchanda, "Intra-oral schwannoma: a case report," *Journal of Clinical and Diagnostic Research*, vol. 8, no. 3, pp. 264-265, 2014.

[56] S. Kumaraswamy, N. Madan, R. Keerthi, and S. Shakti, "Lipomas of oral cavity: case reports with review of literature," *Journal of Maxillofacial and Oral Surgery*, vol. 8, no. 4, pp. 394–397, 2009.

[57] R. Kaur, S. Kler, and A. Bhullar, "Intraoral lipoma: report of 3 cases," *Dental Research Journal*, vol. 8, no. 1, pp. 48–51, 2011, (Isfahan) Winter.

[58] K. Rana, V. Narula, E. K. Bhargava, R. Shankar, and N. Mahajan, "T-cell lymphoma of the oral cavity: case report," *Journal of Clinical and Diagnostic Research*, vol. 9, no. 3, pp. MD03–MD04, 2015.

[59] M. Malaguarnera, M. Giordano, C. Russo et al., "Lymphoma of cheek: a case report," *European Review for Medical and Pharmacological Sciences*, vol. 16, pp. 4–7, 2012.

[60] S. Alirezaei, M. Baharvand, B. Tavakoli, S. Sarikhani, and A. R. Mafi, "Advanced primary lymphoma of oral cavity: report of a case," *Open Journal of Stomatology*, vol. 04, no. 03, pp. 109–114, 2014.

[61] S. I. M. L. Queiroz, G. M. de Assis, V. D. Silvestre, A. R. Germano, and J. S. P. da Silva, "Treatment of oral hemangioma with sclerotherapy: case report," *Jornal Vascular Brasileiro*, vol. 13, no. 3, 2014.

[62] A. Dilsiz, T. Aydin, and N. Gursan, "Capillary hemangioma as a rare benign tumor of the oral cavity: a case report," *Cases Journal*, vol. 2, no. 9, article no. 8622, 2009.

[63] K. A. Kamala, L. Ashok, and G. P. Sujatha, "Cavernous hemangioma of the tongue: a rare case report," *Contemporary Clinical Dentistry*, vol. 5, no. 1, pp. 95–98, 2014.

[64] V. Usha, T. Sivasankari, S. Jeelani, G. S. Asokan, and J. Parthiban, "Lymphangioma of the tongue: a case report and review of literature," *Journal of Clinical and Diagnostic Research*, vol. 8, no. 9, pp. ZD12–ZD14, 2014.

[65] H. Bhayya, D. Pavani, M. L. Avinash Tejasvi, and P. Geetha, "Oral lymphangioma: a rare case report," *Contemporary Clinical Dentistry*, vol. 6, no. 4, pp. 584–587, 2015.

[66] S. Sunil, D. Gopakumar, and B. Sreenivasan, "Oral lymphangioma: case reports and review of literature," *Contemporary Clinical Dentistry*, vol. 3, no. 1, p. 116, 2012.

[67] H. Alan, S. Agacayak, G. Kavak, and A. Ozcan, "Verrucous carcinoma and squamous cell papilloma of the oral cavity: report of two cases and review of literature," *European Journal of Dentistry*, vol. 9, no. 3, pp. 453–456, 2015.

[68] L. A. Goodstein, A. Khan, J. Pinczewski, and V. N. Young, "Symptomatic squamous papilloma of the uvula: report of a case and review of the literature," *Case Reports in Otolaryngology*, vol. 2012, pp. 1-2, 2012.

[69] P. P. Jaju, P. V. Suvarna, and R. S. Desai, "Squamous papilloma: case report and review of literature," *International Journal of Oral Science*, vol. 2, no. 4, pp. 222–225, 2010.

[70] M. Nagaraj, "Verruca vulgaris of the tongue," *Journal of Maxillofacial and Oral Surgery*, vol. 12, no. 3, pp. 329–332, 2013.

[71] A. Ural, S. Arslan, Ş. Ersöz, and B. Değer, "Verruca vulgaris of the tongue: a case report with literature review," *Bosnian Journal of Basic Medical Sciences*, vol. 14, no. 3, pp. 136–138, 2014.

[72] H. Mortazavi, M. Baharvand, and M. Mehdipour, "Oral potentially malignant disorders: an overview of more than 20 entities," *Journal of Dental Research, Dental Clinics, Dental Prospects*, vol. 8, no. 1, p. 14, 2014, Winter.

[73] M. Zargaran, N. Eshghyar, P. B. Vaziri, and H. Mortazavi, "Immunohistochemical evaluation of type IV collagen and laminin-332 γ2 chain expression in well-differentiated oral squamous cell carcinoma and oral verrucous carcinoma: a new recommended cut-off," *Journal of Oral Pathology and Medicine*, vol. 40, no. 2, pp. 167–173, 2011.

[74] A. van Zyl and BK. Bunn, "Clinical features of oral cancer," in *Clinical features of oral cancer*, vol. 67, p. 566, SADJ, Nov 2012.

[75] L. Feller and J. Lemmer, "Oral squamous cell carcinoma: epidemiology, clinical presentation and treatment," *Journal of Cancer Therapy*, vol. 03, no. 04, pp. 263–268, 2012.

[76] H. Mortazavi, S. Hajian, E. Fadavi, S. Sabour, M. Baharvand, and S. Bakhtiari, "ABO blood groups in oral cancer: a first case-control study in a defined group of Iranian patients," *Asian Pacific Journal of Cancer Prevention*, vol. 15, no. 3, pp. 1415–1418, 2014.

[77] N. Shamloo, A. Lotfi, H. R. Motazadian, H. Mortazavi, and M. Baharvand, "Squamous cell carcinoma as the most common lesion of the tongue in Iranians: a 22-year retrospective study," *Asian Pacific Journal of Cancer Prevention*, vol. 17, no. 3, pp. 1415–1419, 2016.

[78] B. Wang, S. Zhang, K. Yue, and X.-D. Wang, "The recurrence and survival of oral squamous cell carcinoma: a report of 275 cases," *Chinese Journal of Cancer*, vol. 32, no. 11, pp. 614–618, 2013.

[79] N. Shamloo, H. Mortazavi, N. Taghavi, and M. Baharvand, "Multifocal epithelial hyperplasia: a forgotten condition in the elderly," *General Dentistry*, vol. 64, no. 5, pp. 72–74, 2016.

[80] B. Ozden, K. Gunduz, O. Gunhan, and F. O. Ozden, "A case report of focal epithelial hyperplasia (Heck's disease) with PCR detection of human papillomavirus," *Journal of Maxillofacial and Oral Surgery*, vol. 10, no. 4, pp. 357–360, 2011.

[81] B. Niebrügge, E.-M. De Villiers, K.-L. Gerlach, I. Franke, and H. Gollnick, "Demonstration of HPV 24 in long-standing Heck's disease with malignant transformation," *European Journal of Dermatology*, vol. 9, no. 6, pp. 477–479, 1999.

30

The Prevalence and Underreporting of Needlestick Injuries among Dental Healthcare Workers in Pakistan

Mehak Pervaiz ®,[1] Ruth Gilbert,[2] and Nasreen Ali ®[3]

[1]*APPNA Institute of Public Health, Jinnah Sindh Medical University, Karachi, Pakistan*
[2]*School of Healthcare Practice, University of Bedfordshire, Putteridge Bury, Luton, Bedfordshire LU2 8LE, UK*
[3]*Institute of Health Research, University of Bedfordshire, Putteridge Bury, Luton, Bedfordshire LU2 8LE, UK*

Correspondence should be addressed to Nasreen Ali; nasreen.ali@beds.ac.uk

Academic Editor: Izzet Yavuz

Needlestick injuries (NSIs) are a major occupational health problem among dental healthcare workers (HCWs) in Pakistan, which places them at a significant risk of acquiring blood-borne infections. However, not all NSIs are reported, leading to an underestimation of the actual prevalence. The harmful impacts of NSIs on the healthcare delivery necessitate an urgent need to measure its actual prevalence. *Objectives.* The aim of this study was to review literature to estimate the prevalence and reporting rates of NSIs among dental-HCWs in Pakistan. *Methods.* 713 potentially relevant citations were identified by electronic databases and hand searching of articles. Nine primary studies were subsequently identified to be included in the review. *Results.* The results of the included studies indicate that the prevalence of NSIs among Pakistani dental-HCWs was between 30% and 73%. The rate of reporting of NSIs was between 15% and 76%, and the most common reason was found to be the lack of awareness regarding the reporting system, or of the need to report NSIs. *Conclusion.* It is evident from the review of the included studies that there is a significantly high prevalence and a low rate of reporting of NSIs among dental-HCWs in Pakistan, suggesting the need to setup an occupational health department in dental settings, for preventing, managing, recording, and monitoring NSIs.

1. Introduction

Globally, an estimated two million healthcare workers (HCWs) experience a needlestick injury (NSI) each year [1] putting them at risk of infectious diseases such as hepatitis B virus (HBV), hepatitis C virus (HCV), and human immunodeficiency virus (HIV) [2, 3]. Globally, more than a third of hepatitis B and hepatitis C cases and approximately 5% of HIV cases result from an NSI [1] despite evidence to show effective infection control policies that can successfully prevent HBV seroconversion and minimise rates of HCV and HIV seroconversion following an NSI [4]. NSIs have also been shown to transmit other bacterial, fungal, or viral infections, including blastomycosis, cryptococcosis, diphtheria, herpes, malaria, mycobacteriosis, and syphilis [5]. It is also reported that in up to 12% of cases, NSIs may also lead to psychiatric morbidity including posttraumatic stress disorder (PTSD) [6]. Furthermore, the presence of blood-contaminated saliva increases the risk of infection with blood-borne viruses or other infectious agents during an NSI [7–9], which can adversely affect both personal and professional life and can restrict career opportunities due to the risk of transmission of blood-borne pathogens to patients [9–11].

In the prevaccination era, the rate of HBV infection amongst dental-HCWs was estimated to be 3–6 times higher than in the general population [12]. Although rates amongst dental-HCWs have fallen in developed countries, in many low- and middle-income countries, vaccine coverage rates remain low and awareness of postexposure prophylaxis (PEP) is poor [13, 14]. The existing evidence base highlights that dental-HCWs appear to be at particularly high risk of NSIs [15–17]. This is mainly due to the use of sharp dental instruments often for multiple injections in the mouth where access and visibility can be poor [9, 18–20].

It is difficult to accurately estimate the global prevalence of NSIs among dental-HCWs due to the underreporting of incidents which is a significant issue in developing countries [21, 22]. Iranian studies have shown that, in some settings, over 80% of dental-HCWs fail to report NSIs [23, 24]. A national community survey which was carried out in 2007-2008 calculated that the prevalence of hepatitis B surface antigen (HBsAg) and hepatitis C virus in Pakistan were 2.5% and 4.8%, respectively, and estimated that there were approximately 13 million chronic hepatitis B and C carriers in the country [25], but this is now outdated. Taking into consideration the evidence on underreporting of NSIs, this figure could potentially be much higher, indicating dental-HCWs in Pakistan are at a particularly high risk of infection following an NSI.

A number of factors for the underreporting of NSIs are presented in the literature and include lack of awareness that NSIs need to be reported [23, 24], lack of awareness of where to report [26, 27], the belief that there is no point in reporting incidents, and unwillingness to report the incident [26]. The fear of getting blamed was also found to be a common reason among dental students [28]. There is, however, a dearth of information on the prevalence, risk factors, and reasons for underreporting NSIs among dental-HCWs in Pakistan despite the high NSI prevalence [17]. Synthesizing existing evidence on the prevalence and risk factors of NSIs and the rate and reasons of underreporting of NSIs among dental-HCWs in Pakistan can potentially underline the existing gaps in the available literature and dental practices that may require further consideration.

2. Aim and Objectives

The aim of this paper is to review the existing literature to determine the prevalence and rate of reporting of NSIs among dental-HCWs in Pakistan.

3. Methodology

3.1. Selection Criteria. Inclusion criteria for relevant studies were as follows:

(1) Primary research studies published in peer-reviewed journals

(2) Studies from Pakistan that sampled dental-HCWs

(3) Studies that reported the prevalence and/or reporting rates of NSIs

(4) Studies published in English between January 2000 and June 2016

4. Search Strategy

The search strategy included electronic database search and hand searching up to 30 June 2016. The electronic databases MEDLINE, Google Scholar, Discover, Cochrane Library, CINAHL, BMC, ScienceDirect, Web of Science, and the Directory of Open Access Journals (DOAJ) were searched using the following key words and Boolean operators: (prevalen* OR occur* OR rate* OR frequency* OR report* OR record*) AND (needle* OR occupation* OR sharp* OR percutaneous) AND (injury* OR trauma* OR wound*) AND (dental worker* OR dental student* OR dental assistant* OR dentist* OR dental staff) AND (Pakistan* OR South Asia* OR developing country*). The titles and abstracts of the papers identified were screened against the inclusion and exclusion criteria. Additional papers were identified from searching Pakistan-based dental journals not indexed in the databases listed above, a citation search of key authors, and screening the reference lists of the papers which passed the screening test for related articles.

5. Data Extraction

Relevant data were extracted from the studies based on the "STROBE" framework criteria for cross-sectional studies [29]. Data were extracted and entered on a Microsoft Excel spreadsheet. The data extraction headings were as follows: author(s), year of publication, journal title, article title, study aim and objectives, study design, participants, study location, sampling technique, study size, data collection method, response rate, descriptive data, data analysis, key results, and conclusions.

6. Quality Appraisal

Following data extraction, the methodological quality and rigour of the included studies were assessed using Boyle's [30] quality assessment framework criteria to evaluate the potential strength of the outcomes. The quality assessment followed a scoring system comprising eight questions, and studies were graded high (7-8 score), moderate (4–6 score), or low (1–3 score) quality based on three main criteria: sampling, measurement, and analysis [30–32]. The sampling framework was applied to all selected studies in a consistent fashion, and the minimum response rate in the reviewed studies was set at 80% [30].

7. Data Analysis

The results were analysed using narrative analysis. A textual approach was used to combine and summarise the findings from different studies and subsequently explain the synthesised findings [33]. It was selected as it systematically evaluates and incorporates the results from across the studies and explores the similarities and dissimilarities between the study findings [34]. Since the included studies demonstrated heterogeneity with regard to their evaluation criteria and study results, performing a meta-analysis was not considered appropriate, as it would have yielded potentially insignificant and misleading results [35]. Furthermore, the data required for performing a meta-analysis were absent in all the reviewed studies [36, 37].

8. Methods of the Review

A review of the abstracts and titles was carried out by all the authors to determine the suitability of the papers and resolve any differences as to whether to include or exclude papers. Mehak Parveiz extracted the data and assessed quality of the data, and Ruth Gilbert and Nasreen Ali cross-checked the extracted data and quality assessment to ensure data accuracy.

9. Results

9.1. Overall Description of the Included and Excluded Studies. A total of 713 potentially relevant citations were identified by electronic and hand searching. Following initial screening of titles and abstracts, 15 duplicate papers were excluded and 686 studies were excluded based on the pre-specified inclusion and exclusion criteria. The full-text of the remaining 12 studies was scrutinized to determine their eligibility for inclusion in the review. Of these, three further articles were excluded as they failed to mention the prevalence or reporting rates of NSIs. As a result, nine primary studies met the inclusion criteria and were included in the review (Figure 1).

9.2. Analysis of Included Studies

9.2.1. Study Design. The nine included studies were conducted in seven different Pakistani cities: Karachi [38, 39], Hyderabad [17, 26], Lahore [40], Jamshoro [41], Quetta [42], Peshawar, and Abbottabad [43, 44]. All the studies had an observational, cross-sectional study design, which quantitatively measured the prevalence of NSIs, whereas only four studies [17, 26, 39, 41] measured the reporting rate of NSIs. All included studies were within the review's inclusion criteria as they were Pakistan-based primary studies reporting the prevalence and/or reporting rate of NSIs among dental-HCWs published between 2009 and 2015 in a peer-reviewed journal in English.

9.2.2. Study Sampling. The study sample sizes ranged from 100 to 800. However, the included studies failed to specify the employed sampling technique, except for Khan et al. [43], which adopted a convenience sampling technique, though no rationale was provided. All studies used questionnaires as their measuring tool.

9.2.3. Response Rate. The response rate ranged from as high as 100% [38–40] to as low as 75% [44]. However, three studies failed to take account of their response rate [17, 42, 43].

9.2.4. Study Population. The gender ratio of the participants was not mentioned in three of the studies [38, 43, 44]. Nonetheless, in other studies [17, 39–42,], on average 53% of the sample were male and 47% were female, making the ratio roughly equal in all studies except for Jan et al. [26], in which 83% of the study participants were male. Almost all studies included dental-HCWs from different job categories including dentists, dental faculty, postgraduates, house officers, undergraduates, assistants, technicians, and paradental staff. However, one study [44] sampled only dentists.

9.2.5. Age Range of Participants. Age of the participants was recorded by only three of the included studies. In two of the studies [39, 42], the majority of the study participants were between 20 and 30 years, whereas in one study [26], 50 participants were 25–35 years old, 73 were 36–45 years old,

and 131 were older than 45 years. Six of the reviewed studies failed to report any information on the age of the participants [17, 38, 40, 41, 43, 44].

9.2.6. Survey Duration. The survey duration was stated by five studies and varied considerably. Survey durations were one month [26], four months [43], nine months [38], and over one year [17, 41]. Four of the selected studies failed to take account of their study period [39, 40, 42, 44]. A full summary of the background information, methodological details, and key findings of the included studies is presented in Table 1.

10. Data Analysis

There were significant variations in the reporting of data on NSI prevalence, rate of reporting, and risk factors, as well as in the data on knowledge and awareness regarding NSIs and dental practices to prevent NSIs. As a result of which it was challenging to compare data across the studies.

10.1. Prevalence of NSIs. The prevalence of NSIs among Pakistani dental-HCWs ranged from 30% [39, 44] to 73% [38] (Table 1). In studies which compared the prevalence rate amongst different groups of dental-HCWs, dental undergraduate students generally experienced the highest rates of NSIs (15–60%) [17, 39, 41], while a lower prevalence of NSIs was observed among the qualified dentists, including dental surgeons, postgraduates, and house officers [17, 39, 41, 42] However, there were variations in the findings; Khan et al. [43] reported almost equal prevalence of NSIs amongst dentists and dental students, while Ikram et al. [38] observed that the majority (42%) of those reporting NSIs were dental house officers. All studies which included dental assistants and technicians showed that they were the group with the lowest rates of NSIs [17, 39, 41], except for one study [26] which reported that 51% of dental technicians had experienced an NSI.

Five studies recorded the number of NSIs experienced by each participant (Table 2). Baig et al. [41] and Gichki et al. [42] recorded that most dental-HCWs who had experienced an NSI experienced just one incident (64%). However, Shahzad et al. [17] and Jan et al. [26] recorded that most dental-HCWs had experienced more than one NSI (67% and 88%, resp.). Furthermore, many participants reported having experienced more than two NSIs [17, 26, 41] with 9% of participants in one study [44] reporting that they experienced more than 10 incidents during their dental career.

10.2. Reporting of NSIs. Only four studies asked participants whether they would report an NSI [17, 26, 38, 41]. Baig et al. [41] recorded the highest underreporting rate (76%); most participants stated that they were unaware of the reporting system. Jan et al. [26] found that 60% of dentists and 92% of dental technicians failed to report injuries. The most common reason for underreporting amongst dentists was the belief that there was no point in reporting incidents (33%), whereas

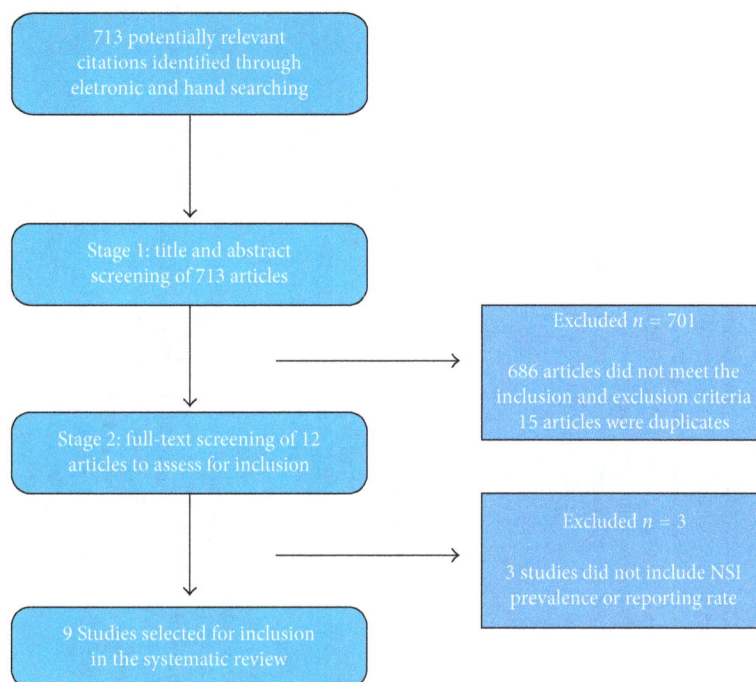

FIGURE 1: Flowchart of search strategy.

amongst dental technicians, it was not knowing where the incident should be reported to, or an unwillingness to report as they were practicing illegally (59%). Shahzad et al. [17] found that 15% of NSIs were not reported, usually because those affected did not know who to report the incident to. Conversely, Malik et al. [39] noted that 28 of the 30 (93%) dental-HCWs who experienced an NSI reported it, thus making it the highest reporting rate observed amongst the included studies.

10.3. Risk Factors for NSIs. A number of different dental procedures appear to put dental-HCWs at risk of sustaining an NSI. NSIs most frequently occurred during needle recapping (33%) [40, 41]. Surgical procedures (28%), drawing blood samples (26%), needle exchange (17%), local anaesthesia administration (9%), and sharps disposal (12%) procedures were also responsible for many NSIs [40, 41]. Jan et al. [26] found that NSIs were most likely to occur during infiltration anaesthesia (43%), followed by general dental procedures (23%) and needle recapping (16%). Malik et al. [39], however, reported that NSIs were most likely to occur whilst disposing of gloves (94%); due to bending needles (92%); or whilst recapping (88%), discarding (69%), separating (64%); or disassembling needles (28%). Meanwhile, Shahzad et al. [17] found that infiltration anaesthesia was responsible for 55% of NSIs and block anaesthesia was responsible for 45%; no other dental procedures were reported to be associated with NSIs.

Only Shahzad et al. [17] investigated which departments had the highest rates of NSIs. The highest prevalence occurred in the oral surgery department (58%), followed by the operative department (18%), while the departments of prosthodontics, orthodontics, and periodontology had the lowest prevalence of NSIs (3% each).

Three studies investigated human factors which may have led to NSIs. Each study reported different factors. Shahzad et al. [17] reported that working hastily was the most common reason for an NSI (42%), followed by fatigue (20%), lack of skill (14%), not wearing gloves (12%), lack of supervision (5%), and the practice of needle resheathing (5%). Baig et al. [41] reported stress as the most common cause of an NSI (43%), followed by work overload (38%), carelessness (8%), and unskilled handling of the instruments (5%), whereas Gichki et al. [42] recorded that negligence among dental-HCWs was the most likely cause of an NSI (20%).

10.4. Hepatitis B Vaccine Coverage. Seven of the reviewed studies calculated HBV vaccine coverage rates among dental-HCWs [17, 26, 38, 40–42, 44]. Rates of vaccine coverage ranged from 46 to 93%. Baig et al. [41] and Ikram et al. [38] reported the highest coverage rates (92% and 93%, resp.). Gichki et al. [42], Ashfaq et al. [40], Mehboob et al. [44], and Shahzad et al. [17] reported vaccine coverage rates of 88%, 87%, 82%, and 68%, respectively. The lowest vaccine coverage rates (57%) were reported by Jan et al. [26]; however, 81% of dentists had received at least one dose of vaccine compared to just 10% of dental technicians.

10.5. Knowledge and Awareness regarding NSIs. Five studies collected information on the awareness of measures to prevent NSIs among dental-HCWs [17, 38–40, 42]. Ikram et al. [38] found that 82% of dental-HCWs had received training regarding the risk of blood-borne infections; 54% felt that training and education were important measures in preventing NSI, and 41% felt that outpatient departments (OPDs) needed to develop specific protocols to protect workers.

TABLE 1: Summary of the included studies.

Serial number	Authors and year of publication	Study location	Research aim and objectives	Study design and time frame	Sample, recruitment method, participant details, characteristics, and response rate	Study outcome measures	Key results	Quality ranking
(1)	Ashfaq et al. (2011) [40]	Lahore Medical and Dental College, Lahore, Pakistan.	To assess the degree of awareness of NSIs among dental health professionals.	Cross-sectional study, questionnaire survey in 2010.	In total, 139 dental health professionals including dental students ($n=55$), graduates ($n=63$), and staff ($n=21$) were sampled (sampling technique was not specified). Participants were of mixed gender: $n=76$ males and $n=63$ females. The response rate was 100%.	Prevalence and frequency of NSI exposures, mechanism of the injury, knowledge of precautionary measures to prevent NSIs, knowledge of first aid management of NSIs, and participant's HBV vaccination status.	In total, 45% ($n=63$) of dental health professionals were exposed to NSIs. NSIs resulted from needle recapping ($n=33$), needle exchange ($n=17$), sharps disposal, ($n=12$) and local anaesthetic administration ($n=9$). A large number of participants were aware of precautionary measures ($n=132$) and first aid management ($n=118$). The HBV vaccine coverage was also high ($n=121$).	Low
(2)	Baig et al. (2014) [41]	Maxillofacial Surgery Department, Liaquat University of Medical and Health Sciences, Jamshoro, Pakistan.	To estimate the risk of NSIs, their frequency, nature, and awareness level of prophylaxis among the students, house officers, and supporting staff of dentistry.	Descriptive cross-sectional study, questionnaire survey from April 2012 to April 2013.	In total, $n=613$ individuals including maxillofacial surgeons (30%, $n=181$), general dentists/supporting staff (3%, $n=21$), house officers (18%, $n=107$) and undergraduate students (49%, $n=298$) were sampled (sampling technique was not stated). The sampled participants were of mixed gender comprising 48% ($n=289$) males and 52% ($n=318$) females. The response rate was 99%.	Prevalence, frequency, and predisposing factors of NSIs, awareness of PEP, and HBV vaccination coverage of dental-HCWs.	A high number of NSIs ($n=776$) were experienced by 60% ($n=363$) of the participants. Of those who experienced an NSI, 40% were students, 38% were dental surgeons, 12% were house officers, and 4% were supporting staff. 64% ($n=233$) of dental-HCWs experienced one NSI, 18% ($n=64$) experienced two NSIs, 12% ($n=42$) experienced three NSIs, and 7% ($n=26$) experienced more than three. NSIs resulted from needle recapping 33% ($n=87$), surgical procedures 28% ($n=73$), or drawing blood samples 26% ($n=69$). The most common reasons behind NSIs among the participants were stress 43% ($n=112$), work overload 38% ($n=99$), carelessness 8% ($n=30$), and unskilled instrument handling 5% ($n=17$). Almost 70% reported NSIs as self-injuries. Overall, almost 76% of NSIs were unreported by dental-HCWs, due to lack of awareness of the reporting system. HBV vaccine coverage was 92%.	Low

TABLE 1: Continued.

Serial number	Authors and year of publication	Study location	Research aim and objectives	Study design and time frame	Sample, recruitment method, participant details, characteristics, and response rate	Study outcome measures	Key results	Quality ranking
(3)	Gichki et al. (2015) [42]	Dental section, Bolan Medical College, Sandeman Provincial Hospital, Quetta, Pakistan.	To assess the knowledge and awareness of NSIs among house officers and dental students.	Observational cross-sectional study, self-administered questionnaire survey. Study period not mentioned.	A total of 100 participants including house officers (29%) and dental students (71%) participated. The age range of the participants was 21–29 years; they were of mixed gender with 44% males and 56% females. The sample recruitment technique as well as the response rate was not mentioned.	Prevalence, frequency, and predisposing factors of NSIs. Knowledge and awareness of the transmission of BBV, availability of vaccines, importance of reporting NSIs, and initiating PEP. Participant's precautionary measures towards NSIs and vaccination status.	A total of 33% of participants experienced an NSI; 21% experienced one NSI and 12% experienced more than one. Good knowledge of the following aspects was reported: NSIs (97%); risk of transmission of BBVs (98%); transmission of pathogens (71%); availability of HBV vaccine (83%); preventing NSIs through needle recapping (69%) and engineering control devices (84%); reporting NSIs (99%); needle recapping technique (61%); and different stages of PEP (60–91%). Knowledge of the risk of HIV transmission through NSIs was the weakest area (13%) and 20% admitted their NSI was due to negligence. 73% of the respondents wore gloves while practicing, 67% avoided the practice of needle recapping, 88% were vaccinated against HBV.	Low
(4)	Ikram et al. (2015) [38]	8 different institutes of Karachi, Pakistan.	To assess the frequency of NSIs and knowledge, attitude, and practice of dental workers towards NSI prevention.	Descriptive cross-sectional study, questionnaire survey from July 2014 to March 2015.	A sample of 800 participants, comprising undergraduates (23%), house officers (25%), faculty (42%), and general dental practitioners (10%), were included. Sampling technique was not stated. The response rate was 100%.	Prevalence of NSIs and the knowledge, attitude, and practices related to NSIs.	In total, 73.1% of participants gave a history of NSI during their dental practice. 92.8% had received HBV vaccine and 73% believed in the effectiveness of the vaccination, whereas only 38.5% believed in the effectiveness of gloves in reducing the occurrence of NSIs. Needle recapping was practiced by 51% of the participants, but 38.3% suggested that it should be avoided, whereas 34.4% and 27.4% suggested careful needle approximation and use of sharps containers, respectively. 70.1% were aware of PEP after an NSI and 82.3% agreed that they were provided with instructions about the risk of infections in their training, but 54.4% suggested the need for training and education, and 40.5% suggested revising protocols in outpatient departments OPDs.	Low

TABLE 1: Continued.

Serial number	Authors and year of publication	Study location	Research aim and objectives	Study design and time frame	Sample, recruitment method, participant details, characteristics, and response rate	Study outcome measures	Key results	Quality ranking
(5)	Jan et al. (2014) [26]	Independent private dental clinics in Hyderabad and Karachi, Pakistan.	To determine the frequency of NSIs among dental-HCWs including dental technicians.	Cross-sectional study, self-administered questionnaire survey during April 2013.	A total of 254 dental-HCWs including qualified dentists ($n = 166$) and dental technicians ($n = 88$) were selected, with no mention of the sampling strategy. The participants were of mixed gender: males ($n = 209$) and females ($n = 45$); from different age groups: 25–35 years old ($n = 50$), 36–45 years old ($n = 73$) and over 45 years old ($n = 131$). The response rate was 92.3%.	Prevalence and frequency of NSIs during the previous year. Reporting rates of NSIs and reasons for underreporting. Also, the knowledge and attitude towards universal precautions.	53% (135) of the 254 participants (qualified dentists and dental technicians) had experienced at least one NSI in the preceding 12 months. Among dentists, 54% experienced at least one NSI; 35% experienced two; and 11% experienced more than two NSIs. Among dental technicians, 51% experienced at least one NSI; 28% experience two; and 21% more than two. Infiltration anaesthesia was the most common procedure causing NSIs (44.4% among dentists and 42% among dental technicians). 59.6% of dentists did not report their NSI; the most common reason given was lack of belief in the reporting system (33.1%), whereas 92% of dental technicians did not report their NSI; the most common reason given was not knowing where to report or did not want to report (59.1%). Dentists (62.6%) had more knowledge about the safety guidelines than dental technicians (8%) and also had a better vaccination coverage (81.3%) than dental technicians (10.2%).	Low
(6)	Khan et al. (2009) [43]	Sardar Begam Dental College, Peshawar, Pakistan.	To evaluate the perception of cross infection in dental practice among dental surgeons and dental students	Descriptive cross-sectional study, survey questionnaire from December 2007 to March 2008.	Total 100 dental-HCWs including 43% dentists (consultants, demonstrators, and house officers) and 57% undergraduate students were sampled through convenience sampling technique. The demographic characteristics and response rate were not mentioned.	Prevalence of NSI, and knowledge and practice of infection control measures.	A total of 35% dental health professionals experienced an NSI during their dental career. The majority of them washed and covered it after allowing it to bleed (85%). Most of the participants also took the patient's medical history (79%) and screened the patient (65%). 65% of dental workers practiced safe disposal, whereas 84% practiced needle resheathing after administering injection, in which one-handed technique was the most common (49%).	Low

TABLE 1: Continued.

Serial number	Authors and year of publication	Study location	Research aim and objectives	Study design and time frame	Sample, recruitment method, participant details, characteristics, and response rate	Study outcome measures	Key results	Quality ranking
(7)	Malik et al. (2012) [39]	Oral surgery department, Dr. Ishrat-ul-Ebad Khan Institute of Oral Health Sciences, Karachi, Pakistan.	Assess knowledge, attitude, and practices relating to NSIs and risk factors among dental practitioners.	Cross-sectional study, survey questionnaire; study period not mentioned.	A total of 100 participants including undergraduates (62%), postgraduates (21%), graduates (13%), and staff (4%) participated, with no identified strategy for sampling. They were of mixed gender: 55% females and 45% males. The majority (85%) were 20–30 years and most (94%) had 1–5 years' experience. The response rate was 100%.	Knowledge, attitude, and practice regarding NSIs, including prevalence and reporting rates.	Of the total 100 participants, 30 experienced an NSI, of which 28 were reported. NSIs were highest among dental students, age group 20–30 years, and practitioners with 1–5 years' experience. The participants were aware of the universal precautions (74%), hepatitis B (98%), hepatitis C, and HIV/AIDS transmission (84%) via NSIs, whereas only 53% were aware of needle-less safety devices. Needle recapping was practiced by 88% and was reported as one of the common reasons for NSIs (88%), along with disposing of gloves (94%). A large number of the participants wore gloves when disposing needles (94%) and manipulating the sharps bin (92%).	Moderate
(8)	Mehboob et al. (2012) [44]	Two teaching hospitals: Khyber College of Dentistry Peshawar, Pakistan, and Ayub Medical College, Abbottabad, Pakistan.	To determine the prevalence and awareness of professional hazards including psychological, musculoskeletal, biological, and allergic problems among dentists.	Cross-sectional study, survey questionnaire- study period not mentioned.	A total of 113 dentists were sampled. The sampling strategy was not specified. The participants included dental graduates (50%) and postgraduate trainees (35%), and the rest were the members or fellows of the college of physicians and surgeons. The majority of the participants (61%) had work experience of less than 5 years. Out of 150, 37 questionnaires were not returned (75% response rate).	The prevalence and frequency of NSIs and the precautions used by dentists during dental treatment.	70% of the participants were exposed to NSIs; 54% experienced less than 5 NSIs; 9.7% experienced 5–10 NSIs; 6.2% had more than 10 NSIs. Only 8.8% of the participants used all precautions during treatment, whereas the majority (85.8%) used a combination of 2 precautions, usually including gloves and masks. 82.3% of participants were vaccinated against HBV.	Low

TABLE 1: Continued.

Serial number	Authors and year of publication	Study location	Research aim and objectives	Study design and time frame	Sample, recruitment method, participant details, characteristics, and response rate	Study outcome measures	Key results	Quality ranking
(9)	Shahzad et al. (2013) [17]	Liaquat Medical University Hospital, Hyderabad, Pakistan.	To identify the risks of NSIs, the participants who sustained them, the circumstances under which they occurred, and how the risk of NSI was minimised among the participants.	Descriptive cross-sectional study, survey questionnaire- from August 2011 to September 2012.	In total, 513 participants including dental students ($n = 325$), house officers ($n = 80$), and paradental staff ($n = 108$), were included in the study. The sampling strategy was not specified. They were of mixed gender: 58% females and 42% males. The response rate was not taken into consideration.	Frequency and reporting rates of NSIs. The type of technique which caused NSIs, the department-wide distribution of NSIs, the different reasons of NSIs, and vaccination status of the participants.	773 total injuries occurred among the participants; 52% were students; 21% were dentists in their first professional year; 10% were paradental staff. 15% of all injuries went unreported. The NSI prevalence was the highest in the oral surgery department (58%), followed by the operative department (18%), and was the lowest in prosthodontics, orthodontics, and periodontology departments (3% each). NSIs most frequently occurred during infiltration anaesthesia (55%), followed by block anaesthesia (44%). The most common reasons for an NSI were hurrying (42%), fatigue (20%), lack of skill (14%), and not wearing gloves (12%). HBV vaccination coverage was 68%.	Low

TABLE 2: Frequency of needlestick injuries amongst dental-HCWs who reported they had experienced at least one NSI.

Study	Number of needlestick injuries				
	1 NSI	>1 NSI	>2 NSIs	<5 NSIs	≥5 NSIs
Baig et al. (2014) [41]	233 (64%)	132 (36%)	68 (19%)	NA	NA
Gichki et al. (2015) [42]	21 (64%)	12 (36%)	NA	NA	NA
Jan et al. (2014)* [26]	16 (12%)	119 (88%)	36 (27%)	NA	NA
Mehboob et al. (2012) [44]	NA	NA	NA	61 (77%)	18 (23%)
Shahzad et al. (2013) [17]	89 (33%)	179 (67%)	121 (45%)	NA	NA

*NSIs were reported in preceding 12 months. NA = not available.

Malik et al. [39] reported good knowledge among dental-HCWs regarding wearing gloves (97%) and universal precautions (74%); however, 88% of participants reported that needles should be recapped or bent needles after use, and only 53% were aware of needle-less safety devices. Ashfaq et al. [40] also found that many dental workers reported they were aware of precautionary measures which could prevent NSIs and transmission of infection (85%). However, Ikram et al. [38] found that only 39% of participants agreed that using surgical gloves would reduce the risk of NSIs, and less than 5% of participants agreed that needles should not be recapped after use. When questioned about strategies to prevent NSIs, only 38% of participants suggested that needles should not be resheathed, 34% suggested that needle approximation should be done carefully, and 27% suggested using sharps containers.

Knowledge and awareness also varied between different groups of dental-HCWs. Jan et al. [26] found 63% of dentists, but only 8% of dental technicians were aware of measures which could be taken to reduce the risk of NSIs, while Gichki et al. [42] found that 76% of house officers and 63% of students were aware needles should not be recapped. Malik et al. [39] found that 98% of dental-HCWs were aware hepatitis B could be transmitted during an NSI, while only 84% were aware HCV and HIV could be transmitted in this way. Similarly, although Gichki et al. [42] reported that 98% of dental-HCWs were aware blood-borne viruses could be transmitted during an NSI, only 13% were aware that HIV could be transmitted during an NSI.

10.6. Dental Practices to Prevent NSIs. Dental practices used to prevent NSIs were also reviewed. One of the main precautions used to prevent an NSI was wearing of gloves; however, there was a wide variation in the proportion of dental-HCWs who reported wearing gloves. Malik et al. [39] found that over 90% of dental-HCWs reported wearing gloves during phlebotomy, while withdrawing a needle from a patient, disposing of the contaminated needle, and when manipulating the sharps bin. Gichki et al. [42] found that 73% of dental-HCWs wore gloves; however, practice varied between students and qualified dental-HCWs (69% of students and 83% of house officers). Similarly, Khan et al. [43] recorded variation in practice between different groups of dental-HCWs (68% of all dental-HCWs wore gloves, 86% of students, and 44% of qualified dentists). Khan et al. [43] also reported that 79% of respondents would change their gloves if

they became dirty during a procedure. Some studies noted that other personal protective equipment was used. Mehboob et al. [44] found that 86% of dental-HCWs used masks and gloves as precautionary measures, but only 9% of dentists used all the recommended universal precautions during dental treatment. Meanwhile, Khan et al. [43] found that 10% of dental-HCWs wore goggles and 90% wore facemasks.

Several studies identified safe disposal of needles as playing an essential role in preventing NSIs. Khan et al. [43] noted that 65% of dental-HCWs reported they disposed of needles safely (60% of qualified dental-HCWs and 68% of students); however, only 16% (23% of qualified dental-HCWs and 11% of students) avoided resheathing needles after injecting local anaesthetic. Similarly, Malik et al. [39] found that only 12% of dental-HCWs avoided recapping needles after use, and approximately a third (36%) avoided separating the needle and syringe before disposal. By contrast, the more recent study by Gichki et al. [40] found that 67% of dental-HCWs did not recap needles after use (63% students and 76% house officers).

11. Discussion

Nine studies were identified which reported data on the prevalence and reporting rates of NSIs amongst dental-HCWs in Pakistan. In each study, the prevalence of NSIs among dental-HCWs in Pakistan was found to be high, ranging from 30% [39] to 73% [38]. The findings were consistent with previous studies from other low- and middle-income countries, including Thailand, Colombia, Saudi Arabia, Iran, Romania, Nigeria, Jordan, and China [13, 22, 45–50]. They also confirmed that dental-HCWs in Pakistan were more likely to experience an NSI than dental-HCWs in developed countries. Only 14% of dentists in Scotland reported that they had experienced an NSI [51], while in UAE, Taiwan, and Australia, approximately 25% of dental-HCWs reported that they had experienced an NSI [10, 52, 53].

From the review, it was evident that many dental-HCWs in Pakistan experience multiple NSIs. Although Baig et al. [41] and Gichki et al. [42] found that most dental-HCWs who had experienced an NSI experienced just one incident (64%), indicating that the incident led to a change in practice; in other studies, many dental-HCWs reported that they had experienced multiple injuries. Consequently, NSIs represent a serious health and safety concern for dental-HCWs. Similarly, other studies conducted in low- and middle-income countries have concluded that over half of dental-HCWs have been exposed to more than one NSI [22, 23, 54]. Furthermore, Jan et al. [26] reported that participants had experienced multiple NSIs in the preceding 12 months, indicating that NSIs remain an ongoing, contemporary risk to dental-HCWs. These findings highlight the need to investigate differences in policies and working practices to identify how rates of NSIs can be effectively reduced in Pakistan and other countries with high rates of injury. Experience appears to be one of a number of factors which play an important role in reducing rates of NSIs. Dental undergraduate students appeared to be more likely to experience an NSI than experienced, qualified dentists. Similarly, the youngest dental-HCWs with the least experience were found to encounter more NSIs than older practitioners with more years of experience [41]. Presumably, this is in part due to a lack of experience when starting clinical practice; however, the heavy clinical load allocated during dental training was also reported to be a reason behind the high rates of NSI among dental students [17]. Dental assistants and technicians reported the lowest rate of NSIs, possibly due to having been in practice longer and having more experience than the other groups of dental-HCWs [17, 39, 41]. However, data from this group were limited, and consequently, it is difficult to draw firm conclusions. These findings were consistent with studies from many other countries, which also reported that dental students were the group most likely to experience an NSI due to their limited experience, skills, and frequent use of sharp instruments [4, 19, 54, 55]. Interestingly, in some settings, experienced or older dental-HCWs were found to be more likely to experience NSIs; in these cases, workload was cited as a key risk factor [52, 56, 57]. Consequently, limited clinical skills, knowledge and experience, and workload all appear to increase the risk of NSIs for dental-HCWs. The evidence highlights the need to review the clinical workload of all dental-HCWs, to prevent work overload, stress, and fatigue, as well as the provision of adequate training and mentoring to reduce the risk of NSIs.

However, data on NSI prevalence are limited in Pakistan, and more robust surveillance data would help to support effective policy development. These studies confirmed that although most NSIs are officially reported in some settings [39, 42], underreporting of NSIs is an ongoing problem in Pakistan with over 75% of NSIs not being reported in some settings [41]. The problem appears to stem from many dental-HCWs being unaware of the reporting system and failing to understand the importance of reporting incidents [17, 41]. Furthermore, some groups of dental-HCWs, such as dental technicians, appear to be particularly reluctant to report NSIs [26]. Poor surveillance of NSIs appears to be a widespread issue. Reporting rates in Pakistan were broadly in-line with rates in other low- and middle-income nations. Studies have shown that more than half of dental-HCWs failed to report their NSIs in Saudi Arabia, Kenya, and India [22, 23, 57] and more than three-quarters of dental-HCWs failed to report NSIs in China, North Jordan, and Iran [22, 23, 57]. Furthermore, in Nigeria, a study from one dental setting found that none of the dental students reported NSIs [27]. Similarly, reasons for underreporting of NSIs included fear of the consequences of infection, stigmatisation and blame, lack of awareness of the need to report

NSIs, and not knowing how or where to report an NSI [23, 24, 27]. These findings highlight a widespread lack of awareness regarding reporting NSIs and indicate the need for further training and guidance to improve reporting rates and strengthen reporting systems.

The included studies also provided insight into which working practices were most likely to result in an NSI. The results revealed that needle recapping or resheathing was the procedure responsible for the greatest number of NSIs [40, 41]. Furthermore, bending a needle prior to disposing it also appeared to be a risk-prone procedure [39]. Similar findings have been reported from other low- and middle-income countries including Iran, India, and China [28, 49, 57]. Despite WHO [50] recommendations that all HCWs should avoid recapping needles or bending, breaking, or manually removing needles before disposal, the majority of dentists in some settings still report resheathing needles [38, 43]. Consequently, to effectively reduce the risk of NSIs, it is essential that working policies and practices are updated to encompass the latest best practice. However, even if policies and protocols are based on best practice guidance, many factors will affect rates of compliance. An individual's practice can be determined by the behavioural theory of health-belief model [58]. Analysis showed that in some settings, a high proportion of dental-HCWs was aware of good practice, such as wearing gloves, safe needle practice, and improved engineering-controlled devices [39, 40, 42–44], whereas it was found to be low in other settings [38]. Likewise, perception of the risk of transmission of infection was found to vary considerably between settings [39, 42], as were hepatitis B vaccine coverage rates [17, 26, 38, 40–42, 44] and understanding of PEP [38, 41, 42]. Consequently, practice and perceived susceptibility which potentially influences decisions to observe precautions was found to be variable between settings. The high prevalence of NSIs, particularly among dental students, indicates a crucial need for dental-HCWs to understand the risk of NSI-associated infections, in order for them to appreciate the importance of complying with the universal precautions and other safe working procedures. Thus, it is essential that education on NSI risks and prevention strategies is included early in the dental course curriculum and repeated regularly as part of ongoing continual professional development (CPD).

The review also highlighted that hepatitis B vaccine coverage was extremely variable both between settings and different groups of dental-HCWs. Therefore, measures should be put in place to ensure that all dental-HCWs have access to affordable hepatitis B immunisation and good coverage rates are achieved amongst all groups of dental professionals. However, since there are no effective vaccines available to protect against HCV and HIV infection, and their treatment is neither affordable nor available in many countries, it is essential that dental-HCWs continue to be aware of the importance of developing good practice to avoid NSIs.

To the best of the authors' knowledge, this is the first systematic review of its kind to highlight the issue of NSIs in dental-HCWs in Pakistan. In absence of the routine collection of accurate data on NSIs, small studies have been useful in highlighting which groups of dental-HCWs are most at risk from NSIs. A major limitation of this systematic review was the low quality of the reviewed studies, thus raising serious quality concerns for the review, which impacts the reliability, credibility, and applicability of the overall results, and consequently the drawn conclusion and recommendations of the review [36]. However, the quality assessment outcome recommends the need for further good-quality studies with robust methodology to increase the transparency, validity, and generalisation of the research outcomes and also highlights gaps in the present literature. Despite these limitations, it can be concluded that a high prevalence of NSIs and low rates of reporting, as well as a lack of awareness of the risks of NSIs, persist in many settings within Pakistan.

12. Conclusion

Reviews of the selected studies suggest that the prevalence of NSIs among dental-HCWs in Pakistan is high while reporting rates are low, suggesting the urgent need to develop educational programmes for all dental-HCWs on the importance of preventing and reporting NSIs. It also indicates the necessity for all dental-HCWs to be able to access a proper occupational health department in all dental settings, to prevent, manage, record, and monitor occupational injuries. There is an urgent need for the development of national guidance protocols to prevent NSIs in Pakistan. Improving health literacy around the risks of NSIs should be accompanied by improving measures to report NSIs. These should incorporate examples of good practice from countries where rates of NSIs have successfully been reduced. However, it is important to note that recommendations for new interventions should take an ecological approach and should be cost-effective for the dental settings since this is crucial for their successful and sustainable application.

References

[1] World Health Organization–WHO, "Occupational health, needlestick injuries," 2016, http://www.who.int/occupational_health/topics/needinjuries/en/.

[2] National Health Services–NHS, "What should I do if I injure myself with a used needle?," 2015, http://www.nhs.uk/chq/Pages/2557.aspx?CategoryID=72.

[3] A. Smith, S. Cameron, J. Bagg, and D. Kennedy, "Management of needlestick injuries in general dental practice," British Dental Journal, vol. 19, no. 12, pp. 645–650, 2001.

[4] M. Gatto, L. Bandini, M. Montevecchi, and L. Checchi, "Occupational exposure to blood and body fluids in a department of oral sciences: results of a thirteen-year surveillance study," The Scientific World Journal, vol. 2013, Article ID 459281, 7 pages, 2013.

[5] Canadian Centre for Occupational Health and Safety–CCOHS, "Needlestick and sharps injuries," 2015, http://www.ccohs.ca/oshanswers/diseases/needlestick_injuries.html.

[6] S. H. Naghavi, O. Shabestari, and J. Alcolado, "Post-traumatic stress disorder in trainee doctors with previous needlestick injuries," Occupational Medicine, vol. 63, no. 4, pp. 260–265, 2013.

[7] J. Ayatollahi, F. Ayatollahi, A. Ardekani et al., "Occupational hazards to dental staff," Dental Research Journal, vol. 9, no. 1, pp. 2–7, 2012.

[8] Centres for Disease Control and Prevention–CDC, "Infection control," 2013, http://www.cdc.gov/oralhealth/infectioncontrol/faq/bloodborne_exposures.html.

[9] H. Rashid, "Needle stick injuries in restorative dentistry: the need for prevention," Journal of Restorative Dentistry, vol. 2, no. 3, p. 157, 2014.

[10] M. Jaber, "A survey of needle sticks and other sharp injuries among dental undergraduate students," International Journal of Infection Control, vol. 7, no. 3, pp. 1–10, 2011.

[11] R. Sharma, S. Rasania, A. Verma, and S. Singh, "Study of prevalence and response to needle stick injuries among health care workers in a Tertiary Care Hospital in Delhi, India," Indian Journal of Community Medicine, vol. 35, no. 1, pp. 74–77, 2010.

[12] S. Alavian and N. Mahboobi, "Hepatitis B infection in dentistry setting needs more attention," Medical Principles and Practice, vol. 20, no. 5, pp. 491-492, 2011.

[13] C. Azodo, O. Ehigiator, and M. Ojo, "Occupational risks and hepatitis B vaccination status of dental auxiliaries in Nigeria," Medical Principles and Practice, vol. 19, no. 5, pp. 364–366, 2010.

[14] V. Singhal, D. Bora, and S. Singh, "Hepatitis B in healthcare workers: Indian scenario," Journal of Laboratory Physicians, vol. 1, no. 2, pp. 41–48, 2009.

[15] W. Kohn, A. Collins, J. Cleveland, J. Harte, K. Eklund, and D. Malvitz, "Guidelines for infection control in dental health-care settings," Morbidity and Mortality Weekly Report-MMWR, vol. 52, no. 17, pp. 1–61, 2003.

[16] D. Kotelchuck, D. Murphy, and F. Younai, "Impact of underreporting on the management of occupational blood-borne exposures in a dental teaching environment," Journal of Dental Education, vol. 68, no. 6, pp. 614–622, 2004.

[17] M. Shahzad, S. Hassan, M. Memon, U. Bashir, and S. Shams, "Needle stick injuries among dental students, house officers and paradental staff working at Liaquat Medical University Hospital, Hyderabad," Pakistan Oral and Dental Journal, vol. 33, no. 1, pp. 23–25, 2013.

[18] F. Younai, D. Murphy, and D. Kotelchuck, "Occupational exposures to blood in a dental teaching environment: results of a ten-year surveillance study," Journal of Dental Education, vol. 65, no. 5, pp. 436–448, 2001.

[19] S. Ebrahimi, N. Shadman, and I. Ghaempanah, "Needlestick injuries in dentists and their assistants in Kerman, Iran: prevalence, knowledge, and practice," Journal of Oral Health and Oral Epidemiology, vol. 2, no. 1, pp. 23–27, 2013.

[20] M. Sawyer, Preventing Needle-Stick Injuries and the Use of Dental Safety Syringes, Work Safe BC-Workers Compensation Board of British Columbia, Richmond, BC, Canada, 2010.

[21] R. Gambhi and V. Kapoor, "Knowledge, awareness and practice regarding needle stick injuries in dental profession in India," International Journal of Preventive Medicine, vol. 6, p. 55, 2015.

[22] Y. Khader, S. Burgan, and Z. Amarin, "Self-reported needle stick injuries among dentists in North Jordan," East Mediterranean Health Journal, vol. 15, no. 1, pp. 185–189, 2009.

[23] M. Askarian and L. Malekmakan, "The prevalence of needle stick injuries in medical, dental, nursing and midwifery students at the university teaching hospitals of Shiraz, Iran," Indian Journal of Medical Sciences, vol. 60, no. 6, pp. 227–232, 2006.

[24] M. Hashemipour and A. Sadeghi, "Needlestick injuries among medical and dental students at the University of Kerman. A questionnaire study," *Journal of dentistry*, vol. 5, no. 2, pp. 71–76, 2007.

[25] H. Qureshi, K. M. Bile, R. Jooma, S. E. Alam, and H. U. Afridi, "Prevalence of hepatitis B and C viral infections in Pakistan: findings of a national survey," *East Mediterranean Health Journal*, vol. 16, no. 15–23, 2010.

[26] S. Jan, T. Akhund, M. Akhtar, and J. Shaikh, "Needle stick injuries among dental health care providers: a survey done at Hyderabad and Karachi," *Pakistan Oral and Dental Journal*, vol. 34, no. 2, pp. 339–343, 2014.

[27] O. Sofola, M. Folayan, O. Denloye, and S. Okeigbemen, "Occupational exposure to bloodborne pathogens and management of exposure incidents in Nigerian Dental Schools," *Journal of Dental Education*, vol. 71, no. 6, pp. 832–837, 2007.

[28] V. K. Pavithran, R. Murali, M. Krishna, A. Shamala, M. Yalamalli, and A. Kumar, "Knowledge, attitude, and practice of needle stick and sharps injuries among dental professionals of Bangalore, India," *Journal of International Society of preventive and Community Dentistry*, vol. 5, no. 5, pp. 406–412, 2015.

[29] "STROBE Statement, STROBE checklists, checklist for case-control studies," 2009, http://www.strobe-statement.org/index.php?id=available-checklists.

[30] M. Boyle, "Guidelines for evaluating prevalence studies," *Evidence Based Mental Health*, vol. 1, no. 2, pp. 37–39, 1998.

[31] L. Barreto, F. Oliveira, S. Nunes et al., "Epidemiologic study of charcot-marie-tooth disease: a systematic review," *Neuro-Epidemiology*, vol. 46, no. 3, pp. 157–165, 2016.

[32] M. Etemadifar, Z. Nasr, B. Khalili, M. Taherioun, and R. Vosoughi, "Epidemiology of neuromyelitis optica in the world: a systematic review and meta-analysis," *Multiple Sclerosis International*, vol. 2015, Article ID 174720, 8 pages, 2015.

[33] J. Popay, H. Roberts, A. Sowden et al., *Guidance on the Conduct of Narrative Synthesis in Systematic Reviews*, Lancaster University, Lancaster, UK, 2006.

[34] R. Ryan, *Cochrane Consumers and Communication Review Group: Data Synthesis and Analysis*, 2013, http://cccrg.cochrane.org/sites/cccrg.cochrane.org/files/uploads/AnalysisRestyled.pdf.

[35] T. Brugha, R. Matthews, Z. Morgan, T. Hill, J. Alonso, and D. Jones, "Methodology and reporting of systematic reviews and meta-analyses of observational studies in psychiatric epidemiology: systematic review," *British Journal of Psychiatry*, vol. 200, no. 6, pp. 446–453, 2012.

[36] A. Boland, G. Cherry, and R. Dickson, *Doing a Systematic Review: a Student's Guide*, SAGE Publications Ltd., London, UK, 2014.

[37] J. Higgins, S. Thompson, J. Deeks, and D. Altman, "Measuring inconsistencies in meta-analysis," *British Medical Journal*, vol. 327, no. 7414, pp. 557–560, 2003.

[38] K. Ikram, H. Siddiqui, S. Maqbool, M. Altaf, and S. Khan, "Frequency of needle stick injury among dental students and dentists in Karachi," *World Journal of Dentistry*, vol. 6, no. 4, pp. 213–216, 2015.

[39] A. Malik, M. Shaukat, and A. Qureshi, "Needle-stick injury: a rising bio-hazard," *Journal of Ayub Medical College Abbottabad*, vol. 24, no. 3-4, pp. 144–146, 2012.

[40] M. Ashfaq, M. Chatha, and A. Sohail, "Awareness of needlestick injuries among the dental health professionals at Lahore Medical and Dental College," *Pakistan Oral and Dental Journal*, vol. 31, no. 2, pp. 255–257, 2011.

[41] M. Baig, S. Baloch, and M. Muslim, "Estimation of risk of needle stick injury and the level of awareness of prophylaxis among the students, house officers and supporting staff of dentistry," *New York Science Journal*, vol. 7, no. 1, pp. 120–123, 2014.

[42] A. Gichki, A. Islam, and W. Murad, "Knowledge and awareness about needle stick injuries among dental students of Bolan Medical College, Quetta," *Pakistan Oral and Dental Journal*, vol. 35, no. 4, pp. 562–566, 2015.

[43] A. Khan, A. Rahim, T. Bangash, M. Chugtai, and Z. Mehboob, "Infection control in dentistry knowledge and practice regarding barrier techniques, post exposure management and prophylaxis–a study," *Pakistan Oral and Dental Journal*, vol. 29, no. 2, pp. 235–240, 2009.

[44] B. Mehboob, M. Khan, A. Fahim-ud-din Khan, and F. Qiam, "Professional hazards among dentists of the two public sector teaching hospitals of Khyber Pakhtunkhwa province of Pakistan," *Pakistan Oral and Dental Journal*, vol. 32, no. 3, pp. 376–380, 2012.

[45] S. Ansari, M. Aldaijy, A. Almijlad et al., "Determining the prevalence and awareness of needlestick injuries among dental health professionals in Riyadh, Saudi Arabia," *International Journal of Current Research*, vol. 7, no. 1, pp. 12102–12105, 2015.

[46] K. Arrieta-Vergara, S. Diaz-Cárdenas, and F. González-Martínez, "Prevalence of occupational accidents and related factors in students of dentistry," *Revista de Salud Publica*, vol. 15, no. 1, pp. 23–31, 2013.

[47] L. Barlean, I. Danila, I. Saveanu, and C. Balcos, "Occupational health problems among dentists in Moldavian Region of Romania," *Revista medico-chirurgicala a Societatii de Medici si Naturalisti din Iasi*, vol. 117, no. 3, pp. 784–788, 2013.

[48] S. Chowanadisai, B. Kukiattrakoon, B. Yapong, and P. Leggat, "Occupational health problems of dentists in Southern Thailand," *International Dental Journal*, vol. 50, no. 1, pp. 36–40, 2000.

[49] S. Shaghagian, A. Golkari, S. Pardis, and A. Rezayi, "Occupational exposure of Shiraz Dental Students to patients' blood and body fluid," *Journal of Dentistry Shiraz University of Medical Sciences*, vol. 16, no. 3, pp. 206–213, 2015.

[50] World Health Organization–WHO, *Best Practices for Injections and Related Procedures Toolkit*, WHO press, Geneva, Switzerland, 2010, http://apps.who.int/iris/bitstream/10665/44298/1/9789241599252_eng.pdf.

[51] P. Leavy, A. Templeton, L. Young, and C. McDonnell, "Reporting of occupational exposures to blood and body fluids in the primary dental care setting in Scotland: an evaluation of current practice and attitudes," *British Dental Journal*, vol. 217, no. 4, p. E7, 2014.

[52] H. Cheng, C. Su, A. Yen, and C. Huang, "Factors affecting occupational exposure to needlestick and sharps injuries among Dentists in Taiwan: a nationwide survey," *PLoS One*, vol. 7, no. 4, article e34911, 2012.

[53] P. Leggat and D. Smith, "Prevalence of percutaneous exposure incidents amongst dentists in Queensland," *Australian Dental Journal*, vol. 51, no. 2, pp. 158–161, 2008.

[54] S. Bindra, K. Reddy, A. Chakrabarty, and K. Chaudhary, "Awareness about needle stick injures and sharps disposal: a study conducted at Army College of Dental Sciences," *Journal of Maxillofacial and Oral Surgery*, vol. 13, no. 4, pp. 419–424, 2014.

[55] Y. Guruprasad and D. Chauhan, "Knowledge, attitude and practice regarding risk of HIV infection through accidental needlestick injuries among dental students of Raichur, India," *National Journal of Maxillofacial Surgery*, vol. 2, no. 2, pp. 152–155, 2011.

31

Early Childhood Caries: Epidemiology, Aetiology, and Prevention

F. Meyer ⓘ and J. Enax

Research Department, Dr. Kurt Wolff GmbH & Co. KG, Bielefeld, Germany

Correspondence should be addressed to F. Meyer; frederic.meyer@drwolffgroup.com

Academic Editor: Ali I. Abdalla

Early childhood caries (ECC) is one of the most prevalent diseases in children worldwide. ECC is driven by a dysbiotic state of oral microorganisms mainly caused by a sugar-rich diet. Additionally, poor oral hygiene or insufficient dental plaque removal leads to the rapid progression of ECC. ECC leads not only to dental destruction and pain with children, but also affects the quality of life of the caregivers. Children with extensive ECC are at high risk to develop caries with the permanent dentition or will have other problems with speaking and/or eating. To prevent ECC, several strategies should be taken into account. Children should brush their teeth with toothpastes containing gentle ingredients, such as mild surfactants and agents showing antiadherent properties regarding oral microorganisms. Parents/caregivers have to help their children with brushing the teeth. Furthermore, remineralizing and nontoxic agents should be included into the toothpaste formulation. Two promising biomimetic agents for children's oral care are amorphous calcium phosphate $[Ca_x(PO_4)_y\, n\, H_2O]$ and hydroxyapatite $[Ca_5(PO_4)_3(OH)]$.

1. Introduction

Early childhood caries (ECC) is still one of the most prevalent diseases in children worldwide. ECC does not only affect children's oral health, but also the general health of children [1, 2]. Not only oral pain, orthodontic problems, and enamel defects, but also problems with eating and speaking can occur as well as an increased risk for caries development in the permanent dentition [3]. Premature loss of primary dentition often leads to orthodontic problems in adult life [4]. Not only children are affected, but also parents will be influenced by this disease being the responsible caregivers [3, 4]. For example, dental problems were shown to be the main reasons for hospitalisation of children in Australia in 2015 [5]. Thus, ECC leads not only to temporary pain, but more importantly has major effects on the quality of life of the family/caregivers including financial and health implications [6, 7]. The aim of this review article is to present the state of the art of the epidemiology, aetiology, characteristics of primary dentition, risk factors, general recommendations, and strategies for prevention of ECC.

2. Background and Epidemiology

As stated before, ECC is still one of the most abundant diseases worldwide. The incidence of ECC among children with deciduous teeth is 1.76 billion (95% CI: 1.26 billion; 2.39 billion) [8]. Interestingly, ECC is not limited to children with a low socioeconomic status (SES) [9, 10]. Recent data, for example, from Australia show a prevalence of more than 50% of 6-year-old children with caries on deciduous teeth [5]. Data from different parts of the world show up to 89.2% of children with ECC in Qatar and 36% in Greece [11, 12]. About the same prevalence (ca. 40%) has been reported in the USA among 2–11 year old children [13]. A recently published study from Germany shows even 10% (up to 26% with initial lesions) of 3-year-old children with ECC and an increase up to about 50% in 6-/7-year-old children [14]. Even though the dmft-index (decayed missing filled teeth) has decreased over time in general [10, 14], the prevalence has not decreased [14]. However, a study from Germany was also able to show different trajectories and an increase of dmft-values when looking at a smaller scale on a regional level [10]. While most of the districts in a midsized German city showed a decrease of dmft, the dmft increased in other districts over time [10]. Milsom et al. described that children with an already existing caries lesion have a 5–6 times higher incidence of developing new caries lesions compared to previously caries-free children [15]. Sleeping problems and insufficient sleep can also be identified as risk factor for ECC, as sleeping problems lead to a more frequent use of night-time bottle use with sugar-sweetened beverages [16–18]. As the role of parents is still unclear with respect to their children developing ECC, several studies have focussed on different associations [19]. Sociocultural and socioeconomic backgrounds of the parents can be found as risk factors for ECC, but parental stress does not show a significant increase in ECC with the children [10, 19, 20]. Not only children, but also their parents should be motivated to take care of the primary dentition to prevent ECC and consequently further caries development in the secondary dentition [21].

3. Aetiology of ECC

Dental caries develops when the dental plaque, a polymicrobial biofilm, is not removed regularly and the diet consists of mainly monosaccharides. Monosaccharides can be metabolized by many of the oral bacteria leading to an increased production of acids which are able to demineralize the enamel [22, 23]. Dental plaque is built on top of the pellicle starting directly after mechanical removal of the biofilm [24, 25]. More than 700 bacterial species/taxa are known in the oral flora [26]. Because the oral habitat consists of many different ecological niches, the relatively high number of different species/taxa can be explained [27]. Oral microorganisms are able to interact with each other and mainly communicate using so-called "quorum sensing" (QS) [28]. Nowadays, it is well known that not only bacteria, but also fungi, such as Candida albicans and the inter-kingdom interactions, can enhance the progression of caries [29, 30]. However, microorganisms grown in polyspecies biofilms are able to produce exopolysaccharides (EPS), also known as extracellular polymeric substances [31, 32]. With the help of the EPS, microorganisms are able to resist antimicrobials that are recently used in toothpastes [32]. Consequently, biofilm formation is not interrupted and together with the absorbed saccharides from the diet leads to a cariogenic dental plaque [33]. The dental plaque on clinically sound enamel of children consists mainly of streptococci and actinomycetes [34]. With a low-sugar diet, these microorganisms are living as commensals in a homeostatic environment controlling each other [35]. As soon as sugars, especially sugary food and beverages, are consumed, the commensal plaque microbiota will absorb these saccharides and metabolize them into acids, mainly lactic acid [36]. This acid production leads to a pH shift from around 7 (neutral) to a pH < 5.5 (acidic) [37]. Acid-tolerant bacteria, mainly mutans streptococci, are able to survive these acidic environments [36]. When oral hygiene habits and nutritional habits do not change, a reduction of highly cariogenic microorganisms (mutans streptococci, Candida spp., and lactobacilli) cannot be achieved [38]. Peterson et al. used next-generation sequencing (NGS) to identify the microbial composition of the dental plaque. They show only slight differences between the biofilms collected from children with and without caries [39]: Streptococcus mitis and Streptococcus sanguinis were found in both groups. Streptococcus was found to be the most abundant genus (>50% of the microorganisms). Veillonella, Granulicatella, Fusobacterium, Neisseria, Campylobacter, Gemella, Abiotrophia, Selenomonas, and Capnocytophaga were also found in abundance between 1 and 10% of the biofilm [39]. Simon-Soro et al. also detected Lactobacillus-species, known as acid-resistant bacteria, associated with caries [40, 41]. Even though the studies described above used NGS strategies, this technique is rapidly developing and recent studies are able to use even more sophisticated models predicting ECC [42]. Teng et al. used in vivo samples from a 3-year cohort study and showed, with the help of mathematical modelling, that S. mutans were not the main trigger for caries, but identified Veillonella spp. and Prevotella spp. instead [43]. Veillonella atypical, V. dispar, and V. parvula as well as Prevotella spp. were identified as bacteria that are mainly responsible for the development of ECC [43].

In conclusion, ECC develops as soon as the dental plaque is not removed adequately and a sugary diet, especially sweetened food and beverages, is consumed. This leads to a changing metabolism with the dental plaque microbiota producing mainly lactic acids that will demineralize the enamel. Prevotella spp. and Veillonella spp. were shown to be microbial risk factors, while together with fungi, bacteria can trigger acid metabolisms and virulence of the microorganisms [29,30,41–43].

4. Characteristics of Deciduous Enamel and Enamel of Permanent Teeth

Enamel is the hardest tissue in the human body. It mainly consists of hydroxyapatite (97%) (HAP), $Ca_5(PO_4)_3(OH)$, which is a calcium phosphate mineral [44–49]. Enamel is highly mineralized and has extraordinary mechanical properties [44, 45, 47, 50, 51]. The interior of a tooth consists of dentin (about 70% HAP and 20% proteins mainly collagen and 10% water), produced by odontoblasts, and the enamel, that is built by ameloblasts. Ameloblasts are restricted to produce enamel one time: ameloblasts produce several proteins and attract calcium and phosphate ions to crystallize these [52, 53]. The enamel of deciduous teeth is built within a significantly shorter period (24 months) than permanent teeth (up to 16 years) [52]. The consequence of the shorter time for enamel development is the formation of a very thin enamel (half the thickness than that of the permanent teeth) and a less organized microstructure [54, 55]. As consequence, acids are able to demineralize deciduous enamel faster than permanent enamel [56–58].

5. Risk Factors

ECC is known to be a multifactorial disease. Sugary food and beverages can lead to a dysbiotic state of the microbial composition causing caries. As ECC is also known as "baby bottle caries," feeding practices are noticed as main risk

TABLE 1: Main ingredients for children's toothpastes (up to 6 years).

Ingredient	Function/comments	References
Silica- or calcium carbonate-based abrasives with low RDA value (RDA: radioactive dentin abrasion)	Plaque removal, gentle cleaning of deciduous teeth	[94]
Hydroxyapatite, ACP-CPP, fluorides in low concentrations	Remineralization	[45, 88]
Hydroxyapatite	Reduction of bacterial adhesion to enamel surfaces due to antiadhesive properties	[82, 84]
Surfactants	Foaming action, due to irritant properties, children's toothpaste should not contain any sodium lauryl sulfate (SLS)	[69]
Preservatives/antimicrobial agents	Due to risk of swallowing, children's toothpaste should not contain any potent antimicrobial agents such as chlorhexidine or triclosan, but mild preservatives (e.g., alkanediols or xylitol as antimicrobial agent)	[69, 95]

factor developing ECC [9, 59, 60]. Here, the upper incisors and molars are affected at first, followed by the molars of the lower jaw and finally the lower jaw incisors [61]. Children sleeping with bottles filled with sweetened tea or milk containing several cariogenic sugars are at high risk for developing ECC. As a consequence of drinking during night time, without clearance of sugars, the oral bacteria will produce lactic acid rapidly, demineralizing the enamel [9, 62]. Nowadays, not only baby bottles, but also several other sweetened juices consumed throughout the day or even at night will enhance the risk to develop caries. ECC is a disease affecting both low-SES families and high-SES families [9, 10]. However, unemployment and migration background can be found as risk factors for spatial disparities in ECC [10]. Other important factors that increase the risk to develop ECC are irregular toothbrushing (mechanical plaque removal) and/or toothbrushing without supervision by any caregivers [63]. Therefore, supervised thorough tooth brushing twice a day should be applied [64].

6. General Recommendations

The primary dentition usually erupts 6 to 8 months after birth [65]. As the oral cavity is highly sensitive, soft touches of the oral mucosa and gingiva should be performed in the early infant life to get the infants used to tooth brushing. Tooth brushing of at least two to three minutes should be performed two times a day by the caregivers as soon as the first tooth erupts [65]. Most dentists recommend to use a "pea-size" amount of a fluoride toothpaste for children, which contain usually not more than 500 ppm fluoride [66]. Additionally, fluoride gels could be used [67]. However, adverse effects like fluorosis need to include assessment of potential adverse effects [67].

7. Biomimetic Concepts and Tooth Brushing to Prevent ECC

It is well known that fluorides and especially fluoridated toothpastes may have a beneficial effect inhibiting caries progression [68]. However, an average caries reduction of 23% compared to a placebo can only be detected using toothpastes containing a minimum of 1000 ppm (0.1%) fluoride. In Europe as well as other parts of the world, toothpastes for children should contain a maximum of 500 ppm (0.05%) fluoride [66, 69]. Toothpastes with more than 1000 ppm fluoride to 1500 ppm fluoride have to be labelled in the EU as "Children of 6 years and younger: Use a pea sized amount for supervised brushing to minimize swallowing. In the case of fluoride intake from other sources consult a dentist or doctor" [70]. Other countries have similar restrictions and warnings. The reason is an enhanced risk for dental fluorosis and skeletal fluorosis due to the accumulation of fluoride from different sources and swallowing the fluoridated toothpaste [66]. Additionally, it is discussed whether fluorides interact with ameloblasts and have negative impact on the enamel formation [53, 71]. Fluorides are mainly functioning due to topical application by enhancing remineralization with calcium and phosphate ions derived from saliva [72]. Consequently, intake of fluoride tablets and fluoridated salts are discussed whether to be effective in caries protection or not [66]. In the past, it was assumed that fluorides lead to the formation of fluoroapatite $[Ca_5(PO_4)_3F]$. This mechanism was thought to make teeth more resistant to acids and protect the enamel. However, only small amounts of fluorapatite can be detected [50,73–75]. Interestingly, fluorotic teeth with higher concentration of fluoride are even less resistant to acids than sound enamel [75–77].

Alternatives to prevent caries and especially ECC in children need to be based on biomimetic strategies. Several products based on different calcium phosphates are already on the market and well studied [78]. Besides others, hydroxyapatite (HAP) $[Ca_5(PO_4)_3(OH)]$ and amorphous calcium phosphates $[Ca_x(PO_4)_y \cdot n\ H_2O]$ stabilized by casein proteins (CPP-ACP) show the most promising results. HAP was identified to be very effective in preventing ECC within a cohort of Japanese children following a 3-year study which showed a reduction of new caries lesions of up to 56% [69, 79]. A recently published randomized, double-blind clinical study shows that microcrystalline HAP is not inferior to fluorides in clinical caries prevention [80]. Besides remineralizing properties that are equal to sodium fluoride [81], HAP-microclusters were shown to reduce dental plaque formation *in situ* and *in vivo* [82–86]. Lelli et al. were able to observe a protective layer on the top of enamel after using HAP-toothpaste *in vivo* [87]. Similar results can be found when using CPP-ACP. This calcium phosphate is also able to remineralize initial enamel lesions equivalent to fluorides [88]. Different studies showed that early lesions can also be remineralized and regressed using CPP-ACP [89] and regarding remineralization identified CPP-ACP to even be superior to a high fluoride containing product (5000 ppm fluoride) [90]. However, others studies have shown contrary results [91, 92].

Besides remineralizing ingredients, toothpastes should have biofilm controlling properties that do not affect children's health [93] (Table 1).

The use of an appropriate toothpaste should be accompanied by twice daily supervised/supported tooth brushing as well as regular visits to the dentist (at least once a year) [96]. With respect to the motor abilities of very young children, brushing should be carried out using electric brushes or manual toothbrushes especially made for children under parental supervision [97]. Even though there are several brushing techniques known, for younger children, the horizontal brushing technique is recommended combined with a 3-minute brushing period [98]. Paediatricians should also check both the oral health and fluoride anamnese of the children while also asking the parents about the child's oral hygiene. Toothbrushes should be replaced every 3 months or when the bristles become frayed with use [99].

8. Conclusion

In additionally to a low sugary diet, children should brush their teeth twice a day under parental supervision and be supported with brushing. The caregivers should especially support very young children (under the age of 3) continuously. Toothpastes should mainly comprise promising remineralizing agents for children's oral care such as calcium phosphates like CPP-ACP or HAP.

Acknowledgments

The authors would like to thank Dr. Barbara Simader, a dentist, for the helpful discussions.

References

[1] R. Naidu, J. Nunn, and E. Donnelly-Swift, "Oral health-related quality of life and early childhood caries among preschool children in Trinidad," *BMC Oral Health*, vol. 16, no. 1, p. 128, 2016.

[2] S. L. Filstrup, D. Briskie, M. da Fonseca, L. Lawrence, A. Wandera, and M. R. Inglehart, "Early childhood caries and quality of life: child and parent perspectives," *Pediatric Dentistry*, vol. 25, no. 5, pp. 431–440, 2003.

[3] J. Abanto, T. S. Carvalho, F. M. Mendes, M. T. Wanderley, M. Bonecker, and D. P. Raggio, "Impact of oral diseases and disorders on oral health-related quality of life of preschool children," *Community Dentistry and Oral Epidemiology*, vol. 39, no. 2, pp. 105–114, 2011.

[4] P. S. Casamassimo, S. Thikkurissy, B. L. Edelstein, and E. Maiorini, "Beyond the dmft: the human and economic cost of early childhood caries," *Journal of the American Dental Association*, vol. 140, no. 6, pp. 650–657, 2009.

[5] S. Chrisopoulos and J. E. Harford, *Oral Health and Dental Care in Australia: Key Facts and Figures 2015*, Australian Institute of Health and Welfare and the University of Adelaide, Canberra, ACT, Australia, 2016.

[6] A. J. Righolt, M. Jevdjevic, W. Marcenes, and S. Listl, "Global-, regional-, and country-level economic impacts of dental diseases in 2015," *Journal of Dental Research*, vol. 97, no. 5, pp. 501–507, 2018.

[7] A. BaniHani, C. Deery, J. Toumba, T. Munyombwe, and M. Duggal, "The impact of dental caries and its treatment by conventional or biological approaches on the oral health-related quality of life of children and carers," *International Journal of Paediatric Dentistry*, vol. 28, no. 2, pp. 266–276, 2017.

[8] T. Vos, A. A. Abajobir, K. H. Abate et al., "Global, regional, and national incidence, prevalence, and years lived with disability for 328 diseases and injuries for 195 countries, 1990–2016: a systematic analysis for the Global Burden of Disease Study," *The Lancet*, vol. 390, no. 10100, pp. 1211–1259, 2016.

[9] H. Colak, C. T. Dulgergil, M. Dalli, and M. M. Hamidi, "Early childhood caries update: a review of causes, diagnoses, and treatments," *Journal of Natural Science, Biology, and Medicine*, vol. 4, no. 1, pp. 29–38, 2013.

[10] F. Meyer, A. Karch, K. M. Schlinkmann et al., "Sociodemographic determinants of spatial disparities in early childhood caries: an ecological analysis in Braunschweig, Germany," *Community Dentistry and Oral Epidemiology*, vol. 45, no. 5, pp. 442–448, 2017.

[11] A. Alkhtib, A. Ghanim, M. Temple-Smith, L. B. Messer, M. Pirotta, and M. Morgan, "Prevalence of early childhood caries and enamel defects in four and five-year old Qatari preschool children," *BMC Oral Health*, vol. 16, p. 73, 2016.

[12] C. J. Oulis, K. Tsinidou, G. Vadiakas, E. Mamai-Homata, A. Polychronopoulou, and T. Athanasouli, "Caries prevalence of 5, 12 and 15-year-old Greek children: a national pathfinder survey," *Community Dental Health*, vol. 29, no. 1, pp. 29–32, 2012.

[13] B. A. Bugis, "Early childhood caries and the impact of current U.S. Medicaid program: an overview," *International Journal of Dentistry*, vol. 2012, Article ID 348237, 7 pages, 2012.

[14] R. Basner, R. M. Santamaría, J. Schmoeckel, E. Schüler, and C. Splieth, *Epidemiologische Begleituntersuchungen zur Gruppenprophylaxe 2016*, DAJ-Deutsche Arbeitsgemeinschaft für Jugendzahnpflege e. V, Bonn, Germany, 2018.

[15] K. M. Milsom, A. S. Blinkhorn, and M. Tickle, "The incidence of dental caries in the primary molar teeth of young children receiving National Health Service funded dental care in practices in the North West of England," *British Dental Journal*, vol. 205, p. E14, 2008.

[16] S. D. Shantinath, D. Breiger, B. J. Williams, and J. E. Hasazi, "The relationship of sleep problems and sleep-associated feeding to nursing caries," *Pediatric Dentistry*, vol. 18, no. 5, pp. 375–378, 1996.

[17] H. Chen, S. Tanaka, K. Arai, S. Yoshida, and K. Kawakami, "Insufficient sleep and incidence of dental caries in deciduous teeth among children in Japan: a population-based cohort study," *Journal of Pediatrics*, pii: S0022-3476(18)30380-9, 2018.

[18] I. Kraljevic, C. Filippi, and A. Filippi, "Risk indicators of early childhood caries (ECC) in children with high treatment needs," *Swiss Dental Journal*, vol. 127, no. 5, pp. 398–410, 2017.

[19] M. Hooley, H. Skouteris, C. Boganin, J. Satur, and N. Kilpatrick, "Parental influence and the development of dental caries in children aged 0–6 years: a systematic review of the literature," *Journal of Dentistry*, vol. 40, no. 11, pp. 873–885, 2012.

[20] S. E. Jabbarifar, N. Ahmady, S. A. R. Sahafian, F. Samei, and S. Soheillipour, "Association of parental stress and early childhood caries," *Dental Research Journal*, vol. 6, no. 2, pp. 65–70, 2009.

[21] K. Narksawat, A. Boonthum, and U. Tonmukayakul, "Roles of parents in preventing dental caries in the primary dentition among preschool children in Thailand," *Asia-Pacific Journal of Public Health*, vol. 23, no. 2, pp. 209–216, 2011.

[22] V. Zijnge, M. B. van Leeuwen, J. E. Degener et al., "Oral biofilm architecture on natural teeth," *PLoS One*, vol. 5, no. 2, article e9321, 2010.

[23] F. Meyer and J. Enax, "Die mundhöhle als ökosystem," *Biologie in Unserer Zeit*, vol. 48, no. 1, pp. 62–68, 2018.

[24] B. Rosan and R. J. Lamont, "Dental plaque formation," *Microbes and Infection*, vol. 2, no. 13, pp. 1599–1607, 2000.

[25] R. Huang, M. Li, and R. L. Gregory, "Bacterial interactions in dental biofilm," *Virulence*, vol. 2, no. 5, pp. 435–444, 2011.

[26] D. Verma, P. K. Garg, and A. K. Dubey, "Insights into the human oral microbiome," *Archives of Microbiology*, vol. 200, no. 4, pp. 525–540, 2018.

[27] X. Xu, J. He, J. Xue et al., "Oral cavity contains distinct niches with dynamic microbial communities," *Environmental Microbiology*, vol. 17, no. 3, pp. 699–710, 2015.

[28] Y.-H. Li and X. Tian, "Quorum sensing and bacterial social interactions in biofilms," *Sensors*, vol. 12, no. 3, pp. 2519–2538, 2012.

[29] H. Sztajer, S. P. Szafranski, J. Tomasch et al., "Cross-feeding and interkingdom communication in dual-species biofilms of *Streptococcus mutans* and *Candida albicans*," *ISME Journal*, vol. 8, no. 11, pp. 2256–2271, 2014.

[30] M. L. Falsetta, M. I. Klein, P. M. Colonne et al., "Symbiotic relationship between *Streptococcus mutans* and *Candida albicans* synergizes virulence of plaque biofilms in vivo," *Infection and Immunity*, vol. 82, no. 5, pp. 1968–1981, 2014.

[31] T. T. More, J. S. Yadav, S. Yan, R. D. Tyagi, and R. Y. Surampalli, "Extracellular polymeric substances of bacteria and their potential environmental applications," *Journal of Environmental Management*, vol. 144, pp. 1–25, 2014.

[32] H. Koo, M. L. Falsetta, and M. I. Klein, "The exopolysaccharide matrix: a virulence determinant of cariogenic biofilm," *Journal of Dental Research*, vol. 92, no. 12, pp. 1065–1073, 2013.

[33] P. Lingstrom, F. O. van Ruyven, J. van Houte, and R. Kent, "The pH of dental plaque in its relation to early enamel caries and dental plaque flora in humans," *Journal of Dental Research*, vol. 79, no. 2, pp. 770–777, 2000.

[34] N. Takahashi and B. Nyvad, "The role of bacteria in the caries process: ecological perspectives," *Journal of Dental Research*, vol. 90, no. 3, pp. 294–303, 2011.

[35] M. Kilian, I. L. C. Chapple, M. Hannig et al., "The oral microbiome—an update for oral healthcare professionals," *British Dental Journal*, vol. 221, no. 10, pp. 657–666, 2016.

[36] R. Touger-Decker and C. van Loveren, "Sugars and dental caries," *American Journal of Clinical Nutrition*, vol. 78, no. 4, pp. 881S–892S, 2003.

[37] I. Struzycka, "The oral microbiome in dental caries," *Polish Journal of Microbiology*, vol. 63, no. 2, pp. 127–135, 2014.

[38] T. Klinke, M. Urban, C. Luck, C. Hannig, M. Kuhn, and N. Kramer, "Changes in *Candida* spp., mutans streptococci and lactobacilli following treatment of early childhood caries: a 1-year follow-up," *Caries Research*, vol. 48, no. 1, pp. 24–31, 2014.

[39] S. N. Peterson, T. Meissner, A. I. Su et al., "Functional expression of dental plaque microbiota," *Frontiers in Cellular and Infection Microbiology*, vol. 4, p. 108, 2014.

[40] A. Simon-Soro, I. Tomas, R. Cabrera-Rubio, M. D. Catalan, B. Nyvad, and A. Mira, "Microbial geography of the oral cavity," *Journal of Dental Research*, vol. 92, no. 7, pp. 616–621, 2013.

[41] A. Simon-Soro and A. Mira, "Solving the etiology of dental caries," *Trends in Microbiology*, vol. 23, no. 2, pp. 76–82, 2015.

[42] E. Hajishengallis, Y. Parsaei, M. I. Klein, and H. Koo, "Advances in the microbial etiology and pathogenesis of early childhood caries," *Cell Host & Microbe*, vol. 32, no. 1, pp. 24–34, 2017.

[43] F. Teng, F. Yang, S. Huang et al., "Prediction of early childhood caries via spatial-temporal variations of oral microbiota," *Cell Host & Microbe*, vol. 18, no. 3, pp. 296–306, 2015.

[44] S. V. Dorozhkin and M. Epple, "Biological and medical significance of calcium phosphates," *Angewandte Chemie International Edition*, vol. 41, no. 17, pp. 3130–3146, 2002.

[45] J. Enax and M. Epple, "Synthetic hydroxyapatite as a biomimetic oral care agent," *Oral Health & Preventive Dentistry*, vol. 16, no. 1, pp. 7–19, 2018.

[46] P. W. Brown and B. Constantz, *Hydroxyapatite and Related Materials*, CRC Press, Boca Raton, FL, USA, 1994.

[47] H. A. Lowenstam and S. Weiner, *On Biomineralization*, Oxford University Press, Oxford, UK, 1989.

[48] M. F. Teaford, M. M. Smith, and M. W. J. Ferguson, *Development, Function and Evolution of Teeth*, Cambridge University Press, Cambridge, UK, 2000.

[49] M. S. Tung and D. Skrtic, "Interfacial properties of hydroxyapatite, fluoroapatite and octacalcium phosphate," *Monographs in Oral Science*, vol. 18, pp. 112–129, 2001.

[50] J. Enax, O. Prymak, D. Raabe, and M. Epple, "Structure, composition, and mechanical properties of shark teeth," *Journal of Structural Biology*, vol. 178, no. 3, pp. 290–299, 2012.

[51] E. D. Yilmaz, S. Bechtle, H. Özcoban, A. Schreyer, and G. A. Schneider, "Fracture behavior of hydroxyapatite nanofibers in dental enamel under micropillar compression," *Scripta Materialia*, vol. 68, no. 6, pp. 404–407, 2013.

[52] K.-J. Moll and M. Moll, *Kurzlehrbuch Anatomie*, Elsevier, New York, NY, USA, 2000.

[53] C. E. Smith, R. Wazen, Y. Hu et al., "Consequences for enamel development and mineralization resulting from loss of function of ameloblastin or enamelin," *European Journal of Oral Sciences*, vol. 117, no. 5, pp. 485–497, 2009.

[54] M. A. De Menezes Oliveira, C. P. Torres, J. M. Gomes-Silva et al., "Microstructure and mineral composition of dental enamel of permanent and deciduous teeth," *Microscopy Research and Technique*, vol. 73, no. 5, pp. 572–577, 2010.

[55] A. Lucchese and E. Storti, "Morphological characteristics of primary enamel surfaces versus permanent enamel surfaces: SEM digital analysis," *European Journal of Paediatric Dentistry*, vol. 12, no. 3, pp. 179–183, 2011.

[56] P. R. Wilson and A. D. Beynon, "Mineralization differences between human deciduous and permanent enamel measured by quantitative microradiography," *Archives of Oral Biology*, vol. 34, no. 2, pp. 85–88, 1989.

[57] M. C. Z. Alcantara-Galeana, R. Contreras-Bulnes, L. E. Rodríguez-Vilchis et al., "Microhardness, structure, and morphology of primary enamel after phosphoric acid, self-etching adhesive, and Er:YAG laser etching," *International Journal of Optics*, vol. 2017, Article ID 7634739, 8 pages, 2017.

[58] C. M. Zamudio-Ortega, R. Contreras-Bulnes, R. J. Scougall-Vilchis, R. A. Morales-Luckie, O. F. Olea-Mejia, and L. E. Rodriguez-Vilchis, "Morphological, chemical and structural characterisation of deciduous enamel: SEM, EDS, XRD, FTIR and XPS analysis," *European Journal of Paediatric Dentistry*, vol. 15, no. 3, pp. 275–280, 2014.

[59] S. Anil and P. S. Anand, "Early childhood caries: prevalence, risk factors, and prevention," *Frontiers in Pediatrics*, vol. 5, p. 157, 2017.

[60] C. A. Feldens, P. H. Rodrigues, G. de Anastacio, M. R. Vitolo, and B. W. Chaffee, "Feeding frequency in infancy and dental caries in childhood: a prospective cohort study," *International Dental Journal*, vol. 68, no. 2, pp. 113–121, 2017.

[61] A. H. Wyne, "Early childhood caries: nomenclature and case definition," *Community Dentistry and Oral Epidemiology*, vol. 27, no. 5, pp. 313–315, 1999.

[62] W. M. Avila, I. A. Pordeus, S. M. Paiva, and C. C. Martins, "Breast and bottle feeding as risk factors for dental caries: a systematic review and meta-analysis," *PLoS One*, vol. 10, no. 11, article e0142922, 2015.

[63] P. Prakash, P. Subramaniam, B. H. Durgesh, and S. Konde, "Prevalence of early childhood caries and associated risk factors in preschool children of urban Bangalore, India: a cross-sectional study," *European Journal of Dentistry*, vol. 6, no. 2, pp. 141–152, 2012.

[64] R. J. Berkowitz, "Causes, treatment and prevention of early childhood caries: a microbiologic perspective," *Journal of the Canadian Dental Association*, vol. 69, no. 5, pp. 304–307, 2003.

[65] "Tooth eruption," *Journal of the American Dental Association*, vol. 137, no. 1, p. 127, 2006.

[66] H. Limeback and C. Robinson, "Fluoride therapy," in *Comprehensive Preventive Dentistry*, pp. 251–282, John Wiley & Sons, Ltd., Hoboken, NY, USA, 2012.

[67] V. C. Marinho, H. V. Worthington, T. Walsh, and L. Y. Chong, "Fluoride gels for preventing dental caries in children and adolescents," *Cochrane Database of Systematic Reviews*, vol. 6, p. CD002280, 2015.

[68] T. Walsh, H. V. Worthington, A. M. Glenny, P. Appelbe, V. C. Marinho, and X. Shi, "Fluoride toothpastes of different concentrations for preventing dental caries in children and adolescents," *Cochrane Database of Systematic Reviews*, vol. 1, p. Cd007868, 2010.

[69] C. V. Loveren, *Toothpastes*, Vol. 23, Karger Publishers, Basel, Switzerland, 2013.

[70] European Academy of Paediatric Dentistry, "Guidelines on the use of fluoride in children: an EAPD policy document," *European Archives of Paediatric Dentistry*, vol. 10, no. 3, pp. 129–135, 2009.

[71] A. L. Bronckers, D. M. Lyaruu, and P. K. DenBesten, "The impact of fluoride on ameloblasts and the mechanisms of enamel fluorosis," *Journal of Dental Research*, vol. 88, no. 10, pp. 877–893, 2009.

[72] J. M. ten Cate, "Review on fluoride, with special emphasis on calcium fluoride mechanisms in caries prevention," *European Journal of Oral Sciences*, vol. 105, no. 5, pp. 461–465, 1997.

[73] J. A. Weatherell, C. Robinson, and A. S. Hallsworth, "Changes in the fluoride concentration of the labial enamel surface with age," *Caries Research*, vol. 6, no. 4, pp. 312–324, 1972.

[74] F. Muller, C. Zeitz, H. Mantz et al., "Elemental depth profiling of fluoridated hydroxyapatite: saving your dentition by the skin of your teeth?," *Langmuir*, vol. 26, no. 24, pp. 18750–18759, 2010.

[75] F. Neues, A. Klocke, F. Beckmann, J. Herzen, J. P. Loyola-Rodriguez, and M. Epple, "Mineral distribution in highly fluorotic and in normal teeth: a synchrotron microcomputer tomographic study," *Materialwissenschaft und Werkstofftechnik*, vol. 40, no. 4, pp. 294–296, 2009.

[76] L. M. Marin, J. A. Cury, L. M. Tenuta, J. E. Castellanos, and S. Martignon, "Higher fluorosis severity makes enamel less resistant to demineralization," *Caries Research*, vol. 50, no. 4, pp. 407–413, 2016.

[77] B. Ogaard, "Effects of fluoride on caries development and progression in vivo," *Journal of Dental Research*, vol. 69, pp. 813–819, 1990.

[78] S. V. Dorozhkin, "Calcium orthophosphates (CaPo4) and dentistry," *Bioceramics Development and Applications*, vol. 6, no. 96, 2016.

[79] K. Kani, M. Kani, A. Isozaki, H. Shintani, T. Ohashi, and T. Tokumoto, "Effect of apatite-containing dentifrices on dental caries in school children," *Journal of Dental Health*, vol. 39, no. 1, pp. 104–109, 1989.

[80] U. Schlagenhauf, K.-H. Kunzelmann, C. Hannig et al., "Microcrystalline hydroxyapatite is not inferior to fluorides in clinical caries prevention: a randomized, double-blind, non-inferiority trial," *bioRxiv*, 2018.

[81] K. Najibfard, K. Ramalingam, I. Chedjieu, and B. T. Amaechi, "Remineralization of early caries by a nano-hydroxyapatite dentifrice," *Journal of Clinical Dentistry*, vol. 22, no. 5, pp. 139–143, 2011.

[82] A. Kensche, C. Holder, S. Basche, N. Tahan, C. Hannig, and M. Hannig, "Efficacy of a mouthrinse based on hydroxyapatite to reduce initial bacterial colonisation in situ," *Archives of Oral Biology*, vol. 80, pp. 18–26, 2017.

[83] I. Harks, Y. Jockel-Schneider, U. Schlagenhauf et al., "Impact of the daily use of a microcrystal hydroxyapatite dentifrice on de novo plaque formation and clinical/microbiological parameters of periodontal health. A randomized trial," *PLoS One*, vol. 11, article e0160142, 2016.

[84] C. Hannig, S. Basche, T. Burghardt, A. Al-Ahmad, and M. Hannig, "Influence of a mouthwash containing hydroxyapatite microclusters on bacterial adherence in situ," *Clinical Oral Investigations*, vol. 17, no. 3, pp. 805–814, 2013.

[85] C. Palmieri, G. Magi, G. Orsini, A. Putignano, and B. Facinelli, "Antibiofilm activity of zinc-carbonate hydroxyapatite nanocrystals against Streptococcus mutans and mitis group Streptococci," *Current Microbiology*, vol. 67, no. 6, pp. 679–681, 2013.

[86] S. A. Hegazy and I. R. Salama, "Antiplaque and remineralizing effects of Biorepair mouthwash: a comparative clinical trial," *Pediatric Dental Journal*, vol. 26, no. 3, pp. 89–94, 2016.

[87] M. Lelli, M. Marchetti, I. Foltran et al., "Remineralization and repair of enamel surface by biomimetic Zn-carbonate hydroxyapatite containing toothpaste: a comparative in vivo study," *Frontiers in Physiology*, vol. 5, p. 333, 2014.

[88] J. Li, X. Xie, Y. Wang et al., "Long-term remineralizing effect of casein phosphopeptide-amorphous calcium phosphate (CPP-ACP) on early caries lesions in vivo: a systematic review," *Journal of Dentistry*, vol. 42, no. 7, pp. 769–777, 2014.

[89] D. L. Bailey, G. G. Adams, C. E. Tsao et al., "Regression of post-orthodontic lesions by a remineralizing cream," *Journal of Dental Research*, vol. 88, no. 12, pp. 1148–1153, 2009.

[90] P. Shen, D. J. Manton, N. J. Cochrane et al., "Effect of added calcium phosphate on enamel remineralization by fluoride in a randomized controlled in situ trial," *Journal of Dentistry*, vol. 39, no. 7, pp. 518–525, 2011.

[91] N. Gupta, C. Mohan Marya, R. Nagpal, S. Singh Oberoi, and C. Dhingra, "A review of casein phosphopeptide-amorphous calcium phosphate (CPP-ACP) and enamel remineralization," *Compendium of Continuing Education in Dentistry*, vol. 37, no. 1, pp. 36–39, 2016.

[92] Y. Wang, J. Li, W. Sun, H. Li, R. D. Cannon, and L. Mei, "Effect of non-fluoride agents on the prevention of dental caries in primary dentition: a systematic review," *PLoS One*, vol. 12, no. 8, article e0182221, 2017.

[93] J. M. ten Cate, "The need for antibacterial approaches to improve caries control," *Advances in Dental Research*, vol. 21, no. 1, pp. 8–12, 2009.

[94] J. Enax and M. Epple, "Die charakterisierung von putzkorpern in zahnpasten," *Deutsche Zahnärztliche Zeitung*, vol. 73, pp. 116–124, 2018.

[95] C. H. Splieth, M. Alkilzy, J. Schmitt, C. Berndt, and A. Welk, "Effect of xylitol and sorbitol on plaque acidogenesis," *Quintessence International*, vol. 40, no. 4, pp. 279–285, 2009.

[96] M. B. Kowash, A. Pinfield, J. Smith, and M. E. Curzon, "Effectiveness on oral health of a long-term health education programme for mothers with young children," *British Dental Journal*, vol. 188, no. 4, pp. 201–205, 2000.

[97] M. Yaacob, H. V. Worthington, S. A. Deacon et al., "Powered versus manual toothbrushing for oral health," *Cochrane Database of Systematic Reviews*, vol. 6, 2014.

[98] M. Muller-Bolla and F. Courson, "Toothbrushing methods to use in children: a systematic review," *Oral Health & Preventive Dentistry*, vol. 11, no. 4, pp. 341–347, 2013.

[99] P. M. Glaze and A. B. Wade, "Toothbrush age and wear as it relates to plaque control," *Journal of Clinical Periodontology*, vol. 13, no. 1, pp. 52–56, 1986.

32

SNP Analysis of Caries and Initial Caries in Finnish Adolescents

Teija Raivisto ⓘ,[1] AnnaMaria Heikkinen,[1] Leena Kovanen,[2] Hellevi Ruokonen,[1] Kaisa Kettunen,[3] Taina Tervahartiala,[1] Jari Haukka,[2,4] and Timo Sorsa[1,5]

[1]Department of Oral and Maxillofacial Diseases, University of Helsinki and Helsinki University Hospital, Helsinki, Finland
[2]Department of Health, National Institute for Health and Welfare, Helsinki, Finland
[3]Institute for Molecular Medicine Finland (FIMM), Helsinki, Finland
[4]Department of Public Health and Clinicum, University of Helsinki, Helsinki, Finland
[5]Department of Dental Medicine, Karolinska Institutet, Huddinge, Sweden

Correspondence should be addressed to Teija Raivisto; teija.raivisto@fimnet.fi

Academic Editor: Gianrico Spagnuolo

Background. Dental caries is the most common infection in the world and is influenced by genetic and environmental factors. Environmental factors are largely known, but the role of genetic factors is quite unknown. The aim was to investigate the genetic background of caries in Finnish adolescents. *Materials and Methods.* This study was carried out at the Kotka Health Center in Eastern Finland. 94 participants aged 15–17 years gave approval for the saliva and DNA analyses. However, one was excluded in DNA analysis; thus, the overall number of participants in analysis was 93. Caries status was recorded clinically and from bite-wing X-rays to all 94 participants. Genomic DNA was extracted by genomic QIAamp® DNA Blood Mini Kit and genotyped for polymorphisms. The results were analyzed using additive and logistic regression models. *Results.* No significant associations between caries and the genes studied were found. However, SNPs in *DDX39B* and *MPO* showed association tendencies but were not statistically significant after false discovery rate (FDR) analysis. SNPs in *VDR, LTA,* and *MMP3* were not statistically significant with initial caries lesions after FDR analysis. *Conclusion.* The present study could not demonstrate statistically significant associations between caries and the genes studied. Further studies with larger populations are needed.

1. Introduction

Dental caries is a common chronic biofilm infection. *Streptococcus mutans* is the primary agent of dental caries; however, its role as a primary pathogen appears less pronounced in populations with prevention programs. In Swedish population, caries-active adolescents were colonized by *Actinomyces, Selenomonas, Prevotella,* and *Capnocytophaga* species [1]. Environmental and socioeconomic factors, reduced salivary flow, tooth structure, and oral dietary and hygienic habits also enhance the caries development and progression. However, there is only a spare information about the effects of genetic background of caries on adolescents [2].

DDX39B (BAT1) belongs to the DEAD-box family of RNA-binding proteins and is encoded in the central human major histocompatibility complex (MHC), which contains numerous genes involved in immune and inflammatory responses. The human leukocyte antigen- (HLA-B-) associated BAT1 is an RNA helicase encoded by the *DDX39B* gene (*BAT1*). BAT1 is shown to be a negative regulator of inflammation [3]. *DDX39B* encodes an RNA helicase known to regulate the expression of two cytokines, such as tumor necrosis factor-alpha (TNF-α) and interleukin-6 (IL-6) [4]. These both cytokines are well known in inflammatory areas. IL-6 acts in both proinflammatory and anti-inflammatory ways, and TNF-α is a monocyte-derived cytotoxin. BAT1 (*D6S81E* and *UAP56*) lies in the central MHC between *TNF* and *HLA-B*, a region containing genes that affect susceptibility to immunopathologic disorders. BAT1 protein may be directly responsible for the genetic association, as antisense studies show that it can downregulate inflammatory cytokines [5].

Myeloperoxidase (MPO) is a peroxidase enzyme. It is most abundantly expressed in neutrophil granulocytes in saliva and is a strong biomarker for both acute and chronic inflammatory conditions. Its main role is to produce hypo-chlorous acid to carry out the antimicrobial activity [6]. MPO also oxidatively activates latent forms of matrix metal-loproteinases (MMPs), especially MMP-8 and MMP-9, and inactivates tissue inhibitors of metalloproteinases (TIMPs) and serpins [7–10].

Lactoferrin is present in or on all mucosal surfaces throughout the body and specifically in saliva. It can act as a host defense protein against *Streptococcus* species operating in the innate arm of the immune system, but also affecting adaptive immunity [11, 12]. Human lactoferrin (HLF) pro-phylaxis significantly decreased the expression levels of in-terferon gamma (IFN-γ), TNF-α, interleukin-1 beta (IL-1β), IL-6, MPO, and nitric oxide synthases (iNOS) [13]. IFN-γ is a cytokine participating in the immune system. IL-1β is also a cytokine present in humans encoded by the *IL1B* gene. The inducible isoform of iNOS is involved in immune response and inflammatory processes.

The aim of this study was to investigate the genetic background related to caries lesions in Finnish adolescents.

2. Materials and Methods

This study was carried out at the Kotka Health Center in Eastern Finland. The sample was collected in 2004-2005 and 2014-2015, comprising 15- to 17-year-old adolescents. Every 15- to 17-year-old living in Kotka was invited to examination in 2004-2005. In 2014-2015, 15- to 17-year-olds were invited to examination according to their individual examination time. The study flow of the participants is described by Heikkinen et al. [14]. This study was approved by the Ethical Committee of the Kymenlaakso Regional Hospital and by the Ethical Committee of the Helsinki and Uusimaa Hospital District (Dnro 260/13/03/00/13). The participants gave written informed consent. Altogether, there were 94 participants who gave their approval for the saliva and DNA analyses. However, in DNA analysis, one was excluded because of discrepant gender check; thus, the overall number of participants in anal-ysis was 93. Caries status (D = at least one caries lesion in per-manent dentition), including initial caries lesions, was recorded clinically and from bite-wing X-rays as well as visible plaque index (VPI) and smoking habits (current smoker/former smoker/nonsmoker) to all adolescents (n = 94).

The selection process of single-nucleotide polymorphisms (SNPs) from caries-related candidate genes, DNA extraction, genotyping, and genotyping quality control have been de-scribed previously [14]. Genotyping success rates ranged from 90.3 to 98.9%. One subject was excluded due to discrepant gender check results.

Genomic DNA was extracted from 300 μl of the saliva samples by genomic QIAamp DNA Blood Mini Kit (Qiagen, Hilden, Germany) and genotyped for polymorphisms. Ge-netic variants for genotyping were selected from the fol-lowing genes of interest: *S100A8, FCGR2A, FCGR2B, IL10, MMP8, MMP3, MMP13, VDR, TLR4, MMP2, MPO, ELANE, IL1A, IL1B, IL1RN, CD28, MMP9, DDX39B, NFKBIL1, LTA, TNF, SOD2, IL6, TLR4, TIMP1,* and *SYN1.*

A logistic regression model was used to model the as-sociation between dichotomic outcome variables (decayed

TABLE 1: General characteristics of the participants with nonmissing DNA sample (n = 94).

Characteristics	n	%	Missing, n
Gender			
Male	47[a]	50.0	
Female	47[a]	50.0	
Caries			
Initial caries lesions	60	68.2	6
No initial caries lesions	28	31.8	
Caries lesions	30	34.5	
No caries lesions	57	65.5	7
Smoking			
Smoking regularly	16	17.2	1
Nonsmokers	77	82.8	

[a]One was excluded because of discrepant gender check; thus, n = 93 the overall number of participants in DNA analysis was 93.

and initial caries) and 63 SNPs in the 93 subjects. An additive effect of SNPs was assumed. For both outcomes, two models were calculated: an unadjusted model with SNP as the only explanatory variable and an adjusted model with VPI, smoking (weekly smoking), and study period (2004-2005/2014-2015). p values for each outcome were corrected for multiple testing using the false discovery rate (FDR) [15, 16]. The significance level was set to FDR q value less than 0.05. All data analyses were carried out using R software version 3.2.2. [17] and SNPassoc package [18].

3. Results

Based on our caries status, of the participants, 30 had at least one caries lesion, 57 did not have any caries lesion, and data were missing from seven patients. Sixty participants had at least one initial caries lesion, 28 did not have any initial caries lesion, and data were missing from six patients. Of all participants, 16 were smoking regularly and 77 were non-smokers. From one patient, information concerning smoking was missing. In DNA analysis, one was excluded because of discrepant gender check; thus, the final number of participants in analysis was 93. General characteristics of the participants are represented in Table 1. SNPs in *DDX39B* (rs7766569, p = 0.03, q = 0.688885) and *MPO* (rs2243828, p = 0.04, q = 0.688885) showed association tendencies, which how-ever remained not statistically significant when corrected for multiple testing by the false discovery rate (FDR). Other studied SNPs did not reveal any associations (Table 2). SNPs in *VDR* (rs2228570, p = 0.01, q = 0.50), *LTA* (rs2009658, p = 0.02, q = 0.50), and *MMP3* (rs650108, p = 0.03, q = 0.61) showed no statistically significant associations after FDR analysis with initial caries lesions (Table 3).

4. Discussion

Dental caries is a multifactorial disease caused by environ-mental factors and behavioral risk factors. These factors in-clude diet, bacterial flora, oral self-care, salivary flow and composition, fluoride exposure, tooth morphology, and ac-cess to dental care. The role of genetic factors on caries risk is still largely unknown but has been investigated in several

TABLE 2: Gene, chromosomal location, and SNPs associated with decayed (D) unadjusted and adjusted values and p values and FDR q values.

Gene	Chr. location	Marker	Allele	OR	Lower	Upper	p value	FDR q value
Unadjusted values								
DDX39B	2807359	RS7766569	G	2.98	1.04	8.5	0.03	0.688885
MPO	56358884	RS2243828	G	2.42	1.04	5.66	0.04	0.688885
VDR	48239835	RS1544410	A	0.46	0.18	1.18	0.08	0.688885
TLR4	120478131	RS11536889	C	2.38	0.74	7.62	0.08	0.688885
ELANE	852104	RS740021	T	8.12	0.69	95.29	0.09	0.688885
Adjusted values by smoking and VPI (visible plaque index)								
DDX39B	2807359	RS7766569	G	3.39	1.1	10.43	0.03	0.71
MPO	56358884	RS2243828	G	2.33	0.97	5.58	0.06	0.71
ELANE	852104	RS740021	T	10.9	0.88	134.6	0.06	0.71
VDR	48239835	RS1544410	A	0.47	0.19	1.18	0.09	0.71
MMP-3	102708787	RS650108	A	2.07	0.89	4.77	0.09	0.71

TABLE 3: Gene, chromosomal location, and SNPs associated with initial caries (i) unadjusted and adjusted values and p values and FDR q values.

Gene	Chr. location	Marker	Allele	OR	Lower	Upper	p value	FDR q value
Unadjusted values								
VDR	48272895	RS2228570	T	2.49	1.18	5.25	0.01	0.66
MMP-3	102708787	RS650108	A	2.24	1.00	5.00	0.04	0.70
LTA	31538244	RS2009658	G	3.78	1.18	12.1	0.04	0.70
NCR3	31564728	RS2736189	T	3.53	1.10	11.3	0.05	0.70
DDX39B	2807359	RS7766569	G	3.33	1.12	9.92	0.06	0.70
Adjusted values by smoking and VPI (visible plaque index)								
VDR	48272895	RS2228570	T	2.68	1.2	5.98	0.01	0.50
LTA	31538244	RS2009658	G	4.00	1.16	13.84	0.02	0.50
MMP-3	102708787	RS650108	A	2.66	1.04	6.8	0.03	0.61
DDX39B	2807359	RS7766569	G	3.07	0.95	9.92	0.05	0.67
NCR3	31564728	RS2736189	T	3.02	0.90	10.13	0.05	0.67

recent studies [2, 19, 20]. Therefore, we aimed to investigate the genetic background related to caries lesions in Finnish adolescents.

Following genes were studied: *S100A8, FCGR2A, FCGR2B, IL10, MMP8, MMP3, MMP13, VDR, TLR4, MMP2, MPO, ELANE, IL1A, IL1B, IL1RN, CD28, MMP9, DDX39B, NFKBIL1, LTA, TNF, SOD2, IL6, TLR4, TIMP1*, and *SYN1*. In the present study, association tendencies between the studied SNPs in *DDX39B* (rs7766569, adjusted OR 3.39, 95% CI 1.10–10.43) and *MPO* (rs2243818, adjusted OR 2.33, 95% CI 0.97–5.58) and dental caries were found; however, statistical significance disappeared after correction for multiple testing (Tables 2 and 3). Furthermore, SNPs in *VDR* (rs2228570), *LTA* (rs2009659), and *MMP3* (rs650108) with initial caries lesions did not remain significant after FDR correction.

In a previous study, a *VDR-FokI* gene polymorphism was associated with dental caries in 12-year-old adolescents in China. Four *VDR* gene polymorphisms were examined, and the other three *VDR* gene polymorphisms (*Bsm* I, *Taq* I, and *Apa* I) showed no statistically significant differences in the caries group compared with the controls [21]. In a Czech study, the *VDR TaqI* gene variant could not be used as a marker for identification of children with increased dental caries risk either [22]. However, according to another study by Cogulu et al. [23], *VDR* gene polymorphisms may be used as a marker for the identification of patients with high caries risk [23].

Several studies have demonstrated that MMPs are involved in dental caries. The release of acids by bacteria rapidly decreases the pH in saliva, and the acidic environment can then activate host-derived pro-MMPs from both dentin and saliva [24]. The importance of MMPs in the development and progression of dentin caries has been studied by Tjäderhane et al. [25]. They found that human MMP-2, MMP-8, and MMP-9 were identified in demineralized dentinal lesions and inhibition of MMPs can reduce dentin caries progression. Host MMPs, activated by bacterial acids, may have a crucial role in the destruction of dentin by caries. *MMP9* and *MMP20* were involved in white spot lesions and early childhood caries development according to the study of Antunes et al. [26]. Lewis et al. [27] investigated SNPs in or near three *MMP* genes (*MMP10, MMP14*, and *MMP16*) for evidence of association with dental caries. Significant evidence of association was seen between two SNPs upstream of *MMP16* with dental caries [27]. The allele frequency of *MMP2, MMP13*, and *TIMP2* was different between caries-affected and caries-free individuals, with significant association for *MMP13* [28]. *MMP2* and *MMP3* genes are likely to be involved in caries [29]. However, we did not find any association between the studied *MMP2, MMP3, MMP8, MMP9*, and *MMP13* SNPs and caries.

The heritability of dental caries varies between 40% and 60% [2, 20, 30]. Wang et al. [31] observed in their studies that

SNPs in three genes, namely, dentin sialophosphoprotein (*DSPP*), aquaporin 5 (*AQP5*), and kallikrein-related peptidase 4 (*KLK4*), showed consistent associations with protection against caries. Genes involved in enamel formation (*AMEX, AMBN, ENAM, TUFT, MMP20*, and *KLK4*), salivary characteristics (*AQP5*), immune regulation, and dietary preferences had the largest impact [27]. *DSPP* gene encodes two principal proteins of the dentin extracellular matrix of the tooth. *AQP5* encodes a series of homologous membrane proteins. *KLK4* is playing a role in enamel mineralization. Two genes, namely, taste 2 receptor member 38 (*TAS2R38*) and taste 1 receptor member (*TAS1R2*), have been identified to be important in taste sensing and to be associated with dental caries risk and/or protection. Dental caries is heritable, and genes affecting susceptibility to caries in the primary dentition may differ from those in permanent teeth [2]. This may help to identify the individuals at risk and enhance the implementation of preventive strategies before the onset of caries [20].

Smoking can be a confounding factor. Tobacco smoking has been found to increase the risk for dental caries [32]. The high rate of restorative treatment may also be explained by poor oral health behaviors [33, 34].

The sample size was quite small in this study of adolescents, and it needs to be acknowledged. Majority of the participants were lost because in Finland, it is difficult to obtain permission from adolescents for a genetic study.

5. Conclusion

In conclusion, no significant associations between SNPs in *DDX39B* and *MPO* genes and dental caries were found in the present study; however, a tendency could be observed, as well as between initial caries and polymorphisms in *VDR, LTA* and *MMP3*. SNPs in other genes were also investigated, but none of these showed a significant relationship, not either for initial caries. Altogether, dental caries is influenced by genetic and environmental factors. Several genes are likely to have influence on dental caries. More studies with larger populations and sample sizes are needed for final conclusion.

Acknowledgments

This work was supported by grants (TYH 2013353, TYH 20144244, and TYH 2016251) from the Helsinki University Hospital Research Foundation, Helsinki, Finland, and the Karolinska Institutet, Stockholm, Sweden.

References

[1] I. D. Johansson, E. Witkowska, B. Kaveh, P. Lif Holgerson, and A. C. Tanner, "The microbiome in populations with a low and high prevalence of caries," *Journal of Dental Research*, vol. 95, no. 1, pp. 80–86, 2016.

[2] X. Wang, J. R. Shaffer, R. J. Weyant et al., "Genes and their effects on dental caries may differ between primary and permanent dentitions," *Caries Research*, vol. 44, no. 3, pp. 277–284, 2010.

[3] R. J. N. Allcock, J. H. Williams, and P. Price, "The central MHC gene, BAT1, may encode a protein that down-regulates cytokine production," *Genes to Cells*, vol. 6, no. 5, pp. 487–494, 2001.

[4] V. R. R. Mendonça, L. C. L. Souza, G. C. Garcia et al., "DDX39B (BAT1), TNF and IL6 gene polymorphisms and association with clinical outcomes of patients with *Plasmodium vivax* malaria," *Malaria Journal*, vol. 13, no. 1, p. 278, 2014.

[5] P. Price, A. M.-L. Wong, D. Williamson et al., "Polymorphisms at positions -22 and -348 in the promoter of the BAT1 gene affect transcription and the binding of nuclear factors," *Human Molecular Genetics*, vol. 13, no. 9, pp. 967–974, 2004.

[6] J. M. Kinkade, S. O. Pember, K. C. Barnes, R. Shapira, J. K. Spitznagel, and L. E. Martin, "Differential distribution of distinct forma of myeloperoxidase in different azurophilic granule subpopulations from human neutrophils," *Biochemical and Biophysical Research Communications*, vol. 114, no. 1, pp. 296–303, 1998.

[7] J. M. Leppilahti, P. A. Hernández-Ríos, J. A. Gamonal et al., "Matrix metalloproteinases and myeloperoxidase in gingival crevicular fluid provide site-specific diagnostic value for chronic periodontitis," *Journal of Clinical Periodontology*, vol. 41, no. 4, pp. 348–356, 2014.

[8] H. Saari, K. Suomalainen, O. Lindy, Y. T. Konttinen, and T. Sorsa, "Activation of latent human neutrophil collagenase by reactive oxygen species and serine proteases," *Biochemical and Biophysical Research Communications*, vol. 171, no. 3, pp. 979–987, 1990.

[9] P. Spallarossa, S. Garibaldi, C. Barisione et al., "Postprandial serum induces apoptosis in endothelial cells: role of polymorphonuclear-derived myeloperoxidase and metalloproteinase-9 activity," *Atherosclerosis*, vol. 198, no. 2, pp. 458–467, 2008.

[10] T. Sorsa, L. Tjäderhane, Y. T. Konttinen et al., "Matrix metalloproteinases: contribution to pathogenesis, diagnosis and treatment of periodontal inflammation," *Annals of Medicine*, vol. 38, no. 5, pp. 306–321, 2006.

[11] D. Legrand, E. Elass, M. Carpentier, and J. Mazurier, "Lactoferrin: a modulator of immune and inflammatory responses," *Cellular and Molecular Life Sciences*, vol. 62, no. 22, pp. 2549–2559, 2005.

[12] D. H. Fine, "Lactoferrin: a roadmap to the borderland between caries and periodontal disease," *Journal of Dental Research*, vol. 94, no. 6, pp. 768–776, 2015.

[13] S. K. Velusamv, D. H. Fine, and K. Velliyagounder, "Prophylatic effect of human lactoferrin against *Streptococcus mutans* bacteremia in lactoferrin knockout mice," *Microbes and Infection*, vol. 16, no. 9, pp. 762–767, 2014.

[14] A. M. Heikkinen, K. Kettunen, L. Kovanen et al., "Inflammatory mediator polymorphisms associate with initial periodontitis in adolescents," *Clinical and Experimental Dental Research*, vol. 2, no. 3, pp. 208–215, 2016.

[15] Y. Benjamini and Y. Hochberg, "Controlling the false discovery rate: a practical and powerful approach to multiple testing," *Journal of the Royal Statistical Society*, vol. 57, no. 1, pp. 289–300, 1995.

[16] M. E. Glickman, S. R. Rao, and M. R. Schultz, "False discovery rate control is a recommended alternative to Bonferroni-type adjustments in health studies," *Journal of Clinical Epidemiology*, vol. 67, no. 8, pp. 850–857, 2014.

[17] R Core Team, *R: A Language and Environment for Statistical Computing*, R Foundation for Statistical Computing, 2017, https://www.R-project.org/.

[18] J. R. Gonzalez, L. Armengol, X. Sole et al., "SNPassoc: an R package to perform whole genome association studies," *Bioinformatics*, vol. 23, no. 5, pp. 644-645, 2007.

[19] J. R. Shaffer, X. Wang, R. S. Desensi et al., "Genetic susceptibility to dental caries on pit and fissure and smooth surfaces," *Caries Research*, vol. 46, no. 1, pp. 38–46, 2012.

[20] S. Wendell, X. Wang, M. Brown et al., "Taste genes associated with dental caries," *Journal of Dental Research*, vol. 89, no. 11, pp. 1198–1202, 2010.

[21] M. Yu, Q. Z. Jiang, Z. Y. Sun, Y. Y. Kong, and Z. Chen, "Association between single nucleotide polymorphisms in vitamin D receptor gene polymorphisms and permanent tooth caries susceptibility to permanent tooth caries in Chinese adolescents," *BioMed Research International*, vol. 2017, Article ID 4096316, 7 pages, 2017.

[22] H. L. Izakovicova, L. P. Borilova, J. Kastovsky et al., "Vitamin D receptor *TaqI* gene polymorphism and dental caries in Czech children," *Caries Research*, vol. 51, no. 1, pp. 7–11, 2017.

[23] D. Cogulu, H. Onay, Y. Ozdemir, G. I. Aslan, F. Ozkinay, and C. Eronat, "The role of vitamin D receptor polymorphisms on dental caries," *Journal of Clinical Pediatric Dentistry*, vol. 40, no. 3, pp. 211–214, 2016.

[24] C. Chaussain-Miller, F. Fiorett, M. Goldberg, and S. Menashi, "The role of matrix metalloproteinases (MMPs) in human caries," *Journal of Dental Research*, vol. 85, no. 1, pp. 22–32, 2006.

[25] L. Tjäderhane, H. Larjava, T. Sorsa, V. J. Uitto, M. Larmas, and T. Salo, "The activation and function of host matrix metalloproteinasas in dentin matrix breakdown in caries lesions," *Journal of Dental Research*, vol. 77, no. 8, pp. 1622–1629, 1998.

[26] L. A. Antunes, L. S. Antunes, E. C. Kuchler et al., "Analysis of the association between polymorphisms in MMP2, MMP3, MMP9, MMP20, TIMP1, and TIMP2 genes with white spot lesions and early childhood caries," *International Journal of Paediatric Dentistry*, vol. 26, no. 4, pp. 310–319, 2016.

[27] D. D. Lewis, J. R. Shaffer, E. Feingold et al., "Genetic association of *MMP10*, *MMP14*, and *MMP16* with dental caries," *International Journal of Dentistry*, vol. 2017, Article ID 8465125, 7 pages, 2017.

[28] P. N. Tannure, E. C. Kuchler, P. Falagan-Lotsch et al., "*MMP13* polymorphism decreases risk for dental caries," *Caries Research*, vol. 46, no. 4, pp. 401–407, 2012.

[29] D. Karayasheva, M. Glushkova, E. Boteva, V. Mitev, and T. Kadiyska, "Association study for the role of matrix metalloproteinases 2 and 3 gene polymorphisms in dental caries susceptibility," *Archives of Oral Biology*, vol. 68, pp. 9–12, 2016.

[30] I. L. Chapple, P. Bouchard, M. G. Cagetti et al., "Interaction of lifestyle, behaviour or systemic diseases with dental caries and periodontal diseases: consensus report of group 2 of the joint EFP/ORCA workshop on the boundaries between caries and periodontal diseases," *Journal of Clinical Periodontology*, vol. 44, pp. S39–S51, 2017.

[31] X. Wang, M. C. Willing, M. L. Marazita et al., "Genetic and environmental factors associated with dental caries in children: the Iowa fluoride study," *Caries Research*, vol. 46, no. 3, pp. 177–184, 2012.

[32] G. Benedetti, G. Campus, L. Strohmenger, and P. Lingström, "Tobacco and dental caries: a systemic review," *Acta Odontologica Scandinavica*, vol. 71, no. 3-4, pp. 363–371, 2013.

[33] T. Tanner, A. Kämppi, J. Päkkilä et al., "Association of smoking and snuffing with dental caries occurrence in a young male population in Finland: a cross-sectional study," *Acta Odontologica Scandinavica*, vol. 72, no. 8, pp. 1017–1024, 2014.

[34] X. Chen, Y. Liu, Q. Yu et al., "Dental caries status and oral health behaviour among civilian pilots," *Aviation, Space, and Environmental Medicine*, vol. 85, no. 10, pp. 999–1004, 2014.

33

Fungal-Host Interaction: Curcumin Modulates Proteolytic Enzyme Activity of *Candida albicans* and Inflammatory Host Response *In Vitro*

Emily Chen,[1] Bruna Benso,[2] Dalia Seleem,[3] Luiz Eduardo Nunes Ferreira ⓘ,[4] Silvana Pasetto,[1] Vanessa Pardi,[1] and Ramiro Mendonça Murata ⓘ[4,5]

[1]*Herman Ostrow School of Dentistry, University of Southern California, Los Angeles, CA, USA*
[2]*School of Dentistry, Pontificia Universidad Católica de Chile, Santiago, Chile*
[3]*College of Dental Medicine, Western University of Health Sciences, Pomona, CA, USA*
[4]*School of Dental Medicine, East Carolina University, Greenville, NC, USA*
[5]*Brody School of Medicine, East Carolina University, Greenville, NC, USA*

Correspondence should be addressed to Ramiro Mendonça Murata; muratar16@ecu.edu

Academic Editor: Timo Sorsa

Current treatments for *Candida albicans* infection are limited due to the limited number of antifungal drugs available and the increase in antifungal resistance. Curcumin is used as a spice, food preservative, flavoring, and coloring agent that has been shown to have many pharmacological activities. Thus, this study evaluated the modulatory effects of curcumin on major virulence factors associated with the pathogenicity of *C. albicans*. The minimum inhibitory concentration (MIC) of curcumin against *C. albicans* (SC5314) was determined. Biofilm formation was quantified and the proteinase and phospholipase secretion was measured. The cytotoxicity was tested in oral fibroblast cells. A cocultured model was used to analyze the gene expression of proinflammatory cytokines (IL-1β, IL-1α, and IL-6) from host cells, as well SAP-1 and PLB-1 by RT-PCR. The MIC was between 6.25 and 12.5 μM, and the activity of proteinase enzyme was significantly decreased in biofilms treated with curcumin. However, proteinase gene expression was not downregulated after curcumin treatment. Furthermore, gene expressions of host inflammatory response, IL-1β and IL-1α, were significantly downregulated after exposure to curcumin. In conclusion, curcumin exhibited antifungal activity against *C. albicans* and modulated the proteolytic enzyme activities without downregulating the gene expression. In host inflammatory response, curcumin downregulated IL-1β and IL-1α gene expression.

1. Introduction

Candida albicans is a prevalent opportunistic fungus that becomes pathogenic in patients with reduced immune competence or in individuals with an imbalance of competing bacterial microflora [1–3]. The pathogenicity of the *Candida* species is attributed to critical virulence factors, such as the ability to evade host defenses, adhere to surfaces (on tissues and medical devices), biofilm formation, and the production of proteolytic enzymes, such as secreted aspartyl proteases (SAP) and phospholipases [4].

Current treatments for *C. albicans* infection consist of topical and systemic pharmaceutical antifungal agents [5].

Antifungal resistance has been increasing due to the limited number of antifungal treatments available and the widespread use of these drugs [6, 7]. Therefore, the discovery of new and effective antifungal therapeutic agents is a necessity. Natural compounds are readily available in many foods and beverages. They are a source of molecules with antimicrobial, anti-inflammatory, and antioxidant potential [8].

Polyphenols are secondary metabolites found in many plants, which have been used for thousands years in traditional herbal remedies due to their diverse biological activities [9]. Protective effects of such flavonoids have been reported against cancer, cardiovascular diseases, diabetes, infectious disease, as well as age-linked conditions, which renders them potential therapeutic agents [10]. Curcumin is a yellow pigment derived from the roots of *Curcuma longa* plants that is commonly used as a spice, food preservative, flavoring, and coloring agent in Asia and India [10–12]. Curcumin has been shown to have many pharmacological activities including antioxidant, anti-inflammatory, antiviral, antitumor, and antibacterial activities [13]. Moreover, curcumin acts as a photosensitizer for photodynamic therapy with clinical application for pharyngotonsillitis, with the proposal to reduce the use of antibiotics [14].

Based on the indexed literature, we hypothesized that curcumin can affect the virulence factors of *Candida albicans* and the host immune response to the pathogen. The aim of this study was to investigate the modulatory effects of curcumin *in vitro* in some virulence factors associated with the pathogenicity of *Candida albicans*. Proteolytic enzyme activities secreted by *C. albicans* were quantified in addition to gene expression of inflammatory cytokines marker of the host in a coculture system. Ultimately, this study explored the mechanisms by which curcumin can modulate the pathogenicity of *Candida albicans* and validated the pharmacological effects of curcumin.

2. Materials and Methods

2.1. Susceptibility Test. Antimicrobial activity of curcumin (Sigma-Aldrich; St. Louis, MO) was tested *in vitro* according to the NCCLS guidelines against *Candida albicans* strain (ATCC SC5314/MYA2876). Curcumin concentrations ranged from 1.5 to 400 μM. Fluconazole (322 μM) (Sigma) and 1% dimethyl sulfoxide (DMSO) (v/v) (Sigma-Aldrich; St. Louis, MO) served as a positive control and vehicle control, respectively. The minimum inhibitory concentration (MIC) was determined using an inoculum of 5×10^3 CFU/ml. *C. albicans* were grown in RPMI-1640 (Lonza, Walkersville, MD) in a 96-well plate, and incubated for 24 h at 37°C in 5% CO_2. After 24 h, the MIC was determined visually, and the minimum fungicidal concentration (MFC) was found by subculturing 20 μl from each concentration above the MIC on Sabouraud dextrose agar (Becton Dickinson, Franklin Lakes, NJ) for 48 hours at 37°C in 5% CO_2 [15].

2.2. Biofilm Assay. One milliliter of 1×10^6 CFU/ml *C. albicans* inoculum was added in each well of a sterile 24-well plate, suspended in yeast nitrogen base medium (Becton Dickinson, Franklin Lakes, NJ) with 50 mM of glucose. The plate was incubated for 24 h (37°C in 5% CO_2) to allow initial biofilm growth and adhesion to the plate surface. Biofilms were then treated every 24 h using curcumin concentrations of 62.5 μM and 125 μM (10x MIC and 20x MIC resp.) for three days. Before each treatment, biofilms were washed with 500 μl of PBS and replenished with 900 μl of fresh medium and 100 μl of curcumin treatments. The 1% ethanol was used as vehicle control, and fluconazole (1 mg/ml) served as a positive control. On the fifth day, biofilms were washed with PBS and the biomass was measured.

PBS (1 mL) was added to each well, and the biofilm was suspended to disrupt the biofilm formation. Viability and

colony formation unit (CFU) of *C. albicans* were determined by plating 20 μl of the suspended biofilm solution on Sabouraud dextrose agar plates (Becton Dickinson, Franklin Lakes, NJ). The plates were incubated for 24 h at 37°C in 5% CO_2, and the number of *C. albicans* colonies was counted. To determine the dry weight of the biofilm sample, *C. albicans* suspended in PBS solution was centrifuged at 10,000 rpm for 5 minutes. The supernatant was discarded and the sample was placed in a speed vacuum to dry for 40 minutes, and dry biofilm mass was determined [16].

2.3. Cell Viability Test. Oral fibroblast cells (ATCC: CRL2014) were cultured in Dulbecco's modified Eagle's medium (DMEM) (Lonza, Walkersville, MD) with 10% fetal bovine serum (FBS, Lonza, Walkersville, MD) at 37°C in 5% CO_2. Fibroblast cells (1×10^5 cells/ml) were first seeded in each well of a 96-well plate in DMEM with 10% FBS, and the plates were incubated for 24 h at 37°C in 5% CO_2. Then, cells were treated with curcumin (1.5–640 μM), and the plates were incubated at 37°C in 5% CO_2 for 24 h. Cell viability was measured by the fluorometric method (Cell Titer Blue, Promega Corp, Madison, WI) in a SpectraMax M5 microplate reader (Molecular Devices Sunnyvale, CA) with 550 nm (Ex)/585 nm (Em) wavelength [17].

2.4. Proteinase and Phospholipase Enzyme Secretion Assay. Proteinase and phospholipase enzyme secretion assays were conducted as previously performed by Santana et al. [15]. Biofilms of *C. albicans* were grown as described before and treated for 72 h using curcumin (62.5 μM and 125 μM) and the standards: phospholipase A2 (Sigma-Aldrich; St. Louis, MO) and trypsin (Lonza, Walkersville, MD) for proteinase assay. The vehicle control was 1% ethanol. *C. albicans* biofilms were sonicated, and the proteinase enzyme activity was determined by mixing the supernatant of the biofilm solution with 1% azocasein at 1 : 9 (v/v) for 1 h at 37°C in 5% CO_2. Then, 500 μl of 10% trichloroacetic acid was added to stop the reaction. The solutions were centrifuged for 5 minutes at 10,000 rpm. The supernatant (500 μl) was combined with 500 μl of NaOH and incubated at 37°C in 5% CO_2 for 15 min. The absorbance was read at 440 nm using a spectrophotometer [5, 13, 17]. The phospholipase enzyme activity is determined by mixing the supernatant of the biofilm solution with phosphatidylcholine substrate for 1 h at 37 °C in 5% CO_2. Absorbance was read in a spectrophotometer at 630 nm [13, 15, 18].

2.5. Coculture Model Quantitative Real-Time PCR. Fibroblast cells (1×10^5 cells/ml) were seeded in a 96-well plate in DMEM medium with 10% FBS and incubated at 37°C in 5% CO_2 for 24 h. The medium was replaced, and *C. albicans* inoculum of 5×10^3 to 2.5×10^3 CFU/ml in DMEM without FBS was added. Fibroblast cells and *C. albicans* were treated with 20 μM and 40 μM (subcytotoxic dose) of curcumin. The plates were incubated for 24 h. The vehicle control tested was 1% ethanol, while fluconazole was the positive control. Total RNA was isolated from fibroblast cells and *C. albicans*. The RNA was purified using the RNeasy MiniKit (Qiagen, Valencia CA) and the RiboPure Yeast Kit (Life Technologies, Carlbad, CA), respectively. A Nano-Photometer P360 (Implen; Westlake Village, CA) was used to quantify the total RNA extracted. Reverse transcription of the RNA into cDNA was carried out using iScript Advanced cDNA synthesis Kit for RT-qPCR (BioRad, Hercules, CA) according to the manufacturer's instructions. Real-time PCR was conducted using iQ SYBR Green Supermix (BioRad, Hercules, CA). The *C. albicans* primers for the genes secreted aspartyl proteinases-1 (SAP-1), phospholipase B-1 (PLB-1), and ACT-1 (housekeeping) at $10\,\mu$M were used [19]. Based on previous analysis using the RT^2 Profiler PCR Array Kit (Qiagen, Valencia CA), the following fibroblast genes were selected: IL1-α (Qiagen Gene ID#: 3552), IL1-β (Qiagen Gene ID#: 3553), IL-6 (Qiagen Gene ID#: 3569), and GADPH (Qiagen Gene ID#: 2597). PCR amplification was performed using $20\,\mu$l of the reaction mix in each of the 96-well plate. The reactions were conducted at 95°C for 3 minutes, followed by 40 cycles of 15 seconds at 95°C and 1 minute at 60°C. After PCR, the melting curve was obtained by incubating the samples at increasing increments of 0.5°C from 55°C to 95°C.

2.6. Statistical Analysis. Data were tested for normal distribution by Shapiro–Wilks' test, and the equivalence of variances were tested by Levene's test. All data were expressed as the mean ± SEM using one-way analysis of variance (ANOVA) and Dunnett's multiple comparison tests in relation to the vehicle. The level of statistical significance was set at 0.05. The lethal dosage (LD_{50}) was found using nonlinear regression analysis by MasterPlex 2010 Reader Fit. PCR analysis was performed using the $\Delta\Delta$Ct method.

3. Results

The MIC for curcumin against *C. albicans* was in a range between $6.25\,\mu$M and $12.5\,\mu$M. The biofilm assay results showed a decrease in the mass of biofilms treated with curcumin ($62.5\,\mu$M and $12.5\,\mu$M) in relation to the vehicle control (Figure 1). However, the results were not statistically significant ($p > 0.05$). Concentrations of curcumin below $40\,\mu$M showed no significant cytotoxicity against oral fibroblast cells when compared to the vehicle (data not shown), and the LD_{50} was $48.75\,\mu$M.

After treatments with curcumin at $62.5\,\mu$M and $125\,\mu$M, there was a significant decrease ($p < 0.05$) in the proteinase and phospholipase enzyme activity when compared to the vehicle (Figures 2(a) and 2(b)). There were no differences in the expression of SAP-1 after exposure to curcumin (Figure 3(a)). The treatment with $10\,\mu$M curcumin significantly increased the PLB-1 gene expression in comparison to the vehicle. However, there was no difference between curcumin at $20\,\mu$M and vehicle (Figure 3(b)). The expression of host inflammatory markers showed a significant downregulation in IL-α and IL1-β with curcumin treatment at $10\,\mu$M and $20\,\mu$M. There were no changes in the expression of IL-6 gene for both curcumin treatments (Figure 4).

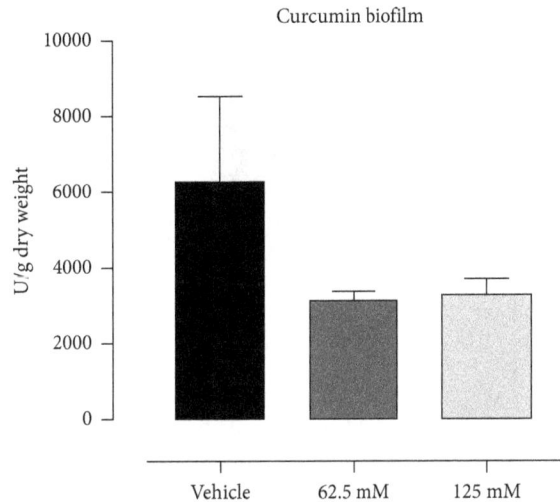

FIGURE 1: Mean and SD of *Candida albicans* biofilm expressed in CFU/grams of dry weight after treatment with curcumin.

4. Discussion

The resistance of *Candida* species to conventional antifungal agents, such as triazoles, represents a major challenge for the treatment of candidiasis especially in individuals with diminished immune response, for example, in HIV patients. Natural compounds are potential therapeutic agents that may be considered for the treatment of fungal infection because of their antimicrobial benefits. Over the past 30 years, the FDA has recognized 69% of 109 small molecules from natural products or derivates as having antimicrobial effects [20].

Curcumin stands as a potential antimicrobial natural compound, which is incorporated as an important traditional remedy spice used by the traditional Asian and Indian culture. However, scientific validation of its antimicrobial efficacy, toxicity effects, and mechanism of action are necessary to establish its safety for therapeutic purposes. Thus, this study demonstrated the curcumin effects on virulence factors of *C. albicans*, including the analysis of gene expression.

Curcumin has been reported to have antifungal activity against various strains of *Candida*, including *Candida albicans* (ATCC 10261), with a minimum inhibitory concentration (MIC) ranging from 250 to 2000 μg/ml (0.68 mM to 5.4 mM) [11, 21]. In this study, we used *C. albicans* SC5314 strain, and the MIC was found in the range of 6.25–$12.5\,\mu$M. *C. albicans* 5314 was used because the genome is fully described, with well-known molecular patterns and phenotypes. In addition, the biofilm formation by this strain is well established in several studies [22, 23].

In the biofilm assay, ten times of MIC concentration ($62.5\,\mu$M and $125\,\mu$M) were tested because biofilms have a denser network of yeasts and hyphal population that are more resistant to drug diffusion than to planktonic counterparts. It was found that both concentrations of curcumin did not significantly reduce the colony formation in the biofilms normalized by the dry weight of the samples. Possible explanation for the lack of the significant CFU reduction/dry weight is that curcumin did not drastically

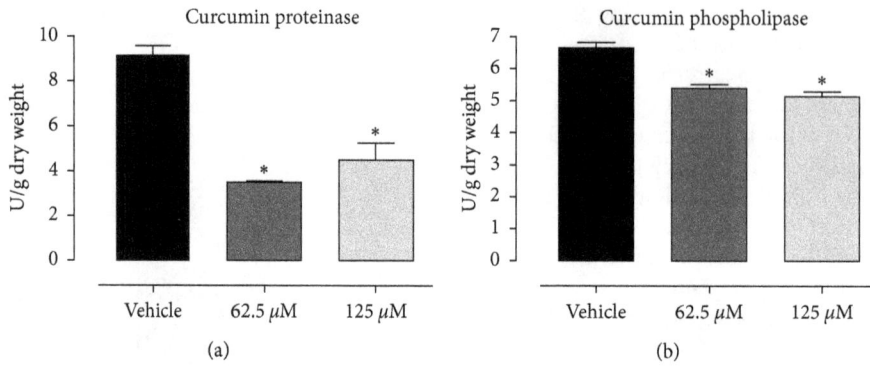

FIGURE 2: Mean and SD of *Candida albicans* proteinase (a) and phospholipase (b) enzyme secretion expressed in U/grams of dry weight after treatment with curcumin (62.5 μM and 125 μM). *Statistical difference in relation to vehicle control, $p < 0.05$, ANOVA, Dunnett's.

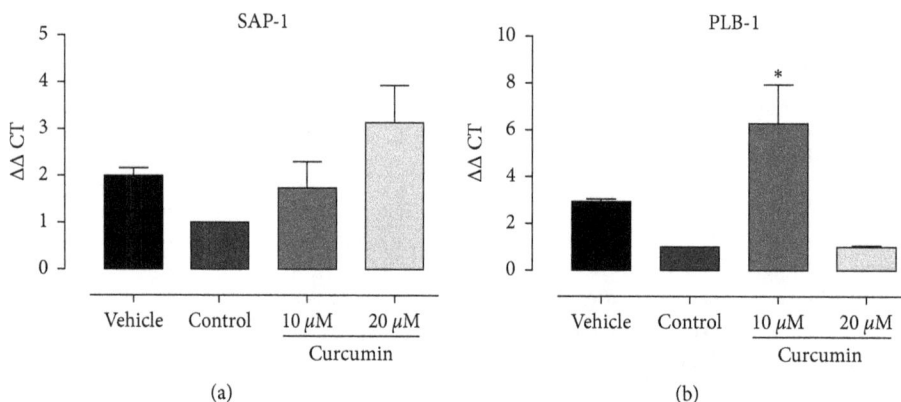

FIGURE 3: Real-time quantitative information about gene expression of SAP-1 (a) and PLB-1 (b) after curcumin treatments (10 μM and 20 μM) in oral fibroblast cells infected by *C. albicans*. *Statistical difference between curcumin treatments and control in comparison with vehicle, $p < 0.05$ ANOVA, Dunnett's.

affect the composition of biofilms. However, this hypothesis needs to be further investigated by studying the polysaccharides and protein composition of the biofilm samples upon treatment with the compound. Similarly, the biofilm's dry weight (data not shown) did not show significant differences among the groups, signifying that the total biomass compositions of all fungal cells, including dead/live cells, were not affected with treatment of any compound.

The lethal dosage or 50% cell viability (LD$_{50}$) was 48.75 μM, which is important to ensure the therapeutic safety level when considering *in vivo* studies as well as human clinical trials. It should also be noted that in coculture models, curcumin has more sensitive and profound effect on the morphology and distribution of fibroblast cells, as this model represents "naked-cells," that have a more susceptible cell response than cells tested under clinically relevant conditions.

Proteinases and phospholipases are enzymes secreted by *Candida albicans* often associated with tissue degradation, hyphal formation, and host invasion, which are critical factors linked to the pathogenicity of *C. albicans* [24, 25]. Proteinase and phospholipase enzyme activities were reduced using curcumin at 62.5 μM and 125 μM. These results suggest that one possible curcumin mechanism of action involves inhibition of proteinase secretion, which is an

important virulence factor [21]. This finding is consistent with the results reported by Neelofar et al. [11], in which curcumin decreased proteinase secretion by 53% in *C. albicans* compared to the vehicle control group.

SAP proteins are often associated with virulence factors able to elicit a destructive effect on the host tissue during mucosal infections, as they facilitate hyphal invasion and activate the degradation of E-cadherin, a major protein present in epithelial cell junction [24, 25]. In this current study, the effect of curcumin on SAP-1 gene expression was analyzed.

There was no significant downregulation in SAP-1 gene expression after treatment curcumin at 10 μM and 20 μM (Figure 3(a)). One possible explanation is based on a negative feedback mechanism modulating gene expression. Gene expression of proteases may play an important role in regulating the enzyme activity of proteases. Thus, as indicated by the significant decrease in proteolytic enzyme activities of phospholipases and proteinases, there may be a negative feedback inhibition regulating their respective gene expression. However, this hypothesis needs to be confirmed through further molecular studies.

The ability of *C. albicans* to attach to the host tissue is considered a key pathogenic characteristic and an important

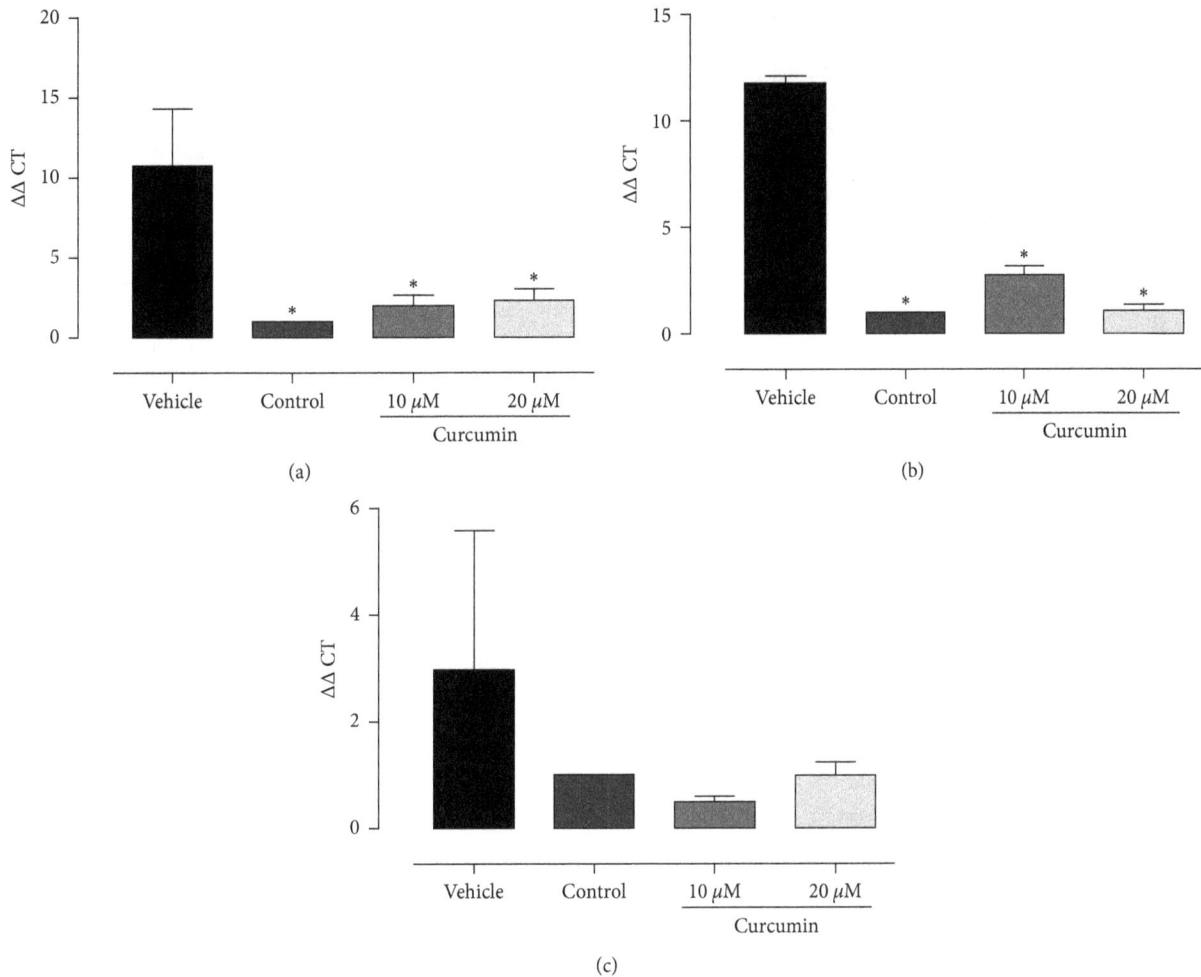

(a)

(b)

(c)

FIGURE 4: Real-time quantitative information about gene expression of IL-1α (a), IL-1β (b), and IL-6 (c). *Statistical difference between curcumin treatments and control in comparison with vehicle, $p < 0.05$, ANOVA, Dunnett's.

virulence factor. Phospholipase B (PLB) proteins were shown to have hydrolytic activity, as they hydrolyze acyl ester bonds in phospholipids and lysophospholipids and catalyze lysophospholipase-transacylase reactions. PLB multigene family encodes for CaPLB5, a putative secretory protein with a predicted GPI-anchor attachment site [26]. The PLB-1 gene expression after curcumin treatment was also evaluated. Although curcumin in lowest concentration increases the expression of PLB-1, this was not reflected in the enzymatic activity.

Host immune defense plays a critical antagonistic role during fungal infections, where the pathogenic state of candidiasis is marked by an increase in the proinflammatory cytokines [27, 28]. Gingival fibroblasts are major actors in the host immune defense against C. albicans infection. Fibroblasts express dectin-1 on the cell surface that recognizes C. albicans and active the inflammatory response by secreting inflammatory cytokines, such as IL-1β, IL-1α, IL-6, and IL-8 [29, 30]. Proinflammatory cytokines play an important role in the pathogenesis of many inflammatory diseases [31]. In this study, the gene expressions of the proinflammatory cytokines, IL1-α, IL1-β, and IL-6, were

analyzed using host oral fibroblast cells infected with C. albicans in a coculture model.

We demonstrated that curcumin can reduce the IL-1α and IL-1β gene expression of fibroblasts exposed to C. albicans infection. Similar results were observed in C. albicans treated with monolaurin [32]. The antiinflammatory property of curcumin is well established and has been demonstrated in different cells [33, 34]. In agreement with our results, curcumin has been reported to block the release of IL-1 in bone marrow stromal cells, colonic epithelial cells, and human articular chondrocytes [35].

These cytokines promote the inflammation by the activation of innate immune response and the induction of cyclooxygenase type 2. Furthermore, these cytokines also increase the expression of adhesion molecules, synthesis of nitric oxide, and the release of other cytokines [36]. However, IL-6 gene expression was not affected after curcumin treatments. In some systemic diseases, the IL-1 blockade reduces the levels of IL-6 [36]. Thus, IL-6 gene expression appears to be more associated with IL-1α and IL-1β levels than with the effects of curcumin.

Curcumin suppressed the production of inflammatory cytokines via regulation of molecular targets and transcription factors [37]. In vascular smooth muscle cells, curcumin inhibits LPS-induced inflammation by suppressing the activation of TLR4, inhibiting phosphorylation of ERK1/2 and p38 MAPK, preventing nuclear translocation of NF-κB, and reducing NADPH-mediated intracellular ROS production [38].

Although gingival fibroblasts are nonprofessional immune cells, they also express other pattern recognition receptors, such as TLRs, that recognizes *C. albicans* molecular patterns [39]. Activation of TLRs leads to activation of transcription factors such as NF-κB and interferon regulatory factors that induces the expression of various proinflammatory cytokines [40]. The downregulation of IL-1α and IL-1β induced by curcumin during the exposure to *C. albicans* could be related to the inhibition of TLR-MAPK/NF-κB pathways. Others anti-inflammatory mechanisms of curcumin in the *C. albicans* infection should be elucidated.

5. Conclusion

Curcumin had a slight antifungal activity against *Candida albicans* (SC5314). Curcumin reduces the proteolytic enzyme activities of phospholipases and SAPs without downregulating the gene expression. Furthermore, curcumin can modulate the host inflammatory response by decreasing gene expression of IL-1β and IL-1α. Future direction for research may involve studying the synergistic effects of curcumin and other conventional therapies on biofilm models. In addition, the curcumin efficacy in *albicans* strains isolated from clinical samples with different virulence profiles should be tested.

Acknowledgments

This research was funded by the National Center for Complementary and Integrative Health (R00AT006507).

References

[1] J. Berman, "*Candida albicans*," *Current Biology*, vol. 22, no. 16, pp. R620–R622, 2002.

[2] L. N. Dovigo, A. C. Pavarina, A. P. D. Ribeiro et al., "Investigation of the photodynamic effects of curcumin against *Candida albicans*," *Photochemistry and Photobiology*, vol. 87, no. 4, pp. 895–903, 2011.

[3] K. H. Neppelenbroek, N. H. Campanha, D. M. P. Spolidorio, L. C. Spolidorio, R. S. Seo, and A. C. Pavarina, "Molecular fingerprinting methods for the discrimination between *C. albicans* and *C. dubliniensis*," *Oral Diseases*, vol. 12, no. 3, pp. 242–253, 2006.

[4] A. Correia, U. Lermann, L. Teixeira et al., "Limited role of secreted aspartyl proteinases Sap1 to Sap6 in *Candida albicans* virulence and host immune response in murine hematogenously disseminated candidiasis," *Infection and Immunity*, vol. 78, no. 11, pp. 4839–4849, 2010.

[5] L. P. Samaranayake and T. W. MacFarlane, *Oral Candidosis*, Wright-Butterworth, London, UK, 1990.

[6] K. D. Hunter, J. Gibson, P. Lockhart, A. Pithie, and J. Bagg, "Fluconazole-resistant Candida species in the oral flora of fluconazole-exposed HIV-positive patients," *Oral Surgery, Oral Medicine, Oral Pathology, Oral Radiology, and Endodontology*, vol. 85, no. 5, pp. 558–564, 1998.

[7] T. C. White, K. A. Marr, and R. A. Bowden, "Clinical, cellular, and molecular factors that contribute to antifungal drug resistance," *Clinical Microbiology Reviews*, vol. 11, no. 2, pp. 382–402, 1998.

[8] C. V. B. Martins, D. L. da Silva, A. T. Neres et al., "Curcumin as a promising antifungal of clinical interest," *Journal of Antimicrobial Chemotherapy*, vol. 63, no. 2, pp. 337–339, 2009.

[9] M. Shahzad, L. Sherry, R. Rajendran, C. A. Edwards, E. Combet, and G. Ramage, "Utilising polyphenols for the clinical management of *Candida albicans* biofilms," *International Journal of Antimicrobial Agents*, vol. 44, no. 3, pp. 269–273, 2014.

[10] Bhawana, R. K. Basniwal, H. S. Buttar, V. K. Jain, and N. Jain, "Curcumin nanoparticles: preparation, characterization, and antimicrobial study," *Journal of Agricultural and Food Chemistry*, vol. 59, no. 5, pp. 2056–2061, 2011.

[11] K. Neelofar, S. Shreaz, B. Rimple, S. Muralidhar, M. Nikhat, and L. A. Khan, "Curcumin as a promising anticandidal of clinical interest," *Canadian Journal of Microbiology*, vol. 57, no. 3, pp. 204–210, 2011.

[12] U. Hani and H. G. Shivakumar, "Solubility enhancement and delivery systems of curcumin a herbal medicine: a review," *Current Drug Delivery*, vol. 11, no. 6, pp. 792–804, 2014.

[13] S. Pasetto, V. Pardi, and R. M. Murata, "Anti-HIV-1 activity of flavonoid myricetin on HIV-1 infection in a dual-chamber in vitro model," *PLoS One*, vol. 9, no. 12, Article ID e115323, 2014.

[14] K. C. Blanco, N. M. Inada, F. M. Carbinatto, A. L. Giusti, and V. S. Bagnato, "Treatment of recurrent pharyngotonsillitis by photodynamic therapy," *Photodiagnosis and Photodynamic Therapy*, vol. 18, pp. 138-139, 2017.

[15] I. L. Santana, L. M. Gonçalves, A. A. de Vasconcellos, W. J. da Silva, J. A. Cury, and A. A. Del Bel Cury, "Dietary carbohydrates modulate *Candida albicans* biofilm development on the denture surface," *PLoS One*, vol. 8, no. 5, Article ID e64645, 2013.

[16] J. O'brien, I. Wilson, T. Orton, and F. Pognan, "Investigation of the Alamar Blue (resazurin) fluorescent dye for the assessment of mammalian cell cytotoxicity," *European Journal of Biochemistry*, vol. 267, no. 17, pp. 5421–5426, 2000.

[17] L. M. Goncalves, A. A. Del Bel Cury, A. Sartoratto, V. L. Garcia Rehder, and W. J. Silva, "Effects of undecylenic acid released from denture liner on Candida biofilms," *Journal of Dental Research*, vol. 91, no. 10, pp. 985–989, 2012.

[18] L. Taniguchi, B. de Fátima Faria, R. T. Rosa et al., "Proposal of a low-cost protocol for colorimetric semi-quantification of secretory phospholipase by *Candida albicans* grown in planktonic and biofilm phases," *Journal of Microbiological Methods*, vol. 78, no. 2, pp. 171–174, 2009.

[19] H. Nalis, S. Kuchaříková, M. Řičicová et al., "Real-time PCR expression profiling of genes encoding potential virulence

factors in *Candida albicans* biofilms: identification of model-dependent and -independent gene expression," *BMC Microbiology*, vol. 10, no. 1, pp. 1–14, 2010.

[20] M. L. Peterson and P. M. Schlievert, "Glycerol monolaurate inhibits the effects of Gram-positive select agents on eukaryotic cells," *Biochemistry*, vol. 45, no. 7, pp. 2387–2397, 2006.

[21] A. Kumar, S. Dhamgaye, I. K. Maurya, A. Singh, M. Sharma, and R. Prasad, "Curcumin targets cell wall integrity via calcineurin-mediated signaling in *Candida albicans*," *Antimicrobial Agents and Chemotherapy*, vol. 58, no. 1, pp. 167–175, 2014.

[22] P. N. Kipanga and W. Luyten, "Influence of serum and polystyrene plate type on stability of *Candida albicans* biofilms," *Journal of Microbiological Methods*, vol. 139, pp. 8–11, 2017.

[23] K. Lagree, H. H. Mon, A. P. Mitchell, and W. A. Ducker, "Impact of surface topography on biofilm formation by *Candida albicans*," *PLoS One*, vol. 13, no. 6, Article ID e0197925, 2018.

[24] J. R. Naglik, D. Moyes, J. Makwana et al., "Quantitative expression of the *Candida albicans* secreted aspartyl proteinase gene family in human oral and vaginal candidiasis," *Microbiology*, vol. 154, no. 11, pp. 3266–3280, 2008.

[25] C. C. Villar, H. Kashleva, C. J. Nobile, A. P. Mitchell, and A. Dongari-Bagtzoglou, "Mucosal tissue invasion by *Candida albicans* is associated with E-cadherin degradation, mediated by transcription factor Rim101p and protease Sap5p," *Infection and Immunity*, vol. 75, no. 5, pp. 2126–2135, 2007.

[26] S. Theiss, G. Ishdorj, A. Brenot et al., "Inactivation of the phospholipase B gene PLB5 in wild-type *Candida albicans* reduces cell-associated phospholipase A2 activity and attenuates virulence," *International Journal of Medical Microbiology*, vol. 296, no. 6, pp. 405–420, 2006.

[27] U. Lermann and J. Morschhauser, "Secreted aspartic proteases are not required for invasion of reconstituted human epithelia by *Candida albicans*," *Microbiology*, vol. 154, no. 11, pp. 3281–3295, 2008.

[28] G. Ramage, K. Vandewalle, B. L. Wickes, and J. L. López-Ribot, "Characteristics of biofilm formation by *Candida albicans*," *Revista Iberoamericana de Micología*, vol. 18, no. 4, pp. 163–170, 2001.

[29] H. Alanazi, A. Semlali, L. Perraud, W. Chmielewski, A. Zakrzewski, and M. Rouabhia, "Cigarette smoke-exposed *Candida albicans* increased chitin production and modulated human fibroblast cell responses," *BioMed Research International*, vol. 2014, Article ID 963156, 11 pages, 2014.

[30] R. Tamai, M. Sugamata, and Y. Kiyoura, "*Candida albicans* enhances invasion of human gingival epithelial cells and gingival fibroblasts by Porphyromonas gingivalis," *Microbial Pathogenesis*, vol. 51, no. 4, pp. 250–254, 2011.

[31] N. Zhang, H. Li, J. Jia, and M. He, "Anti-inflammatory effect of curcumin on mast cell-mediated allergic responses in ovalbumin-induced allergic rhinitis mouse," *Cellular Immunology*, vol. 298, no. 1-2, pp. 88–95, 2015.

[32] D. Seleem, E. Chen, B. Benso, V. Pardi, and R. M. Murata, "In vitro evaluation of antifungal activity of monolaurin against *Candida albicans* biofilms," *PeerJ*, vol. 4, article e2148, 2016.

[33] A. Kumari, D. Dash, and R. Singh, "Curcumin inhibits lipopolysaccharide (LPS)-induced endotoxemia and airway inflammation through modulation of sequential release of inflammatory mediators (TNF-α and TGF-β1) in murine

model," *Inflammopharmacology*, vol. 25, no. 3, pp. 329–341, 2017.

[34] A. Sadeghi, A. Rostamirad, S. Seyyedebrahimi, and R. Meshkani, "Curcumin ameliorates palmitate-induced inflammation in skeletal muscle cells by regulating JNK/NF-kB pathway and ROS production," *Inflammopharmacology*, pp. 1–8, 2018.

[35] P. P. Sordillo and L. Helson, "Curcumin suppression of cytokine release and cytokine storm: a potential therapy for patients with Ebola and other severe viral infections," *In Vivo*, vol. 29, no. 1, pp. 1–4, 2015.

[36] C. A. Dinarello, "Immunological and inflammatory functions of the interleukin-1 family," *Annual Review of Immunology*, vol. 27, no. 1, pp. 519–550, 2009.

[37] E. Sikora, G. Scapagnini, and M. Barbagallo, "Curcumin, inflammation, ageing and age-related diseases," *Immunity & Ageing*, vol. 7, no. 1, p. 1, 2010.

[38] Z. Meng, C. Yan, Q. Deng, D.-f. Gao, and X.-l. Niu, "Curcumin inhibits LPS-induced inflammation in rat vascular smooth muscle cells in vitro via ROS-relative TLR4-MAPK/NF-κB pathways," *Acta Pharmacologica Sinica*, vol. 34, no. 7, pp. 901–911, 2013.

[39] E. Palm, I. Demirel, T. Bengtsson, and H. Khalaf, "The role of toll-like and protease-activated receptors and associated intracellular signaling in Porphyromonas gingivalis-infected gingival fibroblasts," *APMIS*, vol. 125, no. 2, pp. 157–169, 2017.

[40] S. M. Miggin and L. A. O'Neill, "New insights into the regulation of TLR signaling," *Journal of Leukocyte Biology*, vol. 80, no. 2, pp. 220–226, 2006.

34

Antibacterial and Cytotoxic Effects of *Moringa oleifera* (Moringa) and *Azadirachta indica* (Neem) Methanolic Extracts against Strains of *Enterococcus faecalis*

Lucía Arévalo-Híjar,[1] Miguel Ángel Aguilar-Luis ⓘ,[2,3] Stefany Caballero-García,[1] Néstor Gonzáles-Soto,[1] and Juana Del Valle-Mendoza ⓘ[2,3]

[1]School of Odontology, Health Sciences Faculty, Universidad Peruana de Ciencias Aplicadas-UPC, Lima, Peru
[2]Research Center and Innovation of the Faculty of Health Sciences, Universidad Peruana de Ciencias Aplicadas, Av. San Marcos cdra 2, Cedros de Villa, Lima, Peru
[3]Institute of Nutritional Research (IIN), 1885 La Molina Ave., Lima 12, Peru

Correspondence should be addressed to Juana Del Valle-Mendoza; joana.del.valle@gmail.com

Academic Editor: Louis M. Lin

Objective. To evaluate antibacterial and cytotoxic effect of 2 methanolic extracts of *Azadirachta indica* and *Moringa oleifera* against strains of *Enterococcus faecalis* (ATCC 29212) *in vitro*. *Methods.* The methanolic extracts of *Azadirachta indica* and *Moringa oleifera* were prepared *in vitro*. The antibacterial effect of the extracts against *Enterococcus faecalis* was evaluated using the agar diffusion technique. The minimum inhibitory concentration (MIC) was determined using the microdilution method and the cytotoxicity using the cellular line MDCK. *Results.* The methanolic extract with the most antibacterial effect during the first 24 and 48 hours against *Enterococcus faecalis* was *Moringa oleifera*, evidencing a growth inhibition zone of 35.5 ± 1.05 and 44.83 ± 0.98, respectively. The MIC for both extracts was $75 \,\mu g/ml$. The bactericidal effect of the *Azadirachta indica* extract was found at a concentration of $25 \,\mu g/ml$ and a concentration of $75 \,\mu g/ml$ for *Moringa* extract. *Conclusions.* In conclusion, we demonstrated that the methanolic extract of *Azadirachta indica* and *Moringa oleifera* both have an antibacterial effect against *Enterococcus faecalis* strains during the first 24 and 48 hours. None of the extracts exhibited toxicity against the cell lines under low concentrations.

1. Introduction

One of the main objectives of endodontics is root canal disinfection, mainly associated with the colonization of anaerobic bacteria. There are endodontic treatments that fail due to a complex root canal anatomy or antibiotic resistance of some bacterial families, with *Enterococcus faecalis* being the most resistant bacteria reported [1–6].

Various antibacterial agents have been previously studied, and they can be obtained from natural sources or synthetic agents [7]. Furthermore, recent studies have reported the pharmacological properties and high medicinal value of a myriad of natural extracts. Some of these products,

however, have been used empirically, leaving aside the study and determination of its properties [8].

The contemporary field of phytotherapy focuses on the study of plants and its pharmacological properties to treat diseases. *Azadirachta indica* also known as neem and *Moringa oleifera* also known as moringa are both native Indian trees known for their high medicinal values due to their curative properties [9–15]. *A. indica* has analgesic, antifungal, and antibacterial properties and has therefore been used as treatment for gastrointestinal ailments, mouth hygiene, and certain chronic diseases such as diabetes, high blood pressure, and dyslipidemia [16–19]. On the other hand, *M. oleifera* has been reported to have antiviral, antioxidant, antisclerotic, antibacterial, and anti-inflammatory properties. It has been used as treatment for malaria, malnutrition, colon cancer, and myeloma [20].

Even though these plants have been studied to treat the previously mentioned ailments, no research evaluates if time is directly correlated with the antibacterial effect of *A. indica* against *E. faecalis*. On the other hand, there has yet to be any research on the antibacterial effect of *M. oleifera* or its cytotoxicity as a root canal disinfectant.

The objective of this study was to evaluate the antibacterial and cytotoxic properties of methanolic extracts of *A. indica* and *M. oleifera* against some *Enterococcus faecalis* strains (ATCC 29212) *in vitro*.

2. Materials and Methods

2.1. Sample. The sample size was determined with a formula of comparative means using the statistical software Stata® version 12.0. A confidence interval of 95% was considered, and a power of 80% was used. The mean and standard deviation parameters for a group were obtained using a pilot test that was previously run. Finally, a sample of 6 wells per group was established.

2.2. Extract Preparation. Fresh *A. indica* leafs and pulverized *M. oleifera* leafs were obtained from a naturist shop. Both were free of impurities and had a sanitary registry. These products were placed in different containers and were treated with absolute methanol (1 : 2 weight/volume) to be later stored at room temperature for 10 days without sunlight exposure. The solutions were filtered through Whatman paper no. 4 and placed in labeled tubes. A rotatory evaporator was then used at 50°C to separate the methanol by distillation to finally obtain a pure extract. The extracts were stored at 4°C until use.

2.3. Bacterial Cultures. *Enterococcus faecalis* ATCC 29212 was obtained from GenLab Laboratory in Peru, a representative of MicroBiologics Laboratory (USA). The bacteria were cultured in agar BHI (brain heart infusion) in anaerobic conditions at 37°C for 72 hours. 3 to 4 colonies were then isolated and later inoculated in 3 mL of a BHI broth under the same conditions previously mentioned. The cultures were then diluted in a sterile saline solution to reach a McFarland scale density of 0.5, which approximately estimates a concentration of 1.5×10^8 CFU/mL.

2.4. Antimicrobial Activity Evaluation. Antimicrobial activity evaluation was achieved using the well diffusion method [21]. BHI agar was prepared and autoclaved at 121°C for 15 minutes. The agar was left to cool, and then the previously prepared bacterial suspension was inoculated. Finally, we proceeded to add the agar to sterile petri dishes. A sterile cork borer was used to punch 9 mm holes on the agar plate which were then filled with 1000 mL of each methanolic extract. In addition, 2% chlorhexidine was used as the positive control and 1× saline solution as the negative control. The agar plates were incubated at 37°C, and the diameters of the inhibition growth zones were measured during the first 24 and 48 hours in millimeters with a vernier caliper.

2.5. Determination of the Minimum Inhibitory Concentration (MIC). The minimum inhibitory concentration was determined using the microdilution method described by Gupta and Negi [22]. Each methanolic extract underwent serial dilutions (1/2), and each solution was added to the wells in the petri dishes with concentrations ranging from 1.56 to 75 µg/ml. In addition, 2% chlorhexidine was used as the positive control and 1× saline solution as the negative control. The plates were incubated under anaerobic conditions at 37°C for 24 hours. The minimum inhibitory concentration was considered as the minimum concentration of the extract that inhibited bacterial growth.

2.6. Determination of the Minimum Bactericidal Concentration (MBC). The methanolic extract dilutions were added into each well of a 96-well microtiter plate, and then the bacterial suspension was inoculated. The plate was incubated at 37°C for 24 hours. In order to determine the minimum bactericidal concentration (MBC), aliquots were pipetted out of each well and seeded onto the agar. The sample petri dishes were incubated under anaerobic conditions at 37°C for 24 hours. The minimum bactericidal concentration is defined as the minimum concentration required to inhibit any bacterial growth.

2.7. Cytotoxicity Evaluation. Cytotoxicity was evaluated by means of a colorimetric assay based on the reduction of MTT by mitochondrial enzymes [23]. A 96-well microtiter plate was used to culture 1×10^4 cells per well. The plate was then incubated at 37°C in a humid atmosphere of 5% CO_2 for 24 hours. Subsequently, we proceeded to pipette the methanolic extracts *Azadirachta indica* (neem) and *M. oleifera* (moringa) with concentrations ranging from 0 to 100 µg/mL onto the monocellular layer. Each concentration assay had a positive control for cellular viability (culture medium without any extracts). The plates were incubated at 37°C for 6 days, and the morphology of the cells was surveilled daily. The cytotoxic concentration 50 (CC_{50}) is defined as the concentration of a substance required to decrease cellular viability by 50%.

Twenty microliters of MTT solution (3 mg/ml in PBS 1X) was added into each well and then left incubating for 3 hours. The medium was carefully removed to obtain the formazan crystals which were then diluted with 200 µL of DMSO (dimethyl sulfoxide). In order to determine cellular viability, a microplate photometer was used to measure and compare the absorbance of the treated cultures against the nontreated culture. The results were analysed with the computer software Pharm/PCS. The monolayers were observed under the microscope to evaluate any morphological changes.

TABLE 1: *In vitro* antibacterial effect of 2% chlorhexidine and the methanolic extracts of *Moringa oleifera* and *Azadirachta indica* against *Enterococcus faecalis* during the first 24 and 48 hours.

Time	Extracts	Growth inhibition zone (mm)					
		Mean	Standard deviation	Median	Minimum	Maximum	p^*
24 hours	*Azadirachta indica*	33.16	0.75	33.00	32.00	34.00	
	Moringa oleifera	35.50	1.05	35.50	34.00	37.00	<0.01
	Chlorhexidine	19.16	1.33	20.00	17.00	20.00	
48 hours	*Azadirachta indica*	39.83	3.37	42.00	35.00	42.00	
	Moringa oleifera	44.83	0.98	44.50	44.00	46.00	<0.01
	Chlorhexidine	27.00	1.09	27.00	26.00	29.00	

*Kruskal–Wallis test.

2.8. Statistical Analysis. The antibacterial effect was registered in millimeters (mm). It was analysed by means of a nonparametric test, Kruskal–Wallis, with a statistical significance level of 5% for the comparison between *A. indica*, *M. oleifera*, and chlorhexidine. Data were analysed using the statistical package Stata® version 12.0.

3. Results

3.1. Antimicrobial Activity of the Natural Extracts. After the first 24 hours, the methanolic *A. indica* extract generated a growth inhibition zone of 33.16 mm and the extract of *M. oleifera* generated a 35.5 mm zone. At 48 hours, the growth inhibition zones were 38.83 mm and 44.83 mm, respectively. The methanolic extract of *M. oleifera* had a greater antibacterial effect in comparison with chlorhexidine (control group) and the methanolic extract of *A. indica*. Furthermore, statistically significant differences were found for both groups at 24 and 48 hours ($p < 0.01$) (Table 1).

3.2. MIC, MBC, and Bacteriostatic Effect of A. indica and M. oleifera Extracts. The MIC of both the methanolic extracts, *A. indica* and *M. oleifera*, was 75 μg/ml, demonstrating a bacteriostatic concentration up to this value.

Additionally, the bactericidal concentrations for *A. indica* and *M. oleifera* were 25 μg/ml and 75 μg/ml, respectively (Table 2).

3.3. Cytotoxicity of the Methanolic Extracts of A. indica and M. oleifera. The results indicate that the methanolic extracts of *A. indica* and *M. oleifera* inhibit 50% of cellular viability (CC_{50}) at a concentration of 70 μg/ml. Furthermore, none of the extracts produced any adverse effects on the MDCK cellular lines at low concentrations. We observed an indirect correlation between the concentration and cellular viability (Figure 1).

4. Discussion

There are many different types of endodontic infections described. One of them is the persistent root canal infections for which the highly antibiotic-resistant *Enterococcus faecalis* is the main etiologic agent, even amongst patients previously treated for this condition [2]. The pathogenicity of these bacteria includes its capacity to penetrate dentinal

TABLE 2: Bacteriostatic (MIC) and bactericidal (MBC) of 2% chlorhexidine and methanolic extracts of *Moringa oleifera* and *Azadirachta indica* against *Enterococcus faecalis* strains.

Concentrations (μg/ml)	Study groups		
	Azadirachta indica	*Moringa oleifera*	Chlorhexidine
100	—	—	—
75	MIC	MIC/MBC	—
50	—	—	—
25	MBC	—	—
12.5	—	—	MIC
6.25	—	—	—
3.125	—	—	
1.56	—	—	MBC

tubules, its lack of need of other bacteria to survive, its ability to form biofilms in anaerobic and nutrient lacking conditions, and its resistance to acids and alkalis [5, 6, 12]. It is therefore necessary to study new antibacterial agents specific for this bacteria in order to achieve endodontic treatments with a higher success rate and a better prognosis for the tooth.

As a result of the well diffusion method, we were able to determine that the methanolic extracts for *A. indica* and *M. oleifera* had an antibacterial effect against *E. faecalis* during the first 24 and 48 hours. According to Olson and Fahey, the antibacterial effect of *M. oleifera* is due to the chemical compound 4-(4'-O-acetyl-α-L-rhamnopyranosyloxy)-benzylisothiocyanate, whose mechanism of action involves inhibition of essential cellular membrane enzymes [24, 25]. Moreover, Lakshmi et al. mentioned that the active compound responsible for the antibacterial efficacy of *A. indica* is azadirachtin, a cellular membrane synthesis inhibitor [16, 26].

We also found the MIC of the extracts and concluded that no antibacterial effect was evidenced at low concentrations. In 2013, Reyes and Fernández found the MIC of the foliar extract of *A. indica* against *Staphylococcus aureus* to be 35 μg/ml [27]. Muhammad et al. also evaluated the MIC of an aqueous extract of *M. oleifera* against *S. aureus* and found it to be 6.25 μg/ml. This difference could be explained, given the fact that the process of maceration was 3 times the present study, extracting a greater quantity of chemical compounds of *M. oleifera* [28].

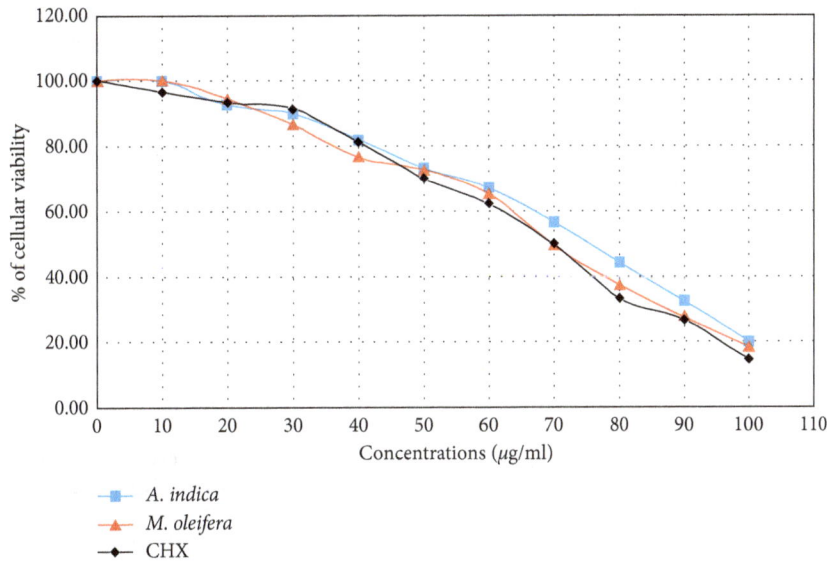

FIGURE 1: Cellular viability evaluation of Jurkat cells against the methanolic extracts of *Moringa oleifera* and *Azadirachta indica* against *Enterococcus faecalis* strains.

The minimum bactericidal concentration for the methanolic extract of *A. indica* was $25\,\mu g/ml$ and $75\,\mu g/ml$ for *M. oleifera* which leads us to conclude that at lower concentrations, *A. indica* has a greater capacity to cause cellular lysis of the bacteria in comparison with *M. oleifera*.

The methanolic extracts of *Azadirachta indica* (neem) and *Moringa oleifera* (moringa) did not show any cytotoxicity against the cellular line of MDCK under low concentrations. Jung evaluated the cytotoxicity of the extract of *M. oleifera* against a cellular line Cos-7 and demonstrated a lack of cytotoxicity even with concentrations of $600\,mg/ml$ [20]. In 2015, Jumba et al. evaluated the cytotoxicity of the methanolic extract of *A. indica* against the cellular line Vero-E6 and determined a CC_{50} of $149\,\mu g/ml$. Despite the difference in these results, the study concludes that the extract stays within a manageable parameter [29].

Additionally, an *in vivo* study with rats showed that none of the subjects suffered any ailment after treatment with *A. indica* extract.

In conclusion, according to this study, *A. indica* and *M. oleifera* demonstrated an antibacterial effect against *E. faecalis* without any toxicity using low concentration. Therefore, they could be considered as alternative antimicrobial agents to use in the root canal therapy field in Odontology. More research is required regarding the cytotoxicity of each of its active components and also its adverse reactions.

The values that were obtained from this study show a direct correlation between the time of exposure to the extract its antibacterial effect. These results are important to continue a line of investigation in relation to fitotherapy applied to Odontology. The purpose of studies in this field is to promote the future creation of treatments based on these natural herbs considering that their use in radicular conduct treatment would lead to a better prognosis.

Disclosure

The manuscript was presented as a thesis in https://repositorioacademico.upc.edu.pe/handle/10757/621020.

Acknowledgments

The study has been supported by the Incentives for Research of the Universidad Peruana de Ciencias Aplicadas (Grant number UPC-COA24-2017) Lima, Peru.

References

[1] M. Ehsani, M. AminMarashi, E. Zabihi, M. Issazadeh, and S. Khafri, "A comparison between antibacterial activity of propolis and aloe vera on *Enterococcus faecalis* (an in vitro study)," *International Journal of Molecular and Cellular Medicine*, vol. 2, no. 3, pp. 110–116, 2013.

[2] F. Benbelaïd, A. Khadir, M. A. Abdoune, M. Bendahou, A. Muselli, and J. Costa, "Antimicrobial activity of some essential oils against oral multidrug-resistant *Enterococcus faecalis* in both planktonic and biofilm state," *Asian Pacific Journal of Tropical Biomedicine*, vol. 4, no. 6, pp. 463–472, 2014.

[3] J. Siqueira and I. Rôças, "Clinical implications and microbiology of bacterial persistence after treatment procedures," *Journal of Endodontics*, vol. 34, no. 11, pp. 1291.e3–1301.e3, 2008.

[4] R. Zan, T. Alacam, I. Hubbezoglu, T. Tunc, Z. Sumer, and O. Alici, "Antibacterial efficacy of super-oxidized water on *Enterococcus faecalis* biofilms in root canal," *Jundishapur Journal of Microbiology*, vol. 9, no. 9, 2016.

[5] V. Zand, M. Lofti, M. H. Soroush, A. A. Abdollahi, M. Sadeghi, and A. Mojadadi, "Antibacterial efficacy of different concentrations of sodium hypochlorite gel and solution

on *Enterococcus faecalis* biofilm," *Iranian Endodontic Journal*, vol. 11, no. 4, pp. 315–319, 2016.

[6] F. Ramezanali, S. Samimi, M. Kharazifard, and F. Afkhami, "The *in vitro* antibacterial efficacy of persian green tea extract as an intracanal irrigant on *Enterococcus faecalis* biofilm," *Iranian Endodontic Journal*, vol. 11, no. 4, pp. 304–308, 2016.

[7] M. Guneser, M. Akbulut, and A. Eldeniz, "Antibacterial effect of chlorhexidine-cetrimide combination, *Salvia officinalis* plant extract and octenidine in comparison with conventional endodontic irrigants," *Dental Materials Journal*, vol. 35, no. 5, pp. 736–741, 2016.

[8] V. Torres and A. Castro, "Fitoterapia," *Revista de Actualización Clínica Médica*, vol. 42, no. 2, pp. 2185–2129, 2014.

[9] P. Chandrappa, A. Dupper, P. Tripathi, R. Arroju, P. Sharma, and K. Sulochana, "Antimicrobial activity of herbal medicines (tulsi extract, neem extract) and chlorhexidine against *Enterococcus faecalis* in Endodontics: an *in vitro* study," *Journal of International Society of Preventive & Community Dentistry*, vol. 5, no. 2, pp. 89–92, 2015.

[10] A. Leone, A. Spada, A. Battezzati, A. Schiraldi, J. Aristil, and S. Bertoli, "Cultivation, genetic, ethnopharmacology, phytochemistry and pharmacology of *Moringa oleifera* leaves: an overview," *International Journal of Molecular Sciences*, vol. 16, no. 12, pp. 12791–12835, 2015.

[11] W. Ghonmode, O. Balsaraf, V. Tambe, K. Saujanya, A. Patil, and D. Kakde, "Comparison of the antibacterial efficiency of neem leaf extracts, grape seed extracts and 3% sodium hypoclorite against *E. feacalis*–an in vitro study," *Journal of International Oral Health*, vol. 5, no. 6, pp. 61–66, 2013.

[12] P. Babaji, K. Jaqtap, H. Lau, N. Bansal, S. Thajuraj, and P. Sondhi, "Comparative evaluation of antimicrobial effect of herbal root canal irrigants *(Morinda citrifolia, Azadirachta indica, Aloe Vera)* with sodium hypochlorite: an *in vitro* study," *Journal of International Society of Preventive and Community Dentistry*, vol. 6, no. 3, pp. 196–199, 2016.

[13] K. Vennila, S. Elanchezhiyan, and S. Ilavarasu, "Efficay of 10% whole *Azadirachta indica* (neem) chip as an adjunct to scaling and root planning in chronic periodontitis: a clinical and microbiology study," *Indian Journal of Dental Research*, vol. 27, no. 1, pp. 15–21, 2016.

[14] A. García, L. Bravo, G. Campos, and D. Medina, "Acción antimicrobiana de la Pterigospermia de *Moringa olifera* sobre los contaminantes del agua y su efecto en el pH, turbidez y crecimiento microbiano," *Revista electrónica de la Facultad de Ingeniería*, vol. 3, no. 1, pp. 11–19, 2015.

[15] J. Rim, K. Ha Lee, D. Ha Shin, S. Sang, and S. Hwang, "Synergistic antimicrobial efficacy of mesoporous ZnO loaded with 4-(α-L-rhamnosyloxy)-benzyl isothiocyanate isolated from the *Moringa oleifera* seed," *Journal of General and Applied Microbiology*, vol. 60, no. 6, pp. 251–255, 2014.

[16] A. Dutta and M. Kundabala, "Comparative anti-microbial efficacy of *Azadirachta indica* irrigant with standard endodontic irrigants: a preliminary study," *Journal of Conservative Dentistry*, vol. 17, no. 2, pp. 133–137, 2014.

[17] S. Chaube, T. Shrivastav, M. Tiwari, S. Prasad, A. Tripathi, and A. Pandey, "Neem (*Azadirachta indica* L.) leaf extract deteriorates oocyte quality by inducing ROS-mediated apoptosis in mammals," *Springerplus*, vol. 3, no. 1, p. 464, 2014.

[18] K. Mistry, Z. Sanghvi, G. Parmar, and S. Shah, "The antimicrobial activity of *Azadirachta indica, Mimusops elengi, Tinospora cardifolia, Ocimum sanctum* and 2% chlorhexidinegluconate on common endodontic pathogens: an *in vitro* study," *European Journal of Dentistry*, vol. 8, no. 2, pp. 172–177, 2014.

[19] V. Kumar and V. Navaratnam, "Neem (*Azadirachta indica*): prehistory to contemporary medicinal uses to humankind," *Asian Pacific Journal of Tropical Biomedicine*, vol. 3, no. 7, pp. 505–514, 2013.

[20] L. Jung, "Soluble extract from *Moringa oleifera* leaves with a new anticancer activity," *PLoS One*, vol. 9, no. 4, Article ID e95492, 2014.

[21] L. Ramirez and D. Marin, "Metodologías para evaluar in vitro la actividad antibacteriana de compuestos de origen vegetal," *Scientia et Technica*, vol. 42, pp. 263–267, 2009.

[22] S. Gupta and P. Negi, "Antibacterial activity of Indian borage (*Plectranthus amboinicus* Benth) leaf extracts in," *Food Systems and Against Natural Microflora in Chicken Meat*, vol. 54, no. 1, pp. 90–102, 2016.

[23] J. Del Valle, T. Pumarola, L. Alzamora, and L. Del Valle, "Antiviral activity of maca (*Lepidium meyenii*) against human influenza virus," *Asian Pacific Journal of Tropical Medicine*, vol. 7, no. 1, pp. 415–420, 2014.

[24] M. Olson and W. Fahey, "Moringa oleifera: un árbol multiusos para las zonas tropicales secas," *Revista Mexicana de Biodiversidad*, vol. 82, no. 4, pp. 1071–1082, 2011.

[25] C. Martin, G. Martín, A. García, T. Fernández, E. Hernández, and J. Puls, "Potenciales aplicaciones de *Moringa oleifera*. una revisión crítica," *Pastos y Forrajes*, vol. 36, no. 2, pp. 137–149, 2013.

[26] T. Lakshmi, V. Krishnan, R. Rajendram, and N. Madhusudhanan, "*Azadirachta indica*: a herbal panacea in dentistry-an update," *Pharmacognosy Reviews*, vol. 9, no. 17, pp. 41–44, 2015.

[27] D. Reyes and R. Fernández, "Efecto biocida *in vitro* del extracto foliar de *Azadirachta indica* en *Staphylococcus* sp y *Pseudomonas* sp," *Salus*, vol. 17, no. 3, pp. 34–41, 2013.

[28] A. A. Muhammad, P. Arulsevan, P. Cheah, F. Abas, and S. Fakurazi, "Evaluation of wound healing properties of bioactive aqueous fraction from *Moringa oleifera* Lam on experimentally induced diabetic animal model," *Drug Design, Development and Therapy*, vol. 10, pp. 1715–1730, 2016.

[29] B. Jumba, C. Anjili, J. Makwali et al., "Evaluation of leishmanicidal activity and cytotoxicity of *Ricinus communis* and *Azadirachta indica* extracts from western Kenya: *in vitro* and *in vivo* assays," *BMC Research Notes*, vol. 8, no. 1, p. 650, 2015.

Permissions

The contributors of this book come from diverse backgrounds, making this book a truly international effort. This book will bring forth new frontiers with its revolutionizing research information and detailed analysis of the nascent developments around the world.

We would like to thank all the contributing authors for lending their expertise to make the book truly unique. They have played a crucial role in the development of this book. Without their invaluable contributions this book wouldn't have been possible. They have made vital efforts to compile up to date information on the varied aspects of this subject to make this book a valuable addition to the collection of many professionals and students.

This book was conceptualized with the vision of imparting up-to-date information and advanced data in this field. To ensure the same, a matchless editorial board was set up. Every individual on the board went through rigorous rounds of assessment to prove their worth. After which they invested a large part of their time researching and compiling the most relevant data for our readers.

The editorial board has been involved in producing this book since its inception. They have spent rigorous hours researching and exploring the diverse topics which have resulted in the successful publishing of this book. They have passed on their knowledge of decades through this book. To expedite this challenging task, the publisher supported the team at every step. A small team of assistant editors was also appointed to further simplify the editing procedure and attain best results for the readers.

Apart from the editorial board, the designing team has also invested a significant amount of their time in understanding the subject and creating the most relevant covers. They scrutinized every image to scout for the most suitable representation of the subject and create an appropriate cover for the book.

The publishing team has been an ardent support to the editorial, designing and production team. Their endless efforts to recruit the best for this project, has resulted in the accomplishment of this book. They are a veteran in the field of academics and their pool of knowledge is as vast as their experience in printing. Their expertise and guidance has proved useful at every step. Their uncompromising quality standards have made this book an exceptional effort. Their encouragement from time to time has been an inspiration for everyone.

The publisher and the editorial board hope that this book will prove to be a valuable piece of knowledge for researchers, students, practitioners and scholars across the globe.

List of Contributors

Jae Won Jang, Hee-Yung Chang, Sung-Hee Pi, Yoon-Sang Kim and Hyung-Keun You
Department of Periodontology, School of Dentistry, Wonkwang University, 344-2 Shinyong-dong, Iksan, Jeonbuk 54538, Republic of Korea

Kujtim Sh. Shala, Linda J. Dula, Teuta Pustina-Krasniqi, Teuta Bicaj, Enis F. Ahmedi, Zana Lila-Krasniqi and Arlinda Tmava-Dragusha
Department of Prosthetic Dentistry, School of Dentistry, Faculty of Medicine, University of Prishtina, Prishtina, Kosovo

R. Lo Giudice and F. G. Cervino
Department of Clinical and Experimental Medicine, Messina University, Policlinico G. Martino, Messina, Italy

Nicita, F. Puleio and A. S. Lizio
Department of Biomedical and Dental Sciences and Morphofunctional Imaging, Messina University, Messina, Italy

A. Alibrandi
Department of Economics, Section of Statistical and Mathematical Sciences, Messina University, Messina, Italy

G. Pantaleo
Department of Neurosciences, Reproductive and Odontostomatological Sciences, Naples Federico II University, Naples, Italy

Francesco Mangano and Renata Bakaj
Department of Medicine and Surgery, University of Insubria, 21100 Varese, Italy

Irene Frezzato and Alberto Frezzato
Private Practice, 45100 Rovigo, Italy

Sergio Montini
Private Practice, 22019 Tremezzo, Italy

Carlo Mangano
Department of Dental Science, Vita Salute S. Raffaele University, 20132 Milan, Italy

Spoorthi Banavar Ravi and Rohit Pandurangappa
School of Dentistry, International Medical University, No. 126, Jalan 19/155B, Bukit Jalil, Kuala Lumpur, Malaysia

Sudarshini Nirupad
Oral Pathology, Dr. Syamala Reddy Dental College Hospital and Research Centre, SGR College Main Road, Marathahalli Post, Bangalore, Karnataka, India

Prashanthi Chippagiri
Faculty of Dentistry, MAHSA University, Kuala Lumpur, Malaysia

Alaa Makke, Abdulwahed Homsi, Montaha Guzaiz and Abdulrahman Almalki
Oral and Maxillofacial Department, Faculty of Dentistry, Umm Al-Qura University, Mecca, Saudi Arabia

Rudyard dos Santos Oliveira, Arlete Maria Gomes Oliveira, JoséLuiz Cintra Junqueira and Francine Kühl Panzarella
Imaging and Oral Radiology, "São Leopoldo Mandic" College, Campus of Campinas, Campinas, SP, Brazil

Trelia Boel
Department of Dental Radiology, Faculty of Dentistry, University of Sumatera Utara, Medan, Indonesia

Ervina Sofyanti and Erliera Sufarnap
Department of Orthodontics, Faculty of Dentistry, University of Sumatera Utara, Medan, Indonesia

Luiza Pereira Dias da Cruz, Robert G. Hill, Xiaojing Chen and David G. Gillam
Oral Bioengineering, Barts and the London School of Medicine and Dentistry, QMUL, London, UK

Manal Almalik
Dental Department, King Fahd Armed Forces Hospital, Jeddah, Saudi Arabia

Abeer Alnowaiser
Pediatric Dentistry Department, Faculty of Dentistry, King Abdulaziz University, Jeddah, Saudi Arabia

Omar El Meligy
Pediatric Dentistry Department, Faculty of Dentistry, King Abdulaziz University, Jeddah, Saudi Arabia Pediatric Dentistry and Dental Public Health Department, Faculty of Dentistry, Alexandria University, Alexandria, Egypt

Jamal Sallam
Ministry of Health, Jeddah, Saudi Arabia

Yusra Balkheyour
King Abdulaziz University, Jeddah, Saudi Arabia

Raidan A. Ba-Hattab
Department of Clinical Dental Sciences, College of Dentistry, Princess Nourah Bint Abdulrahman University, Riyadh, Saudi Arabia

Dieter Pahncke
Department of Operative Dentistry and Periodontology, Dental School, University of Rostock, Rostock, Germany

Manoelito Ferreira Silva-Junior and Maria da Luz Rosário de Sousa
Department of Community Dentistry, Piracicaba Dental School, University of Campinas, Avenue Limeira 901,13414-903 Piracicaba, SP, Brazil

Marília Jesus Batista
Department of Community Health, Faculty of Medicine Jundiaí, R. Francisco Telles,No. 250, Vila Arens II,13202-550 Jundiaí, SP, Brazil

Audrey Peteuil
Instance Régionale d'Éducation et de Promotion de la Santé, 21000 Dijon, France

Corinne Rat
Clinical Research Unit, La Chartreuse Psychiatric Centre, 21033 Dijon, France

Frederic Denis
Clinical Research Unit, La Chartreuse Psychiatric Centre, 21033 Dijon, France UFR Odontology and Public Health Department, 1 Avenue du Maréchal Juin, F-51095 Reims, France EA 75-05 Education, Ethique, Santé, Universit´e François-Rabelais Tours, Faculté de Médecine, 37032 Tours, France

Sahar Moussa-Badran
UFR Odontology and Public Health Department, 1 Avenue du Maréchal Juin, F-51095 Reims,France

Maud Carpentier
Direction de la Recherche Clinique, University Hospital of Dijon, 21079 Dijon, France

Jean-François Pelletier
Department of Psychiatry, Montreal University, Yale Program for Recovery and Community Health, Montreal, Canada

Sebastian Igelbrink
Clinic for Oral and Maxillofacial Surgery, University of Münster, Albert-Schweitzer-Campus 1, 48149 Münster, Germany

Stefan Burghardt, Norbert R. Kübler and Henrik Holtmann
Clinic for Oral and Maxillofacial Surgery, University Clinic of Duesseldorf, Moorenstr 5, 40225 Duesseldorf, Germany

Barbara Michel
Doctor's Practice for Oral and Maxillofacial Surgery, Uhlstraße 97, 50321 Brühl, Germany

Maitreyi Pandya
Oral Medicine and Radiology, Private Practice, New Delhi, India

Anupama N. Kalappanavar and Rajeshwari G. Annigeri
Oral Medicine and Radiology, College of Dental Sciences, Davangere, India

Dhanya S. Rao
Oral Medicine and Radiology, A. J. Institute of Dental Sciences, Mangalore, India

Shivani Kohli
Department of Prosthodontics, Faculty of Dentistry, MAHSA University, Selangor, Malaysia

Aaron Lam Wui Vun, Christopher Daryl Philip, Cassamally Muhammad Aadil and Mahenthiran Ramalingam
Faculty of Dentistry, MAHSA University, Selangor, Malaysia

R. A. G. Khammissa, R. Ballyram, Y. Jadwat, J. Fourie, J. Lemmer and L. Feller
Department of Periodontology and Oral Medicine, Sefako Makgatho Health Sciences University, Medunsa 0204, South Africa

Gianluca Gambarini, Gabriele Miccoli, Gianfranco Gaimari, Deborah Pompei, Andrea Pilloni, Dario Di Nardo and Luca Testarelli
Department of Oral and Maxillofacial Sciences, Sapienza University of Rome, Rome, Italy

Lucila Piasecki
Department of Periodontics and Endodontics, University at Buffalo, Buffalo, NY, USA

Dina Al-Sudani
Department of Restorative Dental Sciences, College of Dentistry, King Saud University, Riyadh, Saudi Arabia

Maria Rita Giuca, Maria Cappè, Elisabetta Carli, Lisa Lardani and Marco Pasini
Department of Surgical, Medical, Molecular Pathology and Critical Area, Dental and Oral Surgery Clinic, Unit of Pediatric Dentistry, University of Pisa, Via Savi 10, 56126 Pisa, Italy

Shaimaa M. Fouda and Fahad A. Al-Harbi
Department of Substitutive Dental Sciences, College of Dentistry, University of Dammam, Dammam 31411, Saudi Arabia

Soban Q. Khan
Department of Clinical Affairs, College of Dentistry, University of Dammam, Dammam 31411, Saudi Arabia

Jorma I. Virtanen
Research Unit of Oral Health Sciences, Department of Community Dentistry, Faculty of Medicine, University of Oulu, 90014 Oulu, Finland
Medical Research Center Oulu, Oulu University Hospital and University of Oulu, Oulu, Finland

Aune Raustia
Medical Research Center Oulu, Oulu University Hospital and University of Oulu, Oulu, Finland
Research Unit of Oral Health Sciences, Department of Prosthetic Dentistry and Stomatognathic Physiology, Faculty of Medicine, University of Oulu, P.O. Box 5281, 90014 Oulu, Finland

Bruno G. S. Casado, Sandra L. D. Moraes, Gleicy F. M. Souza, Juliana R. Souto-Maior and Belmiro C. E. Vasconcelos
School of Dentistry, University of Pernambuco (UPE), Camaragibe, PE, Brazil

Catia M. F. Guerra
School of Dentistry, Pernambuco Federal University (UFPE), Recife, PE, Brazil

Cleidiel A. A. Lemos and Eduardo P. Pellizzer
School of Dentistry, Dental Materials and Prosthodontics, São Paulo State University (UNESP), São Paulo, Araçatuba, Brazil

Ahmed Al-Majid
Clinic of Preventive Dentistry, Periodontology and Cariology, Center of Dental Medicine, University of Zurich, Zurich, Switzerland

Saeed Alassiri and Taina Tervahartiala
Department of Oral and Maxillofacial Diseases, University of Helsinki and Helsinki University Hospital, Helsinki, Finland

Timo Sorsa
Department of Oral and Maxillofacial Diseases, University of Helsinki and Helsinki University Hospital, Helsinki, Finland
Karolinska Institutet, Department of Dental Medicine, Division of Periodontology, Stockholm, Sweden

Nilminie Rathnayake
Karolinska Institutet, Department of Dental Medicine, Division of Periodontology, Stockholm, Sweden

Dirk-Rolf Gieselmann
Institute of Molecular Diagnostics, Dentognostics GmbH, Solingen and Jena, Germany

Carlo Bertoldi, Andrea Forabosco and Luigi Generali
Department of Surgery, Medicine, Dentistry and Morphological Sciences with Transplant Surgery, Oncology and Regenerative Medicine Relevance, University of Modena and Reggio Emilia, Modena, Italy

Michele Lalla
Department of Economics Marco Biagi, University of Modena and Reggio Emilia, Modena, Italy

Davide Zaffe
Department of Biomedical, Metabolic and Neural Sciences, University of Modena and Reggio Emilia, Modena, Italy

Pierpaolo Cortellini
European Research Group on Periodontology (ERGO Perio), Bern, Switzerland

T. M. Kabali
Department of Orthodontics, Paedodontics and Community Dentistry, Muhimbili University of Health and Allied Sciences (MUHAS), Dar-es-Salaam, Tanzania

E. G. Mumghamba
Department of Restorative Dentistry, School of Dentistry, Muhimbili University of Health and Allied Sciences (MUHAS), Dar-es-Salaam, Tanzania

Milaim Sejdini, Sokol Krasniqi, Nora Berisha and Nora Aliu
Faculty of Medicine, Orthodontic Clinic, University of Pristina, Pristina, Kosovo

Agim Begzati
Faculty of Medicine, Paediatric Dentistry Clinic, University of Pristina, Pristina, Kosovo

Sami Salihu
Faculty of Medicine, Maxillofacial Surgery Clinic, University of Pristina, Pristina, Kosovo

Marja-Liisa Laitala, Liina Piipari, Noora Sämpi and Maria Korhonen
Research Unit of Oral Health Sciences, Department of Cariology, Endodontology and Paediatric Dentistry, University of Oulu, Oulu, Finland

Vuokko Anttonen
Research Unit of Oral Health Sciences, Department of Cariology, Endodontology and Paediatric Dentistry, University of Oulu, Oulu, Finland
Medical Research Center, University of Oulu, Oulu University Hospital, Oulu, Finland

Paula Pesonen
Research Unit of Oral Health Sciences, University of Oulu, Oulu, Finland

Tiina Joensuu
Kuopio University Hospital, Kuopio, Finland

Aqdar A. Akbar and Mohammad Y. Sabti
Department of General Dental Practice, Kuwait University, Kuwait City, Kuwait

Noura Al-Sumait and Hanan Al-Yahya
Ministry of Health, Kuwait City, Kuwait

Muawia A. Qudeimat
Department of Developmental and Preventive Sciences, Kuwait University, Kuwait City, Kuwait

Da In Kim
School of Dentistry, Faculty of Medicine and Dentistry, University of Alberta, ECHA, 11405-87 Avenue, Edmonton, AB, Canada T6G 1C9

Manuel O. Lagravère
School of Dentistry, Faculty of Medicine and Dentistry, University of Alberta, Edmonton, AB, Canada T6G 1C9

Hamed Mortazavi, Maryam Baharvand, Somayeh Rahmani and Soudeh Jafari
Department of Oral Medicine, School of Dentistry, Shahid Beheshti University of Medical Sciences, Tehran, Iran

Yaser Safi
Department of Oral and Maxillofacial Radiology, School of Dentistry, Shahid Beheshti University of Medical Sciences, Tehran, Iran

Mehak Pervaiz
APPNA Institute of Public Health, Jinnah Sindh Medical University, Karachi, Pakistan

Ruth Gilbert
School of Healthcare Practice, University of Bedfordshire, Putteridge Bury, Luton, Bedfordshire LU2 8LE, UK

Nasreen Ali
Institute of Health Research, University of Bedfordshire, Putteridge Bury, Luton, Bedfordshire LU2 8LE, UK

T. M. Kabali
Department of Orthodontics, Paedodontics and Community Dentistry, Muhimbili University of Health and Allied Sciences (MUHAS), Dar-es-Salaam, Tanzania

E. G. Mumghamba
Department of Restorative Dentistry, School of Dentistry, Muhimbili University of Health and Allied Sciences (MUHAS), P.O. Box 65014, Dar-es-Salaam, Tanzania

F. Meyer and J. Enax
Research Department, Dr. Kurt Wolff GmbH and Co. KG, Bielefeld, Germany

Teija Raivisto, AnnaMaria Heikkinen, Hellevi Ruokonen and Taina Tervahartiala
Department of Oral and Maxillofacial Diseases, University of Helsinki and Helsinki University Hospital, Helsinki, Finland

Timo Sorsa
Department of Oral and Maxillofacial Diseases, University of Helsinki and Helsinki University Hospital, Helsinki, Finland
Department of Dental Medicine, Karolinska Institutet, Huddinge, Sweden

Leena Kovanen
Department of Health, National Institute for Health and Welfare, Helsinki, Finland

Jari Haukka
Department of Health, National Institute for Health and Welfare, Helsinki, Finland
Department of Public Health and Clinicum, University of Helsinki, Helsinki, Finland

Kaisa Kettunen
Institute for Molecular Medicine Finland (FIMM), Helsinki, Finland

Emily Chen, Silvana Pasetto and Vanessa Pardi
Herman Ostrow School of Dentistry, University of Southern California, Los Angeles, CA, USA

Bruna Benso
School of Dentistry, Pontificia Universidad Católica de Chile, Santiago, Chile

Dalia Seleem
College of Dental Medicine, Western University of Health Sciences, Pomona, CA, USA

Luiz Eduardo Nunes Ferreira
School of Dental Medicine, East Carolina University, Greenville, NC, USA

Ramiro Mendonça Murata
School of Dental Medicine, East Carolina University, Greenville, NC, USA
Brody School of Medicine, East Carolina University, Greenville, NC, USA

Lucía Arévalo-Híjar, Stefany Caballero-García and Néstor Gonzáles-Soto
School of Odontology, Health Sciences Faculty, Universidad Peruana de Ciencias Aplicadas-UPC, Lima, Peru

Miguel Ángel Aguilar-Luis
Research Center and Innovation of the Faculty of Health Sciences, Universidad Peruana de Ciencias Aplicadas, Av. San Marcos cdra 2, Cedros de Villa, Lima, Peru
Institute of Nutritional Research (IIN), 1885 La Molina Ave., Lima 12, Peru

Juana Del Valle-Mendoza
Research Center and Innovation of the Faculty of Health Sciences, Universidad Peruana de Ciencias Aplicadas, Av. San Marcos cdra 2, Cedros de Villa, Lima, Peru
Institute of Nutritional Research (IIN), 1885 La Molina Ave., Lima 12, Peru

Index